Cancer Genes

(Volume 1)

Edited by

Satish Ramalingam
Department of Genetic Engineering, School of
Bioengineering
SRM Institute of Science and Technology
Kattankulathur-603203
India

Cancer Genes (Volume 1)

Editor: Satish Ramalingam

ISBN (Online): 978-981-5080-29-2

ISBN (Print): 978-981-5080-30-8

ISBN (Paperback): 978-981-5080-31-5

© 2023, Bentham Books imprint.

Published by Bentham Science Publishers Pte. Ltd. Singapore. All Rights Reserved.

First published in 2023.

need for a court order if at any point you breach any terms of this License Agreement. In no event will any delay or failure by Bentham Science Publishers in enforcing your compliance with this License Agreement constitute a waiver of any of its rights.

3. You acknowledge that you have read this License Agreement, and agree to be bound by its terms and conditions. To the extent that any other terms and conditions presented on any website of Bentham Science Publishers conflict with, or are inconsistent with, the terms and conditions set out in this License Agreement, you acknowledge that the terms and conditions set out in this License Agreement shall prevail.

Bentham Science Publishers Pte. Ltd.
80 Robinson Road #02-00
Singapore 068898
Singapore
Email: subscriptions@benthamscience.net

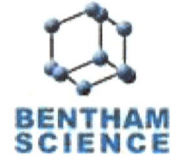

BENTHAM SCIENCE

CONTENTS

FOREWORD

The collection of diseases known as cancer has been recognized as a deadly disease for more than 4000 years. Amazing improvements in the treatment of cancer have occurred in the past century. Still, however, understanding the molecular basis of cancers' origins remains incomplete. Neoplasms are complex diseases that involve mutations or aberrant expression of dozens of genes. The pace of cancer genetics research has expanded exponentially following the sequencing of the human genome. While a tremendous boon for cancer researchers, there have been numerous missed opportunities because the overwhelming numbers of papers published make it nearly impossible for any cancer researcher to keep up.

Dr. Satish Ramalingam and colleagues provide this extensive compendium of cancer genes. The catalog summarizes key data which implicates each gene in one or more cancers and summarizes key studies that explore each mechanism of action. The organization, by the chromosomes on which the genes are encoded, allows both experts and neophytes to cross-reference and facilitate their research objective(s).

The monograph is a compendious primer that will be a valuable resource for cancer biologists, clinical oncologists and students engaging in basic discovery, translational research, or clinical treatment of cancer.

Danny R. Welch, PhD
University of Kansas Cancer Center
Kansas City, Kansas, USA

PREFACE

Cancer incidence is rising and has become a leading cause of death in many cities worldwide. It is well documented that cancer initiation and progression depend on the genes expressed in the cell's genome. It is imperative to understand the genetics of this dreaded disease to win the war against it. As we attempted to understand the latest update about all cancer-related genes in all the chromosomes, we noticed a clear lacuna because no books cover all the important genes that play a role in cancer presented chromosome-wise for easy understanding. We have decided to fill the gap and compiled most of the genes that are identified to play an important role in cancer. We delve into the world of cancer-causing genes and their location on each chromosome. This book will provide valuable mechanistic insights about the mutations and dysregulation of cancer genes that provide an advantage for cancer cell survival during each stage of tumorigenesis. This volume provides a comprehensive overview of the cancer-causing genes located on chromosomes 1-12 and serves as an invaluable resource for researchers, medical professionals, and anyone interested in the genetic basis of cancer.

Satish Ramalingam
Department of Genetic Engineering, School of Bioengineering
SRM Institute of Science and Technology
Kattankulathur-603203
India

List of Contributors

Abhishek Mitra
Department of Genetic Engineering, School of Bioengineering, SRM Institute of Science and Technology, Kattankulathur, India 603203

Aishwarya Raja
Department of Genetic Engineering, School of Bioengineering, SRM Institute of Science and Technology, Kattankulathur, India 603203

Anindita Menon
Department of Genetic Engineering, School of Bioengineering, SRM Institute of Science and Technology, Kattankulathur, India 603203

Harini Hariharan
Department of Genetic Engineering, School of Bioengineering, SRM Institute of Science and Technology, Kattankulathur, India 603203

Muthu Vijai Bharath Vairamani
Department of Genetic Engineering, School of Bioengineering, SRM Institute of Science and Technology, Kattankulathur, India 603203

Ravi Gor
Department of Genetic Engineering, School of Bioengineering, SRM Institute of Science and Technology, Kattankulathur, India 603203

Satish Ramalingam
Department of Genetic Engineering, School of Bioengineering, SRM Institute of Science and Technology, Kattankulathur, India 603203

Saurav Panicker
Department of Genetic Engineering, School of Bioengineering, SRM Institute of Science and Technology, Kattankulathur, India 603203

Sayooj Madhusoodanan
Department of Genetic Engineering, School of Bioengineering, SRM Institute of Science and Technology, Kattankulathur, India 603203

Shivani Singh
Department of Genetic Engineering, School of Bioengineering, SRM Institute of Science and Technology, Kattankulathur, India 603203

Sivasankari Ramadurai
Department of Genetic Engineering, School of Bioengineering, SRM Institute of Science and Technology, Kattankulathur, India 603203

Thilaga Thirugnanam
Department of Genetic Engineering, School of Bioengineering, SRM Institute of Science and Technology, Kattankulathur, India 603203

Yamini Chandrapraksh
Department of Genetic Engineering, School of Bioengineering, SRM Institute of Science and Technology, Kattankulathur, India 603203

CHAPTER 1

Chromosome 1

Ravi Gor[1], **Saurav Panicker**[1] and **Satish Ramalingam**[1,*]

[1] *Department of Genetic Engineering, School of Bioengineering, SRM Institute of Science and Technology, Kattankulathur, India*

Abstract: Chromosome 1 is the largest human chromosome, constituting approximately 249 million base pairs. Chromosome 1 is the largest metacentric chromosome, with "p" and "q" arms of the chromosome almost similar in length. Chromosome 1 abnormalities or inclusion of any mutations leads to developmental defects, mental, psychological, cancer, *etc*., among the most common diseases. $1/10^{th}$ of the genes in chromosome 1 have been reported its involvement in cancer growth and development. These cancer genes result from chromosomal rearrangement, fusion genes, somatic mutations, point mutation, gene insertion, gene deletion, and many more. Some of these cancer-causing genes appear to be involved in cancer more often, and other novel genes are also enlisted in this chapter.

Keywords: Cancer, Developmental defects, Fusion gene, Gene, Gene insertion, Gene deletion, Metacentric, Mutation, p-arm, Point mutation, Psychological, q-arm, Somatic mutation.

1. INTRODUCTION

Chromosomes are the large chunk of hereditary material that carries information from four nucleotides. This together makes a list of instructions for making proteins, regulatory elements, and other nucleotides required to maintain the growth and normal development of the cells. A human cell constitutes 22 pairs of autosomes and two sex chromosomes, one from each parent. Chromosome 1 is the largest human chromosome, with about 249 million long DNA base pairs, representing about 8% of the total DNA in cells. Chromosome 1 likely contains 2000 to 2100 genes that function cooperatively to achieve the existence of a well-functioning cell. Since we know there are approximately more than 2000 genes coded in chromosome 1 alone, we take a deep look into how many are reported to be involved in cancer disease. The Atlas of Cancer Genetics and Cytogenetics in Oncology and Haematology is a freely available database where all the inform-

---

* **Corresponding author Satish Ramalingam**: Department of Genetic Engineering, School of Bioengineering, SRM Institute of Science and Technology, Kattankulathur, India; E-mail: rsatish76@gmail.com

ation about the genes involved or has been reported for the cancer disease is updated regularly.

The list involves the proteins, microRNA, long non-coding RNA, *etc.*, which are now included in the list. Among the 2000 genes on chromosome 1, 1/10th of its dynamic cancer growth and development have been reported. Out of these many genes, we have listed here some t, some top-notch genes that are repeatedly coming into the limelight and showing involvement in cancer.

1.1. MUC1: Mucin-1 Chromosome 1; 1q22

MUC1 protein is widely studied, and its expression is increased in various cancer types like breast, pancreatic, colon, *etc.* Human MUC1 protein is translated as a long single polypeptide, which auto cleaves into two subunits resulting in the formation of a non-covalent heterodimer. The MUC1-N subunit is expressed at the cell surface by forming a complex with the MUC1-C cytoplasmic subunit located in the cytoplasm [1]. Under typical situations, this assembly helps define polarity and create a protective mucous barrier in specialized organs, gastrointestinal and respiratory tracts, or lumen lining ducts. In a different scenario of stress conditions, the cell's polarity is lost, and the MUC1 protein is now positioned everywhere. MUC1-C cytoplasm domain is a 72 amino acid-long polypeptide and consists of various motifs which play an essential role in signaling. One of the binding motifs is CQC which is necessary to form a MUC1-C oligomer. The oligomerization process is critical for transporting MUC1-C to the nucleus and further its interaction with importin β, which helps transport MUC1-C to the nucleus. Inside the nucleus, MUC1-C associates with p53, β-catenin/TCF4, estrogen receptor α [ERα], NF-κB p65, and STATs. In MUC1-C, phosphorylation of the YEKV site induces the binding of β-catenin to the SAGNGGSSLS sequence. This stabilizes the β- catenin and activates Wnt target genes, such as *cyclin D1* and CTFG. The cytoplasm subunit MUC1-C interacts with receptor tyrosine kinases [*e.g.*, ErbB1- 4] and participates in downstream signaling pathways activating EGFR, FGFR3, PDGFRβ, and Met [2, 3]. MUC1-C tail domain also starts EZH2 and BMI1 in triple-negative breast cancer epigenetic reprogramming. MUC1-C interacts with MYC and selectively activates the MTA1 and MBD3 genes. These are components of NuRD signaling. This results in the activation of the NuRD complex and drives dedifferentiation and reprogramming of triple Negative Breast Cancer Cells [4].

1.2. NTRK1: Neurotrophic receptor Tyrosine Kinase-1 Location: Chromosome 1; 1q23.3

NTRK1 encodes a Tropomyosin receptor kinase [Trk]; these tyrosine kinases are membrane-bound and activated by neurotrophins. Some neutrophils which activate the receptors are Brain-derived neurotrophic factor [BDNF], nerve growth factor [NGF], neurotrophin-3, and neurotrophin-4. Neutrophine signaling results in cell proliferation, survival, the fate of the neural precursor's cell, programmed cell death, *etc* [5]. As the Trk receptors are activated by the neurotrophins, their function independent of the neurotrophins is also reported, which makes them an oncogene. The fusion of the tropomyosin gene with the locus of the extracellular locus of the Trk gene leads to the constitutive expression of the Trk gene, which results in continuous cellular proliferation [6]. Higher expression of the neurotrophins is a clear indication of the progression of cancer and decreases the survival of the patients [7].

1.3. PBX1: Pre-B-Cell Leukemia Transcription Factor-1 Chromosome 1; 1q23.3

PBX1 (Fig. **1**) encodes a protein involved as a transcription factor and belongs to the PBX homeobox family. A fusion protein E2A-PBX1 is produced by the translocation of the t(1;19) (q23.3;p13). This chimeric protein contains transcriptional activation domains from E2A and the homeodomain of PBX1. This complex will disrupt the transcriptional regulation of genes under PBX1 control [8]. Fusion protein E2A-PBX1 has been reportedly associated with pre-B-Cell acute lymphoblastic leukemia. Overexpression of the chimeric protein E2A-PBX1 positive cells in mice has shown hyper-phosphorylation of PLCγ2, which is essential in the proliferation. Its binding has been located to understand the mechanism behind the E2A-PBX1 for enhancing the proliferation using bioinformatics analysis. It has been found that the chimeric protein binds to the kinases located upstream of the PLCγ2 gene, that is, ZAP70, LCK, and SYK. Expression of these kinases helps in the phosphorylation of the PLCγ2 and further its involvement in the proliferation [9]. The E2A-PBX1 fusion protein is also detected in non-small cell lung cancer, shows a standard genetic change, and can be used as a biomarker for the early detection of the disease [10].

1.4. ABL2: Tyrosine Protein Kinase ABL2 Chromosome 1; 1q25.2

ABL2 is a tyrosine-protein kinase that activates the cell's survival, invasion, angiogenesis and growth. ABL2 shows overlapping functions with its family member ABL1. A consistent increase in the expression of ABL2 has been reported in advanced high-grade renal, colorectal, and pancreatic tumors. This shows the direct involvement of the ABL2 in the tumor progression [11 - 13]. Reduced expression of ABL2 in non-small cell lung cancer lines reduced cell growth [14]. In the case of other solid tumors like invasive breast carcinoma, lung squamous cell carcinoma, *etc.*, ABL2 showed higher amplification and higher mRNA expression in the cell, which correlates to the aggressiveness of the solid tumors [15].

Chromosome 1

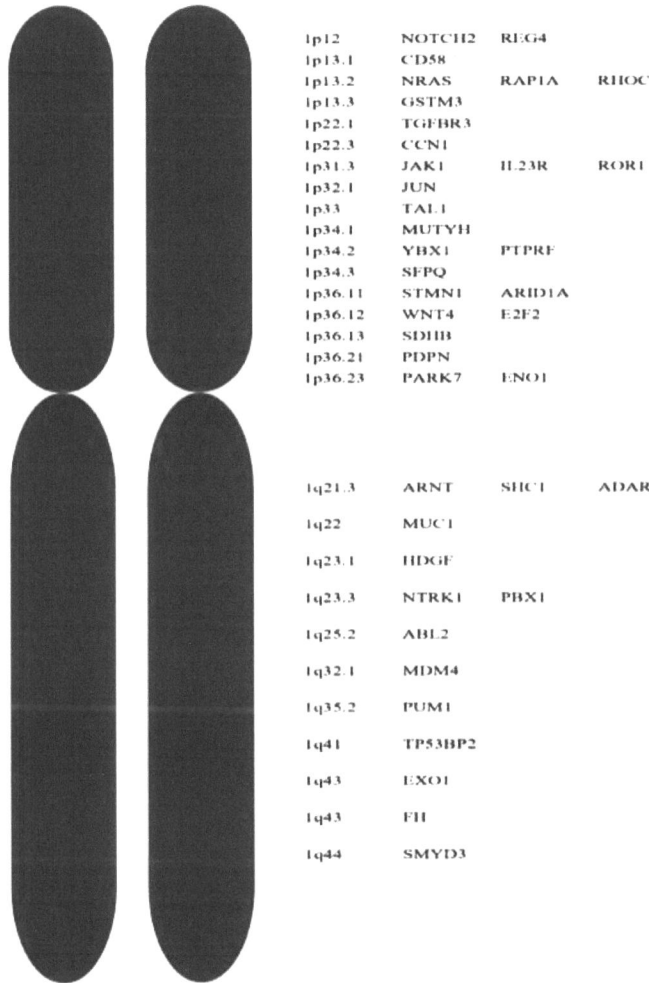

1p12	NOTCH2	REG4	
1p13.1	CD58		
1p13.2	NRAS	RAP1A	RHOC
1p13.3	GSTM3		
1p22.1	TGFBR3		
1p22.3	CCN1		
1p31.3	JAK1	IL23R	ROR1
1p32.1	JUN		
1p33	TAL1		
1p34.1	MUTYH		
1p34.2	YBX1	PTPRF	
1p34.3	SFPQ		
1p36.11	STMN1	ARID1A	
1p36.12	WNT4	E2F2	
1p36.13	SDHB		
1p36.21	PDPN		
1p36.23	PARK7	ENO1	
1q21.3	ARNT	SHC1	ADAR
1q22	MUC1		
1q23.1	HDGF		
1q23.3	NTRK1	PBX1	
1q25.2	ABL2		
1q32.1	MDM4		
1q35.2	PUM1		
1q41	TP53BP2		
1q43	EXO1		
1q43	FH		
1q44	SMYD3		

Fig. (1). This figure displays the loci of the genes from Chromosome 1 whose roles in cancer have been explained in this chapter. Sayooj Madhusoodanan designs this diagram.

1.5. Notch2: Neurogenic Locus Notch Homolog Protein-2 Chromosome 1; 1p12

Notch signaling is juxtracrine signaling which is also called contact-dependent signaling. Here, the Notch receptor physically contacts the ligand molecules from a member of the Delta, Serrate, and lag2 [DSL] family of proteins. Notch signaling is widely studied in cancer disease progression; out of the four subtypes of the Notch receptors, Notch2 is commonly found overexpressed in different types of cancer. The typical role of notch signaling in cell growth, survival, deciding the cell's fatal, maintaining stemness, metastasis, and epithelial to mesenchymal transitional [16]. A recent study in breast cancer found that Notch2 signaling helps maintain breast cancer cell dormancy and safe mobilization to the bone microenvironment. These cancer cells compete with the Hematopoietic Stem Cells in the bone marrow in the endosteal niche made by N- cadherin-positive osteoblasts called SNPs. In this area, the cell remains in the dormant state until a significant change in cellular activity. Disrupting the notch2 signaling pathway makes the dormant cell divide and metastasize to a distant organ,s and the cancer relapse again. This shows the involvement of the notch2 signaling in maintaining the stemness properties of cancer and increases the cancer relapse after the treatment [17]. Notch2 has demonstrated its crucial role in regulating self-renewal and tumorigenicity in hepatocellular carcinoma cells [18]. Cancer stem cell-based gene expression studies have shown a novel gene signature of GSK3B [high], β-catenin [high], and notch2 [low] shown to correlate with a better patient survival rate [19]. Overall Notch2 expression is found to be high in cancer. It also indicates its involvement in maintaining the cancer cell's stem cell properties and increases the disease's prognosis.

1.6. NRAS: NRAS Proto-Oncogene Chromosome 1; 1p13.2

NRAS gene (Fig. **1**) belongs to the family of RAS oncogenes. N-Ras protein is a GTPase and acts like a switch turned on and off by GTP and GDP molecules. Oncogenic mutation in the ras gene prevents GTP hydrolysis, resulting in constitutively active RAS protein and downstream signaling. In human melanoma cells, it is found that NRAS plays an essential role in protecting the cell from apoptosis. Most likely, it is done through activation of PKB/Akt *via* phosphoino-sitide 3' [PI3]-kinase. Ras protein is also involved in maintaining the proliferation of cells by applying the Ras-Raf-mitogen-activated Protein kinase [MAPK] pathway [20]. This is how the NRAS oncogene shows its importance in tumorgenicity in different types of cancer like melanoma, leukemia, skin cancer, colorectal cancer, acute myeloid leukemia, thyroid, neuroblastoma, bladder cancer, *etc*.

1.7. JUN: Jun Proto-Oncogene Chromosome 1; 1p32.1

JUN (Fig. **1**). encodes a protein c-jun similar to the v-jun protein [from avian sarcoma virus 17] and can induce oncogenic transformation in the targeted cells. C-Jun protein plays a vital role in the formation of transcription factors, which is essential in the various downstream processes, including proliferation, differentiation, Oncogenic Transformation, and Apoptosis. C-Jun protein forms a heterodimer with the Fos protein to form the transcription factor Activator Protein-1 [AP-1] [21 - 23]. c-Jun protein is the first cellular oncogene found to be overexpressed in human breast cancer. Knockdown c-June reduces memosphere formation, cell migration, and invasion. While the expression of c- Jun induces expansion of SCF and CCL5 for directly increasing the cellular migration and mammosphere expansion [24]. Tumor angiogenesis and further metastasis is the higher risk for the disease prognosis. C-Jun protein was found to play an essential role in the proliferation and angiogenesis of breast cancer [25].

1.8. TAL1: T-Cell Acute Lymphocytic Leukemia Protein-1 Chromosome 1; 1p33

T-cell acute lymphoblastic leukemia 1[TAL1], also known as Stem Cell Leukemia [SCL,] is a class II basic helix-loop-helix [bHLH] family of transcription factors and plays a critical role in the regulation of hematopoiesis [26]. TAL1 has an independent DNA binding motif and can bind to the other proteins to form significant transcription factors to regulate prior downstream example; the TAL1 p protein forms a heterodimer with E-proteins, binds to the E-box DNA-binding motif, ding motif, and holds several genes such as HBA [27, 28]. Ectopic overexpression of TAL1 is observed in most cases of T-Cell Acute Myeloid Leukemia. One of the researches, a transgenic mouse model with TAL1 misexpression in the thymus, shows that overexpressing TAL1 alone can play a transforming role. The tumorigenesis is drastically increased by co-expressing the catalytic domain of casein kinase IIalpha [CKIIalpha]. The higher expression of the TAL1 protein competes with the E-proteins and eventually leads to tumor formation. E-protein functions as a counter role to suppress the tumor, competing with the TAL-1 to form a heterodimer, does not allow the regular expression of the E-protein to repress the tumor formation and increases the ability of a transformed cell to create a tumor [27, 29]. Other studies have shown that TAL1 interactions with rising LMO1 oncogene the thymocyte progenitors inhibit the later differentiation of the cells. This makes the cell surface with the T-cell receptor and respective T-cell antigen receptor signaling. These conditions favor the NOTCH1 mutations and lead to the emergence of self-renewing leukemia-initiating cells in T-ALL [30].

1.9. JAK1: Jenus Kinase-1 Chromosome 1; 1p31.3

Janus kinase 1 [JAK1] encodes a class of protein-tyrosine kinases, which phosphorylates STAT proteins. The combination of the JAK1 and their downstream STAT proteins is essential in cytokine signaling, cancer development, and tissue homeostasis. JAK1 is critical for cancer progression and metastasis. JAK1 activation leads to phosphorylation of the STAT3, which targets FOS, and MAP3K8 which promotes tumorsphere formation and migration of cells. Also, loss of JAK1 prevents metastasis in an ERBB2-induced mammary cancer model [31]. JAK1 is a dependent predictor for poor prognosis in non-small cell lung cancer [32].

1.10. SFPQ: Splicing Factor, Proline and Glutamine-Rich Chromosome 1; 1p34.3

SFPQ codes for a splicing factor proline and glutamine-rich; this protein has one DNA binding domain and two RNA binding domains for regulating gene expression. Recent data have shown the role of SFPQ in prostate cancer; here, SFPQ promotes the expression of androgen receptor variant 7. This results in the worst prognosis of prostate cancer in patients [33]. In Epithelial Ovarian Cancer [EOC,] SFPQ in complex with p54^{nrb} binds and regulates the activity of the splicing factor SRSF2. SRSF2 is a critical factor for the caspase-9 alternative splicing regulation. The SFPQ/p54^{nrb} complex prevents Smovementifrom binding to caspase- 9 RNA and favors the production of an anti-apoptotic isoform that increases cell survival and chemoresistance. Downregulation of SFPQ/p54^{nrb} allows binding of SRSF2 to caspase-9 RNA and leads to increased expression of caspase-9 pro-apoptotic isoform, which induces cell death [34]. Not much research is done on the SFPQ gene and its mechanism involved in cancer maintenance and progression, which opens up a new area of research horizon and new opportunities the understand cancer [35].

1.11. ARNT: Aryl Hydrocarbon Translocator Chromosome 1; 1q21.3

The ARNT gene produces an aryl hydrocarbon receptor nuclear translocator; it is essential for the translocation of a ligand-bound subunit from the cytosol to the nucleus. In Hepatocellular Carcinoma [HCC], ARNT is found to negatively regulate Cyclin-E1, CDK2, Fos, and Jun, positively regulating CDKN1C, CNK-N2A, CDKN2B, MAPK11, and MAPK14. It shows its regulation of significant cell cycle checkpoints and supports the growth of performing proteins to increase growth. ARNT is an essential regulator in HCC growth and metastasis and can be used further as a prognostic detection marker in the case of HCC patients [36]. Also, ARNT expression is only required in the early phase of the tumor than late tumor growth [37]. In the late stage of colorectal tumor growth, ARNT expression is reduced, and the fibronectin/integrin β1/FAK signaling axis is upregulation. This complex signaling promotes epithelial-mesenchymal transition [EMT] and tumor metastasis. This also suggests that the expression of the ARNT in human colorectal cancer is inversely proportional to the cancer stage [38].

1.12. REG4: Regenerating Islet-Derived Protein-4 Chromosome 1; 1p12

Regenerating family member 4 [REG4] are lectin-like proteins involved in pancreatic, gastric, intestinal, and hepatic cell proliferation and differentiation [39]. Abnormal expression of REG4 is associated with the growth, resistance to apoptosis, adhesion, and survival of tumor cells. REG4 is upregulated in human colorectal carcinoma. This increase has also shown a significant increase in the expression of anti-apoptotic genes like Bcl-2, Bcl-XL, and survival. To further contribute to the cancer progression in the early stage of the disease, REG4 activates the EGFR/Akt/AP-1 signaling pathways in Colorectal Cancer [CRC]. Activation of genes responsible for cell growth and antiapoptotic protein increases the tumor growth potential with a poor prognosis of CRC [40]. REG4 is under control of the GATA6 expression, this signaling cascade promotes the tumorigenicity of colon cancer cells [41]. REG4 expression is also found to be an independent prognostic marker for relapse of prostate cancer after prostatectomy [42].

1.13. CD58: Cluster of Differentiation 58 Chromosome 1; 1p13.1

CD58 is a cell surface marker used to identify the population of cells in a tumor that shows self-renewal capabilities, and possesses an essential role in metastasis, tumorigenesis, recurrence, and treatment resistance in colorectal cancer. Upregulation of the Wnt/β-catenin pathway activates CD58 and promotes the colorectal tumor-initiating cell self-renewal and tumor-initiating ability. Dkk-3 is a negative regulator of the Wnt pathway, upregulation of the Wnt pathway is done *via* the degradation of Dkk-3 by CD58 [43].

1.14. RAP1A: Ras-Related Protein Rap-1A Chromosome 1; 1p13.2

RAP1A encodes a member of the Ras family of small GTPases. RAP1A is overexpressed in most esophageal squamous cell carcinoma [ESCC] and correlates with lymph node metastasis. In vitro studies have also indicated RAP1A to function as a promoter for esophageal cancer cell migration and invasion through matrix metalloproteinase 2. RAP1A can also be used as a prognostic marker for the diagnosis of ESCC [44]. RAP1A expression is higher in the breast cancer cell line and also plays a vital role in the invasiveness of breast cancer. RAP1A also interacts with LPA1 and regulates LPA-induced breast cancer cell migration [45].

1.15. GSTM3: Glutathione S-Transferase M3C Chromosome 1; 1p13.3

GSTM3 has been reported as being dysregulated in different cancers, such as lung cancer [46], colorectal cancer [47, 48], and prostate cancer [49]. Overexpression of GSTM3 protein expression is considered a marker of regional node metastasis in colon cancer [47]. In cervical cancer, the protein expression of GSTM3 consistently increases during tumor growth. Interaction of GSTM3 is found with the TRAF6, which activates the downstream pathway of the mitogen-activated protein kinase [MAPK]. It shows GSTM3, involving tumor progression *via* repressing apoptotic processes and activating cell proliferation constantly. GSTM3 was also found to interact with the HPV18 E7, an oncoprotein and a diagnostic marker for cervical cancer. GSTM3 and HPV18 E7 complex contribute to the survival of the cell. Overall, GSTM3, with its interaction withproteins increase tumor growth and reduce apoptosis, proliferation, and survival [50].

1.16. YBX1: Y-Box Binding Protein Chromosome 1; 1p34.2

YBX1 gene codes for Y-box binding protein one. It is involved in the proliferation of cells and has been reported to be overexpressed in various cancers. In the case of bladder cancer, overexpressing YBX1 correlates with the overexpression of Glut1, HK2, Pfk1, and LDHA. All these enzymes play a critical role in the glycolysis pathway, and YBX1 promotes the glycolysis pathway in bladder cancer which, in turn, promotes tumor growth. YBX1 regulates Myc and HIF1α expression in bladder cancer to promote glycolysis [51]. YBX1 is involved in Renal cell carcinoma [RCC] tumor stages and metastasis. YBX1 interacts with G3BP1, and these complexes upregulate the SPP1, which activates the NF-kB signaling pathway. [52] YBX1 activated various drug resistance-related genes, ABCB1, MYC, BCL2, CD49f, CD44, MVP/LRP, TOP2A, and androgen receptors. Overexpression of YBX1 and nuclear localization has increased the grade of tumors and poor outcomes in patients. YBX1 nuclear localization and expression have led to the dysregulation of genes involved in drug resistance, malignancy, uncontrolled cell proliferation, and immortalization in cancer [53].

1.17. STMN1: Stahmin-1 Chromosome 1; 1p36.11

STMN1, also called Stathmin-1, is a cytosolic phosphoprotein that regulates cellular microtubule dynamics and is also known to have oncogenic activity. STMN1 is highly expressed in hepatocellular carcinoma [HCC] and is associated with higher histology grade, vascular invasion, and shorter survival time in patients. STMN1 overexpression showed increased cell proliferation, migration, drug resistance, and cancer stem cell properties. STMN1 triggers the hepatocyte growth factor [HGF]/MET signal pathway and allows the HCC cells to get transformed into the hepatic stellate cells [HSC] cells; this makes the tumor more aggressive [54]. Higher expression of STMN1 is associated with vascular invasion and poor prognosis in lung squamous cell carcinoma [LSCC] [55]. Immunohistochemical analysis of STMN1 in gastric patients has shown the tumor to be chemoresistance with a poor prognosis [56]. Overexpression of STMN1 is correlated with poor prognosis and promotes cell migration and proliferation in oesophageal squamous cell carcinoma [57]. Current research has shown STMN1 involvement in the cancer progression and poor prognosis of disease, a detailed study to understand the molecular mechanism behind the protein needs to be done for better-targeted therapy.

1.18. WNT4: WNT Family Member 4 Chromosome 1; 1p36.12

WNT4 is upregulated in serum and tissues of colorectal cancer [CRC], contributing to epithelial to mesenchymal transition [EMT]. It also activates fibroblasts by activating the WNT4/β-catenin pathway. The WNT4/β-catenin/Ang2 pathway also induces angiogenesis in the CRC. Increased serum levels of WNT4 can be used as a potential biomarker for CRC diagnosis [58]. WNT4 is also reported to promote cell proliferation in breast and gastric cancer growth [59, 60].

1.19. E2F2: Transcription Factor E2F2 Chromosome 1; 1p36.12

E2F2 expression is more in non-small cell lung cancer [NSCLC] than in the normal tissues; reduction in its expression results in reduced viability and colony formation. It has been found that E2F2 is related to poor prognosis in NSCLC patients, and it could be a promising marker for diagnosis [61]. E2F2 is also used as a potential biomarker and target for ovarian cancer [62]. Overexpressing E2F2 with its repressor miR-99a has resulted in the resurrection of tumorigenicity and cell migration [63]. These are some contradictory results showing E2F2 in supporting cancer growth compared to the other research on tumor suppressor function [64].

1.20. PARK7: Parkinson Disease Protein-7 Chromosome 1; 1p36.23

PARK7 [DJ-1] is upregulated in various cancer types, suggesting a potential role in the pathogenesis of cancer; survival was reported to modulate oncoproteins expression and tumor suppressors. In colorectal cancer, PARK7 increases GLI1, GLI2, and PTCH1 protein expression, which is involved in the hedgehog signaling pathway. It also activates Wnt signaling in colorectal cancer by upregulating PLAGL,2, which increases BMP; this results in β-catenin accumulation and transcription of TCF, which enhances the Wnt signaling [65]. PARK7 is also reported to suppress apoptosis; in prostate cancer, PARK7 inhibits tumor.

Necrosis factor-related apoptosis-inducing ligand [TNFSF10] [66]. In laryngeal carcinoma cells, apoptosis is inhibited by the expression of surviving by PARK7; surviving inhibits apoptotic proteins and induces the proliferation of cells [67] PARK7 also inhibits autophagy by interacting with MEP3K1/PARK7 complex that suppresses JNK activity and transcription of Beclin-1 [68]. PARK7 is a positive regulator for the Androgen Receptor [AR], and its increase in expression leads to independent and metastatic prostate cancer [69]. PARK7 works with multiple proteins to reduce tumor suppressor activity, apoptosis, and autophagy and promote tumor growth.

1.21. ARID1A: AT-Rich Interaction Domain-1A Chromosome 1; 1p36.11

AT-rich interaction domain 1A [ARID1A] codes for an SWI/SNF family of proteins; they regulate the transcription of various genes by alteration of chromatin structure. ARID1A is mutated in different tumor types, including clear-cell ovarian and endometroid [45.2%], gastric [18.7], bladder [18.6%], hepatocellular [13.7], colorectal [9.4%], melanoma [11.5%], lung [8.2], pancreatic [3.6%], and breast cancer [2.5%] [70]. Gynecological cancer showed the highest frequency of ARID1A mutation; it has been found that the mutation co-occurs with PIK3CA or PTEN mutations in the human tumor sample. This suggests that the shutdown of these pathways with ARID1A loss in function drives cancer [70]. Loss of the APC gene is the major initiator for colon cancer initiation, but the inactivation of ARID1A does not drive; instead inactivates the tumor formation in the APC- mutant mouse models. This shows a possible oncogenic role of ARID1A in promoting the formation of loss of the APC gene, which drives colon cancer [71].

1.22. ENO1: Enolase-1 Chromosome 1; 1p36.23

ENO1 gene encodes an alpha-enolase enzyme, its upregulation in multiple cancer has been reported, and overexpression is involved in tumor cell proliferation and metastasis. Overexpression of ENO1 has enhanced gastric cancer proliferation and metastasis through the protein kinase B [AKT] signaling pathway [72]. In pancreatic ductal adenocarcinoma, overexpression of ENO1 correlates with the clinical stage, lymph node metastasis, and poor prognosis [73]. ENO1 overex-pression is a potent promoter of colorectal cancer development and metastasis by regulating the AMPK/mTOR pathway [74]. ENO1 is a potential prognostic marker in glioma is shown to promote cell growth, migration, and invasion [75].

1.23. SMYD3: SET and MYND Domain-Containing Protein-3 Chromosome 1; 1q44

SET and MYND domain-containing protein 3 [SMYD3] is a lysine methyltransferase. Overexpression of SMYD3 results in cell proliferation, migration, and invasion in non-small cell lung cancer [NSCLC] [76]. SMYD3 high expression correlates with the malignant characteristics of hepatocellular carcinoma [HCC]. It is found that SMYD3 is bound to the CDK2 and MMP2 promoter and increased H3K4me3 modification at the corresponding promoters to promote gene transcription of the respective genes [77]. SMYD3 drives epigenetic upregulation of the MMP-9 protein and facilitates cancer invasion characteristics. In oesophageal squamous cell carcinoma, SMYD3 enhances tumorigenicity *via* EZR and LOXL2 transcription [78], which are involved in proliferation, migration, and invasion [79]. SMYD3 epigenetic modification is also seen in ovarian cancer progression. SMYD3 binds to the promoter of CDKN2A and downregulates it by triple methylation H4K29me3 to reduce tumor proliferation. Another hand, apoptosis is reduced by binding to the BIRC3 promoter and upregulating the BIRC3 with triple-methylating H3K4me3. It shows that SMYD3 acts as an epigenetic regulator with triple methylation H4K20 /H3K4 in ovarian cancer for upregulating and downregulating the genes [80].

1.24. TP53BP2: Tumor Suppressor p53 Binding Protein-2 Chromosome 1; 1q41

TP53BP2 gene encodes an apoptosis-stimulating protein of the p53 [ASPP] family of p53 interacting proteins, also called ASPP2. ASPP2 expression is correlated with pituitary tumor proliferation and invasion. ASPP2, ki- 67, and nucleostemin may be potent clinical markers to detect invasive pituitary adenomas [81].

1.25. PDPN: Podoplanin Chromosome 1; 1p36.21

Podoplanin [PDPN] is a transmembrane receptor glycoprotein that is upregulated on transformed cells, contributing to cancer progression. PDPN expression induces Rho-associated coiled-coil kinase [ROCK] activity to promote squamous cell carcinoma survival and expansion of the colony [82]. In thyroid cancer, PDPN regulates the expression of ezrin, radixin, and moesin in association with MMP2 and MMP9, which promotes epithelial-mesenchymal transition [EMT] and invasiveness [83].

1.26. SHC1: SHC Adaptor Protein-1 Chromosome 1; 1q21.3

SHC1 gene encodes for three distinct isoforms p46SHC, p52SHC, and p66SHC. Out of these three isoforms, p52SHC is a critical isoform that drives breast cancer initiation, progression, and development [84]. In breast cancer, SHC1 elevates STAT3 levels, reduces STAT1 levels to result in intrinsic immune suppression, and reduces the sensitivity to immunotherapy. This shows how cleverly SHC1 regulates the expression of STAT proteins to achieve immune suppression in breast cancer [85].

1.27. MDM4: Mouse Double Minute-4 Chromosome 1; 1q32.1

MDM4, also known as HDMx [human MDMX], is a negative regulator of the tumor suppressor of p53. MDM4 has a p53 binding domain at the N-terminus and binds at the transcriptional activation domain of the p53 protein. Along with MDM4, MDM2 also plays a vital role in the negative regulation of the p53 protein. The C-terminal of the MDM4 domain has a RING finger domain which interacts with the MDM2 protein and regulates p53 expression further by inhibiting the latter degradation [86]. MDM4 gene is reported higher in multiple types of cancer, and its face was first reported in malignant gliomas [87]. Overexpression of MDM4 and MDM2 enhances the Circulating Tumor Cell Phenotype and directly involves cancer metastasis [88]. A recent finding has shown exciting facts about the two isoforms of the MDM4 due to alternate splicing and its downstream actions. MDM4-S, an alternately spliced variant of MDM4 excluding exon-6, contributes less to Breast cancer development, whereas the other isoform MDM4-FL, which includes the exon-6, increases the progression of breast cancer [89]. In the case of Multiple Human Melanoma cells, exon6 skipping has decreased the MDM4 expression, and further melanoma growth is also reduced [90].

1.28. ADAR: Adenosine Deaminases Acting on RNA Chromosome 1; 1q21.3

Adenosine deaminases acting on RNA [ADAR] catalyze the conversion of adenosine to inosine in double-stranded RNA. Their change results in a change in codons after transcription. ADAR1-mediated editing for the DHFR target gene in breast cancer enhances cell proliferation and resistance to methotrexate [91]. RNA modification of AZINI promotes its function as an oncogene by inhibiting the tumor suppressor activities of antizyme, tumor growth, metastasis, and recurrence of hepatocellular cancer [92]. ADAR1 lead RNA editing emerged as a driver of cancer progression, genomic amplification, and inflammatory cytokine release, and combining these stimulate multiple myeloma progression and resistance to therapeutics [93]. ADAR1 overexpression is a cause of apoptosis, growth inhibition, and S-phase arrest; ADAR1 modifies many sites in the BLCAP YXXQ domain to promote cervical cancer [94].

1.29. HDGF: Hepatoma-Derived Growth Factor Chromosome 1; 1q23.1

Overexpression of HDGF is seen in ovarian cancer and correlates with ovarian cancer growth. HDGF is released in the environment by the cancer cell. It stimulates the phosphorylation of ERK1/2 and P38, which enhances cellular migration,n [95]. Downregulation of the HDGF gene relates to cell migration and invasion inhibition *via* epithelial-mesenchymal transition [EMT], MMP2, and MMP9 signaling pathways. Which refers indirectly to the HDGF involvement in prostate cancer progression *via* these downregulated signaling pathways [96]. HDGF and DDX5 complex activates β-catenin to promote carcinogenesis and progression of endometrial cancer [EC] [97].

1.30. MUTYH: mutY DNA Glycosylase Chromosome 1; 1p34.1

A mutation in the MUTYH gene causes an autosomal recessive familial adenomatous polyposis-2 [FAP2]. MUTYH codes for a DNA glycosylase involved in oxidative DNA damage repair. MUTYH and OG, G1, another base excision repair pathway member, help repair the post-DNA replication repair of G: C to T: A transversion mutation due to oxidative damage in the replication process [98]. MUTYH increases the DNA damage in the oxidative-rich environment of the cancer cells. MUTYH association polyposis [MAP] occurs due to mutation in the MUTYH gene and is found to be because of genetics and hereditary phenomenon [99].

1.31. SDHB: Succinate Dehydrogenase Iron-Sulfur Subunit B Chromosome 1; 1p36.13

Succinate Dehydrogenase complex iron-sulfur subunit B is an essential gene for producing a subunit for the Succinate Dehydrogenase enzyme [SDH]. It is common in the citric acid cycle and oxidative phosphorylation. The presence of succinate stabilizes a protein hypoxia-inducible factor [HIF] and turns on or off further cell division and angiogenesis based on the oxygen availability in the environment. Mutation in this gene is frequently observed in various tumors and leads to a poor prognosis [100].

1.32. EXO1: Exonuclease-1 Chromosome 1; 1q43

EXO1 encodes a protein exonuclease 1 with 5' to 3' exonuclease activity, and RNase H activity. Overexpression of EXO1 is associated with cell proliferation, clonogenicity in Hepatocellular Carcinoma [HCC] [101]. Mutation in EXO1 is related to different cancer. These common point mutations are reported. Some reported SNP with cancers are rs756251971 in exon for colorectal cancer, rs41-50000 in intron for pancreatic cancer, rs1776148 in exon for oral cancer, and many more SNPs correlate to the hereditary form of EXO1 mutation and their correlation for various types of cancer [102 - 107].

1.33. FH: Fumarate Hydratase Chromosome 1; 1q43

The FH gene provides instructions to make Fumarate Hydratase, also known as fumarase enzyme. It plays a vital role in the citric acid cycle for the conversion of fumarate to malate. Mutation in the FH gene may cause cells to lose the ability to use oxygen and grow; this is advantageous for abnormal and cancer cells. Mutation in the FH gene is found in Hereditary leiomyomatosis and renal cell cancer [HLRCC] inheriting cancer [108]. These patients have an increased risk of kidney cancer and tumor in the skin and uterus [35]. Loss of FH function leads to the reprogramming of cells for better survival, activating oncogenic cascades. Accumulating fumarate is toxic to a cell, creating oxidative stress conditions. To escape from the oxidative stress condition and avoid cell senescence, antioxidant programs in the cell are triggered by NRF2 *via* succinate KEAP1. All these contribute to further. Transforming the cellular mechanism to live in a stressful environment becomes a transformed cell [109].

1.34. RHOC: RAS Homolog Gene Family Member C Chromosome 1; 1p13.2

RHOC gene encodes a Rho family of small GTPases, it was first reported to be overexpressed, and it is a significant correlate with the poor prognosis of patients with pancreatic ductal adenocarcinoma [110]. Similar upregulation of RHOC is recorded in ovarian carcinoma. RHOC is also involved in the progression of prostate cancer by activating essential proteins and activating a cascade of pathways. RHOC activates Pyk2, FAK, MAPK, and Akt, following the upregulation of MMP2 and MMP9 to promote tumor metastasis in prostate cancer [111, 112].

1.35. TGFBR3: Transforming Growth Factor-Beta Receptor-3 Chromosome 1; 1p22.1

TGFBR3 is a tumor-promoting gene in mesenchymal-stem-like triple-negative breast cancer (Fig. **1**). TGFBR3 reduces the expression of integrin-α2 and promotes cell migration, invasion and invasion tumorigenicity [113]. Bladder urothelial carcinoma [BUC] accounts for more than 90% of bladder cancer. TGFBR3 expression also increases as the tumor progresses and supports the tumor with motility, invasion, and cell growth [114]. TGFBR3 expression positively correlates with the ki-67 expression, which corresponds to cell proliferation in the case of oesophageal squamous cell carcinoma [ESCC] and results in poor prognosis [115]. A negative role of TGFBR3 is also reported in breast cancer and renal cell carcinoma, where the decrease in expression has improved the carcinogenesis, and its involvement has suppressed accumulated growth [116, 117].

1.36. CCN1: CCN Family Member-1 Chromosome 1; 1p22.3

CCN1 protein is associated with the Heregulin-induced breast cancer migration and metastasis and also increases tumor angiogenesis likely by interacting with αvβ3 integrin receptor [118, 119]. CCN1-positive breast cancer cells were shown to regulate fibroblast production of MMP1, resulting in increased breast cell migration and invasion [120]. Hedgehog signaling has also upregulated CCN1 expression and results in increased vascularity and spontaneous metastasis of breast cancer [121]. CCN1 overexpression in the glioma cell line resulted in phosphorylation of GSK3β and accumulated nuclear translocation of β-catenin, leading to activation of the β-catenin-TCF/Lef-1 signaling pathway. CCN1 overexpression also leads to activating the phosphatidylinositol-3-kinase/Akt signaling pathway. Activation of these pathways leads to inhibition of the pro-apoptotic protein, Bad [122].

1.37. IL23R: Interleukin 23 Receptor Chromosome 1; 1p31.3

Expression of IL23R is correlated with the possession of stem-like potential in esophageal squamous cell carcinoma; these activated compounds promote cancer growth and make cells resistant to radiation therapy [123]. IL23R, combined with IL-12R β2, creates homeostasis within tumor cells and tumor-infiltrating lympho-cytes, affecting the prognosis of patients with laryngeal cancer [124].

1.38. ROR1: Receptor Tyrosine kinase-Like Orphan Receptor-1 Chromosome 1; 1p31.3

ROR1 is a tyrosine kinase receptor with altered expression in different cancers, including ovarian, colon, lung, lymphoma, skin, pancreatic, bladder, uterus, prostate, and adrenal cancer. Higher expression of ROR1 is also associated with higher levels of activated AKT or CREB; these activated compounds promote cancer growth. Overall, ROR1 is more expressed in the poorly differentiated with high-grade histology than in tumors with low-grade histology showing its oncogenicity in the developed stage of cancer [125]. Ovarian cancer showed increased expression of ROR1 protein and is found to be involved in spheroid formation; tumor growth enhances tumor capacity for engraftment. ROR1 silencing has also reduced Bmi-1 expression, an oncogene that regulates CSC self-renewal. ROR1 silencing has also inhibited the expression level of EMT markers like vimentin, N-cadherin, and SNAIL-1/2 [126]. ROR1 is reported as a novel therapeutic target for patients with endometrial cancer. Further research and investigation on the actual molecular partners involved in endometrial cancer patients need to be studied for better treatment of the disease [127].

1.39. PTPRF: Protein Tyrosine Phosphatase Receptor Type-F Chromosome 1; 1p34.2

Protein Tyrosine Phosphatase Receptor Type F belongs to the protein tyrosine phosphatase family of proteins, which helps regulate cell growth, differentiation, and oncogenic transformation. PTPRF has shown its involvement in regulating Wnt signaling in colorectal cancer. The code is accomplished by controlling the endocytosis of the LRP6 receptor in colorectal cancer [128].

1.40. PUM1: Pumilio-1 Chromosome 1; 1q35.2

Pumilio-1 is an RNA Binding Protein and a post-transcriptional suppressor and is a member of the PUF family. PUM1 functions by targeting a specific sequence at a 3' untranslated region. PUM1 is reported as an oncogene, and its overexpression is involved in the proliferation, migration, invasion, and inhibiting cell apoptosis in Ovarian cancer [129]. Another research in Pancreatic Ductal adenocarcinoma [PDAC] showed PUM1 overexpression had decreased p-PERK, p- EIF2A, and ATF4 in MIA PaCa-2 cells, thus indicating the inactivating the PERK/eIF2/ATF4 signaling pathway [130]. In the case of non-small cell lung cancer [NSCLC], PUM1 suppresses the MicroRNA-411-5p, a tumor suppressor gene that indicates PUM1's oncogenic effect in the NSCLC [131]. A recent publication by Gor *et al.* shows that PUM1 expression is higher in colon cancer and colon cancer metastasis tissues and cell lines compared to normal colon tissues and normal colon cell lines, respectively. Overexpressing PUM1 resulted in increases in colonies, migration, and colonospheroid formation [132]. A phytochemical Morin is reported to inhibit colon cancer growth by inhibiting the PUM1 expression [133].

CONCLUSION

Chromosome 1 is the highly dense chromosome due to the occurrence of the gene after every 14.2 Mega Base (MB) of DNA. Genes supporting the growth, development, angiogenesis, *etc.*, are enlisted. Various gene abnormalities are seen here, including gene fusion, mutation, *etc.* In chromosome 1, the negative regulator of the p53 gene, *i.e.*, MDM4, resides, and its dysregulation affects the function of the p53 gene, which supports the normal cell to become a cancerous cell. Other essential genes and abnormalities that help cancer involve the WNT4,

JAK1, NRAS, *etc.*, some crucial proteins in the cell's normal functioning. Specific gene fusion genes also reside in this chromosome, like E2A- PBX1, helping at the gene regulation level for all the downstream genes involved under this DNA binding protein. Overexpression has supported the higher expression of the responsible proliferative genes in the case of pre-B-Cell acute lymphoblastic leukemia. Various other genes involving cell signaling, proliferation, *etc.*, are also present, and their dysregulation is reported in multiple.

Cancer types include the RAS family of an oncogene, JAK1, WNT4, *etc.* This shows the critical genes residing on chromosome 1 with their gene mutations or other changes that have been shown to support the development and growth of cancer in various ways, like regulating the tumor-suppressor gene, enhancing the proliferative cell cycle, *etc.*

REFERENCES

[1]   Kufe D. Oncogenic function of the MUC1 receptor subunit in gene regulation. Oncogene 2010; 29(42): 5663-6.
        [http://dx.doi.org/10.1038/onc.2010.334] [PMID: 20711235]

[2]   Kufe DW. Mucins in cancer: function, prognosis and therapy. Nat Rev Cancer 2009; 9(12): 874-85.
        [http://dx.doi.org/10.1038/nrc2761] [PMID: 19935676]

[3]   Behrens ME, Grandgenett PM, Bailey JM, *et al.* The reactive tumor microenvironment: MUC1 signaling directly reprograms transcription of CTGF. Oncogene 2010; 29(42): 5667-77.
        [http://dx.doi.org/10.1038/onc.2010.327] [PMID: 20697347]

[4]   Hata T, Rajabi H, Takahashi H, *et al.* MUC1-C activates the NuRD complex to drive dedifferentiation of triple-negative breast cancer cells. Cancer Res 2019; 79(22): 5711-22.
        [http://dx.doi.org/10.1158/0008-5472.CAN-19-1034] [PMID: 31519689]

[5]   Huang EJ, Reichardt LF. Trk receptors: roles in neuronal signal transduction. Annu Rev Biochem 2003; 72(1): 609-42.
        [http://dx.doi.org/10.1146/annurev.biochem.72.121801.161629] [PMID: 12676795]

[6]   Nakagawara A. Trk receptor tyrosine kinases: A bridge between cancer and neural development. Cancer Lett 2001; 169(2): 107-14.
        [http://dx.doi.org/10.1016/S0304-3835(01)00530-4] [PMID: 11431098]

[7]   Antunes LCM, Cartell A, de Farias CB, Bakos RM, Roesler R, Schwartsmann G. Tropomyosin-Related Kinase Receptor and Neurotrophin Expression in Cutaneous Melanoma Is Associated with a Poor Prognosis and Decreased Survival. Oncology 2019; 97(1): 26-37.
        [http://dx.doi.org/10.1159/000499384] [PMID: 31071716]

[8]   LeBrun DP, Cleary ML. Fusion with E2A alters the transcriptional properties of the homeodomain protein PBX1 in t (1; 19) leukemias. Oncogene. 1994; 9(6): 1641-7.

[9]   Duque-Afonso J, Lin CH, Han K, *et al.* E2A-PBX1 remodels oncogenic signaling networks in B- cell precursor acute lymphoid leukemia. Cancer Res 2016; 76(23): 6937-49.
        [http://dx.doi.org/10.1158/0008-5472.CAN-16-1899] [PMID: 27758892]

[10]   Mo ML, Chen Z, Zhou HM, *et al.* Detection of E2A-PBX1 fusion transcripts in human non-small-cell lung cancer. J Exp Clin Cancer Res 2013; 32(1): 29.
        [http://dx.doi.org/10.1186/1756-9966-32-29] [PMID: 23688269]

[11]   Behbahani TE, Thierse C, Baumann C, *et al.* Tyrosine kinase expression profile in clear cell renal cell carcinoma. World J Urol 2012; 30(4): 559-65.

[http://dx.doi.org/10.1007/s00345-011-0767-z] [PMID: 21969129]

[12]   Crnogorac-Jurcevic T, Efthimiou E, Nielsen T, *et al.* Expression profiling of microdissected pancreatic adenocarcinomas. Oncogene 2002; 21(29): 4587-94.
       [http://dx.doi.org/10.1038/sj.onc.1205570] [PMID: 12085237]

[13]   Chen G, Yuan SSF, Liu W, *et al.* Radiation-induced assembly of Rad51 and Rad52 recombination complex requires ATM and c-Abl. J Biol Chem 1999; 274(18): 12748-52.
       [http://dx.doi.org/10.1074/jbc.274.18.12748] [PMID: 10212258]

[14]   Yuan BZ, Jefferson AM, Popescu NC, Reynolds SH. Aberrant gene expression in human non small cell lung carcinoma cells exposed to demethylating agent 5-aza-2'-deoxycytidine. Neoplasia 2004; 6(4): 412-9.
       [http://dx.doi.org/10.1593/neo.03490] [PMID: 15256063]

[15]   Greuber EK, Smith-Pearson P, Wang J, Pendergast AM. Role of ABL family kinases in cancer: from leukaemia to solid tumours. Nat Rev Cancer 2013; 13(8): 559-71.
       [http://dx.doi.org/10.1038/nrc3563] [PMID: 23842646]

[16]   Aster JC, Pear WS, Blacklow SC. The Varied Roles of Notch in Cancer. Annu Rev Pathol 2017; 12(1): 245-75.
       [http://dx.doi.org/10.1146/annurev-pathol-052016-100127] [PMID: 27959635]

[17]   Capulli M, Hristova D, Valbret Z, *et al.* Notch2 pathway mediates breast cancer cellular dormancy and mobilisation in bone and contributes to haematopoietic stem cell mimicry. Br J Cancer 2019; 121(2): 157-71.
       [http://dx.doi.org/10.1038/s41416-019-0501-y] [PMID: 31239543]

[18]   Wu WR, Zhang R, Shi XD, Yi C, Xu LB, Liu C. Notch2 is a crucial regulator of self-renewal and tumorigenicity in human hepatocellular carcinoma cells. Oncol Rep 2016; 36(1): 181-8.
       [http://dx.doi.org/10.3892/or.2016.4831] [PMID: 27221981]

[19]   Bauer L, Langer R, Becker K, *et al.* Expression profiling of stem cell-related genes in neoadjuvant-treated gastric cancer: a NOTCH2, GSK3B and β-catenin gene signature predicts survival. PLoS One 2012; 7(9): e44566.
       [http://dx.doi.org/10.1371/journal.pone.0044566] [PMID: 22970250]

[20]   Eskandarpour M, Kiaii S, Zhu C, Castro J, Sakko AJ, Hansson J. Suppression of oncogenicNRAS by RNA interference induces apoptosis of human melanoma cells. Int J Cancer 2005; 115(1): 65-73.
       [http://dx.doi.org/10.1002/ijc.20873] [PMID: 15688405]

[21]   Zhang Y, Pu X, Shi M, *et al.* c-Jun, a crucial molecule in metastasis of breast cancer and potential target for biotherapy. Oncol Rep 2007; 18(5): 1207-12.
       [http://dx.doi.org/10.3892/or.18.5.1207] [PMID: 17914574]

[22]   Vogt PK. Jun, the oncoprotein. Oncogene 2001; 20(19): 2365-77.
       [http://dx.doi.org/10.1038/sj.onc.1204443] [PMID: 11402333]

[23]   Shaulian E, Karin M. AP-1 as a regulator of cell life and death. Nat Cell Biol 2002; 4(5): E131-6.
       [http://dx.doi.org/10.1038/ncb0502-e131] [PMID: 11988758]

[24]   Jiao X, Katiyar S, Willmarth NE, *et al.* c-Jun induces mammary epithelial cellular invasion and breast cancer stem cell expansion. J Biol Chem 2010; 285(11): 8218-26.
       [http://dx.doi.org/10.1074/jbc.M110.100792] [PMID: 20053993]

[25]   Vleugel MM, Greijer AE, Bos R, van der Wall E, van Diest PJ. c-Jun activation is associated with proliferation and angiogenesis in invasive breast cancer. Hum Pathol 2006; 37(6): 668-74.
       [http://dx.doi.org/10.1016/j.humpath.2006.01.022] [PMID: 16733206]

[26]   Porcher C, Chagraoui H, Kristiansen MS. SCL/TAL1: a multifaceted regulator from blood development to disease. Blood 2017; 129(15): 2051-60.
       [http://dx.doi.org/10.1182/blood-2016-12-754051] [PMID: 28179281]

[27]   Sanda T, Leong WZ. TAL1 as a master oncogenic transcription factor in T-cell acute lymphoblastic leukemia. Exp Hematol 2017; 53: 7-15.
[http://dx.doi.org/10.1016/j.exphem.2017.06.001] [PMID: 28652130]

[28]   Kassouf MT, Hughes JR, Taylor S, *et al.* Genome-wide identification of TAL1's functional targets: Insights into its mechanisms of action in primary erythroid cells. Genome Res 2010; 20(8): 1064-83.
[http://dx.doi.org/10.1101/gr.104935.110] [PMID: 20566737]

[29]   Kelliher MA, Seldin DC, Leder P. Tal-1 induces T cell acute lymphoblastic leukemia accelerated by casein kinase IIalpha. EMBO J 1996; 15(19): 5160-6.
[http://dx.doi.org/10.1002/j.1460-2075.1996.tb00900.x] [PMID: 8895560]

[30]   Tremblay M, Tremblay CS, Herblot S, *et al.* Modeling T-cell acute lymphoblastic leukemia induced by the *SCL* and *LMO1* oncogenes. Genes Dev 2010; 24(11): 1093-105.
[http://dx.doi.org/10.1101/gad.1897910] [PMID: 20516195]

[31]   Wehde BL, Rädler PD, Shrestha H, Johnson SJ, Triplett AA, Wagner KU. Janus Kinase 1 Plays a Critical Role in Mammary Cancer Progression. Cell Rep 2018; 25(8): 2192-2207.e5.
[http://dx.doi.org/10.1016/j.celrep.2018.10.063] [PMID: 30463015]

[32]   Liu D, Huang Y, Zhang L, Liang DN, Li L. Activation of Janus kinase 1 confers poor prognosis in patients with non-small cell lung cancer. Oncol Lett 2017; 14(4): 3959-66.
[http://dx.doi.org/10.3892/ol.2017.6690] [PMID: 28989534]

[33]   Takayama K ichi, Suzuki T, Fujimura T, et al. Dysregulation of spliceosome gene expression in advanced prostate cancer by RNA-binding protein PSF. Proceedings of the National Academy of Sciences of the United States of America 2017; 114: 10461–10466.

[34]   Pellarin I, Dall'Acqua A, Gambelli A, *et al.* Splicing factor proline- and glutamine-rich (SFPQ) protein regulates platinum response in ovarian cancer-modulating SRSF2 activity. Oncogene 2020; 39(22): 4390-403.
[http://dx.doi.org/10.1038/s41388-020-1292-6] [PMID: 32332923]

[35]   Trpkov K, Hes O, Agaimy A, *et al.* Fumarate hydratase-deficient renal cell carcinoma is strongly correlated with fumarate hydratase mutation and hereditary leiomyomatosis and renal cell carcinoma syndrome. Am J Surg Pathol 2016; 40(7): 865-75.
[http://dx.doi.org/10.1097/PAS.0000000000000617] [PMID: 26900816]

[36]   Liang Y, Li WW, Yang BW, *et al.* Aryl hydrocarbon receptor nuclear translocator is associated with tumor growth and progression of hepatocellular carcinoma. Int J Cancer 2012; 130(8): 1745-54.
[http://dx.doi.org/10.1002/ijc.26166] [PMID: 21544813]

[37]   Shi S, Yoon DY, Hodge-Bell K, Huerta-Yepez S, Hankinson O. Aryl hydrocarbon nuclear translocator (hypoxia inducible factor 1β) activity is required more during early than late tumor growth. Mol Carcinog 2010; 49(2): 157-65.
[http://dx.doi.org/10.1002/mc.20585] [PMID: 19824022]

[38]   Huang CR, Lee CT, Chang KY, *et al.* Down-regulation of ARNT promotes cancer metastasis by activating the fibronectin/integrin β1/FAK axis. Oncotarget 2015; 6(13): 11530-46.
[http://dx.doi.org/10.18632/oncotarget.3448] [PMID: 25839165]

[39]   Hartupee JC, Zhang H, Bonaldo MF, Soares MB, Dieckgraefe BK. Isolation and characterization of a cDNA encoding a novel member of the human regenerating protein family: Reg IV. Biochim Biophys Acta Gene Struct Expr 2001; 1518(3): 287-93.
[http://dx.doi.org/10.1016/S0167-4781(00)00284-0] [PMID: 11311942]

[40]   Bishnupuri KS, Luo Q, Murmu N, Houchen CW, Anant S, Dieckgraefe BK. Reg IV activates the epidermal growth factor receptor/Akt/AP-1 signaling pathway in colon adenocarcinomas. Gastroenterology 2006; 130(1): 137-49.
[http://dx.doi.org/10.1053/j.gastro.2005.10.001] [PMID: 16401477]

[41]   Kawasaki Y, Matsumura K, Miyamoto M, *et al.* REG4 is a transcriptional target of GATA6 and is

essential for colorectal tumorigenesis. Sci Rep 2015; 5(1): 14291.
[http://dx.doi.org/10.1038/srep14291] [PMID: 26387746]

[42]   Ohara S, Oue N, Matsubara A, *et al.* Reg IV is an independent prognostic factor for relapse in patients with clinically localized prostate cancer. Cancer Sci 2008; 99(8): 1570-7.
[http://dx.doi.org/10.1111/j.1349-7006.2008.00846.x] [PMID: 18754868]

[43]   Xu S, Wen Z, Jiang Q, *et al.* CD58, a novel surface marker, promotes self-renewal of tumor-initiating cells in colorectal cancer. Oncogene 2015; 34(12): 1520-31.
[http://dx.doi.org/10.1038/onc.2014.95] [PMID: 24727892]

[44]   Wang K, Li J, Guo H, *et al.* MiR-196a binding-site SNP regulates RAP1A expression contributing to esophageal squamous cell carcinoma risk and metastasis. Carcinogenesis 2012; 33(11): 2147-54.
[http://dx.doi.org/10.1093/carcin/bgs259] [PMID: 22859270]

[45]   Alemayehu M, Dragan M, Pape C, *et al.* β-Arrestin2 regulates lysophosphatidic acid-induced human breast tumor cell migration and invasion *via* Rap1 and IQGAP1. PLoS One 2013; 8(2): e56174.
[http://dx.doi.org/10.1371/journal.pone.0056174] [PMID: 23405264]

[46]   Ye Z, Song H, Higgins JPT, Pharoah P, Danesh J. Five glutathione s-transferase gene variants in 23,452 cases of lung cancer and 30,397 controls: meta-analysis of 130 studies. PLoS Med 2006; 3(4): e91.
[http://dx.doi.org/10.1371/journal.pmed.0030091] [PMID: 16509765]

[47]   Meding S, Balluff B, Elsner M, *et al.* Tissue-based proteomics reveals FXYD3, S100A11 and GSTM3 as novel markers for regional lymph node metastasis in colon cancer. J Pathol 2012; 228(4): 459-70.
[http://dx.doi.org/10.1002/path.4021] [PMID: 22430872]

[48]   Loktionov A, Watson MA, Gunter M, Stebbings WSL, Speakman CTM, Bingham SA. Glutathione--transferase gene polymorphisms in colorectal cancer patients: interaction between GSTM1 and GSTM3 allele variants as a risk-modulating factor. Carcinogenesis 2001; 22(7): 1053-60.
[http://dx.doi.org/10.1093/carcin/22.7.1053] [PMID: 11408349]

[49]   Medeiros R, Vasconcelos A, Costa S, *et al.* Metabolic susceptibility genes and prostate cancer risk in a southern European population: The role of glutathione S-transferases GSTM1, GSTM3, and GSTT1 genetic polymorphisms. Prostate 2004; 58(4): 414-20.
[http://dx.doi.org/10.1002/pros.10348] [PMID: 14968442]

[50]   Checa-Rojas A, Delgadillo-Silva LF, Velasco-Herrera MC, *et al.* GSTM3 and GSTP1: novel players driving tumor progression in cervical cancer. Oncotarget 2018; 9(31): 21696-714.
[http://dx.doi.org/10.18632/oncotarget.24796] [PMID: 29774096]

[51]   Xu L, Li H, Wu L, Huang S. YBX1 promotes tumor growth by elevating glycolysis in human bladder cancer. Oncotarget 2017; 8(39): 65946-56.
[http://dx.doi.org/10.18632/oncotarget.19583] [PMID: 29029484]

[52]   Wang Y, Su J, Wang Y, *et al.* The interaction of YBX1 with G3BP1 promotes renal cell carcinoma cell metastasis *via* YBX1/G3BP1-SPP1- NF-κB signaling axis. J Exp Clin Cancer Res 2019; 38(1): 386.
[http://dx.doi.org/10.1186/s13046-019-1347-0] [PMID: 31481087]

[53]   Kuwano M, Shibata T, Watari K, Ono M. Oncogenic Y-box binding protein-1 as an effective therapeutic target in drug-resistant cancer. Cancer Sci 2019; 110(5): 1536-43.
[http://dx.doi.org/10.1111/cas.14006] [PMID: 30903644]

[54]   Zhang R, Gao X, Zuo J, *et al.* STMN1 upregulation mediates hepatocellular carcinoma and hepatic stellate cell crosstalk to aggravate cancer by triggering the MET pathway. Cancer Sci 2020; 111(2): 406-17.
[http://dx.doi.org/10.1111/cas.14262] [PMID: 31785057]

[55]   Bao P, Yokobori T, Altan B, *et al.* High STMN1 Expression is Associated with Cancer Progression and Chemo-Resistance in Lung Squamous Cell Carcinoma. Ann Surg Oncol 2017; 24(13): 4017-24.

[http://dx.doi.org/10.1245/s10434-017-6083-0] [PMID: 28933054]

[56]   Bai T, Yokobori T, Altan B, *et al.* High STMN1 level is associated with chemo-resistance and poor prognosis in gastric cancer patients. Br J Cancer 2017; 116(9): 1177-85.
       [http://dx.doi.org/10.1038/bjc.2017.76] [PMID: 28334732]

[57]   Ni PZ, He JZ, Wu ZY, *et al.* Overexpression of Stathmin 1 correlates with poor prognosis and promotes cell migration and proliferation in oesophageal squamous cell carcinoma. Oncol Rep 2017; 38(6): 3608-18.
       [PMID: 29039594]

[58]   Yang D, Li Q, Shang R, *et al.* WNT4 secreted by tumor tissues promotes tumor progression in colorectal cancer by activation of the Wnt/β-catenin signalling pathway. J Exp Clin Cancer Res 2020; 39(1): 251.
       [http://dx.doi.org/10.1186/s13046-020-01774-w] [PMID: 33222684]

[59]   Zhu Y, Zhang B, Gong A, *et al.* Anti-cancer drug 3,3′-diindolylmethane activates Wnt4 signaling to enhance gastric cancer cell stemness and tumorigenesis. Oncotarget 2016; 7(13): 16311-24.
       [http://dx.doi.org/10.18632/oncotarget.7684] [PMID: 26918831]

[60]   Brisken C, Hess K, Jeitziner R. Progesterone and overlooked endocrine pathways in breast cancer pathogenesis. Endocrinology 2015; 156(10): 3442-50.
       [http://dx.doi.org/10.1210/en.2015-1392] [PMID: 26241069]

[61]   Chen L, Yu JH, Lu ZH, Zhang W. E2F2 induction in related to cell proliferation and poor prognosis in non-small cell lung carcinoma. Int J Clin Exp Pathol 2015; 8(9): 10545-54.
       [PMID: 26617764]

[62]   Zhou Q, Zhang F, He Z, Zuo MZ. E2F2/5/8 serve as potential prognostic biomarkers and targets for human ovarian cancer. Front Oncol 2019; 9: 161.
       [http://dx.doi.org/10.3389/fonc.2019.00161] [PMID: 30967995]

[63]   Feliciano A, Garcia-Mayea Y, Jubierre L, *et al.* miR-99a reveals two novel oncogenic proteins E2F2 and EMR2 and represses stemness in lung cancer. Cell Death Dis 2017; 8(10): e3141.
       [http://dx.doi.org/10.1038/cddis.2017.544] [PMID: 29072692]

[64]   Opavsky R, Tsai SY, Guimond M, *et al.* Specific tumor suppressor function for E2F2 in Myc-induced T cell lymphomagenesis. Proc Natl Acad Sci USA 2007; 104(39): 15400-5.
       [http://dx.doi.org/10.1073/pnas.0706307104] [PMID: 17881568]

[65]   Zhou J, Liu H, Zhang L, *et al.* DJ-1 promotes colorectal cancer progression through activating PLAGL2/Wnt/BMP4 axis. Cell Death Dis 2018; 9(9): 865.
       [http://dx.doi.org/10.1038/s41419-018-0883-4] [PMID: 30158634]

[66]   Hod Y. Differential control of apoptosis by DJ-1 in prostate benign and cancer cells. J Cell Biochem 2004; 92(6): 1221-33.
       [http://dx.doi.org/10.1002/jcb.20159] [PMID: 15258905]

[67]   Shen Z, Jiang Z, Ye D, Xiao B, Zhang X, Guo J. Growth inhibitory effects of DJ-1-small interfering RNA on laryngeal carcinoma Hep-2 cells. Med Oncol 2011; 28(2): 601-7.
       [http://dx.doi.org/10.1007/s12032-010-9474-7] [PMID: 20300974]

[68]   Ren H, Fu K, Mu C, Li B, Wang D, Wang G. DJ-1, a cancer and Parkinson's disease associated protein, regulates autophagy through JNK pathway in cancer cells. Cancer Lett 2010; 297(1): 101-8.
       [http://dx.doi.org/10.1016/j.canlet.2010.05.001] [PMID: 20510502]

[69]   Balk SP. Androgen receptor as a target in androgen-independent prostate cancer. Urology 2002; 60(3) (Suppl. 1): 132-8.
       [http://dx.doi.org/10.1016/S0090-4295(02)01593-5] [PMID: 12231070]

[70]   Kadoch C, Hargreaves DC, Hodges C, *et al.* Proteomic and bioinformatic analysis of mammalian SWI/SNF complexes identifies extensive roles in human malignancy. Nat Genet 2013; 45(6): 592-601.
       [http://dx.doi.org/10.1038/ng.2628] [PMID: 23644491]

[71]   Mathur R, Alver BH, San Roman AK, *et al.* ARID1A loss impairs enhancer-mediated gene regulation and drives colon cancer in mice. Nat Genet 2017; 49(2): 296-302.
[http://dx.doi.org/10.1038/ng.3744] [PMID: 27941798]

[72]   Sun L, Lu T, Tian K, *et al.* Alpha-enolase promotes gastric cancer cell proliferation and metastasis *via* regulating AKT signaling pathway. Eur J Pharmacol 2019; 845: 8-15.
[http://dx.doi.org/10.1016/j.ejphar.2018.12.035] [PMID: 30582908]

[73]   Yin H, Wang L, Liu HL. ENO1 Overexpression in Pancreatic Cancer Patients and Its Clinical and Diagnostic Significance 2018.
[http://dx.doi.org/10.1155/2018/3842198]

[74]   Zhan P, Zhao S, Yan H, *et al.* α-enolase promotes tumorigenesis and metastasis *via* regulating AMPK/mTOR pathway in colorectal cancer. Mol Carcinog 2017; 56(5): 1427-37.
[http://dx.doi.org/10.1002/mc.22603] [PMID: 27996156]

[75]   Song Y, Luo Q, Long H, *et al.* Alpha-enolase as a potential cancer prognostic marker promotes cell growth, migration, and invasion in glioma. Mol Cancer 2014; 13(1): 65.
[http://dx.doi.org/10.1186/1476-4598-13-65] [PMID: 24650096]

[76]   Li J, Zhao L, Pan Y, *et al.* SMYD3 overexpression indicates poor prognosis and promotes cell proliferation, migration and invasion in non-small cell lung cancer. Int J Oncol 2020; 57(3): 756-66.
[http://dx.doi.org/10.3892/ijo.2020.5095] [PMID: 32705243]

[77]   Wang Y, Xie B, Lin W, *et al.* Amplification of SMYD3 promotes tumorigenicity and intrahepatic metastasis of hepatocellular carcinoma *via* upregulation of CDK2 and MMP2. Oncogene 2019; 38(25): 4948-61.
[http://dx.doi.org/10.1038/s41388-019-0766-x] [PMID: 30842588]

[78]   Cock-Rada AM, Medjkane S, Janski N, *et al.* SMYD3 promotes cancer invasion by epigenetic upregulation of the metalloproteinase MMP-9. Cancer Res 2012; 72(3): 810-20.
[http://dx.doi.org/10.1158/0008-5472.CAN-11-1052] [PMID: 22194464]

[79]   Zhu Y, Zhu MX, Zhang XD, *et al.* SMYD3 stimulates EZR and LOXL2 transcription to enhance proliferation, migration, and invasion in esophageal squamous cell carcinoma. Hum Pathol 2016; 52: 153-63.
[http://dx.doi.org/10.1016/j.humpath.2016.01.012] [PMID: 26980013]

[80]   Jiang Y, Lyu T, Che X, Jia N, Li Q, Feng W. Overexpression of SMYD3 in ovarian cancer is associated with ovarian cancer proliferation and apoptosis *via* methylating H3K4 and H4K20. J Cancer 2019; 10(17): 4072-84.
[http://dx.doi.org/10.7150/jca.29861] [PMID: 31417652]

[81]   Ma L, Chen ZM, Li XY, Wang XJ, Shou JX, Fu XD. Nucleostemin and ASPP2 expression is correlated with pituitary adenoma proliferation. Oncol Lett 2013; 6(5): 1313-8.
[http://dx.doi.org/10.3892/ol.2013.1562] [PMID: 24179515]

[82]   Krishnan H, Rayes J, Miyashita T, *et al.* Podoplanin: An emerging cancer biomarker and therapeutic target. Cancer Sci 2018; 109(5): 1292-9.
[http://dx.doi.org/10.1111/cas.13580] [PMID: 29575529]

[83]   Sikorska J, Gaweł D, Domek H, Rudzińska M, Czarnocka B. Podoplanin (PDPN) affects the invasiveness of thyroid carcinoma cells by inducing ezrin, radixin and moesin (E/R/M) phosphorylation in association with matrix metalloproteinases. BMC Cancer 2019; 19(1): 85.
[http://dx.doi.org/10.1186/s12885-018-5239-z] [PMID: 30654768]

[84]   Wright KD, Miller BS, El-Meanawy S, *et al.* The p52 isoform of SHC1 is a key driver of breast cancer initiation. Breast Cancer Res 2019; 21(1): 74.
[http://dx.doi.org/10.1186/s13058-019-1155-7] [PMID: 31202267]

[85]   Ahn R, Sabourin V, Bolt AM, *et al.* The Shc1 adaptor simultaneously balances Stat1 and Stat3 activity to promote breast cancer immune suppression. Nat Commun 2017; 8(1): 14638.

[http://dx.doi.org/10.1038/ncomms14638] [PMID: 28276425]

[86]   Tanimura S, Ohtsuka S, Mitsui K, Shirouzu K, Yoshimura A, Ohtsubo M. MDM2 interacts with MDMX through their RING finger domains. FEBS Lett 1999; 447(1): 5-9.
[http://dx.doi.org/10.1016/S0014-5793(99)00254-9] [PMID: 10218570]

[87]   Riemenschneider MJ, Büschges R, Wolter M, et al. Amplification and overexpression of the MDM4 (MDMX) gene from 1q32 in a subset of malignant gliomas without TP53 mutation or MDM2 amplification. Cancer Res. 1999; 59(24): 6091-6.

[88]   Gao C, Xiao G, Piersigilli A, Gou J, Ogunwobi O, Bargonetti J. Context-dependent roles of MDMX (MDM4) and MDM2 in breast cancer proliferation and circulating tumor cells. Breast Cancer Res 2019; 21(1): 5.
[http://dx.doi.org/10.1186/s13058-018-1094-8] [PMID: 30642351]

[89]   Haupt S, Vijayakumaran R, Miranda PJ, Burgess A, Lim E, Haupt Y. The role of MDM2 and MDM4 in breast cancer development and prevention. J Mol Cell Biol 2017; 9(1): 53-61.
[http://dx.doi.org/10.1093/jmcb/mjx007] [PMID: 28096293]

[90]   Dewaele M, Tabaglio T, Willekens K, *et al.* Antisense oligonucleotide–mediated MDM4 exon 6 skipping impairs tumor growth. J Clin Invest 2015; 126(1): 68-84.
[http://dx.doi.org/10.1172/JCI82534] [PMID: 26595814]

[91]   Nakano M, Fukami T, Gotoh S, Nakajima M. A-to-I RNA editing up-regulates human dihydrofolate reductase in breast cancer. J Biol Chem 2017; 292(12): 4873-84.
[http://dx.doi.org/10.1074/jbc.M117.775684] [PMID: 28188287]

[92]   Chen L, Li Y, Lin CH, *et al.* Recoding RNA editing of AZIN1 predisposes to hepatocellular carcinoma. Nat Med 2013; 19(2): 209-16.
[http://dx.doi.org/10.1038/nm.3043] [PMID: 23291631]

[93]   Lazzari E, Mondala PK, Santos ND, *et al.* Alu-dependent RNA editing of GLI1 promotes malignant regeneration in multiple myeloma. Nat Commun 2017; 8(1): 1922.
[http://dx.doi.org/10.1038/s41467-017-01890-w] [PMID: 29203771]

[94]   Chen W, He W, Cai H, *et al.* A-to-I RNA editing of BLCAP lost the inhibition to STAT3 activation in cervical cancer. Oncotarget 2017; 8(24): 39417-29.
[http://dx.doi.org/10.18632/oncotarget.17034] [PMID: 28455960]

[95]   Giri K, Pabelick CM, Mukherjee P, Prakash YS. Hepatoma derived growth factor (HDGF) dynamics in ovarian cancer cells. Apoptosis 2016; 21(3): 329-39.
[http://dx.doi.org/10.1007/s10495-015-1200-7] [PMID: 26612514]

[96]   Yang F, Yu N, Wang H, *et al.* Downregulated expression of hepatoma-derived growth factor inhibits migration and invasion of prostate cancer cells by suppressing epithelial-mesenchymal transition and MMP2, MMP9. PLoS One 2018; 13(1): e0190725.
[http://dx.doi.org/10.1371/journal.pone.0190725] [PMID: 29300772]

[97]   Liu C, Wang L, Jiang Q, *et al.* Hepatoma-Derived Growth Factor and DDX5 Promote Carcinogenesis and Progression of Endometrial Cancer by Activating β-Catenin. Front Oncol 2019; 9: 211.
[http://dx.doi.org/10.3389/fonc.2019.00211] [PMID: 31032220]

[98]   Wood ML, Dizdaroglu M, Gajewski E, Essigmann JM. Mechanistic studies of ionizing radiation and oxidative mutagenesis: genetic effects of a single 8-hydroxyguanine (7-hydro-8-oxoguanine) residue inserted at a unique site in a viral genome. Biochemistry 1990; 29(30): 7024-32.
[http://dx.doi.org/10.1021/bi00482a011] [PMID: 2223758]

[99]   Kashfi SMH, Golmohammadi M, Behboudi F, Nazemalhosseini-Mojarad E, Zali MR. MUTYH the base excision repair gene family member associated with colorectal cancer polyposis. Gastroenterol Hepatol Bed Bench 2013; 6 (Suppl. 1): S1-S10.
[PMID: 24834277]

[100] SDHB gene - Genetics Home Reference - NIH, https://ghr.nlm.nih.gov/gene/SDHB (accessed July 15,

2020).

[101] Dai Y, Tang Z, Yang Z, *et al.* EXO1 overexpression is associated with poor prognosis of hepatocellular carcinoma patients. Cell Cycle 2018; 17(19-20): 2386-97.
[http://dx.doi.org/10.1080/15384101.2018.1534511] [PMID: 30328366]

[102] Bayram S, Akkız H, Bekar A, Akgöllü E, Yıldırım S. The significance of Exonuclease 1 K589E polymorphism on hepatocellular carcinoma susceptibility in the Turkish population: a case–control study. Mol Biol Rep 2012; 39(5): 5943-51.
[http://dx.doi.org/10.1007/s11033-011-1406-x] [PMID: 22205538]

[103] Tsai MH, Tseng HC, Liu CS, *et al.* Interaction of Exo1 genotypes and smoking habit in oral cancer in Taiwan. Oral Oncol 2009; 45(9): e90-4.
[http://dx.doi.org/10.1016/j.oraloncology.2009.03.011] [PMID: 19515603]

[104] Alimirzaie S, Mohamadkhani A, Masoudi S, *et al.* Mutations in known and novel cancer susceptibility genes in young patients with pancreatic cancer. Arch Iran Med 2018; 21(6): 228-33.
[PMID: 29940740]

[105] Sun X, Zheng L, Shen B. Functional alterations of human exonuclease 1 mutants identified in atypical hereditary nonpolyposis colorectal cancer syndrome. Cancer res. 2002; 62(21): 6026-30.

[106] Hsu NY, Wang HC, Wang CH, et al. Lung cancer susceptibility and genetic polymorphisms of Exo1 gene in Taiwan. Anticancer Res. 2009; 29(2): 725-30.

[107] Keijzers G, Bakula D, Petr M, *et al.* Human exonuclease 1 (EXO1) regulatory functions in DNA replication with putative roles in cancer. Int J Mol Sci 2018; 20(1): 74.
[http://dx.doi.org/10.3390/ijms20010074] [PMID: 30585186]

[108] Lehtonen HJ, Kiuru M, Ylisaukko-Oja SK, *et al.* Increased risk of cancer in patients with fumarate hydratase germline mutation. J Med Genet 2006; 43(6): 523-6.
[http://dx.doi.org/10.1136/jmg.2005.036400] [PMID: 16155190]

[109] Schmidt C, Sciacovelli M, Frezza C. Fumarate hydratase in cancer: A multifaceted tumour suppressor. Semin Cell Dev Biol 2020; 98: 15-25.
[http://dx.doi.org/10.1016/j.semcdb.2019.05.002] [PMID: 31085323]

[110] Suwa H, Ohshio G, Imamura T, *et al.* Overexpression of the rhoC gene correlates with progression of ductal adenocarcinoma of the pancreas. Br J Cancer 1998; 77(1): 147-52.
[http://dx.doi.org/10.1038/bjc.1998.23] [PMID: 9459160]

[111] Horiuchi A, Imai T, Wang C, *et al.* Up-regulation of small GTPases, RhoA and RhoC, is associated with tumor progression in ovarian carcinoma. Lab Invest 2003; 83(6): 861-70.
[http://dx.doi.org/10.1097/01.LAB.0000073128.16098.31] [PMID: 12808121]

[112] Iiizumi M, Bandyopadhyay S, Pai S. RhoC promotes metastasis but not growth of prostate tumor. Cancer Research 2008; 68.

[113] Jovanović B, Beeler JS, Pickup MW, *et al.* Transforming growth factor beta receptor type III is a tumor promoter in mesenchymal-stem like triple negative breast cancer. Breast Cancer Res 2014; 16(4): R69.
[http://dx.doi.org/10.1186/bcr3684] [PMID: 24985072]

[114] Liu XL, Xiao K, Xue B, *et al.* Dual role of TGFBR3 in bladder cancer. Oncol Rep 2013; 30(3): 1301-8.
[http://dx.doi.org/10.3892/or.2013.2599] [PMID: 23835618]

[115] Zhang X, Chen Y, Li Z, Han X, Liang Y. TGFBR3 is an independent unfavourable prognostic marker in oesophageal squamous cell cancer and is positively correlated with Ki☐67. Int J Exp Pathol 2020; 101(6): 223-9.
[http://dx.doi.org/10.1111/iep.12380] [PMID: 33146446]

[116] Dong M, How T, Kirkbride KC, *et al.* The type III TGF-β receptor suppresses breast cancer

progression. J Clin Invest 2007; 117(1): 206-17.
[http://dx.doi.org/10.1172/JCI29293] [PMID: 17160136]

[117]   Nishida J, Miyazono K, Ehata S. Decreased TGFBR3/betaglycan expression enhances the metastatic abilities of renal cell carcinoma cells through TGF-β-dependent and -independent mechanisms. Oncogene 2018; 37(16): 2197-212.
[http://dx.doi.org/10.1038/s41388-017-0084-0] [PMID: 29391598]

[118]   Tsai MS, Hornby AE, Lakins J, Lupu R. Expression and function of CYR61, an angiogenic factor, in breast cancer cell lines and tumor biopsies. Cancer res. 2000; 60(20): 5603-7.

[119]   Espinoza I, Menendez JA, Kvp CM, Lupu R. CCN1 promotes vascular endothelial growth factor secretion through αvβ3 integrin receptors in breast cancer. J Cell Commun Signal 2014; 8(1): 23-7.
[http://dx.doi.org/10.1007/s12079-013-0214-6] [PMID: 24338441]

[120]   Nguyen N, Kuliopulos A, Graham RA, Covic L. Tumor-derived Cyr61(CCN1) promotes stromal matrix metalloproteinase-1 production and protease-activated receptor 1-dependent migration of breast cancer cells. Cancer Res 2006; 66(5): 2658-65.
[http://dx.doi.org/10.1158/0008-5472.CAN-05-2082] [PMID: 16510585]

[121]   Harris LG, Pannell LK, Singh S, Samant RS, Shevde LA. Increased vascularity and spontaneous metastasis of breast cancer by hedgehog signaling mediated upregulation of cyr61. Oncogene 2012; 31(28): 3370-80.
[http://dx.doi.org/10.1038/onc.2011.496] [PMID: 22056874]

[122]   Xie D, Yin D, Tong X, *et al.* Cyr61 is overexpressed in gliomas and involved in integrin-linked kinase-mediated Akt and β-catenin-TCF/Lef signaling pathways. Cancer Res 2004; 64(6): 1987-96.
[http://dx.doi.org/10.1158/0008-5472.CAN-03-0666] [PMID: 15026334]

[123]   Zhou Y, Su Y, Zhu H, *et al.* Interleukin-23 receptor signaling mediates cancer dormancy and radioresistance in human esophageal squamous carcinoma cells *via* the Wnt/Notch pathway. J Mol Med (Berl) 2019; 97(2): 177-88.
[http://dx.doi.org/10.1007/s00109-018-1724-8] [PMID: 30483821]

[124]   Tao Y, Tao T, Gross N, *et al.* Combined Effect of IL-12Rβ2 and IL-23R Expression on Prognosis of Patients with Laryngeal Cancer. Cell Physiol Biochem 2018; 50(3): 1041-54.
[http://dx.doi.org/10.1159/000494515] [PMID: 30355949]

[125]   Zhang S, Chen L, Wang-Rodriguez J, *et al.* The onco-embryonic antigen ROR1 is expressed by a variety of human cancers. Am J Pathol 2012; 181(6): 1903-10.
[http://dx.doi.org/10.1016/j.ajpath.2012.08.024] [PMID: 23041612]

[126]   Zhang S, Cui B, Lai H, *et al.* Ovarian cancer stem cells express ROR1, which can be targeted for anti–cancer-stem-cell therapy. Proc Natl Acad Sci USA 2014; 111(48): 17266-71.
[http://dx.doi.org/10.1073/pnas.1419599111] [PMID: 25411317]

[127]   Liu D, Gunther K, Enriquez LA, *et al.* ROR1 is upregulated in endometrial cancer and represents a novel therapeutic target. Sci Rep 2020; 10(1): 13906.
[http://dx.doi.org/10.1038/s41598-020-70924-z] [PMID: 32807831]

[128]   Müller T, Choidas A, Reichmann E, Ullrich A. Phosphorylation and free pool of β-catenin are regulated by tyrosine kinases and tyrosine phosphatases during epithelial cell migration. J Biol Chem 1999; 274(15): 10173-83.
[http://dx.doi.org/10.1074/jbc.274.15.10173] [PMID: 10187801]

[129]   Guan X, Chen S, Liu Y, Wang L, Zhao Y, Zong ZH. PUM1 promotes ovarian cancer proliferation, migration and invasion. Biochem Biophys Res Commun 2018; 497(1): 313-8.
[http://dx.doi.org/10.1016/j.bbrc.2018.02.078] [PMID: 29428722]

[130]   Dai H, Shen K, Yang Y, *et al.* PUM1 knockdown prevents tumor progression by activating the PERK/eIF2/ATF4 signaling pathway in pancreatic adenocarcinoma cells. Cell Death Dis 2019; 10(8): 595.

[http://dx.doi.org/10.1038/s41419-019-1839-z] [PMID: 31395860]

[131] Xia LH, Yan QH, Sun QD, Gao YP. MiR-411-5p acts as a tumor suppressor in non-small cell lung cancer through targeting PUM1. Eur Rev Med Pharmacol Sci 2018; 22(17): 5546-53.
[http://dx.doi.org/10.26355/eurrev_201809_15816] [PMID: 30229827]

[132] Gor R, Sampath SS, Lazer LM, Ramalingam S. RNA binding protein PUM1 promotes colon cancer cell proliferation and migration. Int J Biol Macromol 2021; 174: 549-61.
[http://dx.doi.org/10.1016/j.ijbiomac.2021.01.154] [PMID: 33508364]

[133] Gor R, Saha L, Agarwal S, *et al.* Morin inhibits colon cancer stem cells by inhibiting PUM1 expression in vitro. Med Oncol 2022; 39(12): 251.
[http://dx.doi.org/10.1007/s12032-022-01851-4] [PMID: 36224472]

CHAPTER 2

Chromosome 2

Thilaga Thirugnanam[1], Saurav Panicker[1] and **Satish Ramalingam[1,*]**

[1] *Department of Genetic Engineering, School of Bioengineering, SRM Institute of Science and Technology, Kattankulathur, India*

Abstract: The human chromosome 2 was formed by a head-to-head fusion mutation caused by two chromosomes of our ancestors. The gorilla and chimpanzee contain 48 chromosomes in contrast to 46 chromosomes in humans. Ten million years ago, the two chromosomes of apes underwent telomere-to-telomere fusion that gave rise to human chromosome 2. Apart from the exciting history, the human chromosome 2 is involved in various genetic conditions caused due to chromosomal deletions and duplications, leading to SATB2 (Special AT-rich sequence-binding protein 2)-associated syndrome, MBD5 (Methyl-CpG-binding domain 5)-associated neurodevelopmental disorder, 2q37 deletion syndrome, partial trisomy 2, myelodysplastic syndrome as well as cancer. These mutations cause different human abnormalities, such as craniofacial anomalies, cleft palate, genitourinary tract anomalies, microcephaly, hypotonia, heart defects, anemia, and myeloid malignances. This chapter discusses 50 genes of human chromosome 2 involved in various cancer types.

Keywords: Cancer, CFLAR, Leukemia, Metastasis, MYCN, RALB, RAS, REL, RHOB, Tumor.

1.1. APOB - APOLIPOPROTEIN B CHROMOSOME 2; 2p24.1

APOB encoding apolipoprotein B is a glycoprotein involved in composing and distributing lipids, and mutations in this gene translate a shortened protein causing hypocholesterolemia and familial hypobetalipoproteinemia [1]. APOB is involved in liver cancer in which the gene is mutated [2]. APOB was inactivated in hepatocellular carcinoma, which correlated to poor prognosis [2]. APOB gene signature was associated with other verified signature genes in hepatocellular carcinoma samples showing that silencing of APOB was related to poor prognosis in hepatocellular carcinoma [2]. Network analysis results showed that the activity

---

* **Corresponding author Satish Ramalingam**: Department of Genetic Engineering, School of Bioengineering, SRM Institute of Science and Technology, Kattankulathur, India; E-mail: rsatish76@gmail.com

of low-APOB was linked to increased certain regulators necessary for metastasis and oncogenesis and decreased tumor suppressors compared to high-APOB activity in the progression of hepatocellular carcinoma [2].

1.2. BOLL - BOULE HOMOLOG, RNA BINDING PROTEIN CHROMOSOME 2; 2q33.1

BOLL gene (Fig. 1) comes under DAZ or Deleted in Azoospermia gene family is the parent gene and plays a role in spermatogenesis [3]. BOLL was involved in colorectal cancer, where the expression of this gene was upregulated [3]. BOLL promoter was more methylated in colorectal cancer tissues than in normal tissues [3]. Also, BOLL was highly expressed in colorectal cancer cell lines, which led to the proliferation and migration of these cancer cells and increased the number of cells in the S-phase of the cell cycle [3]. These observations indicated that BOLL has an oncogenic property with increased promoter methylation, particularly in colorectal cancer [3]. BOLL could be a potential prognostic cancer for colorectal cancer [3].

1.3. BUB1 - BUB1 MITOTIC CHECKPOINT SERINE/THREONINE KINASE CHROMOSOME 2; 2q13

BUB1 is a serine/threonine kinase that plays a role in cell cycle checkpoint in mitosis. It localizes along with other proteins involved in the spindle checkpoint to the kinetochore during chromosome congression [4]. Upregulation of BUB1 led to augmentation of phosphorylation of SMAD2 protein and cell proliferation in liver cancer tissues compared to normal liver tissues suggesting that BUB1 might have the diagnostic potential of liver cancer [5]. The role of BUB1 in glioblastoma was also reported, where it was overexpressed and led to cell proliferation and tumor development *in vivo* and *in vitro* [6]. It also serves as a poor prognostic factor due to its increased expression in patients with glioblastoma [6].

1.4. CCL20 - C-C MOTIF CHEMOKINE LIGAND 20 CHROMOSOME 2; 2q36.3

CCL20 is involved in various types of cancers. The expression of CCL20 was induced by interleukin-1β, which activated signaling pathways in non-small cell lung cancer, where it was upregulated compared to normal samples of lung cells. This resulted in the proliferation and migration of lung cancer cells [7]. CCL20 can serve as a therapeutic target for non-small cell lung cancer [7]. CCL20 was highly expressed in breast cancer patients, which led to reduced survival of these patients [8]. Expression of CCL20 also led to bone metastasis in breast cancer, where it increased the activity of nuclear factors, such as kappa-B and osteoprotegerin in osteoblastic cells and breast cancer cells and suggest that CCL20 has therapeutic potential in breast cancer bone metastasis [8].

1.5. CFLAR - CASP8 AND FADD-LIKE APOPTOSIS REGULATOR CHROMOSOME 2; 2q33.1

CFLAR, an anti-apoptotic protein homologous to caspase-8 commonly known as c-FLIP or Cellular FLICE-like Inhibitory Protein, plays a major role in inhibiting tumor necrosis factor-α (TNF- α) and TNF-related apoptotic factors and apoptosis during chemotherapy [9]. CFLAR, or c-FLIP, was upregulated in various cancers such as cervical cancer, hepatocellular cancers, head and neck squamous cell carcinoma, and colorectal cancers [9]. c-FLIP also plays a role in non-Hodgkin lymphomas (NHLs), where the expression of c-FLIP could assist in finding the progression of tumors and prognosis of NHLs [10]. c-FLIP inhibits the ligands of death receptors during chemotherapy, causing resistance in cancer cells [10].

1.6. CREB1 - CAMP RESPONSIVE ELEMENT BINDING PROTEIN 1 CHROMOSOME 2; 2q33.3

CREB1 is a transcription factor that controls the proliferation of cells by phosphorylation and dephosphorylation [11], which is targeted by miRNAs in different cancers, such as colorectal, breast, gastric, and ovarian cancer serving as a potential target to treat cancer [12]. miR-122 was one of the miRNAs that targeted CREB1 in bladder cancer in which CREB1 was overexpressed in bladder cancer cell lines and tissues, and miR-122 regulated the expression of *CREB1,* leading to cell invasion and cell proliferation which further could serve as a potential target for bladder cancer [11]. *CREB1,* along with miR-373, was induced by norepinephrine led to colon cancer cell's invasion, proliferation, and metastasis [13].

1.7. CTLA4 - CYTOTOXIC T-LYMPHOCYTE ASSOCIATED PROTEIN 4 CHROMOSOME 2; 2q33.2

CTLA-4 (Fig. 1) is a glycoprotein that plays a significant role in the immune response. It is expressed on the membranes of T cells to inhibit T cell division and is also involved in the cell cycle and cytokinesis [14]. Expression of CTLA-4 with single nucleotide polymorphisms (SNPs) was observed in various cancers such as melanoma, hepatocellular carcinoma, colorectal cancer, cervical cancer, renal cell carcinoma, *etc* [14]. An SNP in exon 1 of CTLA-4 leads to a threonine-to-alanine (A/G) exchange [15]. When this SNP in breast cancer was compared to normal breast, the incidence of the GG genotype was reduced in patients with breast cancer. Also, the AA genotype was correlated to the tumor size, indicating that CTLA-4 polymorphism promotes tumor formation [15].

Chromosome 2

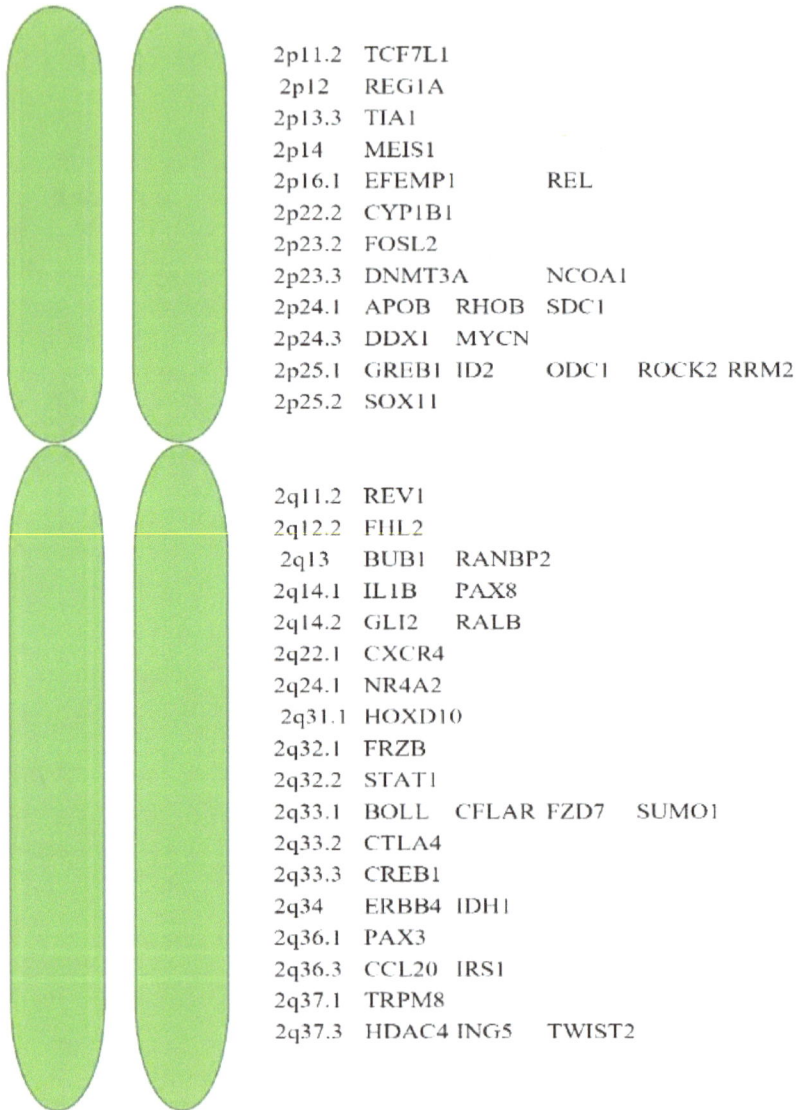

Locus	Genes				
2p11.2	TCF7L1				
2p12	REG1A				
2p13.3	TIA1				
2p14	MEIS1				
2p16.1	EFEMP1		REL		
2p22.2	CYP1B1				
2p23.2	FOSL2				
2p23.3	DNMT3A		NCOA1		
2p24.1	APOB	RHOB	SDC1		
2p24.3	DDX1	MYCN			
2p25.1	GREB1	ID2	ODC1	ROCK2	RRM2
2p25.2	SOX11				
2q11.2	REV1				
2q12.2	FHL2				
2q13	BUB1	RANBP2			
2q14.1	IL1B	PAX8			
2q14.2	GLI2	RALB			
2q22.1	CXCR4				
2q24.1	NR4A2				
2q31.1	HOXD10				
2q32.1	FRZB				
2q32.2	STAT1				
2q33.1	BOLL	CFLAR	FZD7	SUMO1	
2q33.2	CTLA4				
2q33.3	CREB1				
2q34	ERBB4	IDH1			
2q36.1	PAX3				
2q36.3	CCL20	IRS1			
2q37.1	TRPM8				
2q37.3	HDAC4	ING5	TWIST2		

Fig. (1). This figure displays the loci of the genes from Chromosome 2 whose roles in cancer have been explained in this chapter. Sayooj Madhusoodanan designed this diagram.

1.8. CXCR4 - C-X-C MOTIF CHEMOKINE RECEPTOR 4 CHROMO-SOME 2; 2q22.1

CXCR4 is a chemokine member of the heterotrimeric G-coupled proteins super-family, involved in various cellular mechanisms binding specifically to another chemokine, CXCL12, or stromal cell-derived factor 1 (SDF-1) [16]. CXCR4 is also expressed in different cancers, where it helps in the migration and proliferation of cancer cells [16]. In breast cancer, CXCR4 binds to SDF-1, where SDF-1 promotes the formation of blood vessels in the tumor by signaling the endothelial cells [16]. This interaction also led to breast cancer metastasis, where the cells reach organs that produce more chemokines [16]. Also, upregulation of CXCR4 resulted in metastasis of breast cancer cells to bones as bone cells generate SDF-1 [16].

1.9. CYP1B1 - CYTOCHROME P450 FAMILY 1 SUBFAMILY B MEMBER 1 CHROMOSOME 2; 2p22.2

CYP1B1 (Fig. 1) is a member of the CYP1 family produced in normal cells but upregulated in tumors [17]. CYP1B1 is involved in the metabolism of carcinogens forming DNA adducts [17]. This gene is primarily upregulated in cancers induced by hormones such as prostate, breast, and ovary tumors and promotes the proliferation of cells in breast and endometrial cancer cells [17]. CYP1B1 increased the expression of β-catenin, leading to the induction of Wnt/β-catenin signaling in cancer cells, increasing cancer cell proliferation [17]. Also, CYP1B1 increased the expression of E-cadherin repressors resulting in metastasis of cancer cells by inducing epithelial-mesenchymal transition (EMT). Therefore, CYP1B1 plays an essential role in promoting cancer [17].

1.10. DDX1 – DEAD-BOX HELICASE 1 CHROMOSOME 2; 2p24.3

DDX1 encoding for DEAD-box helicase-1 protein belongs to the DEAD-box helicase family, which is involved in various physiological processes, such as the synthesis of ribosomes and tRNA, processing of miRNA and mRNA, and DNA repair [18]. DDX1 also plays a role in cancer, which was upregulated in retino-blastoma and neuroblastoma tumors [18]. DDX1 induced transcription of genes involved in stem cells, especially in chromosome 12p and Cyclin-D2, resulting in the formation of testicular tumors [18]. Also, DDX1 is involved in colorectal cancer. The knock-out of the DDX1 gene in LoVo cells led to the inhibition of marker genes of cancer stem cells, particularly the *LGR5* gene indicating the significance of DDX1 in inducing tumorigenesis of colorectal cancer cells [18].

1.11. DNMT3A - DNA METHYL TRANSFER ASE 3 ALPHA CHROMOSOME 2; 2p23.3

DNMT3A (Fig. 1) is one of the genes involved in DNA methyl transfer ase activity and DNA methylation of CpG islands during embryogenesis by de novo methylation [19]. It has a conserved protein of 130-kDa size in vertebrates such as mice and humans and forms dimers and tetramers in the nucleus [19]. DNMT3A is involved in cancers such as lymphoid and myeloid neoplasms and acute myeloid leukemia (AML), where this gene is mutated [19]. R882, one of the highly mutated sites in DNMT3A in AML, led to a gain of function in DNMT3A [20]. Mutations in DNMT3A, especially R882H, caused a change in the methylation of CpG sites, but there was no change in 5- methyl-cytosine in AML [20]. Also, DNMT3A disrupted methylation in CpG islands of the promoter regions [20].

1.12. EFEMP1 - EGF CONTAINING FIBULIN EXTRACELLULAR MATRIX PROTEIN 1 CHROMOSOME 2; 2p16.1

EFEMP1 is a member of fibulin, an extracellular matrix protein that retains the stability of basal laminae and extracellular matrix [21]. EFEMP1 plays a role in cancer where the upregulation of this gene leads to adhesion, invasion, and proliferation of cervical cancer cells, which is also correlated to VEGF expression [21]. The expression of this gene was reduced in pleomorphic glioma, breast cancer, and nasopharyngeal carcinoma, which resulted in the suppression of metastasis and invasion of tumor cells [21]. EFEMP1 is also involved in ovarian cancer. The upregulation of this gene in ovarian cancer tissues was linked to the metastasis of lymph nodes, decreased differentiation of cells, high stage, and a low prognostic value, indicating that EFEMP1 has a therapeutic value for ovarian cancer [21].

1.13. EPCAM - EPITHELIAL CELL ADHESION MOLECULE CHRO-MOSOME 2; 2p21

EpCAM is a glycoprotein located on the cell surface that plays a role in cell-cell adhesion and is expressed in normal and cancer epithelial cells [22]. EpCAM is a weak adhesion molecule compared to E-Cadherin, indicating that cells with EpCAM have a weak connection between the cells [22]. It also regulates the integrity of epithelial cells and the binding of claudins by changing the structure and function of tight junctions between the cells [22]. EpCAM is highly expressed in the colon with increased proliferation and decreased differentiation of cells [22]. This property is also seen in human embryonic stem cells serving as a surface marker in these cells [22]. The role of EpCAM is observed in colon cancer, which induces the proliferation and metastasis of colon cancer cells and tumor progression [23].

1.14. ERBB4 - ERB-B2 RECEPTOR TYROSINE KINASE 4 CHROMO-SOME 2; 2q34

ERBB4 is a glycoprotein belonging to the receptor tyrosine kinases subfamily with tyrosine kinase property and is involved in triggering kinase activity, dimerization of receptors, regulated intramembrane proteolysis and induction of phosphoinositide 3-kinase/Akt and mitogen-activated protein kinase pathways [24]. The expression of ERBB4 decreased in ER-positive breast cancer cells and cleaved in *in vivo* breast cancer tissues [24]. ERBB4 and the epidermal growth factor-induced cell proliferation and cell division [25]. ERBB4 is highly expressed in various cancers, such as breast, head, and neck squamous cell carcinoma, bladder cancer, and gastric cancer [25]. Furthermore, upregulation of ERBB4 in gastric cancer correlated to poor prognosis [25].

1.15. FHL2 - FOUR AND A HALF LIM DOMAINS 2 CHROMOSOME 2; 2q12.2

FHL2 belongs to the member of the LIM-only protein family. The gene encodes for four-and-a-half LIM-only proteins, which expresses in specific cells, including the heart, colon, kidney, prostate, lung, pancreas, stomach, and cortex [26]. In addition, FHL2 said differently in various cancers, such as ovarian, colon, and breast cancers, and melanoma showed upregulation of FHL2. In contrast, in rhabdomyosarcoma, prostate cancer, and hepatocellular carcinoma, FHL2 is expressed in lower levels as a tumor suppressor [26]. Overexpression of FHL2 was observed in cervical cancer cell lines and tissues where it was induced the proliferation of cells inhibited apoptosis through AKT/mTOR pathway, indicating that FHL2 can have a potential prognostic value for cervical cancer [27].

1.16. FOSL2 - FOS LIKE 2, AP-1 TRANSCRIPTION FACTOR SUBUNIT CHROMOSOME 2; 2p23.2

FOSL2 is a member of an AP-1 transcription factor involved in pathological, physiological, and developmental events, especially in the establishment of bone [28]. Upregulation of FOSL2 influenced the TGF-β, a cytokine in systemic sclerosis [28]. FOSL2 is involved in maintaining the synthesis and structuring of the extracellular matrix [28]. Upregulation of FOSL2 resulted in the migration of non-small cell lung carcinoma cells by inducing TGF-β signaling through the binding of Smad3 protein, which then led to the acetylation of Smad3 by P300 protein [28]. This indicated that FOSL2 has therapeutic potential in non-small cell lung carcinoma [28]. FOSL2 also plays a role in colorectal cancer, where the expression of FOSL2 leads to metastasis serving as a prognostic marker for colorectal cancer [29].

1.17. FRZB - FRIZZLED RELATED PROTEIN CHROMOSOME 2; 2q32.1

FRZB belongs to the family of secreted frizzled-related proteins involved in embryo development through Wnt signaling [30]. FRZB inhibited genes responsible for Wnt/β-catenin signalings, such as cyclooxygenase and MMP3, to maintain the structure of cartilage and the density and opacity of cortical bones [30]. FRZB suppressed the proteinase activity of MPP3 protein by interacting using the netrin-like domain in FRZB, which is responsible for binding Wnt proteins [30]. Expression of FRZB is required for metastasis in renal cancer, where it functions as an oncogene [30]. FRZB is also involved in hepatocellular carcinoma, where upregulation of FRZB leads to metastasis of bone when paired with hepatocellular carcinoma indicating that FRZB is essential for hepatocellular carcinoma bone metastasis [30].

1.18. FZD7 - FRIZZLED CLASS RECEPTOR 7 CHROMOSOME 2; 2q33.1

FZD7, a transmembrane protein, binds to the Wnt receptor and controls the Wnt signaling pathways, including canonical and non-canonical pathways [31]. FZD7 is involved in various types of cancers where upregulation of FZD7-induced Wnt signaling pathway resulting in the progression of cancer [31]. FZD7 also plays a role in hepatocellular carcinoma and colorectal and breast cancers, where it follows the canonical pathway of Wnt/β-catenin signaling. In contrast, FZD7 influenced the non-canonical pathway of Wnt/PCP signaling in colon cancer by upregulating RhoA expression [31]. In addition, FZD7 induced the growth of gastric cancer cells, and in patients with gastric cancer, especially in the late-stage of cancer, FZD7 was upregulated. The overall survival of patients was poor [31].

1.19. GREB1 - GROWTH REGULATING ESTROGEN RECEPTOR BINDING 1 CHROMOSOME 2; 2p25.1

GREB1 is involved in various types of cancers, such as breast cancer with ER-positive cells, and GREB1 is regulated by estrogen receptor α for proliferation of cells in a hormone-dependent manner [32]. GREB1 produces three different isoforms, such as GREB1a, GREB1b, and GREB1c, with co-regulatory functions [32]. GREB1a isoform expression increased the expression of genes regulated by estrogen receptors [32]. Furthermore, expression of GREB1a or GREB1b led to reduced proliferation of breast carcinoma cell lines with ER-positive and ER-negative cells [32]. These results indicated that GREB1 function even without estrogen receptors [32]. GREB1b and GREB1c isoforms expression were elevated in breast tissue during metastasis, suggesting that GREB1 isoforms function in a specific manner [32].

1.20. GLI2 - GLI FAMILY ZINC FINGER 2 CHROMOSOME 2; 2q14.2

GLI2 belongs to the family of transcription factors involved in developing the pituitary gland and forebrain by regulating the Sonic Hedgehog signaling pathway

[33]. Mutations, such as nonsense and frameshift in GLI2 led to various abnormalities and deficiencies, such as defects in the face and pituitary hormones, partial penetrance, polydactyly, and diabetes insipidus [33]. GLI2 is involved in gastric cancer. Bioinformatics analysis showed the expression of GLI2 increased in gastric cancer tissues compared to normal gastric tissues resulting in poor overall survival and progression-free survival of gastric cancer patients [34]. GLI2 regulated the cancer stem cells by interacting and inducing the expression of platelet-derived growth factor beta [PDGFRB] in gastric cancer cells [34].

1.21. HDAC4 - HISTONE DEACETYLASE 4 CHROMOSOME 2; 2q37.3

HDAC4 belongs to a class of HDAC proteins that forms complexes with transcriptional repressor proteins [35]. HDAC4 is involved in DNA damage response by suppressing p21, a cyclin-dependent kinase inhibitor using transcription factors, such as p53 and Sp1 in cancer cells [35]. HDAC4 is expressed in different cancers, such as breast, ovarian, cervical, colorectal, glioma, and prostate cancers [35]. In colon cancer, HDAC4 inhibited the p21 protein and induced the progression of cancer cells [35]. Expression of HDAC4 was increased in gastric cancer cell lines and tissues, which led to a proliferation of cells and increased ATP levels and colony formation [35]. Like colon cancer, HDAC4 suppressed the expression of p21 in the gastric cancer cell line indicating that HDAC4 induces cell growth by inhibiting p21 in gastric cancer [35].

1.22. HOXD10 - HOMEOBOX D10 CHROMOSOME 2; 2q31.1

HOXD10 is one of the HOX genes that belong to the family of transcription factors involved in the function of stem cells and the growth of embryonic cells [36]. HOXD genes play a role in different cancers, such as lung cancer, leukemia, and breast cancer, where the expression of these genes differs from normal cells [36]. Expression of HOXD10 was observed in colorectal cancer where decreased expression of HOXD10 and upregulation of Ras homolog family member C were associated with overexpression of microRNA-10b, and HOXD10 was targeted by microRNA-10b [37]. Also, HOXD10 levels were reduced in tumor tissues of lymph nodes with metastatic activity compared to tumor tissues without metastatic properties [37].

1.23. ID2 - INHIBITOR OF DNA BINDING 2 CHROMOSOME 2; 2p25.1

ID proteins are a group of proteins that regulate stem cells and are involved in tumor formation, where it controls angiogenesis and regeneration of cells [38]. ID2 is one of the proteins in the ID proteins group which plays a role in angiogenesis in tumor and glioma stem cell activity [38]. A study elucidated the mechanism of angiogenesis and stem cell property where ID2 hampered the Von

Hippel Lindau (VHL) complex by interacting with the complex, which in turn blocked the degradation of hypoxia-inducible factor 2 alpha (HIF2α) induced by ubiquitin in brain tumor cells under hypoxic condition [38]. In addition, ID2-induced breast cancer metastasis to the brain where bone morphogenetic protein 7 (BMP7) produced by astrocytes led to overexpression of ID2 [39].

Higher levels of ID2 indicated that patients with breast cancer have a higher chance of reoccurring metastasis in the brain [39].

1.24. IDH1 - ISOCITRATE DEHYDROGENASE (NADP (+)) 1 CHROMOSOME 2; 2q34

IDH1 encodes isocitrate dehydrogenase-1 protein, where the gene is frequently mutated in tumors of secondary glioblastomas [40]. A report showed that IDH1 was 70% mutated at amino acid 132 in glioblastomas formed from secondary glioblastoma, oligodendrogliomas, and astrocytoma WHO graded I and II [40]. The role of mutated IDH1 R132H was studied *in vivo* and *in vitro*, where expression of IDH1 R132H mutation in astrocytes led to a decrease in NADPH and an increase in [R]-2-hydroxygluturate, growth, and proliferation of cells [41]. IDH1 R132H mutant, platelet-derived growth factor A (PDGFA), and loss of genes responsible for the cell cycle, led to the can be rewritten as formation of glioma in *in vivo* model [41].

1.25. IL1B - INTERLEUKIN 1 BETA CHROMOSOME 2; 2q14.1

Interleukin 1 beta encoded by IL1B belongs to the family of cytokines IL-1, a proinflammatory cytokine expressed in various cell types, such as skin, dendritic cells, blood monocytes, microglial cells in the brain, and macrophages [42]. The expression of IL1B occurs during the entry of foreign agents that induces pattern-associated molecular patterns and damage-associated molecular patterns [42]. Furthermore, IL1B was expressed in breast cancer tissues where breast cancer cells that metastasized to the bone had increased levels of IL1B, indicating that expression of IL1B led to metastasis [42]. Besides metastatic properties, IL1B was also associated with tumor growth and invasion [42]. The prognostic value of IL1B in breast cancer was poor [42].

1.26. ING5 - INHIBITOR OF GROWTH FAMILY MEMBER 5 CHROMOSOME 2; 2q37.3

ING5 encodes for inhibitor of growth family 5 belonging to the family of inhibitor growth factor (ING) proteins and has a type-II tumor suppressor property [43]. ING5 forms a complex with mini-chromosome maintenance proteins responsible for replication [43]. ING5 role was reported in pancreatic cancer where ING5 was downregulated by interacting with microRNA-196a leading to higher invasion and proliferation and reduced apoptosis of cells [43]; in colorectal cancer, upregulation of ING5 showed the reduced population of cells and colony formation and apoptosis through p53 [43]. In addition, binding p21 and p300 with ING5 in the nucleus induced cell cycle arrest and apoptosis in head and neck squamous cell carcinoma (HNSCC). In gastric, colorectal cancers, and HNSCC, ING5 nuclear expression decreased [43].

1.27. IRS1- INSULIN RECEPTOR SUBSTRATE 1 CHROMOSOME 2; 2q36.3

IRS1 is a cytoplasmic protein that serves as a substrate for insulin-like growth factor 1 receptor and insulin receptor to regulate these signaling pathways [44]. IRS1 controls the activities of insulin-like growth factor 1 and insulin receptors, such as anti-apoptosis, cell proliferation, and glucose homeostasis, by a cascade of downstream effector responses from the activated receptors [44]. Also, decreased expression of IRS1 is linked to resistance to insulin, especially in skeletal muscle [44]. IRS1 is also responsible for human cancers, where the activated form of IRS1 causes cancer, such as colorectal cancer [44]. A report on the relationship between IRS1 expression and exercise in colorectal cancer patients has shown that physical activities like exercise aid the cancer patient's survival, where IRS1 expression was less [44].

1.28. MEIS1 - MEIS HOMEOBOX 1 CHROMOSOME 2; 2p14

MEIS1 belongs to the TALE [Transcription activator-like effector] family of transcription factors containing the homeodomain, which induces the transcription of genes by binding to Hox transcription factors [45]. MEIS1 blocked the formation of reactive oxygen species in hematopoietic stem cells by inducing HIF1α and 2α proteins [45]. MEIS1 is involved in the proliferation of myeloid leukemia cells, suppression of proliferation of cardiomyocytes and neonatal cells by increasing the expression of CDK inhibitors such as Arf and Cdkn1a, and increased expression in neuroblastoma [45]. In non-small cell lung cancer, decreased expression of MEIS1 suppressed the proliferation of cells by regulating CDK inhibitors for the progression of the cell cycle and might serve as a therapeutic target for non-small cell lung cancer [45].

1.29. MYCN - MYCN PROTO-ONCOGENE, BHLH TRANSCRIPTION FACTOR CHROMOSOME 2; 2p24.3

MYCN belongs to the member of the MYC family and is involved in various activities by expressing genes responsible for proliferation, metastasis, regeneration, angiogenesis, survival, and pluripotency but inhibits the transcription of genes responsible for immune surveillance, differentiation, and cell cycle arrest [46]. Expression of MYCN damaged the integrity of the extracellular matrix, leading to cell invasion and migration [46]. MYCN also induced the integrin signaling protein, focal adhesion kinase resulting in an elevation in metastasis and migration of tumor cells [46]. In neuroblastoma, MYCN intensified the condition by overexpressing SKp2 and CDK4 proteins and regulating TP53 inducible nuclear protein 1, which made CDK2 bypass the suppression of the p21 protein [46].

1.30. NCOA1 - NUCLEAR RECEPTOR COACTIVATOR 1 CHROMO-SOME 2; 2p23.3

NCOA1 belongs to the family of p160 SRC proteins that plays a role in the transcription of genes and chromatin remodeling. It induces the formation of complex transcription factors by binding to transcription factors and nuclear hormone receptors [47]. NCOA1 is involved in cancers such as breast cancer, where there was upregulation of NCOA1 in breast tumors with HER2 proteins [47]. NCOA1 plays a role in the metastasis and invasion of breast cancer cells, where NCOA1 increases the expression of genes responsible for migration, metastasis, aggression, and epithelial and mesenchymal transition by binding and activating various transcription factors [47]. Upregulation of NCOA1 in breast cancer cells and mouse models with mammary tumors activated the expression of CSF1 to promote metastasis and growth of cancer [47].

1.31. NR4A2 - NUCLEAR RECEPTOR SUBFAMILY 4 GROUP A MEMBER 2 CHROMOSOME 2; 2q24.1

NR4A2 is a transcription factor belonging to the orphan nuclear receptor super-family and plays a role in the pathways of dopaminergic neurons [48]. NR4A2 is also involved in fatty acid and glucose metabolism [48]. The expression of NR4A2 was observed in colorectal cancer, where NR4A2 was activated by prostaglandin E2 (PGE2), resulting in the upregulation of NR4A2 in colon cancer cells [48]. NR4A2 suppressed apoptosis-inducing genes responsible for fatty acid oxidation by interacting with the Nurr77-binding response element (NBRE) [48]. This led to the survival of colon cancer cells [48]. NR4A2 is also involved in cervical. In cancer where Notch signaling decreased the expression of NR4A2, the development of cervical cancer cells was increased [49].

1.32. ODC1 - ORNITHINE DECARBOXYLASE 1 CHROMOSOME 2; 2p25.1

ODC1 is an oncogene and rate-limiting enzyme in polyamines' metabolism [50].

ODC1 was observed in various colorectal, breast, endometrial, and prostate cancers where ODC1 was overexpressed and associated with poor survival [50]. In gastric cancer, ODC1 regulates polyamine metabolism and isoflavones' binding with the enzymes involved in polyamine synthesis [50]. In hepatocellular carcinoma (HCC) cells and tissues, ODC1 was overexpressed [50]. Downregulation of ODC1 in HCC cells resulted in cell cycle arrest and suppression of migration, the proliferation of HCC cells by changing the acidotic microenvironment, and regulating the AKT/GSK3β/ β-catenin pathway [50].

1.33. PAX3 - PAIRED BOX 3 CHROMOSOME 2; 2q36.1

PAX3 is a transcription factor that belongs to the family of paired box proteins, and the gene encodes for paired box 3 protein [51]. PAX3 binds with other proteins, and forms homodimers and heterodimers during the transcription of genes [51]. Apart from activating genes, PAX3 has other functions, such as inhibiting transcription by interacting with co-repressors and stimulating protein-protein interaction [51]. PAX3 plays a significant role in muscle development and neural tube formation during embryogenesis [51]. PAX3 is also involved in different tumors derived from the neural tube and neural crest lineages, including neurofibroma, glioblastoma, Ewing's sarcoma, melanoma, medulloblastoma, and malignant nerve sheath tumor [51]. Also, PAX3 is involved in osteosarcoma, gastric and breast cancers [51].

1.34. PAX8 - PAIRED BOX 8 CHROMOSOME 2; 2q14.1

PAX8 is a transcription factor that encodes for paired box 8 protein and is involved in cellular events such as mitosis and embryogenesis [52]. PAX8 is also involved in cancer, where upregulation of this gene leads to an increase in cell proliferation by inducing the expression of genes responsible for the cell cycle including Cyclin B1 and Aurora B [52]. Expression of PAX8 was increased in ovarian and endometrial cancers, where PAX8 expression was associated with an increased chance of recurrence and death of the patients [52]. In stomach cancer, PAX8 was overexpressed in cancer tissues where this gene regulated SOX13, altering the expression of cell cycle proteins, including Cyclin B1 and Aurora B, and inducing the development of tumors in stomach cancer [52].

1.35. RALB - RAS LIKE PROTO-ONCOGENE B CHROMOSOME 2; 2q14.2

RALB is a member of the superfamily of RAS proteins and is involved in different cancers such as the bladder, colon, skin, pancreatic, lung, and prostate [53]. RALB is essential for metastasis, proliferation, invasion of cancer cells, and maintaining human tumors [53]. RALB plays a role in pancreatic cancer, forming invadopodium to promote metastasis and invasion of pancreatic cancer cells [53]. Higher expression of RALB was found in bladder cancer cell lines where phosphorylation of RALB by protein kinase C was required to promote metastasis of bladder cancer cells [53]. In colorectal cancer, RALB-induced growth of colorectal cancer is in an anchorage-independent manner by binding with SEC5, a protein that is required for migration and exosome formation [53].

1.36. RANBP2 - RAN BINDING PROTEIN 2 CHROMOSOME 2; 2q13

RANBP2 encoding for RAN binding protein 2 (Fig. **1**), also known as Nup358, belongs to the nucleoporin family containing nuclear pore complex proteins [54]. RANBP2 protein is present mainly in the cytoplasm but, during mitosis, localized from the cytoplasm to mitotic spindle microtubules and kinetochore in the nucleus [54]. It also possesses a pleiotropic function showing multiple effects [54]. Down-modulating RANBP2 resulted in abnormal chromosome alignment, cell cycle arrest at the G2/M phase, apoptosis, and mitotic defects [54]. RANBP2 plays a vital role in cancer as a tumor suppressor and oncogene [54]. RANBP2 is essential for the survival of colorectal cancer as the downregulation of this gene leads to apoptosis, delay, and defects in mitosis in BRAF-like colorectal cancer [55].

1.37. REG1A - REGENERATING FAMILY MEMBER 1 ALPHA CHROMOSOME 2; 2p12

REG1A encoding for regenerating protein 1 alpha belongs to the superfamily of calcium-dependent lectins, and as the name suggests, it is involved in regeneration [56]. REG1A was first found as an endogenous growth factor in pancreatic islet beta cells [57]. REG1A plays a role in the mucous of the gastrointestinal tract involving cell proliferation and tissue regeneration [57]. As a growth factor, REG1A is also involved in inflammation, where it reduces epithelial apoptosis [56]. The function of REG1A is observed in different cancers such as gastric, cutaneous melanoma, lung, hepatocellular carcinoma, pancreatic, colorectal, esophageal bladder, and breast cancers [56, 57]. In gastric cancer, REG1A showed angiogenesis and anti-apoptotic properties where even overexpression inhibited cell viability and invasion of gastric cancer cells [56].

1.38. REL - REL PROTO-ONCOGENE, NF-KB SUBUNIT CHROMO-SOME 2; 2p16.1

REL or c-REL is a transcription factor belonging to the family of nuclear factor k-light-chain enhancer of activated B cells [58]. c-Rel protein has a conserved Rel domain which is homologous to members of the NF-kB family involved in DNA binding, inhibitor interaction, dimerization, and nuclear localization [58]. Rel is also engaged in nuclear shuttling, signaling cascades induced by receptors, post-translational modifications, and stability of REL mRNA [58]. Increased levels of nuclear c-Rel protein were observed in cancers such as B-cell lymphoma in lower levels and 50% of classical Hodgkin lymphoma [59]. c-Rel also plays a role in nuclear localization, which is linked to cancers such as activated B-cell-like (ABC) and germinal center B-cell-like (GCB) diffuse large B-cell lymphomas (DLCBL) [59].

1.39. REV1 - REV1 DNA DIRECTED POLYMERASE CHROMOSOME 2; 2q11.2

REV1 belongs to the Y family of DNA polymerases involved in DNA repair and translesion synthesis [60]. Mutations in human REV1 were observed in single nucleotide polymorphism in different cancer types and tumors [61]. In addition, hREV1 is involved in human glioma pathogenesis [60]. REV1 upregulation and deletion play a role in cytotoxicity, tumor generation, chemoresistance, and muta-genesis induced by carcinogens [60, 61]. In m6G lesions, upregulation of REV1 enhances the activity of DNA polymerases such as Pol δ–Pol ζ resulting in mutagenesis induced by *N*-methyl-*N*-nitrosourea (MNU) [61]. During starvation in cancer cells, REV1 modified by SUMOylating, releases its binding partner, p53 leading to increased expression of p53 and apoptosis in melanoma and breast cancer cells [60].

1.40. RHOB - RAS HOMOLOG FAMILY MEMBER B CHROMOSOME 2; 2p24.1

RhoB is one among the Rho proteins belonging to the Ras superfamily that activates various pathways, such as vesicle trafficking, gene regulation, and reorganization of the cytoskeleton involving cell migration, growth control, cell adhesion, and differentiation [62]. RhoB protein is found in the plasma mem-brane, nucleus, vesicles, and endosomes [62]. RhoB protein acts as a molecular switch and is modified by post-translation modifications such as geranylgerany-lation, farnesylation, and prenylation to perform different functions [62]. For instance, RhoB helps in the survival of endothelial cells by modulating the phosphorylation of AKT and AKT/PKB nuclear trafficking in endothelial cells [62]. The function zoning of RhoB in cancer is related to the generation of the tumor by promoting cell migration, proliferation, invasion, and angiogenesis [62].

1.41. ROCK2 – RHO-ASSOCIATED COILED-COIL CONTAINING PROTEIN KINASE 2 CHROMOSOME 2; 2p25.1

ROCK2 plays a role in interacting with small GTPases in the Rho subfamily to perform various functions, such as reorganization of the cytoskeleton, including tumor invasion, cell movement, and focal adhesion [63]. ROCK2 is involved in multiple tumors, such as lung, colon, and liver cancers, for pathogenesis, metastasis, tumor progression, and invasion of cancer cells [63]. In colorectal cancer, ROCK2 was upregulated compared to non-cancer cells, leading to tumor invasion, and overexpression of ROCK2. Triggered cell proliferation, metastasis, and invasion in gastric cancer [63]. Also, in breast cancer, ROCK2 was upregulated, which was related to the overall sur-vival of cancer cells [63]. In contrast, in colorectal carcinoma, suppression of ROCK2 led to the accumu-lation and invasion of colorectal carcinoma cells [64].

1.42. RRM2 - RIBONUCLEOTIDE REDUCTASE REGULATORY SUBUNIT M2 CHROMOSOME 2; 2p25.1

RRM2 is a rate-limiting enzyme consisting of a ribonucleotide reductase complex involved in forming dNTPs [65]. RRM2 expression levels are associated with the cell cycle, where higher levels of RRM2 were observed in the S-phase of the cell cycle [65]. RRM2 also controls the activity of ribonucleotide reductase, a nucleo-tide metabolism enzyme, during the cell cycle [66]. Expression of RRM2 in cancer is associated with angiogenesis and epithelial-mesenchymal transition of cancer cells [66]. RRM2 is also involved in promoting cancers where upregulation of RRM2 was observed in melanoma, clear-cell renal cell carcinoma, and gastric carcinoma [65]. RRM2 was also overexpressed in non-small cell lung carcinoma cell lines and tissues of tumors which was correlated with low survival and poor prognostic outcomes [65].

1.43. SDC1 – SYNDECAN 1 CHROMOSOME 2; 2p24.1

SDC1 belongs to the family of transmembrane proteins, heparan sulfate proteo-glycan [67]. It is a cell surface protein adheres to the microenvironment to regulate cell interaction and morphology [67]. SDC1 is expressed in various cells, such as mesenchymal, epithelial cells, mature plasma, and immature B cells in hematopoietic tissues [67]. Across various mammalian cells, growth factors such as essential fibroblast growth factor and tumor growth factor- β maintain SDC1 expression [67]. In different cancers, SDC1 is abnormally expressed to induce cancer cell metastasis, proliferation, angiogenesis, and cell invasion, and the expression is also linked to the deteriorating effect of chemoresistance [67]. Downregulation of SDC1 in epithelial cells resulted in metastasis linked to poor prognosis [67].

1.44. SOX11 – SRY-BOX TRANSCRIPTION FACTOR 11 CHROMOSO-ME 2; 2p25.2

SOX11 is a transcription factor belonging to the SOXC family and is involved in the regeneration, development, homeostasis of tissue, and reprogramming of cell fate [68]. SOX11 found in the nucleus is related to the small primary tumor, low-grade tumor, prolonged overall survival, and metastasis of non-lymph nodes [68]. DNA methylation in cancer cells such as high-grade tumors and low-grade endometrial cancer inhibited SOX11 expression, which was related to the instability of microsatellites and methylation of the MutL homolog 1 (MLH1) gene [68]. In mantle cell lymphoma, SOX11 serves as an oncogene and a marker for mantle cell lymphoma diagnosis. SOX11 expression was upregulated in medulloblastoma and malignant breast tumors and downregulated in prostate cancer tissues [68].

1.45. STAT1 - SIGNAL TRANSDUCER AND ACTIVATOR OF TRANS-CRIPTION 1 CHROMOSOME 2; 2q32.2

STAT1 protein is part of the interferon signaling pathway. It is triggered by growth factors, cytokines, and hormones to perform various functions, such as suppression of cell growth, maintenance of cell differentiation, and stimulation of cell death and the immune system [69]. STAT1 induces transcription of specific genes, such as interferon regulatory factor 1, low molecular mass polypeptide, and antigen peptide transporter, after translocating into the nucleus in the activated protein form [69]. STAT1 acts as a tumor suppressor where the loss of expression of STAT1 was observed in cancers such as colorectal, gastric, esophageal, lung, breast cancers, and melanoma [69]. Overexpression of STAT1 resulted in positive clinical responses in cancer patients such as breast, and gastrointestinal cancers, hepatocellular carcinoma, and melanoma [69].

1.46. SUMO1 - SMALL UBIQUITIN-LIKE MODIFIER 1 CHROMOSOME 2; 2q33.1

SUMO1 belongs to the family of ubiquitin-like proteins responsible for post-translational modifications, and SUMO1 accumulation in cells influences substrate stability and subcellular localization, affecting transcription [70]. SUMO1 is also involved in tumor formation. In glioblastoma, SUMO1 expression leads to tumor progression [70]. SUMO1 promotes epithelial-to-mesenchymal transition through the NF-kB signaling pathway in liver, breast, and ovarian cancers and tumors [70]. In non-small cell lung cancer, upregulation of SUMO1 led to NF-kB expression, pathological tumor node metastasis, tumor differentiation, lymphatic metastasis, invasion, and colony formation of non-small cell lung carcinoma cell lines, whereas inhibition of SUMO1 resulted in suppression of invasion, colony formation and NF-kB expression [70].

1.47. TCF7L1 - TRANSCRIPTION FACTOR 7 LIKE 1 CHROMOSOME 2; 2p11.2

TCF7L1 is a transcription factor belonging to the family of T cell factor/ Lymphoid enhancer factor. It serves as a DNA binding protein by interacting with β-catenin, a regulator of the Wnt signaling pathway [71]. TCF7L1 is also involved in cancer, where overexpression of TCF7L1 was observed in high-grade tumors and related to poor cancer survival [71]. In gastric cancer, overexpression of TCF7L1 modulated aerobic glycolysis and antioxidant activity using nuclear factor erythroid 2-related factor 2 (NRF2), which induced cell proliferation [71]. In addition, upregulation of TCF7L1 was associated with poor prognosis of breast cancer; meanwhile, downregulation of TCF7L1 resulted in metastasis and tumor development. Also, TCF7L1 promoted cell proliferation in colorectal cancer [71].

1.48. TIA1 - TIA1 CYTOTOXIC GRANULE ASSOCIATED RNA BINDING PROTEIN CHROMOSOME 2; 2p13.3

TIA1, encoding for T-cell intracellular antigen 1, is an RNA-binding protein responsible for various cellular functions in the cytoplasm and nucleus, such as the metabolism of RNA [72]. TIA1 is also a tumor suppressor, responsible for cancer progression and carcinogenesis. It binds to various mRNA required for aberrant processes in cancer, such as cell metastasis, invasion, immune evasion, apoptosis, cell proliferation, and angiogenesis [72]. TIA1 modulates alternative splicing of the Fas receptor to induce cell apoptosis [72]. Also, knocking down TIA1 induced tumor growth, invasion, and cell proliferation [72]. In colorectal cancer, TIA1 maintained angiogenesis, expression of vascular endothelial growth factor [VEGF] isoform, and drug resistance to bevacizumab [72].

1.49. TRPM8 - TRANSIENT RECEPTOR POTENTIAL CATION CHANNEL SUBFAMILY M, MEMBER 8 CHROMOSOME 2; 2q37.1

TRPM8 is one of the transient receptor potential [TRP] ion channels required for pancreatic cancer [73]. TRPM8 expression is responsible for cell migration, cell Viability and proliferation of pancreatic cancer cells [73]. Expression of TRPM8 resulting in differentiation of epithelial cells in prostate cancer is dependent on androgen as androgens determined TRPM8 localization in normal and cancer cells of the prostate [73]. In addition, depletion of TRPM8 expression is associated with androgen-independent pancreatic cancer [73]. In the first stage of pancreatic cancer, TRPM8 was overexpressed, and as the disease progressed to the late stages, TRPM8 expression decreased [73]. Due to this change in expression, TRPM8 serves as a prognostic marker for pancreatic cancer [73].

1.50. TWIST2 - TWIST FAMILY BHLH TRANSCRIPTION FACTOR 2 CHROMOSOME 2; 2q37.3

TWIST2 belongs to the family of an essential helix-loop-helix transcription factor responsible for cell differentiation in embryogenesis. Twist proteins suppress mesenchymal cells of bone and muscle cell differentiation, which results in epithelial-to-mesenchymal transition inducing neural crest cell migration [74]. TWIST2 is also involved in tumorigenesis as TWIST2 was upregulated in several solid tumors, cancer cell lines, and tissues such as kidney cancer [74]. Also, TWIST2 expression suppressed early senescence in cancer cells and induced metastasis, epithelial-to-mesenchymal transition, and cancer invasion [74]. TWIST2 was upregulated in kidney cell lines and cancer tissues which then induced cell migration, proliferation, invasion, tumor growth, and suppressed apoptosis [74].

CONCLUSION

The human chromosome 2 has a fascinating history behind it. However, specific genes in the human chromosome 2 undergo mutations and cause severe health conditions. This chapter consolidates the cancer genes present in human chromosome 2.

REFERENCES

[1]   Whitfield AJ, Barrett PHR, van Bockxmeer FM, Burnett JR. Lipid disorders and mutations in the APOB gene. Clin Chem 2004; 50(10): 1725-32.
[http://dx.doi.org/10.1373/clinchem.2004.038026] [PMID: 15308601]

[2]   Lee G, Jeong YS, Kim DW, *et al.* Clinical significance of APOB inactivation in hepatocellular carcinoma. Exp Mol Med 2018; 50(11): 1-12.
[http://dx.doi.org/10.1038/s12276-018-0174-2] [PMID: 30429453]

[3]   Kang KJ, Pyo JH, Ryu KJ, *et al.* Oncogenic Role of BOLL in Colorectal Cancer. Dig Dis Sci 2015; 60(6): 1663-73.
[http://dx.doi.org/10.1007/s10620-015-3533-z] [PMID: 25605553]

[4]   Johnson VL, Scott MIF, Holt SV, Hussein D, Taylor SS. Bub1 is required for kinetochore localization of BubR1, Cenp-E, Cenp-F and Mad2, and chromosome congression. J Cell Sci 2004; 117(8): 1577-89.
[http://dx.doi.org/10.1242/jcs.01006] [PMID: 15020684]

[5]   Zhu LJ, Pan Y, Chen XY, Hou PF. BUB1 promotes proliferation of liver cancer cells by activating SMAD2 phosphorylation. Oncol Lett 2020; 19(5): 3506-12.
[http://dx.doi.org/10.3892/ol.2020.11445] [PMID: 32269624]

[6]   Yu H, Zhang S, Ibrahim AN, Deng Z, Wang M. RETRACTED: Serine/threonine kinase BUB1 promotes proliferation and radio-resistance in glioblastoma. Pathol Res Pract 2019; 215(8): 152508.
[http://dx.doi.org/10.1016/j.prp.2019.152508] [PMID: 31272759]

[7]   Wang B, Shi L, Sun X, Wang L, Wang X, Chen C. Production of CCL 20 from lung cancer cells induces the cell migration and proliferation through PI 3K pathway. J Cell Mol Med 2016; 20(5): 920-

9.
[http://dx.doi.org/10.1111/jcmm.12781] [PMID: 26968871]

[8]   Lee SK, Park KK, Kim HJ, *et al*. Human antigen R-regulated CCL20 contributes to osteolytic breast cancer bone metastasis. Sci Rep 2017; 7(1): 9610.
[http://dx.doi.org/10.1038/s41598-017-09040-4] [PMID: 28851919]

[9]   Safa AR. c-FLIP, a master anti-apoptotic regulator. Exp Oncol 2012; 34(3): 176-84.
[PMID: 23070002]

[10]   Valente G, Manfroi F, Peracchio C, *et al*. cFLIP expression correlates with tumour progression and patient outcome in non-Hodgkin lymphomas of low grade of malignancy. Br J Haematol 2006; 132(5): 560-70.
[http://dx.doi.org/10.1111/j.1365-2141.2005.05898.x] [PMID: 16445828]

[11]   Guo L, Yin M, Wang Y. CREB1, a direct target of miR-122, promotes cell proliferation and invasion in bladder cancer. Oncol Lett 2018; 16(3): 3842-8.
[http://dx.doi.org/10.3892/ol.2018.9118] [PMID: 30127997]

[12]   Yang Q, Yu W, Han X. Overexpression of microRNA-101 causes anti-tumor effects by targeting CREB1 in colon cancer. Mol Med Rep 2019; 19(4): 3159-67.
[http://dx.doi.org/10.3892/mmr.2019.9952] [PMID: 30816471]

[13]   Han J, Jiang Q, Ma R, *et al*. Norepinephrine-CREB1-miR-373 axis promotes progression of colon cancer. Mol Oncol 2020; 14(5): 1059-73.
[http://dx.doi.org/10.1002/1878-0261.12657] [PMID: 32118353]

[14]   Zhao Y, Yang W, Huang Y, Cui R, Li X, Li B. Evolving Roles for Targeting CTLA-4 in Cancer Immunotherapy. Cell Physiol Biochem 2018; 47(2): 721-34.
[http://dx.doi.org/10.1159/000490025] [PMID: 29794465]

[15]   Ghaderi A, Yeganeh F, Kalantari T, *et al*. Cytotoxic T lymphocyte antigen-4 gene in breast cancer. Breast Cancer Res Treat 2004; 86(1): 1-7.
[http://dx.doi.org/10.1023/B:BREA.0000032918.89120.8e] [PMID: 15218356]

[16]   Xu C, Zhao H, Chen H, Yao Q. CXCR4 in breast cancer: oncogenic role and therapeutic targeting. Drug Des Devel Ther 2015; 9: 4953-64.
[PMID: 26356032]

[17]   Kwon YJ, Baek HS, Ye DJ, Shin S, Kim D, Chun YJ. CYP1B1 enhances cell proliferation and metastasis through induction of EMT and activation of Wnt/β-catenin signaling *via* Sp1 upregulation. PLoS One 2016; 11(3): e0151598.
[http://dx.doi.org/10.1371/journal.pone.0151598] [PMID: 26981862]

[18]   Tanaka K, Ikeda N, Miyashita K, Nuriya H, Hara T. DEAD box protein DDX 1 promotes colorectal tumorigenesis through transcriptional activation of the *LGR5* gene. Cancer Sci 2018; 109(8): 2479-89.
[http://dx.doi.org/10.1111/cas.13661] [PMID: 29869821]

[19]   Brunetti L, Gundry MC, Goodell MA. DNMT3A in Leukemia. Cold Spring Harb Perspect Med 2017; 7(2): a030320.
[http://dx.doi.org/10.1101/cshperspect.a030320] [PMID: 28003281]

[20]   Ley TJ, Ding L, Walter MJ, *et al*. DNMT3A mutations in acute myeloid leukemia. N Engl J Med 2010; 363(25): 2424-33.
[http://dx.doi.org/10.1056/NEJMoa1005143] [PMID: 21067377]

[21]   Yin X, Fang S, Wang M, Wang Q, Fang R, Chen J. EFEMP1 promotes ovarian cancer cell growth, invasion and metastasis *via* activated the AKT pathway. Oncotarget 2016; 7(30): 47938-53.
[http://dx.doi.org/10.18632/oncotarget.10296] [PMID: 27351229]

[22]   Schnell U, Cirulli V, Giepmans BNG. EpCAM: Structure and function in health and disease. Biochim Biophys Acta Biomembr 2013; 1828(8): 1989-2001.
[http://dx.doi.org/10.1016/j.bbamem.2013.04.018] [PMID: 23618806]

[23]   Liang KH, Tso HC, Hung SH, *et al.* Extracellular domain of EpCAM enhances tumor progression through EGFR signaling in colon cancer cells. Cancer Lett 2018; 433: 165-75.
[http://dx.doi.org/10.1016/j.canlet.2018.06.040] [PMID: 29981429]

[24]   Hollmén M, Liu P, Kurppa K, *et al.* Proteolytic processing of ErbB4 in breast cancer. PLoS One 2012; 7(6): e39413.
[http://dx.doi.org/10.1371/journal.pone.0039413] [PMID: 22761786]

[25]   Xu J, Gong L, Qian Z, Song G, Liu J. ERBB4 promotes the proliferation of gastric cancer cells *via* the PI3K/Akt signaling pathway. Oncol Rep 2018; 39(6): 2892-8.
[http://dx.doi.org/10.3892/or.2018.6343] [PMID: 29620274]

[26]   Cao CY, Mok SWF, Cheng VWS, Tsui SKW. The FHL2 regulation in the transcriptional circuitry of human cancers. Gene 2015; 572(1): 1-7.
[http://dx.doi.org/10.1016/j.gene.2015.07.043] [PMID: 26211626]

[27]   Jin X, Jiao X, Jiao J, Zhang T, Cui B. Increased expression of FHL2 promotes tumorigenesis in cervical cancer and is correlated with poor prognosis. Gene 2018; 669: 99-106.
[http://dx.doi.org/10.1016/j.gene.2018.05.087] [PMID: 29800735]

[28]   Wang J, Sun D, Wang Y, *et al.* FOSL2 positively regulates TGF-β1 signalling in non-small cell lung cancer. PLoS One 2014; 9(11): e112150.
[http://dx.doi.org/10.1371/journal.pone.0112150] [PMID: 25375657]

[29]   Li S, Fang X, Wang X, Fei B. Fos-like antigen 2 (FOSL2) promotes metastasis in colon cancer. Exp Cell Res 2018; 373(1-2): 57-61.
[http://dx.doi.org/10.1016/j.yexcr.2018.08.016] [PMID: 30114390]

[30]   Huang J, Hu W, Lin X, Wang X, Jin K. FRZB up-regulated in hepatocellular carcinoma bone metastasis. Int J Clin Exp Pathol 2015; 8(10): 13353-9.
[PMID: 26722540]

[31]   Li G, Su Q, Liu H, *et al.* Frizzled7 promotes epithelial-to-mesenchymal transition and stemness *via* activating canonical Wnt/β-catenin pathway in gastric cancer. Int J Biol Sci 2018; 14(3): 280-93.
[http://dx.doi.org/10.7150/ijbs.23756] [PMID: 29559846]

[32]   Haines CN, Braunreiter KM, Mo XM, Burd CJ. GREB1 isoforms regulate proliferation independent of ERα co-regulator activities in breast cancer. Endocr Relat Cancer 2018; 25(7): 735-46.
[http://dx.doi.org/10.1530/ERC-17-0496] [PMID: 29695586]

[33]   Wang JX, Zhou JF, Huang FK, *et al.* GLI2 induces PDGFRB expression and modulates cancer stem cell properties of gastric cancer. Eur Rev Med Pharmacol Sci 2017; 21(17): 3857-65.
[PMID: 28975979]

[34]   França MM, Jorge AAL, Carvalho LRS, *et al.* Novel heterozygous nonsense GLI2 mutations in patients with hypopituitarism and ectopic posterior pituitary lobe without holoprosencephaly. J Clin Endocrinol Metab 2010; 95(11): E384-91.
[http://dx.doi.org/10.1210/jc.2010-1050] [PMID: 20685856]

[35]   Kang ZH, Wang CY, Zhang WL, *et al.* Histone deacetylase HDAC4 promotes gastric cancer SGC-7901 cells progression *via* p21 repression. PLoS One 2014; 9(6): e98894.
[http://dx.doi.org/10.1371/journal.pone.0098894] [PMID: 24896240]

[36]   Hakami F, Darda L, Stafford P, Woll P, Lambert DW, Hunter KD. The roles of HOXD10 in the development and progression of head and neck squamous cell carcinoma (HNSCC). Br J Cancer 2014; 111(4): 807-16.
[http://dx.doi.org/10.1038/bjc.2014.372] [PMID: 25010866]

[37]   Wang Y, Li Z, Zhao X, Zuo X, Peng Z. miR-10b promotes invasion by targeting HOXD10 in colorectal cancer. Oncol Lett 2016; 12(1): 488-94.
[http://dx.doi.org/10.3892/ol.2016.4628] [PMID: 27347170]

[38]   Lee SB, Frattini V, Bansal M, *et al.* An ID2-dependent mechanism for VHL inactivation in cancer. Nature 2016; 529(7585): 172-7.
[http://dx.doi.org/10.1038/nature16475] [PMID: 26735018]

[39]   Kijewska M, Viski C, Turrell F, *et al.* Using an in-vivo syngeneic spontaneous metastasis model identifies ID2 as a promoter of breast cancer colonisation in the brain. Breast Cancer Res 2019; 21(1): 4.
[http://dx.doi.org/10.1186/s13058-018-1093-9] [PMID: 30642388]

[40]   Yan H, Parsons DW, Jin G, *et al.* IDH1 and IDH2 mutations in gliomas. N Engl J Med 2009; 360(8): 765-73.
[http://dx.doi.org/10.1056/NEJMoa0808710] [PMID: 19228619]

[41]   Philip B, Yu DX, Silvis MR, *et al.* Mutant IDH1 Promotes Glioma Formation In Vivo. Cell Rep 2018; 23(5): 1553-64.
[http://dx.doi.org/10.1016/j.celrep.2018.03.133] [PMID: 29719265]

[42]   Tulotta C, Ottewell P. The role of IL-1B in breast cancer bone metastasis. Endocr Relat Cancer 2018; 25(7): R421-34.
[http://dx.doi.org/10.1530/ERC-17-0309] [PMID: 29760166]

[43]   Yang XF, Shen DF, Zhao S, *et al.* Expression pattern and level of ING5 protein in normal and cancer tissues. Oncol Lett 2019; 17(1): 63-8.
[PMID: 30655738]

[44]   Hanyuda A, Kim SA, Martinez-Fernandez A, *et al.* Survival Benefit of Exercise Differs by Tumor IRS1 Expression Status in Colorectal Cancer. Ann Surg Oncol 2016; 23(3): 908-17.
[http://dx.doi.org/10.1245/s10434-015-4967-4] [PMID: 26577117]

[45]   Li W, Huang K, Guo H, Cui G. Meis1 regulates proliferation of non-small-cell lung cancer cells. J Thorac Dis 2014; 6(6): 850-5.
[PMID: 24977012]

[46]   Huang M, Weiss WA. Neuroblastoma and MYCN. Cold Spring Harb Perspect Med 2013; 3(10): a014415.
[http://dx.doi.org/10.1101/cshperspect.a014415] [PMID: 24086065]

[47]   Qin L, Wu YL, Toneff MJ, *et al.* NCOA1 directly targets M-CSF1 expression to promote breast cancer metastasis. Cancer Res 2014; 74(13): 3477-88.
[http://dx.doi.org/10.1158/0008-5472.CAN-13-2639] [PMID: 24769444]

[48]   Holla VR, Wu H, Shi Q, Menter DG, DuBois RN. Nuclear orphan receptor NR4A2 modulates fatty acid oxidation pathways in colorectal cancer. J Biol Chem 2011; 286(34): 30003-9.
[http://dx.doi.org/10.1074/jbc.M110.184697] [PMID: 21757690]

[49]   Sun L, Liu M, Sun GC, *et al.* Notch signaling activation in cervical cancer cells induces cell growth arrest with the involvement of the nuclear receptor NR4A2. J Cancer 2016; 7(11): 1388-95.
[http://dx.doi.org/10.7150/jca.15274] [PMID: 27471554]

[50]   Ye Z, Zeng Z, Shen Y, *et al.* ODC1 promotes proliferation and mobility via the AKT/GSK3β/β-catenin pathway and modulation of acidotic microenvironment in human hepatocellular carcinoma. OncoTargets Ther 2019; 12: 4081-92.
[http://dx.doi.org/10.2147/OTT.S198341] [PMID: 31239700]

[51]   Boudjadi S, Chatterjee B, Sun W, Vemu P, Barr FG. The expression and function of PAX3 in development and disease. Gene 2018; 666: 145-57.
[http://dx.doi.org/10.1016/j.gene.2018.04.087] [PMID: 29730428]

[52]   Bie LY, Li N, Deng WY, Lu XY, Guo P, Luo SX. RETRACTED ARTICLE: Evaluation of PAX8 expression promotes the proliferation of stomach Cancer cells. BMC Mol Cell Biol 2019; 20(1): 61.
[http://dx.doi.org/10.1186/s12860-019-0245-9] [PMID: 31881968]

[53] Yan C, Theodorescu D. RAL GTpases: Biology and potential as therapeutic targets in cancer. Pharmacol Rev 2018; 70(1): 1-11.
[http://dx.doi.org/10.1124/pr.117.014415] [PMID: 29196555]

[54] Wong RW, D'Angelo M. Linking Nucleoporins, Mitosis, and Colon Cancer. Cell Chem Biol 2016; 23(5): 537-9.
[http://dx.doi.org/10.1016/j.chembiol.2016.05.004] [PMID: 27203373]

[55] Vecchione L, Gambino V, Raaijmakers J, *et al.* A vulnerability of a subset of colon cancers with potential clinical utility. Cell 2016; 165(2): 317-30.
[http://dx.doi.org/10.1016/j.cell.2016.02.059] [PMID: 27058664]

[56] Qiu YS, Liao GJ, Jiang NN. DNA methylation-mediated silencing of regenerating protein 1 alpha (REG1A) affects gastric cancer prognosis. Med Sci Monit 2017; 23: 5834-43.
[http://dx.doi.org/10.12659/MSM.904706] [PMID: 29222406]

[57] Sato Y, Marzese DM, Ohta K, *et al.* Epigenetic regulation of REG1A and chemosensitivity of cutaneous melanoma. Epigenetics 2013; 8(10): 1043-52.
[http://dx.doi.org/10.4161/epi.25810] [PMID: 23903855]

[58] Kober-Hasslacher M, Schmidt-Supprian M. The unsolved puzzle of C-rel in B cell lymphoma. Cancers (Basel) 2019; 11(7): 941.
[http://dx.doi.org/10.3390/cancers11070941] [PMID: 31277480]

[59] Hunter JE, Leslie J, Perkins ND. c-Rel and its many roles in cancer: an old story with new twists. Br J Cancer 2016; 114(1): 1-6.
[http://dx.doi.org/10.1038/bjc.2015.410] [PMID: 26757421]

[60] Shim HS, Wei M, Brandhorst S, Longo VD. Starvation promotes REV1 SUMOylation and p53-dependent sensitization of melanoma and breast cancer cells. Cancer Res 2015; 75(6): 1056-67.
[http://dx.doi.org/10.1158/0008-5472.CAN-14-2249] [PMID: 25614517]

[61] Sasatani M, Xi Y, Kajimura J, *et al.* Overexpression of Rev1 promotes the development of carcinogen-induced intestinal adenomas *via* accumulation of point mutation and suppression of apoptosis proportionally to the Rev1 expression level. Carcinogenesis 2017; 38(5): 570-8.
[http://dx.doi.org/10.1093/carcin/bgw208] [PMID: 28498946]

[62] Ju J, Gilkes D. Rhob: Team oncogene or team tumor suppressor? Genes (Basel) 2018; 9(2): 67.
[http://dx.doi.org/10.3390/genes9020067] [PMID: 29385717]

[63] Yi H, Wang K, Jin H, *et al.* Overexpression of rho-associated coiled-coil containing protein kinase 2 is correlated with clinical progression and poor prognosis in breast cancer. Med Sci Monit 2018; 24: 4776-81.
[http://dx.doi.org/10.12659/MSM.908507] [PMID: 29990315]

[64] Libanje F, Raingeaud J, Luan R, *et al.* ROCK 2 inhibition triggers the collective invasion of colorectal adenocarcinomas. EMBO J 2019; 38(14): e99299.
[http://dx.doi.org/10.15252/embj.201899299] [PMID: 31304629]

[65] Yang Y, Li S, Cao J, Li Y, Hu H, Wu Z. RRM2 regulated by LINC00667/miR-143-3p signal is responsible for non-small cell lung cancer cell progression. OncoTargets Ther 2019; 12: 9927-39.
[http://dx.doi.org/10.2147/OTT.S221339] [PMID: 31819489]

[66] Mazzu YZ, Armenia J, Chakraborty G, *et al.* A novel mechanism driving poor-prognosis prostate cancer: Overexpression of the DNA repair gene, ribonucleotide reductase small subunit M2 (RRM2). Clin Cancer Res 2019; 25(14): 4480-92.
[http://dx.doi.org/10.1158/1078-0432.CCR-18-4046] [PMID: 30996073]

[67] Akl MR, Nagpal P, Ayoub NM, *et al.* Molecular and clinical profiles of syndecan-1 in solid and hematological cancer for prognosis and precision medicine. Oncotarget 2015; 6(30): 28693-715.
[http://dx.doi.org/10.18632/oncotarget.4981] [PMID: 26293675]

[68]   Shan T, Uyar DS, Wang LS, *et al.* SOX11 hypermethylation as a tumor biomarker in endometrial cancer. Biochimie 2019; 162: 8-14.
[http://dx.doi.org/10.1016/j.biochi.2019.03.019] [PMID: 30935961]

[69]   Zhang Y, Liu Z. STAT1 in cancer: friend or foe? Discov Med 2017; 24(130): 19-29.
[PMID: 28950072]

[70]   Ke C, Zhu K, Sun Y, Ni Y, Zhang Z, Li X. SUMO1 promotes the proliferation and invasion of non-small cell lung cancer cells by regulating NF-κB. Thorac Cancer 2019; 10(1): 33-40.
[http://dx.doi.org/10.1111/1759-7714.12895] [PMID: 30393970]

[71]   Zhang B, Wu J, Cai Y, Luo M, Wang B, Gu Y. TCF7L1 indicates prognosis and promotes proliferation through activation of Keap1/NRF2 in gastric cancer. Acta Biochim Biophys Sin (Shanghai) 2019; 51(4): 375-85.
[http://dx.doi.org/10.1093/abbs/gmz015] [PMID: 30811526]

[72]   Liu Y, Liu R, Yang F, *et al.* miR-19a promotes colorectal cancer proliferation and migration by targeting TIA1. Mol Cancer 2017; 16(1): 53.
[http://dx.doi.org/10.1186/s12943-017-0625-8] [PMID: 28257633]

[73]   Grolez G, Gkika D. TRPM8 puts the chill on prostate cancer. Pharmaceuticals (Basel) 2016; 9(3): 44.
[http://dx.doi.org/10.3390/ph9030044] [PMID: 27409624]

[74]   Zhang HJ, Tao J, Sheng L, *et al.* Twist2 promotes kidney cancer cell proliferation and invasion by regulating ITGA6 and CD44 expression in the ECM-receptor interaction pathway. OncoTargets Ther 2016; 9: 1801-12.
[PMID: 27099513]

CHAPTER 3

Chromosome 3

Saurav Panicker[1] and **Satish Ramalingam**[1,*]

[1] *Department of Genetic Engineering, School of Bioengineering, SRM Institute of Science and Technology, Kattankulathur, India*

Abstract: Myriad genes in the genome have been implicated in cancer. However, a focused compilation of genes from the same chromosome would provide a valuable detailed yet succinct catalog for researchers, advantageous in quickly understanding the leading roles played by these genes in cancer. This chapter fulfills the above aim of furnishing a pocket dictionary- like a concise yet meticulous explanation of many genes from Chromosome 3, describing these genes' functional essentialities in various cancers. Such a judicious collection of genes from a single chromosome is probably the first of its kind. The multiple inputs in this chapter from Chromosome 3 include oncogenes (BCL6, RAF1), tumor suppressor genes (SRGAP3, FHIT), transcription factors (FOXP1, MITF), fusion genes (MECOM), and many other types. With approximately 1085 genes spanning 198 million base pairs, Chromosome 3 constitutes 6.5% of the total DNA.

Keywords: Ductal carcinoma, Glioma, Leukemia, Melanoma, MicroRNA, Neuroblastoma, Oncogene, Oncoprotein, Prostate cancer, Stem cells, Tumorigenesis.

1. INTRODUCTION

Chromosome 3 consists of 198 million base pairs. Hence, chromosome 3 roughly symbolizes 6.5% of the total deoxyribonucleic acid in 1 cell. Chromosome 3 is a metacentric chromosome closely associated with many congenital disabilities including deafness. Let us take a deeper look at some of the genes from Chromosome 3 that have been reported in cancer.

1.1. BCL6: B-Cell Lymphoma 6 Chromosome 3; 3q27.3

After BCL6 discovery in B-cell lymphomas, BCL-6 was widely regarded as an oncogene [1]. The BCL-6 locus undergoes translocations in diffuse large B-cell

* **Corresponding author Satish Ramalingam**: Department of Genetic Engineering, School of Bioengineering, SRM Institute of Science and Technology, Kattankulathur, India; E-mail: rsatish76@gmail.com

Satish Ramalingam (Ed.)

lymphomas [DLBCL] [1]. Such translocations cause the promoter switch of the BCL-6 coding region [1]. BCL6 can initiate tumorigenesis through the suppression of DNA damage checkpoints [1]. BCL6 has been under current scrutiny to consider it a prospective drug target [1]. BCL6 has been reported in solid and hematological cancers [1]. BCL6 gene expression is essential for NSCLC cell survival [1].

1.2. RAF1: Rapidly Accelerated Fibrosarcoma, Chromosome 3; 3p25.2

RAF1 codes for c-RAF (Fig. **1**). RAF1 impacts cellular migratory potentials, cell cycle, apoptosis, and senescence [2]. In the RASRAF- MEK-MAPK cellular signaling pathways, RAF1 has a significant effect [2]. RAF1 can be used as a prognostic marker in NSCLC patient's post-therapy [2]. RAF functions as a cellular oncogene. Even metastasis and invasive potential can be determined from the oncogenic hits in RAF [including RAF1] [2, 3].

1.3. TFG: Tropomyosin-Receptor Kinase Fused Gene Chromosome 3; 3q12.2

TFG fusion proteins have been described to cause tumorigenesis [4]. The function of this TFG protein in cancer has had paradoxical reports; some reports state that TFG could function as a tumor suppressor, while others say that TFG could serve as an oncoprotein [4]. TFG has been implicated in metastatic melanoma with a tumor suppressor function [5]. TFG has been identified as a mutational hotspot that could hold clinical significance for diagnosing and treating metastatic melanoma [5].

1.4. SRGAP3: SLIT-ROBO Rho GTPase-Activating Protein 3 Chromosome 3; 3p25.3

SRGAP3 gene (Fig. **1**) codes for an enzyme that regulates actin and microtubule dynamics [6]. SRGAP3 is a negative modulator of Rac1 [6]. SRGAP3 functions as a tumor suppressor in mammary epithelial cells [6]. SRGAP3 expression is depleted in breast cancer cells [6]. SRGAP3 under expression would promote anchorage-independent growth of breast cancer cells [6]. Lower levels of SRGAP3 expression have been reported in osteosarcomas and invasive breast carcinomas [7].

1.5. GATA2: GATA Binding Protein 2 Chromosome 3; 3q21.3

GATA2 is a crucial endothelial transcription factor that regulates Androgen Receptor [AR] activity [8]. GATA2 has been linked with the progression of prostate cancer in an AR-dependent and independent manner [8]. GATA2 hyper-expression in prostate cancer rapidly augments proliferation, drug resistance, and metastatic invasion [8]. GATA2 is a prominent factor for the marked aggressiveness in prostate cancer and, henceforth, could be a suitable target for novel drug therapies [8].

Chromosome 3

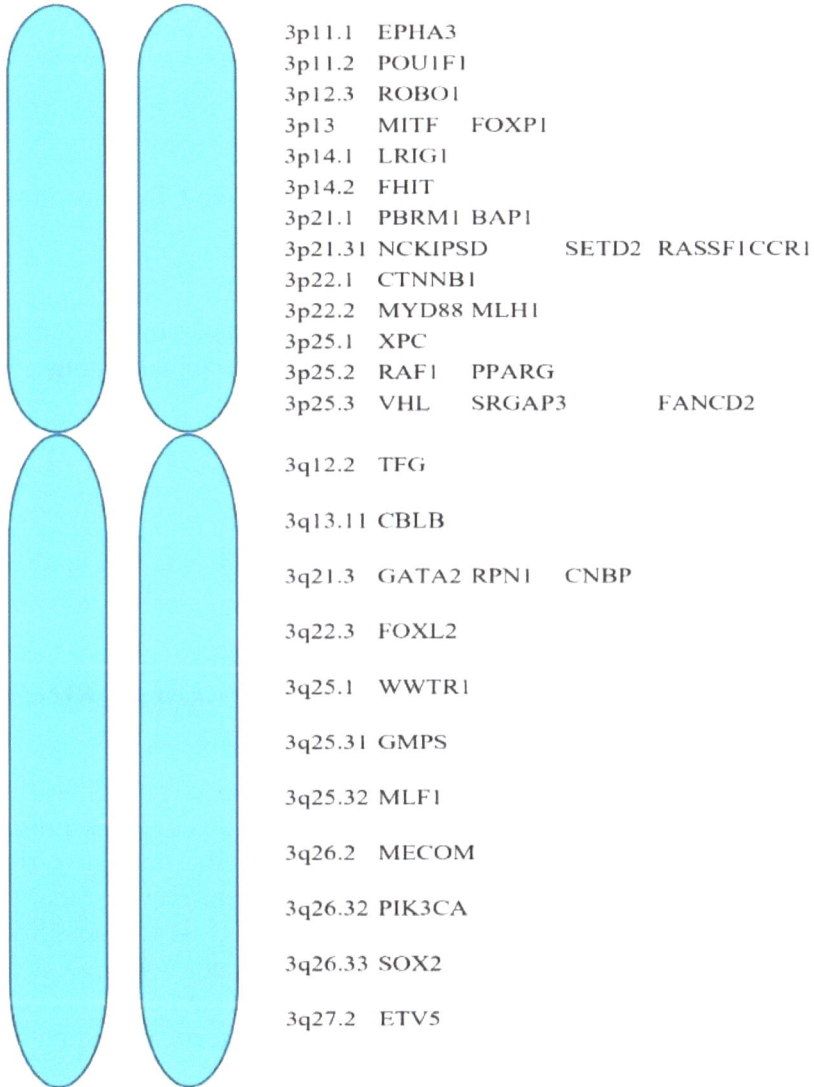

Locus	Genes
3p11.1	EPHA3
3p11.2	POU1F1
3p12.3	ROBO1
3p13	MITF FOXP1
3p14.1	LRIG1
3p14.2	FHIT
3p21.1	PBRM1 BAP1
3p21.31	NCKIPSD SETD2 RASSF1CCR1
3p22.1	CTNNB1
3p22.2	MYD88 MLH1
3p25.1	XPC
3p25.2	RAF1 PPARG
3p25.3	VHL SRGAP3 FANCD2
3q12.2	TFG
3q13.11	CBLB
3q21.3	GATA2 RPN1 CNBP
3q22.3	FOXL2
3q25.1	WWTR1
3q25.31	GMPS
3q25.32	MLF1
3q26.2	MECOM
3q26.32	PIK3CA
3q26.33	SOX2
3q27.2	ETV5

Fig. (1). This figure displays the loci of the genes from Chromosome 3 whose roles in cancer have been explained in this chapter. Sayooj Madhusoodanan designs this diagram.

1.6. RPN1: Ribophorin I Chromosome 3; 3q21.3

Chromosome translocations at RPN1 (Fig. **1**) have been reported in AML [Acute Myeloid Leukemia] patients [9]. Inversions at the RPN1 gene (Fig. **1**) have also been observed in AML and other hematological malignancies [10]. RPN1 gene is also used as a reference gene for the discovery of other oncogenes in the lung [NSCLC] and kidney tumors [clear cell renal cell tumors] [11, 12]. Transcriptome variations in RPN1 are relatively lesser [11]. Using RPN1 as a reference gene could aid the data normalization for future gene discoveries related to cancer [11].

1.7. CNBP: Cellular Nucleic Acid-Binding Protein Chromosome 3; 3q21.3

CNBP regulates matrix metalloproteinases. CNBP overexpression has been associated with tumorigenesis [13]. CNBP modulates other genes that support tumorigenesis [13]. CNBP can increase the expression of inflammatory cytokines that, in turn, support tumorigenesis in the tumor microenvironment [13].

1.8. FHIT: Fragile Histidine Triad Diadenosine Triphosphatase Chromosome 3; 3p14.2

FHIT is a tumor suppressor gene that is inactivated in multiple cancers [14] (Fig. **1**). The primary function of FHIT is to repress tumorigenic initiations by acting as a guardian to the genome [14]. FHIT inactivation has been considered an essential step in tumorigenic initiation [14].

1.9. PPARG: Peroxisome Proliferator-Activated Receptor Gamma Chromosome 3; 3p25.2

Contrasting theories and evidence have been shown regarding the tumorigenic role of PPARG. Nevertheless, PPARG is still considered a prominent gene in bladder cancer and colorectal cancer [15]. PPARG has been strongly implicated in colorectal carcinogenesis [16]. PPARG is a nuclear receptor that reregulates the transcription of inflammation factors [16]. Even T cells and dendritic cells express PPARG [16]. PPARG is expressed in colon tumors, though it is not directly correlated with prognosis [16]. PPARG is a significant player in cellular homeostasis [15]. PPARG has been implicated in other cancers, including breast, prostate, and lung cancer [15].

1.10. MECOM: MDS1 and EVI1 Complex Locus Chromosome 3; 3q26.2

MECOM codes for a protein that is vital in regulating hematopoietic stem cells, including epigenetic modifications (Fig. **1**). The chromosomal rearrangement t [3, 7] [q26;q21] causes an exchange between MECOM and CDK6 genes in myeloid neoplasm [17]. MECOM expression is higher in MECOM-rearranged pediatric malignant neoplastic patients [17]. MECOM expression has also been assessed for prognostic value in glioblastoma multiforme [18].

1.11. MITF – Melanocyte Inducing Transcription Factor Chromosome 3; 3p13

Missense mutations in MITF have been linked to melanoma, renal cell carcinoma, and pancreatic cancer [19]. MITF germline mutations have been studied in cancer [19, 20]. MITF has been suggested to function as an oncogene in melanoma while it activates the HIF1A pathway in renal cancer [20]. E318K missense mutation in MITF has been under focus in MITF mutation-related cancers [19]. MITF germline mutations remain a strong point for research in pancreatic cancer, kidney cancer, and melanoma.

1.12. FOXP1: Forkhead Box Protein P1 Chromosome 3; 3p13

FOXP1 is a transcription factor involved in the proper development of lympho-cytes [21]. FOXP1 can function either as a tumor suppressor protein or an oncoprotein in different tumors [21]. In B cell lymphoma, FOXP1 is an oncogene that augments tumor cell survival pathways, whereas in T cell lymphoma, FOXP1 is a tumor suppressor protein [21]. The role of FOXP1 was investigated in untreated primary breast cancer, and it was found that FOXP1 inversely affects the migration of Tumor Infiltrating Lymphocytes [21]. FOXP1 has been suggested to function as a tumor suppressor in NSCLC, endometrial, colorectal, and prostate cancers [21]. FOXP1 undergoes rearrangements in various lympho-mas, often resulting in its overexpression [22].

1.13. PBRM1: Polybromo-1 Chromosome 3; 3p21.1

PBRM1 gene was widely mutated in clear cell renal cell carcinomas [clear cell Renal Cell Carcinoma] [23, 24]. The PBRM1 gene is supposed to function as a tumor suppressor gene in various cancers [23, 24]. Deletions in the 3p region are frequent in ccRCC, often resulting in the loss of the PBRM1 gene [23]. PBRM1 mutations in renal cancer results in loss of protein [23]. PBRM1 and VHL mutations can happen simultaneously in renal cancer [23]. PBRM1 mutations can cause hypoxia, without VHL loss [23]. The PBRM1 gene is c potential biomarker for immunotherapy in ccRCC [24]. PBRM1 mutant NSCLC patients did not show any improvement in post-ICB therapy [Immune Checkpoint Blockade] [24].

1.14. BAP1: BRCA1 Associated Protein 1 Chromosome 3; 3p21.1

BAP1 germline mutations can lead to skin melanocytic tumors [25]. Germline BAP1 mutations were also identified in some mesothelioma patients [25]. The BAP1 gene was identified while investigating a 3p21 locus highly mutated in uveal melanomas and mesotheliomas [25]. BAP1 mutations in uveal melanoma patients had a higher chance of hereditary cancer [25]. Cancer therapies targeting BAP1 mutations have been proposed while some of them are being tested in clinical trials, and not all BAP1 mutations have been fully characterized [26].

1.15. NCKIPSD: NCK Interacting Protein with SH3 Domain Chromosome 3; 3p21.31

t [3, 11] [p21;q23] KMT2A/NCKIPSD is a translocation discovered in t- AML [27]. This translocation involved the MLL gene [27]. This translocation was the only cytogenetic anomaly revealed in a t-AML patient who had previously undergone treatment for ALL [28]. This MLL fusion gene was considered a novel MLL fusion gene when it was first cloned and identified in 2000 [28].

During its initial discovery, NCKIPSD protein was proposed to play a role in signal transduction [29].

1.16. SETD2: Set Domain Containing 2 Chromosome 3; 3p21.31

SETD2 is an H3K6 histone methyltransferase that is mutated in a variety of cancers [30]. Oncogenic mutations in SETD2 have been documented in various cancer, including epithelial, CNS [central Nervous system], and liquid cancers [30]. Studies suggest that SETD2's oncogenic mutations are clinically relevant for the onset of specific ccRCC subsets [30]. High-grade gliomas and acute leukemias have registered SETD2 mutations [30]. Since oncogenic mutations in epigenetic regulators have been associated with multiple cancers, focusing on SETD2 for drugging the epigenome could be ideal, provided its role in tumor initiation [31].

1.17. CTNNB1 Gene: Catenin Beta 1 Chromosome 3; 3p22.1

CTNNB1 gene codes for the beta-catenin protein [32] (Fig. **1**). Beta-catenin is an essential molecule in the Wnt signaling pathway that is important for APC regulation [32]. Mutations in the 3rd exon of beta-catenin have been found to play a role in tumorigenesis [32]. Exon 3 was primarily under observation for studying the mutational hotspots in CTNNB1 [32, 33]. Exon 3 deletion mutation in CTNNB1 was related to colorectal metastasis. Significant oncogenic CTNNB1 genomic alterations have been detected in endometrial, liver, and colorectal cancer [33].

1.18. MYD88: Myeloid Differentiation Primary Response 88 Chromosome 3; 3p22.2

MyD88 is described as a signaling adaptor in TLR [Toll Like Receptor] signaling [34]. MyD88 is an important molecule in innate immune signaling. MyD88 mutations have been found in Primary central nervous system lymphoma [PCNSL] [35]. NF-kB and JAK/STAT3 pathways are induced by MyD88 [35]. MyD88 was shown to support colorectal carcinogenesis [36]. L265P missense mutation in MyD88 has been reported in numerous cases of large B-cell lymphoma [37].

1.19. CBLB: Cbl Proto-Oncogene B Chromosome 3; 3q13.11

The CBLB gene's oncogenic functionality in various subsets of lung cancer was tested to distinguish between its roles in squamous cell carcinoma and adenocarcinoma [38]. CBLB regulates the NK cells [natural killer] and CD 8 T-cells [39]. CBLB mutations have been identified in solid tumors [40]. CBLB mutations in various tumors have been classified and described in TCGA [the Cancer genome Atlas] [40].

1.20. FOXL2: Forkhead Box Protein L2 Chromosome 3; 3q22.3

FOXL2 is responsible for granulosa cell tumors [41]. Different theories still exist on whether FOXL2 is a tumor suppressor gene or not [41]. miR-937 inhibited gastric cancer metastasis by downregulating FOXL2 [41]. STAT3- FOXL2 pathway might play an essential role in HeLa cell's growth, elucidating that FOXL2 might have a role in cervical cancer [41]. FOXL2 has been studied before in cervical cancer to know its effects on apoptosis [42].

1.21. WWTR1: WW Domain Containing Transcription Regulator 1 Chromosome 3; 3q25.1

WWTR1 operates on the cytoskeleton and cell migration properties [43]. WWT-R1 can support metastasis by enhancing cancer cell survival and drug-resistance properties [43]. Hippo 61ignalling and WWTR1 are suggested to play a role in gastric cancer invasion [43]. WWTRI is meant to be a prognostic and metastatic marker for gastric cancer [gastric cardia adenocarcinoma] [43]. WWTR1 plays a vital role in supporting the proliferation of colorectal cancer cells [44].

1.22. GMPS: Guanine Monophosphate Synthase Chromosome 3; 3q25.31

GMPS is a significant player in p53 deubiquitylation and p53 stabilization [45]. GMPS expression is significantly higher in invasive ductal and mucinous carcinoma [45]. GMPS is a cogent molecular agent responsible for rapid tumorigenicity in malignant melanoma [46]. In malignant melanoma, GMPS further supports the invasive tumor potential of melanoma cells [46]. GMPS displays a higher expression pattern in metastatic melanoma [46]. Upregulation of GMPS is observed during melanoma's rapid tumor progression [46]. Angustmycinmediated GMPS inhibition reduces the tumorigenic invasiveness of malignant melanoma [46].

1.23. MLF1: Myeloid Leukemia Factor 1 Chromosome 3; 3q25.32

MLF1 inhibits C/EBPα, modulates myeloid differentiation, and controls leukemogenesis [47]. MLF1 was discovered from a fusion gene named NPM- MLF1 detected in AML patients [47]. MLF1 is expressed in multipotent progenitor cells; hence, MLF1 mutation can cause an aberration, leading to leukemogenesis [48]. T [3, 5] [q25.1; q34] is the rearrangement that forms the NPM- MLF1 fusion protein in myelodysplastic syndrome [MDS] [48].

1.24. PIK3CA: Phosphatidylinositol-4,5-Bisphosphate 3-Kinase Catalytic Subunit Alpha Chromosome 3; 3q26.32

Missense mutations in PIK3CA have been detected in various tumors [49]. The tumors in which PIK3CA mutations have been identified comprise breast cancer, endometrial cancer, skin cancer, lung cancer, colorectal cancer, thyroid cancer, head and neck cancer, brain tumors, pituitary tumors, and so many more [49]. PIK3CA is one of the most frequently mutated genes in several cancer types [49]. These mutations are oncogenic [50]. PIK3CA is essential for proper cellular growth [51]. PIK3CA mutations indicate poor prognosis in solid cancers [52].

1.25. SOX2: Sex-Determining Region Y [SRY]-Box Rranscription Factor 2 Chromosome 3; 3q26.33

SOX2 is a crucial pluripotency factor concerned with conferring stemness in cancer stem cells [CSC] [53]. SOX2-positive tumor cells were responsible for tumor relapse in ovarian cancer because these cells possessed an aggressive tumor-initiating capability [53]. SOX2 was upregulated in glioma stem cells of high-grade gliomas [53]. Owing to the high expression of SOX2 in CSCs in many cancers, it's concluded that SOX2 is a decisive factor in promoting t the stemness of CSCs [53]. Therapies related to targeting SOX2 have been discussed recently [53].

1.26. ETV5: ETS Variant Transcription Factor 5 Chromosome 3; 3q27.2

ETV5 has been implicated in neuroblastoma [54]. ETV5 expression in neuroblastoma enhances tumor migration and invasiveness [54]. ETV5 knockdown inhibited tumor proliferation in neuroblastoma [54]. Ovarian cancers have upregulated ETV5 [55]. ETV5 overexpression is in papillary thyroid carcinoma [PTC] [56]. ETV5 is crucial for PTC tumor growth and tumor cell proliferation [56]. ETV5 modulates TWIST1 in PTC [56].

1.27. EIF4A2: Eukaryotic Translation Initiation Factor 4A, Isoform 2 Chromosome 3; 3q27.3

EIF4A2 expression brings about major translation changes in breast cancer cells, often resulting in a malignant phenotype [57]. In normal cells, EIF4A2 is vital to microRNA [miR] mediated translation repression [58]. EIF4A2 is very important for binding mRNA to the ribosome for accurate translation initiation [59]. EIF4A2 is one among many fusion partners of BCL6 in diffuse large B-cell lymphomas [DLBL] [60]. EIF42 is a potent prognostic assessment marker in NSCLC [60, 61]. EIF4A2 is upregulated in colorectal cancer, and its high expression predicts poor prognosis for patients [59].

1.28. LPP: Lipoma Preferred Partner Chromosome 3; 3q27.3-q28

LPP plays a critical role in the induction of tumor invasion and metastasis [62]. LPP controls cell migration and cell adhesion properties [62]. LPP is required for breast cancer metastasis because it is active in regulating breast cancer cell migration [62]. The discovery of LPP was from a fusion transcript that comprised the fusion of LPP with HMGA2 [62]. LPP interacts with alpha-actinin and serves as a crucial marker for tumor cell migration and invasion [63]. LPP promotes invadopodia formation [63].

1.29. RASSF1: Ras Association Domain-Containing Protein 1 Chromosome 3; 3p21.31

RASSF1 is a frequently inactivated tumor suppressor gene in pancreatic ductal adenocarcinoma [PDAC] [64]. CpG island methylation of RASSF1 was the cause of RASSFI inactivation in PDAC. RASSF1 methylation did not determine the prognosis [64]. RASSF1 hypermethylation was detected in the majority of PDAC cases [64]. RASSF1 is a tumor suppressor gene that blocks the RAS pathway [64]. RASSF1 displayed copy number variations in PDAC [64]. RASSF1 has isoforms ranging from A-G, and all these isoforms [formed by alternative splicing] have been underreported for their methylation patterns in various cancers [64, 65]. RASSF1 gene undergoes methylation-based inactivation in breast and lung cancers [65].

1.30. MLH1: MutL Homolog 1 Chromosome 3; 3p22.2

MLH1 is a DNA mismatch repair gene [MMR] [66]. Germline mutations in MLH1 increase the chances of colorectal cancer [66]. Mutations in MMR genes [including MLH1] that cause cancer are categorized under Lynch Syndrome [66]. A large proportion of Lynch syndrome cases result from MLH1 mutations [66]. MLH1 mutations were also associated with gastric cancer [66]. Families carrying germline MLH1 deletions had carriers in their second and third generations [67]. New MLH1 mutations have been associated with bowel cancers [68].

1.31. VHL: Von Hippel-Lindau Chromosome 3; 3p25.3

VHL is a prominent tumor suppressor gene widely known to be highly mutated in renal cancers [69]. VHL directly regulates the HIF [Hypoxia Inducible Factor] for controlling the hypoxia pathway [70]. Germline mutation of VHL causing its inactivation results in VHL hereditary cancer [71]. Genomic alterations in the VHL gene involving promoter methylation, LOH, and other somatic or germline mutations have been implicated in renal carcinogenesis [70]. VHL mutations have been the hallmark of both hereditary and sporadic ccRCC [clear cell Renal cell carcinoma]. VHL mutations are concerned with both solid and cystic ccRCC [69].

1.32. XPC: Xeroderma Pigmentosum Complementation Group C [XP Complex Subunit C] Chromosome 3; 3p25.1

XPC is a DNA repair gene [72]. Mutations in XPC cause xeroderma pigmentosum [72]. This disorder can further exacerbate skin cancer [72]. XPC mutations [especially deletions] produce an aberrantly spliced XPC mRNA, adversely affecting the nucleotide excision repair function and increasing the risk for cancer [72]. The correlation of XPC polymorphisms with prostate cancer predisposition has been investigated in Iranian patients. However, a negative correlation was the outcome [73]. The role of XPC has been recently investigated in colorectal cancer and is elucidated to have a conspicuous prediction factor for colorectal cancer [74].

1.33. FANCD2: Fanconi Anemia Complementation Group D2 Protein Chromosome 3; 3p25.3

FANCD2 is essential for DNA damage responses [75]. FANCD2 expression has been explored in breast cancer along with BRCA1 presentation [76]. Earlier reports had corroborated FANCD2 expression levels to be linked with sporadic breast cancer susceptibility [77]. In secretory breast carcinoma [SBC], high levels of FANCD2 expression and low ubiquitination levels were linked to poor patient outcomes [76]. Breast cancer patients with FANCD2 expression had a decreased disease-free survival [DFS] [76]. FANCD2 ubiquitination can be used independently for prognostic prediction in SBC [76].

1.34. POU1F1: POU Class 1 Homeobox 1 Chromosome 3; 3p11.2

POU1F1, also known as Pit-1, transcriptionally modulates mammary Prolactin [PRL] [78]. POU1F1 transfection had elevated PRL levels *in vitro* [78]. POU1F1 expression is higher in breast tumor tissues compared to its expression in normal tissue [78]. POU1F1 can impact tumor cell proliferation through its effects on cyclin D-1 [78]. This evidence suggests that more focus should be given to POU1F1 in breast-invasive ductal carcinomas [78]. POU1F1 gene mutations can lead to pituitary hormone disorders [79].

1.35. EPHA3: EPH Receptor A3 Chromosome 3; 3p11.1

EPHA3 is a receptor tyrosine kinase [80]. Genome sequencing studies have deciphered oncogenic mutations in EPHA3 [80]. These EPHA3 oncogenic mutations adversely affect the tumor suppressor function of EPHA3 in lung cancer [80]. Deletions in EPHA3 have been observed in lung cancer [80]. In Leukemia, promoted hypermethylation of EPHA3 results in its silencing [80]. EPHA3 is repeatedly mutated in colon cancer [81]. EPH pathway deregulation supports colorectal tumorigenesis [81].

1.36. ROBO1: Roundabout Guidance Receptor 1 Chromosome 3; 3p12.3

ROBO1 belongs to the immunoglobulin protein family [82]. ROBO1 can be employed in precise molecular subtyping of prostate cancer [82]. ROBO1 has a tumor suppressor function [82]. ROBO1 expression decreases during prostate cancer progression [82]. When prostate cancer reaches the metastatic stage, ROBO1 expression is lost [82]. ROBO1 alters the cellular metabolic cascades and supports the Warburg effect in osteosarcoma [83]. ROBO1 is upregulated in osteosarcoma [83].

1.37. LRIG1: Leucine-Rich Repeats and Immunoglobulin-Like Domains 1 Chromosome 3; 3p14.1

LRIG1 expression in colorectal cancer displayed a lot of heterogeneity [84]. LRIG1 ubiquitinylates ERBB receptors to modulate ERBB expression [84]. LRIG1 downregulates ERBB [84]. LRIG1 is upregulated in prostate cancer [85]. LRIG1 is a pleiotropic tumor suppressor gene that inhibits c-Myc and ERBB in prostate cancer [85]. Androgen receptor signalling transactivates LRIG1 [85]. The tumor suppressor function of LRIG1 is vital in inhibiting tumor regeneration [85].

1.38. ADAMTS9: ADAM Metallopeptidase with Thrombospondin Type 1 Motif 9 Chromosome 3; 3p14.1

ADAMTS9 is a tumor suppressor in colorectal and gastric cancer [86, 87]. ADAMTS9 arrested Akt activation in colorectal cancer in-vitro [86]. ADAMTS9 expression was repressed due to promoter methylation in colorectal cancer [86]. ADAMTS9 transfection in-vitro retarded cell proliferation [86]. ADAMTS9 impedes the Akt/mTOR pathways in gastric cancer to suppress the oncogenic 66ignalling that promotes gastric cancer progression [87]. ADAMTS9 functions in tumor suppression of multiple myeloma, nasopharyngeal carcinoma, and esophageal squamous cell carcinoma [86].

1.39. WNT5A: Wnt Family Member 5A. Chromosome 3; 3p14.3

Wnt5a regulates Noncanonical Wnt signalling cascades [88]. Wnt5a is pivotal in regulating stem cells' various properties, including self-renewal, differentiation, and proper development [88]. The abnormal expression of Wnt5a contributes to the development of cancer stem cells [88]. The mechanistic insights into the roles of Wnt5a signaling in breast cancer stem cells and ovarian cancer stem cells have been elucidated [88]. Wnt5a has heterogenous roles in tumorigenesis – Wnt5a can inhibit or augment carcinogenesis [88]. Further investigations into the crosstalk of Wnt5a-regulated pathways with other pathways will explicate newer therapeutic strategies to target cancer stem cells.

1.40. CCR1: C-C Motif Chemokine Receptor 1 Chromosome 3; 3p21.31

CCR1 is expressed by the cells belonging to the myeloid lineage [89]. CCR1 is implied to have a salient role in determining the colonization step of colorectal cancer metastasis [90]. Early stages of liver colonization are indicated by an increase in CCR1 expression [90]. CCR1 supports tumor aggressiveness and angiogenesis [89]. The recruitment of myeloid cells into the tumor sites is decided by the CCR1 face [89]. Lymphocyte recruitment and infiltration into the tumor site are regulated by CCR1 [89].

CONCLUSION

Chromosome 3 has been under scrutiny since the 1980s for studying related congenital anomalies and other genetic disorders caused by chromosomal abnormalities in chromosome 3. With specific reference to cancer, this chapter has elaborately recapitulated the significant contributions of various genes from chromosome 3 in tumorigenesis. Clear cell renal carcinoma is one primary type of cancer that can arise from genetic anomalies in chromosome 3. Other solid cancers have also been associated with genetic instability on chromosome 3. However, as undoubtedly evident, more research must be conducted to unravel cancers affiliated with aberrations on chromosome 3. Admittedly, this chapter will be beneficial to revisit through the voluminous cutting-edge knowledge regarding various genes published in the past decades after numerous investigations.

REFERENCES

[1]   Cardenas MG, Oswald E, Yu W, Xue F, MacKerell AD Jr, Melnick AM. The expanding role of the BCL6 oncoprotein as a cancer therapeutic target. Clin Cancer Res 2017; 23(4): 885-93.
[http://dx.doi.org/10.1158/1078-0432.CCR-16-2071] [PMID: 27881582]

[2]   Tian H, Yin L, Ding K, *et al.* Raf1 is a prognostic factor for progression in patients with non-small cell lung cancer after radiotherapy. Oncol Rep 2018; 39(4): 1966-74.
[http://dx.doi.org/10.3892/or.2018.6277] [PMID: 29484414]

[3]   Maurer G, Tarkowski B, Baccarini M. Raf kinases in cancer–roles and therapeutic opportunities. Oncogene 2011; 30(32): 3477-88.
[http://dx.doi.org/10.1038/onc.2011.160] [PMID: 21577205]

[4]   Chen Y, Tseng S-H. Targeting tropomyosin-receptor kinase fused gene in cancer. Anticancer Res 2014; 34(4): 1595-600.
[PMID: 24692687]

[5]   Dutton-Regester K, Aoude LG, Nancarrow DJ, *et al.* Identification of TFG (TRK-fused gene) as a putative metastatic melanoma tumor suppressor gene. Genes Chromosomes Cancer 2012; 51(5): 452-61.
[http://dx.doi.org/10.1002/gcc.21932] [PMID: 22250051]

[6]   Lahoz A, Hall A. A tumor suppressor role for srGAP3 in mammary epithelial cells. Oncogene 2013; 32(40): 4854-60.
[http://dx.doi.org/10.1038/onc.2012.489] [PMID: 23108406]

[7]   Kazanietz MG, Caloca MJ. The Rac GTPase in Cancer: From Old Concepts to New Paradigms. Cancer Res 2017; 77(20): 5445-51.
[http://dx.doi.org/10.1158/0008-5472.CAN-17-1456] [PMID: 28807941]

[8]   Rodriguez-Bravo V, Carceles-Cordon M, Hoshida Y, Cordon-Cardo C, Galsky MD, Domingo-Domenech J. The role of GATA2 in lethal prostate cancer aggressiveness. Nat Rev Urol 2017; 14(1): 38-48.
[http://dx.doi.org/10.1038/nrurol.2016.225] [PMID: 27872477]

[9]   Shearer BM, Sukov WR, Flynn HC, Knudson RA, Ketterling RP. Development of a dual-color, double fusion FISH assay to detect RPN1/EVI1 gene fusion associated with inv(3), t(3;3), and ins(3;3) in patients with myelodysplasia and acute myeloid leukemia. Am J Hematol 2010; 85(8): 569-74.
[http://dx.doi.org/10.1002/ajh.21746] [PMID: 20556821]

[10]   De Braekeleer E, Douet-Guilbert N, Basinko A, *et al.* Conventional cytogenetics and breakpoint distribution by fluorescent *in situ* hybridization in patients with malignant hemopathies associated with inv(3)(q21;q26) and t(3;3)(q21;q26). Anticancer Res 2011; 31(10): 3441-8.
[PMID: 21965759]

[11]   Krasnov GS, Oparina NY, Dmitriev AA, *et al.* RPN1, a new reference gene for quantitative data normalization in lung and kidney cancer. Mol Biol 2011; 45(2): 211-20.
[http://dx.doi.org/10.1134/S0026893311020129]

[12]   Senchenko VN, Anedchenko EA, Kondratieva TT, *et al.* Simultaneous down-regulation of tumor suppressor genes RBSP3/CTDSPL, NPRL2/G21 and RASSF1A in primary non-small cell lung cancer. BMC Cancer 2010; 10(1): 75.
[http://dx.doi.org/10.1186/1471-2407-10-75] [PMID: 20193080]

[13]   Lee E, Lee TA, Yoo HJ, Lee S, Park B. CNBP controls tumor cell biology by regulating tumor-promoting gene expression. Mol Carcinog 2019; 58(8): 1492-501.
[http://dx.doi.org/10.1002/mc.23030] [PMID: 31087358]

[14]   Kiss DL, Baez W, Huebner K, Bundschuh R, Schoenberg DR. Impact of FHIT loss on the translation of cancer-associated mRNAs. Mol Cancer 2017; 16(1): 179.
[http://dx.doi.org/10.1186/s12943-017-0749-x] [PMID: 29282095]

[15]   Lv S, Wang W, Wang H, Zhu Y, Lei C. PPARγ activation serves as therapeutic strategy against bladder cancer *via* inhibiting PI3K-Akt signaling pathway. BMC Cancer 2019; 19(1): 204.
[http://dx.doi.org/10.1186/s12885-019-5426-6] [PMID: 30845932]

[16]   Villa AL, Parra RS, Feitosa MR, et al. PPARG expression in colorectal cancer and its association with staging and clinical evolution. Acta Cir Bras. 2020; 35(7): e202000708.

[17]   Capela de Matos RR, Othman MAK, Ferreira GM, *et al.* Molecular approaches identify a cryptic MECOM rearrangement in a child with a rapidly progressive myeloid neoplasm. Cancer Genet 2018; 221: 25-30.
[http://dx.doi.org/10.1016/j.cancergen.2017.12.002] [PMID: 29405993]

[18]   Hou A, Zhao L, Zhao F, *et al.* Expression of MECOM is associated with unfavorable prognosis in glioblastoma multiforme. OncoTargets Ther 2016; 9: 315-20.
[PMID: 26834490]

[19]   Gromowski T, Masojć B, Scott RJ, *et al.* Prevalence of the E318K and V320I MITF germline mutations in Polish cancer patients and multiorgan cancer risk-a population-based study. Cancer Genet 2014; 207(4): 128-32.
[http://dx.doi.org/10.1016/j.cancergen.2014.03.003] [PMID: 24767713]

[20]   Bertolotto C, Lesueur F, Giuliano S, *et al.* A SUMOylation-defective MITF germline mutation predisposes to melanoma and renal carcinoma. Nature 2011; 480(7375): 94-8.
[http://dx.doi.org/10.1038/nature10539] [PMID: 22012259]

[21]   De Silva P, Garaud S, Solinas C, *et al.* FOXP1 negatively regulates tumor infiltrating lymphocyte migration in human breast cancer. EBioMedicine 2019; 39: 226-38.
[http://dx.doi.org/10.1016/j.ebiom.2018.11.066] [PMID: 30579865]

[22]   Koon HB, Ippolito GC, Banham AH, Tucker PW. FOXP1: a potential therapeutic target in cancer. Expert Opin Ther Targets 2007; 11(7): 955-65.
[http://dx.doi.org/10.1517/14728222.11.7.955] [PMID: 17614763]

[23]   Brugarolas J. PBRM1 and BAP1 as novel targets for renal cell carcinoma. Cancer J 2013; 19(4): 324-32.
[http://dx.doi.org/10.1097/PPO.0b013e3182a102d1] [PMID: 23867514]

[24]   Zhou H, Liu J, Zhang Y, et al. PBRM1 mutation and preliminary response to immune checkpoint blockade treatment in non-small cell lung cancer. NPJ Precis Oncol. 2020; 4: 6.

[25]   Carbone M, Yang H, Pass HI, Krausz T, Testa JR, Gaudino G. BAP1 and cancer. Nat Rev Cancer 2013; 13(3): 153-9.
[http://dx.doi.org/10.1038/nrc3459] [PMID: 23550303]

[26]   Okonska A, Felley-Bosco E. BAP1 Missense Mutations in Cancer: Friend or Foe? Trends Cancer 2019; 5(11): 659-62.
[http://dx.doi.org/10.1016/j.trecan.2019.09.006] [PMID: 31735283]

[27]   Meyer C, Burmeister T, Gröger D, *et al.* The MLL recombinome of acute leukemias in 2017.

Leukemia 2018; 32(2): 273-84.
[http://dx.doi.org/10.1038/leu.2017.213] [PMID: 28701730]

[28]   Sano K, Hayakawa A, Piao JH, Kosaka Y, Nakamura H. Novel SH3 protein encoded by the AF3p21 gene is fused to the mixed lineage leukemia protein in a therapy-related leukemia with t(3;11) (p21;q23). Blood 2000; 95(3): 1066-8.
[http://dx.doi.org/10.1182/blood.V95.3.1066.003k11_1066_1068] [PMID: 10648423]

[29]   Hayakawa A, Matsuda Y, Daibata M, Nakamura H, Sano K. Genomic organization, tissue expression, and cellular localization ofAF3p21, a fusion partner ofMLL in therapy-related leukemia. Genes Chromosomes Cancer 2001; 30(4): 364-74.
[http://dx.doi.org/10.1002/gcc.1102] [PMID: 11241789]

[30]   Fahey CC, Davis IJ. SETting the Stage for Cancer Development: SETD2 and the Consequences of Lost Methylation. Cold Spring Harb Perspect Med 2017; 7(5): a026468.
[http://dx.doi.org/10.1101/cshperspect.a026468] [PMID: 28159833]

[31]   Li J, Duns G, Westers H, Sijmons R, van den Berg A, Kok K. SETD2: an epigenetic modifier with tumor suppressor functionality. Oncotarget 2016; 7(31): 50719-34.
[http://dx.doi.org/10.18632/oncotarget.9368] [PMID: 27191891]

[32]   Gao C, Wang Y, Broaddus R, Sun L, Xue F, Zhang W. Exon 3 mutations of *CTNNB1* drive tumorigenesis: a review. Oncotarget 2018; 9(4): 5492-508.
[http://dx.doi.org/10.18632/oncotarget.23695] [PMID: 29435196]

[33]   Kim S, Jeong S. Mutation Hotspots in the β-Catenin Gene: Lessons from the Human Cancer Genome Databases. Mol Cells 2019; 42(1): 8-16.
[PMID: 30699286]

[34]   MYD88 - an overview | ScienceDirect Topics, https://www.sciencedirect.com/topics/immunology-and-microbiology/myd88 (accessed 24 December 2020).

[35]   Cai Q, Fang Y, Young KH. Primary Central Nervous System Lymphoma: Molecular Pathogenesis and Advances in Treatment. Transl Oncol 2019; 12(3): 523-38.
[http://dx.doi.org/10.1016/j.tranon.2018.11.011] [PMID: 30616219]

[36]   Zhu G, Cheng Z, Huang Y, *et al.* MyD88 mediates colorectal cancer cell proliferation, migration and invasion *via* NF-κB/AP-1 signaling pathway. Int J Mol Med 2020; 45(1): 131-40.
[PMID: 31746347]

[37]   Yu X, Li W, Deng Q, *et al. MYD88* L265P Mutation in Lymphoid Malignancies. Cancer Res 2018; 78(10): 2457-62.
[http://dx.doi.org/10.1158/0008-5472.CAN-18-0215] [PMID: 29703722]

[38]   Li P, Liu H, Zhang Z, *et al.* Expression and Comparison of Cbl-b in Lung Squamous Cell Carcinoma and Adenocarcinoma. Med Sci Monit 2018; 24: 623-35.
[http://dx.doi.org/10.12659/MSM.908076] [PMID: 29384143]

[39]   Liyasova MS, Ma K, Lipkowitz S. Molecular pathways: cbl proteins in tumorigenesis and antitumor immunity-opportunities for cancer treatment. Clin Cancer Res 2015; 21(8): 1789-94.
[http://dx.doi.org/10.1158/1078-0432.CCR-13-2490] [PMID: 25477533]

[40]   Daniels SR, Liyasova M, Kales SC, *et al.* Loss of function Cbl-c mutations in solid tumors. PLoS One 2019; 14(7): e0219143.
[http://dx.doi.org/10.1371/journal.pone.0219143] [PMID: 31260484]

[41]   Han Y, Wu J, Yang W, Wang D, Zhang T, Cheng M. New STAT3-FOXL2 pathway and its function in cancer cells. BMC Mol Cell Biol 2019; 20(1): 17.
[http://dx.doi.org/10.1186/s12860-019-0206-3] [PMID: 31221094]

[42]   Liu X-L, Meng Y-H, Wang J-L, Yang BB, Zhang F, Tang SJ. FOXL2 suppresses proliferation, invasion and promotes apoptosis of cervical cancer cells. Int J Clin Exp Pathol 2014; 7(4): 1534-43.
[PMID: 24817949]

[43]   Wei J, Wang L, Zhu J, *et al.* The Hippo signaling effector WWTR1 is a metastatic biomarker of gastric cardia adenocarcinoma. Cancer Cell Int 2019; 19(1): 74.
[http://dx.doi.org/10.1186/s12935-019-0796-z] [PMID: 30976198]

[44]   Lu X. Lentivirus-mediated RNA interference targeting WWTR1 in human colorectal cancer cells inhibits cell proliferation *in vitro* and tumor growth *in vivo*. Oncol Rep 2012; 2.
[http://dx.doi.org/10.3892/or.2012.1751]

[45]   Reddy BA, van der Knaap JA, Bot AGM, *et al.* Nucleotide biosynthetic enzyme GMP synthase is a TRIM21-controlled relay of p53 stabilization. Mol Cell 2014; 53(3): 458-70.
[http://dx.doi.org/10.1016/j.molcel.2013.12.017] [PMID: 24462112]

[46]   Bianchi-Smiraglia A, Wawrzyniak JA, Bagati A, *et al.* Pharmacological targeting of guanosine monophosphate synthase suppresses melanoma cell invasion and tumorigenicity. Cell Death Differ 2015; 22(11): 1858-64.
[http://dx.doi.org/10.1038/cdd.2015.47] [PMID: 25909885]

[47]   Nakamae I, Kato J, Yokoyama T, Ito H, Yoneda-Kato N. Myeloid leukemia factor 1 stabilizes tumor suppressor C/EBPα to prevent Trib1-driven acute myeloid leukemia. Blood Adv 2017; 1(20): 1682-93.
[http://dx.doi.org/10.1182/bloodadvances.2017007054] [PMID: 29296815]

[48]   Matsumoto N, Yoneda-Kato N, Iguchi T, *et al.* Elevated MLF1 expression correlates with malignant progression from myelodysplastic syndrome. Leukemia 2000; 14(10): 1757-65.
[http://dx.doi.org/10.1038/sj.leu.2401897] [PMID: 11021751]

[49]   Samuels Y, Waldman T. Oncogenic mutations of PIK3CA in human cancers. Curr Top Microbiol Immunol 2010; 347: 21-41.
[http://dx.doi.org/10.1007/82_2010_68] [PMID: 20535651]

[50]   Ligresti G, Militello L, Steelman LS, *et al.* PIK3CA mutations in human solid tumors: Role in sensitivity to various therapeutic approaches. Cell Cycle 2009; 8(9): 1352-8.
[http://dx.doi.org/10.4161/cc.8.9.8255] [PMID: 19305151]

[51]   Madsen RR, Vanhaesebroeck B, Semple RK. Cancer-Associated PIK3CA Mutations in Overgrowth Disorders. Trends Mol Med 2018; 24(10): 856-70.
[http://dx.doi.org/10.1016/j.molmed.2018.08.003] [PMID: 30197175]

[52]   Alqahtani A, Ayesh HSK, Halawani H. PIK3CA Gene Mutations in Solid Malignancies: Association with Clinicopathological Parameters and Prognosis. Cancers (Basel) 2019; 12(1): 93.
[http://dx.doi.org/10.3390/cancers12010093] [PMID: 31905960]

[53]   Mamun MA, Mannoor K, Cao J, Qadri F, Song X. SOX2 in cancer stemness: tumor malignancy and therapeutic potentials. J Mol Cell Biol 2020; 12(2): 85-98.
[http://dx.doi.org/10.1093/jmcb/mjy080] [PMID: 30517668]

[54]   Mus LM, Lambertz I, Claeys S, *et al.* The ETS transcription factor ETV5 is a target of activated ALK in neuroblastoma contributing to increased tumour aggressiveness. Sci Rep 2020; 10(1): 218.
[http://dx.doi.org/10.1038/s41598-019-57076-5] [PMID: 31937834]

[55]   Llauradó M, Majem B, Castellví J, *et al.* Analysis of gene expression regulated by the ETV5 transcription factor in OV90 ovarian cancer cells identifies FOXM1 overexpression in ovarian cancer. Mol Cancer Res 2012; 10(7): 914-24.
[http://dx.doi.org/10.1158/1541-7786.MCR-11-0449] [PMID: 22589409]

[56]   Puli OR, Danysh BP, McBeath E, *et al.* The Transcription Factor ETV5 Mediates BRAFV600E-Induced Proliferation and TWIST1 Expression in Papillary Thyroid Cancer Cells. Neoplasia 2018; 20(11): 1121-34.
[http://dx.doi.org/10.1016/j.neo.2018.09.003] [PMID: 30265861]

[57]   Modelska A, Turro E, Russell R, *et al.* The malignant phenotype in breast cancer is driven by eIF4A1-mediated changes in the translational landscape. Cell Death Dis 2015; 6(1): e1603-3.
[http://dx.doi.org/10.1038/cddis.2014.542] [PMID: 25611378]

[58]   Meijer HA, Kong YW, Lu WT, *et al.* Translational repression and eIF4A2 activity are critical for microRNA-mediated gene regulation. Science 2013; 340(6128): 82-5.
[http://dx.doi.org/10.1126/science.1231197] [PMID: 23559250]

[59]   Chen ZH, Qi JJ, Wu QN, *et al.* Eukaryotic initiation factor 4A2 promotes experimental metastasis and oxaliplatin resistance in colorectal cancer. J Exp Clin Cancer Res 2019; 38(1): 196.
[http://dx.doi.org/10.1186/s13046-019-1178-z] [PMID: 31088567]

[60]   Yoshida S, Kaneita Y, Aoki Y, Seto M, Mori S, Moriyama M. Identification of heterologous translocation partner genes fused to the BCL6 gene in diffuse large B-cell lymphomas: 5'-RACE and LA – PCR analyses of biopsy samples. Oncogene 1999; 18(56): 7994-9.
[http://dx.doi.org/10.1038/sj.onc.1203293] [PMID: 10637510]

[61]   Shaoyan X, Juanjuan Y, Yalan T, Ping H, Jianzhong L, Qinian W. Downregulation of EIF4A2 in non-small-cell lung cancer associates with poor prognosis. Clin Lung Cancer 2013; 14(6): 658-65.
[http://dx.doi.org/10.1016/j.cllc.2013.04.011] [PMID: 23867391]

[62]   Ngan E, Kiepas A, Brown CM, Siegel PM. Emerging roles for LPP in metastatic cancer progression. J Cell Commun Signal 2018; 12(1): 143-56.
[http://dx.doi.org/10.1007/s12079-017-0415-5] [PMID: 29027626]

[63]   LPP is a Src substrate required for invadopodia formation and efficient breast cancer lung metastasis | Nature Communications, https://www.nature.com/articles/ncomms15059 (accessed 26 December 2020).

[64]   Amato E, Barbi S, Fassan M, *et al.* RASSF1 tumor suppressor gene in pancreatic ductal adenocarcinoma: correlation of expression, chromosomal status and epigenetic changes. BMC Cancer 2016; 16(1): 11.
[http://dx.doi.org/10.1186/s12885-016-2048-0] [PMID: 26754001]

[65]   Reeves ME, Firek M, Chen ST, Amaar Y. The RASSF1 Gene and the Opposing Effects of the RASSF1A and RASSF1C Isoforms on Cell Proliferation and Apoptosis. Mol Biol Int 2013; 2013: 1-9.
[http://dx.doi.org/10.1155/2013/145096] [PMID: 24327924]

[66]   Dowty JG, Win AK, Buchanan DD, *et al.* Cancer risks for MLH1 and MSH2 mutation carriers. Hum Mutat 2013; 34(3): 490-7.
[http://dx.doi.org/10.1002/humu.22262] [PMID: 23255516]

[67]   Momma T, Gonda K, Akama Y, *et al.* MLH1 germline mutation associated with Lynch syndrome in a family followed for more than 45 years. BMC Med Genet 2019; 20(1): 67.
[http://dx.doi.org/10.1186/s12881-019-0792-0] [PMID: 31046708]

[68]   A novel MLH1 mutation in a Japanese family with Lynch syndrome associated with small bowel cancer | Human Genome Variation, https://www.nature.com/articles/s41439-018-0013-y (accessed 27 December 2020).

[69]   Kim E, Zschiedrich S. Renal Cell Carcinoma in von Hippel–Lindau Disease—From Tumor Genetics to Novel Therapeutic Strategies. Front Pediatr 2018; 6: 16.
[http://dx.doi.org/10.3389/fped.2018.00016] [PMID: 29479523]

[70]   Cowey CL, Rathmell WK. VHL gene mutations in renal cell carcinoma: Role as a biomarker of disease outcome and drug efficacy. Curr Oncol Rep 2009; 11(2): 94-101.
[http://dx.doi.org/10.1007/s11912-009-0015-5] [PMID: 19216840]

[71]   Kim WY, Kaelin WG. Role of *VHL* gene mutation in human cancer. J Clin Oncol 2004; 22(24): 4991-5004.
[http://dx.doi.org/10.1200/JCO.2004.05.061] [PMID: 15611513]

[72]   Khan SG, Muniz-Medina V, Shahlavi T, *et al.* The human XPC DNA repair gene: arrangement, splice site information content and influence of a single nucleotide polymorphism in a splice acceptor site on alternative splicing and function. Nucleic Acids Res 2002; 30(16): 3624-31.
[http://dx.doi.org/10.1093/nar/gkf469] [PMID: 12177305]

[73]   Kahnamouei S, Narouie B, Sotoudeh M, *et al.* Association of XPC Gene Polymorphisms with Prostate Cancer Risk. Clin Lab 2016; 62(06/2016): 1009-15.
[http://dx.doi.org/10.7754/Clin.Lab.2015.150914] [PMID: 27468562]

[74]   Hu LB, Chen Y, Meng XD, Yu P, He X, Li J. Nucleotide Excision Repair Factor XPC Ameliorates Prognosis by Increasing the Susceptibility of Human Colorectal Cancer to Chemotherapy and Ionizing Radiation. Front Oncol 2018; 8: 290.
[http://dx.doi.org/10.3389/fonc.2018.00290] [PMID: 30109214]

[75]   Komatsu H, Masuda T, Iguchi T, *et al.* Clinical Significance of *FANCD2* Gene Expression and its Association with Tumor Progression in Hepatocellular Carcinoma. Anticancer Res 2017; 37(3): 1083-90.
[http://dx.doi.org/10.21873/anticanres.11420] [PMID: 28314268]

[76]   Feng L, Jin F. Expression and prognostic significance of Fanconi anemia group D2 protein and breast cancer type 1 susceptibility protein in familial and sporadic breast cancer. Oncol Lett 2019; 17(4): 3687-700.
[http://dx.doi.org/10.3892/ol.2019.10046] [PMID: 30881493]

[77]   Barroso E, Milne RL, Fernández LP, *et al.* FANCD2 associated with sporadic breast cancer risk. Carcinogenesis 2006; 27(9): 1930-7.
[http://dx.doi.org/10.1093/carcin/bgl062] [PMID: 16679306]

[78]   Ben-Batalla I, Seoane S, Macia M, *et al.* The Pit-1/Pou1f1 transcription factor regulates and correlates with prolactin expression in human breast cell lines and tumors. Endocr Relat Cancer 2010; 17(1): 73-85.
[http://dx.doi.org/10.1677/ERC-09-0100] [PMID: 19808898]

[79]   Turton JPG, Reynaud R, Mehta A, *et al.* Novel mutations within the POU1F1 gene associated with variable combined pituitary hormone deficiency. J Clin Endocrinol Metab 2005; 90(8): 4762-70.
[http://dx.doi.org/10.1210/jc.2005-0570] [PMID: 15928241]

[80]   Zhuang G, Song W, Amato K, *et al.* Effects of cancer-associated EPHA3 mutations on lung cancer. J Natl Cancer Inst 2012; 104(15): 1183-98.
[http://dx.doi.org/10.1093/jnci/djs297] [PMID: 22829656]

[81]   Andretta E, Cartón-García F, Martínez-Barriocanal Á, *et al.* Investigation of the role of tyrosine kinase receptor EPHA3 in colorectal cancer. Sci Rep 2017; 7(1): 41576.
[http://dx.doi.org/10.1038/srep41576] [PMID: 28169277]

[82]   Parray A, Siddique HR, Kuriger JK, *et al.* ROBO1, a tumor suppressor and critical molecular barrier for localized tumor cells to acquire invasive phenotype: Study in African-American and Caucasian prostate cancer models. Int J Cancer 2014; 135(11): 2493-506.
[http://dx.doi.org/10.1002/ijc.28919] [PMID: 24752651]

[83]   Zhao SJ, Shen YF, Li Q, *et al.* SLIT2/ROBO1 axis contributes to the Warburg effect in osteosarcoma through activation of SRC/ERK/c-MYC/PFKFB2 pathway. Cell Death Dis 2018; 9(3): 390.
[http://dx.doi.org/10.1038/s41419-018-0419-y] [PMID: 29523788]

[84]   Ljuslinder I, Golovleva I, Palmqvist R, *et al.* LRIG1 expression in colorectal cancer. Acta Oncol 2007; 46(8): 1118-22.
[http://dx.doi.org/10.1080/02841860701426823] [PMID: 17851870]

[85]   Li Q, Liu B, Chao HP, *et al.* LRIG1 is a pleiotropic androgen receptor-regulated feedback tumor suppressor in prostate cancer. Nat Commun 2019; 10(1): 5494.
[http://dx.doi.org/10.1038/s41467-019-13532-4] [PMID: 31792211]

[86]   Chen L, Tang J, Feng Y, *et al.* ADAMTS9 is Silenced by Epigenetic Disruption in Colorectal Cancer and Inhibits Cell Growth and Metastasis by Regulating Akt/p53 Signaling. Cell Physiol Biochem 2017; 44(4): 1370-80.
[http://dx.doi.org/10.1159/000485534] [PMID: 29186710]

[87]   Du W, Wang S, Zhou Q, *et al.* ADAMTS9 is a functional tumor suppressor through inhibiting AKT/mTOR pathway and associated with poor survival in gastric cancer. Oncogene 2013; 32(28): 3319-28.
[http://dx.doi.org/10.1038/onc.2012.359] [PMID: 22907434]

[88]   Zhou Y, Kipps TJ, Zhang S. Wnt5a Signaling in Normal and Cancer Stem Cells. Stem Cells Int 2017; 2017: e5295286.

[89]   Rodero MP, Auvynet C, Poupel L, Combadière B, Combadière C. Control of both myeloid cell infiltration and angiogenesis by CCR1 promotes liver cancer metastasis development in mice. Neoplasia 2013; 15(6): 641-IN13.
[http://dx.doi.org/10.1593/neo.121866] [PMID: 23730212]

[90]   Akram IG, Georges R, Hielscher T, Adwan H, Berger MR. The chemokines CCR1 and CCRL2 have a role in colorectal cancer liver metastasis. Tumour Biol 2016; 37(2): 2461-71.
[http://dx.doi.org/10.1007/s13277-015-4089-4] [PMID: 26383527]

CHAPTER 4

Chromosome 4

Anindita Menon[1], Ravi Gor[1], Saurav Panicker[1] and Satish Ramalingam[1,*]

[1] *Department of Genetic Engineering, School of Bioengineering, SRM Institute of Science and Technology, Kattankulathur, India*

Abstract: Chromosome 4 represents around 6 percent of the total DNA in the cell with 191 million DNA base pairs. Genetic changes in chromosome 4, such as somatic mutation, and chromosomal rearrangement like translocation, gene deletion, *etc.*, have been reported to develop several types of cancer. This includes leukemias, multiple myeloma, oesophageal squamous cell carcinoma, prostate cancer, breast cancer, bladder cancer, *etc.* In this chapter, we have listed genes residing in chromosome 4, which further frequently support cancer development, progression, and metastasis.

Keywords: Bladder cancer, Breast cancer, Cancer, Gene deletion, Leukemia, Metastasis, Multiple myeloma, Oesophageal squamous cell carcinoma, Prostate cancer, Somatic mutation, Translocation.

1.1. AAA2 - AORTIC ANEURYSM, FAMILIAL ABDOMINAL 2 CHROMOSOME 4; 4q31

AAA2 is associated with an abdominal aortic aneurysm. ATPase family AAA domain-containing protein 2 (ATAD2) is related to many cellular processes, such as cell proliferation, invasion, and migration. Knocking of this gene in HeLa and SiHa cells showed a reduction in the capacity for invasion and migration and inhibited growth and clonogenic potential in these cell lines [1]. This gene is also a therapeutic target in various tumors, and profiling reveals dysregulation of ATAD2 specifically in Oesophageal Squamous Cell Carcinoma (ESCC). In-vivo experiments showed the suppressive effect of siRNA-mediated ATAD2 silencing on tumor growth in nude mice. Thus, downregulating the gene restrains the malignant phenotype of ESCC through inhibition of the Hedgehog signaling pathway [2].

* **Corresponding author Satish Ramalingam**: Department of Genetic Engineering, School of Bioengineering, SRM Institute of Science and Technology, Kattankulathur, India; E-mail: rsatish76@gmail.com

1.2. ABCG2- ATP BINDING CASSETTE SUBFAMILY G MEMBER DOMAIN 29 CHROMOSOME 4; 4q34.1

They are a member of the ADAM family and are membrane-anchored proteins that structurally are similar to snake venom disintegrins with implicated biological processes involving cell-cell and cell-matrix interaction, including fertilization, muscle development, and neurogenesis. This protein encodes a gene highly expressed in the testis and is involved in spermatogenesis—alternate splicing results in multiple transcript variants. ADAM29 has been a susceptible locus with risk factors in breast cancer under genome-wide significance. Transcript expression was found more in breast cancer tissue than in normal tissue. They may be a prognostic marker for human breast cancer and a novel therapeutic target [3].

1.3. AFF1- AF4/FMR2 FAMILY MEMBER 1 CHROMOSOME 4; 4Q21.3-q 22.1

This gene (Fig. 1) encodes a member of the AF4/ lymphoid nuclear protein related to the Fragile X syndrome family of proteins, which have been implicated in human childhood lymphoblastic leukemia, fragile X chromosome, intellectual disability, and ataxia. Members of this family have three conserved domains N- the terminal homology domain, the AF4/ lymphoid nuclear protein domain, and a C- terminal homology domain. The protein regulates RNA polymerase II- mediated transcription through elongation and chromatin remodeling functions. The translocation of genes results in fusion genes. These fusion genes may be due to genetic and environmental factors [4].

1.4. AFP-ALPHA-FETOPROTEIN CHROMOSOME 4; 4q13.3

AFP is a type of plasma protein produced in the yolk sac and the liver during fetal life. AFP expression in adults is associated with hepatocarcinoma and teratoma and has prognostic value for managing advanced gastric cancer. However, hereditary persistence of alpha-fetoprotein is also found, but these individuals show no obvious pathology. The protein is thought to be the fetal counterpart of serum albumin. The AFP and albumin genes are both present in tandem in the same transcriptional orientation on chromosome 4. AFP is found in monomeric, dimeric, and trimeric forms. They also bind to copper, nickel, fatty acids, and bilirubin. The level of AFP in amniotic fluid can be used to measure renal loss of protein to screen spina bifida and anencephaly, which are disorders that are caused due to improper development of neural tubes. DNA methylation of its promoter is the driving mechanism of such overexpression(>400ng/ml). These tumors show a distinct phenotype characteristic, such as poor differentiation, enrichment of progenitor features and enhanced proliferation [5]. AFP concentration in blood serum is the most specific tumor marker for screening and diagnostic methods [6].

Chromosome 4

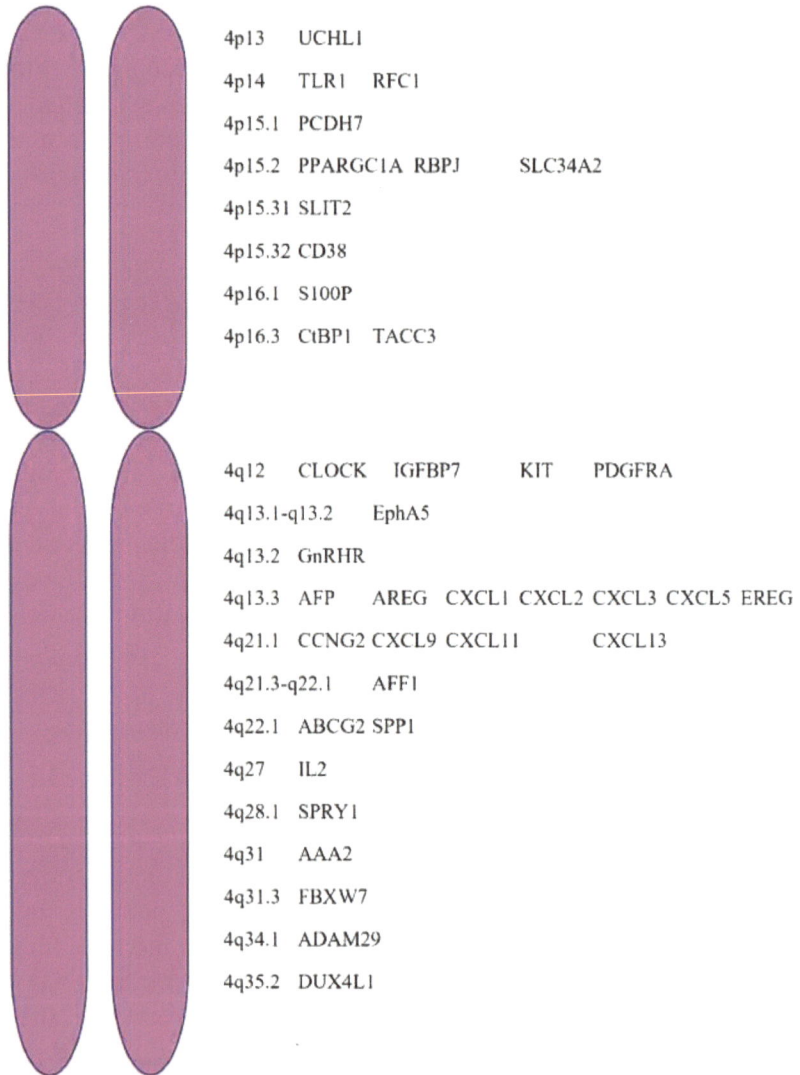

4p13	UCHL1			
4p14	TLR1	RFC1		
4p15.1	PCDH7			
4p15.2	PPARGC1A	RBPJ	SLC34A2	
4p15.31	SLIT2			
4p15.32	CD38			
4p16.1	S100P			
4p16.3	CtBP1	TACC3		

4q12	CLOCK	IGFBP7	KIT	PDGFRA
4q13.1-q13.2	EphA5			
4q13.2	GnRHR			
4q13.3	AFP	AREG CXCL1 CXCL2 CXCL3 CXCL5 EREG		
4q21.1	CCNG2 CXCL9 CXCL11	CXCL13		
4q21.3-q22.1	AFF1			
4q22.1	ABCG2 SPP1			
4q27	IL2			
4q28.1	SPRY1			
4q31	AAA2			
4q31.3	FBXW7			
4q34.1	ADAM29			
4q35.2	DUX4L1			

Fig. (1). This figure displays the loci of the genes from Chromosome 4 whose roles in cancer have been explained in this chapter. Sayooj Madhusoodanan designs this diagram.

1.5. AREG- AMPHIREGULIN CHROMOSOME 4; 4q13.3

The protein encoded by this gene (Fig. **1**) is a member of the epidermal growth factor family. It is an autocrine growth factor as a mitogen for astrocytes, Schwann cells, and fibroblasts. It is related to the epidermal growth factor and transforming growth factor-alpha. The protein interacts with the receptor present, promotes average epithelial cell growth, and inhibits aggressive carcinoma. They function in mammary cells, oocyte formation, and bone tissue development. They are seen to be overexpressed in many cancers, including gastric cancer. However, its role is unknown. They possessed an oncogenic property that could serve as a target for gastric cancer therapy [7].

1.6. CCNG2- CYCLIN G2 CHROMOSOME 4; 4q21.1

It is a cyclin-dependent protein kinase whose activities are regulated by cyclins and inhibitors. 8 species of cyclins are reported in mammals with a conserved amino acid sequence of about 90 residues, also known as a cyclin box. The amino acid of cyclin G is conserved among mammals. Cyclin G1 and G2 contain a destabilization suggesting that they are highly regulated. microRNA-1246 (miRNA-1246), which is a serum biomarker for breast cancer cell line MDA-MB-231 cells [8], Pancreatic cell line Panc1 [9], and Colorectal cancer line HCT-116 and LOVO [10]. They suppress the target gene cyclin- G2 expression level that indicates functional significance. Treatment with this exosome can enhance the viability, migration, and chemotherapy resistance to non-malignant HMLE cells [8].

1.7. CD38 CHROMOSOME 4: 4p15.32

The protein encoded by this gene (Fig. **1**) is a non-lineage-restricted type II transmembrane glycoprotein. It synthesizes as well as hydrolyzes cyclic adenosine 5'diphosphate ribose, which is a calcium ion mobilizing messenger. They have both intercellular and extracellular functions for the protein. The enzymatic process of CD38 results from its immunosuppressive environment, which increases the immune resistance in tumor cells, growth rate, and rates of proliferation [11].

1.8. CLOCK- CLOCK CIRCADIAN REGULATOR CHROMOSOME 4; 4q12

This is a protein encoded by the gene (Fig. **1**) in the regulation of circadian rhythm. The transcription factor of the basic helix-loop-helix contains histone acetyltransferase activity. The central loop consists of Bmal1: CLOCK heterodimer driving expression of repressor. The effect of dexamethasone on cell cycle and tumor growth is mediated by this CLOCK gene and can be used to control cancer progression [12]. They are associated with the development of tumors. Levels of Bmal1, a type of circadian clock gene, were downregulated in Pancreatic Cancer and are closely correlated with the clinicopathology features of patients [13].

1.9. CXLC1- C-X-C MOTIF CHEMOKINE LIGAND 1 CHROMOSOME 4; 4q13.3

They encode for the CXC subfamily of chemokines. The encoded protein is a growth factor signaling G-protein coupled receptor. They play a significant role in inflammation and are chemo-attractants in the case of neutrophils. Expression of this protein leads to the growth and progression of certain kinds of tumors. Alternate splicing results in coding and non-coding variants. They are chemotactic cytokines that regulate breast cancer progression and related chemoresistance. The prognostic of CXL1 expression has yet to be fully characterized. Fibroblasts are important cellular components of the tumor microenvironment and indicate cell-type sources in breast tumors [14].

1.10. CXCL 2- C-X-C MOTIF CHEMOKINE LIGAND 2 CHROMOSOME 4; 4q13.3

It also belongs to the chemokine superfamily involved in immunoregulatory and inflammatory processes. They are divided based on arrangements of N-terminal cysteine residue of the mature peptide. They express at sites of inflammation and suppress hematopoietic progenitor cell proliferation. Colon cancer cells showed increased expression in CXL2. CPT-11-R LoVo cells displayed significantly increased intercellular protein levels in CXL2 and CXCR2 [15].

1.11. CXCL3- C-X-C MOTIF CHEMOKINE LIGAND 3 CHROMOSOME 4; 4q13.3

The encoded protein is a secreted growth factor that signals *via* G-protein receptor CXC receptor 2. They play a role in inflammation and are chemoattractants for neutrophils. An elevated level of CXCR2 was detected in DU145, LNCaP, and RWPE-1, and CXCL3 was detected in PC-3 and RWPE-1. Protein expression in tissue microarray was consistent in the case of prostate cancer metastasis. CXCL3 and CXCR2 were overexpressed in prostate cancer cells which may have many roles in progression and metastasis [16]. They are thought to have an important role in tumor initiation and invasion, but little information is known in the case of hepatocellular carcinoma. Knockdown of *CXCL3* inhibited CD133$^+$ self-renewal and tumorigenesis. The serum CXCL3 level was higher in HCC patients' samples than in healthy individuals [17].

1.12. CXCL5- C-X-C MOTIF CHEMOKINE LIGAND 5 CHROMOSOME 4; 4q13.3

The gene (Fig. 1) encodes a protein member of the chemokine family. Chemokines recruits and activate leukocytes that are classified by function or structure. They bind to G-protein coupled receptor chemokine receptor 2 to recruit neutrophils that increase angiogenesis and remodel connective tissue. They could serve as a potential biomarker but is still controversial as a prognostic biomarker [18]. They are profiling the soluble factors from conditioned media that are identified as a candidate to induce metastatic colonization in the bone while inhibiting its receptor CXCR2 with an antagonist that blocks the proliferation of metastatic cancer cells. Recombinant protein CXCL5 is sufficient to promote breast cancer cell proliferation and colonization in bone [19].

1.13. CXCL9- C-X-C MOTIF CHEMOKINE LIGAND 9 CHROMOSOME 4; 4q21.1

They encode a protein that is known to be involved in T-cell trafficking. The encoded protein binds to the CXC motif chemokine 3 and is a chemoattractant for lymphocytes but not neutrophils. Transcriptional regulation of CXCL9 is a multi-step process that involves many TFs, of which signal transducer and activator of transcription (STAT1) and nuclear factor κB (NF- κB) are the two most well-characterized members. Gene mutation of STAT1 and blocking of the JAK/STAT pathway can reduce CXCL9 expression. They have a role in CXCL9 in different types of tumors but have a contradictory role in tumor progression [20]. CCL5 and CXCL9 are correlated even with T-cell infiltration across several cancer types [21]. The function of CXCL9 promotes prostate cancer progression by inhibiting T-cell cytokine [22].

1.14. CXCL11- C-X-C MOTIF CHEMOKINE LIGAND 11 CHROMO-SOME 4: 4q21.1

Chemokines are primarily basic and structurally similar to molecules known to traffic various types of leukocytes through interaction with a subset of transmembrane G-protein-coupled receptors. They are important in development, homeostasis, and are even shown to function in our immune system. CXCL11 was highly expressed in different solid tumors and also controls tumor growth. CXCL11- induced cell migration was sensitive to CXCR3 antagonist, CXCR7 antagonist, CCX771, or both. CXCL11 system showed cell type-specific organization, which is not due to the difference in expression levels or subcellular location of its receptors [23]. DOC (docetaxel), a chemotherapeutic agent, modifies the expression of HMGb1 and CXCL11, leading to the infiltration of $CD8^+$ in the tumor microenvironment. The release was checked by flow cytometry, immunofluorescence, and western blot. DOC enhances the HGMB1 and CXCL11 that, shown to improve anti-tumor efficacy, which may be helpful in NSCLC patients [24].

1.15.   CXCL13- C-X-C MOTIF CHEMOKINE LIGAND 13 CHROMO-SOME 4; 4q21.1

It is a B lymphocyte chemoattractant that preferentially promotes the migration of B lymphocytes stimulated by calcium influx and chemotaxis in BLR-1 cells. They were later independently cloned and named Angie, an antimicrobial peptide and CXC chemokine that was strongly expressed in the spleen, lymph nodes, and Peyer's patch follicles. CXCL13 and CXCR5 are key chemotactic factors that play a significant role in deriving cancer cell biology. This signaling axis greatly contributes to the development and progression of several human cancers [25]. It is well established that CXCL13 and its receptor G-protein-coupled receptor (GPCR) play a fundamental role in inflammatory, infectious and immune responses. CXCL13 exerts importance in lymphoid neogenesis, which was implicated in the pathogenesis of several autoimmune diseases and inflammatory conditions. CXCL13:CXCR5 axis orchestrates cell-cell interactions regulating infiltration of lymphocytes within the tumor microenvironment, thereby determining responsiveness to cytotoxic and immune-targeted therapies [26].

1.16. CTBP1- C-TERMINAL BINDING PROTEIN 1 CHROMOSOME 4; 4p16.3

This is a code for a protein binding C-terminus of adenovirus E1A proteins. Phosphoprotein is a repressor of transcription and drives cellular proliferation. The protein and product of the second closely related gene, CtBP2, dimerize. These corepressor proteins are often altered due to loss or gain of function, leading to the imbalance of transcription. They could impact the future development of new cancer diagnoses, prognoses, and therapies [27]. Integrated correlation of gene expression in breast cancer patients with a nuclear level of CtBP and LSD1 reveals new therapeutic vulnerability [28] CtBP2 is elevated in ovarian cancers and can be used as a therapeutic strategy for High-grade Serous Ovarian Cancer (HGSOC) [29].

1.17. DUX4L1- DOUBLE HOMEOBOX 4 LIKE 1 CHROMOSOME 4; 4q35.2

This gene is located in the D4Z4 repeat array in the sub-telomeric region of chromosome 4q. D4Z4 repeat is polymorphic in length, and a similar repeat is also found in chromosome 10. D4Z4 repeat has an open reading frame that encodes the homeobox. Contraction of microsatellite repeat causes autosomal facioscapulohumeral muscular dystrophy. 15 genes were reported in squamous cell carcinoma in non or never smokers, and DUX4L1 was enlisted [30].

1.18. EPHA5- ERYTHROPOIETIN PRODUCING HEPATOCELLULAR RECEPTOR A5 CHROMOSOME 4; 4Q13.1- q13.2

This belongs to the ephrin receptor subfamily of the protein tyrosine kinase family. They mediate developmental events, particularly in the nervous system [31]. This family's receptor has a single kinase domain and extracellular region with Cys-rich domain and 2 fibronectin type III repeats. Based on their extracellular domain and affinities to bind, ephrin-A and ephrin-B are classified into 2 groups. The association between EphA5 expression, clinicopathological parameters, HER2 status, and Ki-67 proliferation was analyzed. Expression was detected in all mon tumor gastric epithelia but was found to be expressed differentially in gastric cancer samples. EphA5 may be a potential therapeutic target with clinical utility as a marker in lymph node metastasis in gastric cancer [32]. Role in oesophageal squamous cell carcinoma, was seen to enhance invasion and migration *via* epithelial-mesenchymal transition by activating the Wnt/ β-catenin pathway [33].

1.19. EREG- EPIREGULIN CHROMOSOME 4; 4q13.3

They encode a secreted peptide hormone and are members of the Epidermal Growth Family of proteins. They encode ligands of the EGFR and structurally erb-b2 receptor tyrosine kinase 4 (ERBB4) [34]. They are involved in inflammation, wound healing, maturation of oocytes, and proliferation. EREG is several putative transcriptional targets in KRAS-mutant NSCLC cells and bronchial epithelial cells expressing ectopic mutants. EREG is remarkably upregulated in Cancer Associated Fibroblast with higher T stage, deeper invasion, and worst pattern of Invasion in Oral Squamous Cell Carcinoma and predicted shorter overall survival [35].

1.20. FBXW7- F-BOX WD REPEAT DOMAIN CONTAINING 7 CHROMOSOME 4; 4q31.3

They encode for the F-box family of proteins characterized by 40 amino acid motifs. F-box constitutes 1 of the 4 subunits of a ubiquitin-protein complex called SCFs and functions in phosphorylation-dependent ubiquitination. They contain leucine-rich repeats, and Fbxs contain protein-protein interaction modules or non-recognizable motifs. They are found to be frequently mutated in many cancers, although studies show the tumor suppressive capacity of FBXW7 in tumor cells and the host microenvironment suppress cancer metastasis. In human breast cancer patients, there was an association between FBXW7 and serum CCL2 expression in peripheral blood [36].

1.21. GNRHR- GONADOTROPIN-RELEASING HORMONE RECEPTOR CHROMOSOME 4; 4q13.2

They encode for a receptor type 1 gonadotropin-releasing hormone which belongs to the 7 transmembrane G-protein coupled receptor family. They are expressed on pituitary gonadotropin cells as well as lymphocytes—breast, ovary, and prostate. Activation of receptors results in the release of luteinizing hormone (LH) and follicular stimulating hormone (FSH), and defects can lead to Hypogonadotropic Hypogonadism. GnRHR expression is deficient in gastric cancer and is a poor prognostic factor but an essential factor in the development of Gastric Cancer [37]. Cetrorelix acetate (CTX) treatment can improve therapy in human adreno-cortical carcinoma by direct action in GnRHR-positive cancer cells inducing apoptosis or reducing gonadotropin release directing towards a healthy adrenal gene expression profile [38].

1.22. IGFBP7- INSULIN-LIKE GROWTH FACTOR BINDING PROTEIN 7 CHROMOSOME 4; 4q12

They encode a member of the IGF family and regulate the availability of both body fluids and tissues. They bind to IGF I and II with relatively low affinity. They stimulate prostacyclin production and cell adhesion. They have been known to create many cancer types, and their biological function in various types of thyroid carcinoma that remain poorly understood. Expression is decreased in FTC and ATC. It may represent a promising biomarker and therapeutic target [39]. Putative TGFβ-target IGFBP7 was identified as a tumor stroma marker of epithelial cancers and as a tumor antigen in mesenchyme-derived sarcomas.

In epithelial cells, IGFPB7 can promote anchorage-independent growth in malignant mesenchymal cells and epithelial cells with an EMT phenotype when IGFBP7 is expressed by tumor cells and can induce colony formation in colon cancer cells co-cultured with IGFBP7-expressing CAFs by a paracrine tumor stroma interaction [40].

1.23. IL2- INTERLEUKIN 2 CHROMOSOME 4; 4q27

The protein encoded by the gene is secreted cytokinin, which is essential in the proliferation of both T and B lymphocytes. The receptor is a heterotrimeric complex whose gamma chain relates to IL4 and IL7. Gene in mature thymocytes is monoallelic, representing an unusual regulatory mode for the control over expression in a single gene. IL2 regulates lymphocytes which led to a new direction in cancer immunotherapy. Monotherapy has been demonstrated that maintain cancer regression and was approved for renal carcinoma treatment but was found to be inefficient in improving patient's survival rates [41].

1.24. KIT- KIT PROTO-ONCOGENE RECEPTOR TYROSINE KINASE CHROMOSOME 4; 4q12

The gene encoded the homolog of proto-oncogene c-kit and was the first identified as a cellular homolog of the sarcoma viral oncogene. They have been identified as stem cell factor transmembrane receptors. The mutation leads to the gastrointestinal stromal tumor, leukemia. They control important cellular mechanisms such as proliferation, migration, and survival. Receptor tyrosine kinase transmits the signal *via* signal transduction. KIT protein is found in the cell membrane of cell types where the stem cell attaches and then activates the protein inside the cell by adding a cluster of oxygen and phosphorous atoms. Regulation of development and function of cell types like germ cells, hematopoietic stem cells, and mast cells. Mutant forms of KIT were found to be sensitive to imatinib which illustrated mutation analysis in patients. Mutation analysis of critical exons is relatively inexpensive and economically justified [42].

1.25. MUC7- MUCIN 7 CHROMOSOME 4; 4q13.3

They encode small salivary mucin that is in a secreted form. They facilitate the clearance of bacteria in the oral cavity and aid in mastication, speech, and swallowing. They are composed of 23 Amino Acid and have antimicrobial and antibacterial activity. The most common allele contains repeats and is associated with susceptibility to asthma. It has emerged in the placenta of mammals with multiple sites for glycosylation. PTS repeats have recurrently evolved under adaptive constraints under positive selection in primate lineage [43].

1.26. PCDH7- PROTOCADHERIN 7 CHROMOSOME 4; 4p15.1

PCDH7 belongs to a subfamily of the cadherin superfamily. Gene encodes an extracellular domain that contains 7 cadherin repeats. This gene is an integral membrane protein that is thought to function in cell recognition and adhesion. They act as a tumor suppressor in several human cancers and remain inactive in most cancers, including bladder cancers. PCDH7 expression in Non-Muscle Invasive Bladder Cancer and normal bladder epithelial tissues were studied. Expression of PCDH7 was significantly low in normal epithelial cells of bladder tissues which showed that it could be a potential biomarker for testing primary NMIBC [44]. The Androgen receptor greatly enriched the upstream of the PCDH7 gene. Expression of PCDH7 was decreased while methylation of PCDH7 was increased in Androgen Independent Prostate Cancer (AIPC) when compared to Androgen Dependent Prostate Cancer (ADPC) cells. DNA methyltransferase inhibitor suppressed methylation and increased the mRNA and protein levels of PCDH7 [45].

1.27. PDGFRA- PLATELET-DERIVED GROWTH FACTOR RECEPTOR ALPHA CHROMOSOME 4;4q12

Gene encodes cell surface tyrosine kinase receptors for the members of the PDGF family. They are mitogens for cells of mesenchymal origin. They play roles in organ development, wound healing, and the progression of tumors. Mutations of this gene showed a role in idiopathic hypereosinophilic syndrome, gastrointestinal tumors, and a wide range of cancer. C-kit immunohistochemical and c-kit PDGFRA were studied in triple-negative breast cancers. PDGFRA gene mutations were seen in exons 12 and 18. C-kit expressions were frequently found in triple-negative breast cancers [46].

1.28. PPARGC1A- PEROXISOME PROLIFERATOR-ACTIVATED RECEPTOR GAMMA COACTIVATOR 1 ALPHA CHROMOSOME 4; 4p15.2

It is a transcriptional coactivator that regulates genes in energy metabolism. This protein interacts with PPAR gamma, permitting the protein's interaction with multiple transcription factors. This protein interacts with and controls the activities of cAMP response element binding protein (CREB) and nuclear respiratory factors (NRF). The direct link between external physiological stimuli and regulating Mitochondrial biogenesis, which is a significant factor in regulating muscle fiber type determination.

They may be involved in controlling BP and regulating cellular cholesterol homeostasis. PPARGC1A was the topmost overexpressed in all three non-small cell lung cancer patients. Upregulation was seen in metastatic lung cancer cell lines to the brain [47].

1.29. RASSF6- RAS ASSOCIATION DOMAIN FAMILY MEMBER 6 CHROMOSOME 4; 4q13.3

Gene encodes a member of RASSF members of the family from the core of the highly conserved tumor suppressor network. The protein encoded by the gene induces apoptosis. The genomic region is also linked to susceptible viral bronchiolitis. RASSF are tumor suppressors that are downregulated during the development of cancer. Best characterized by RASSF1A, which is downregulated by methylation of the promoter in most of the tumor. RASSF6 was downregulated and associated with a poor prognosis of gastric cancer, which was shown by LOH and cDNA microarrays [48].

1.30. RBPJ- RECOMBINANT SIGNAL BINDING PROTEIN FOR IMMUNOGLOBIN KAPPA J REGION CHROMOSOME 4; 4p15.2

This is a transcription regulator in the Notch signaling pathway. The protein acts as a repressor that doesn't bind to Notch protein and an activator when bound to Notch protein. Function in recruiting chromatin remodeling as they contain histone deacetylase or histone acetylases to Notch signaling genes. Recombination of RBPJ and MAML are new therapeutic targets for pancreatic cancer and small cell lung cancer (SCLC). Signaling was by Hedgehog and Notch pathways. Inhibition of RBPJ MAML3 reduced proliferation and invasiveness *via* the reduction of matrix metalloproteinase [47].

1.31. RFC1- REPLICATION FACTOR C SUBUNIT 1 CHROMOSOME 4; 4p14

This is a five-subunit DNA polymerase accessory protein, which is a DNA-dependent ATPase that is required for DNA replication and repair. They act as a primer recognition factor as larger subunits act as an activator of DNA polymerase, bind to the 3' end of primers, and promote synthesis in both strands. They also have a major role in telomere stability. They are biologically active in many malignant forms of cancers and show a major role in proliferation, progression, invasion, and metastasis. Based on the cellular and histological characteristics of tumors, they can act as an oncogene or tumor suppressor gene [49].

1.32. S100P- S100 CALCIUMBINDING PROTEIN P CHROMOSOME 4; 4p16.1

They belong to the family of S100 that contains 2 EF-hand calcium-binding motifs. These proteins are localized in the cytoplasm and nucleus in many cells.

They regulate many cellular processes, such as the progression and differentiation of the cell cycle. The rest of the S100 genes are present in chromosome 1. They play a significant role in the etiology of prostate cancers. S100P is a marker for differentiating cancer cells from normal cells. They are originally isolated from the placenta and were found to express in the rhythmic hormonal fluctuations within the uterine wall. It may have a close association with embryonic implantation and developing embryos. Increasingly recognized as potential diagnostic and therapeutic targets [50]. S100P has a dual role in gastric cancer. It acts as an oncogenic factor in E-cadherin loss as well as acts as a tumor suppressor in an E-cadherin setting [51].

1.33. SLC34A2- SOLUTE CARRIER FAMILY 34 MEMBER 2 CHROMOSOME 4; 4p15.2

The SLC34A2 gene instructs protein type II sodium phosphate cotransporter that plays a role in phosphate homeostasis. These proteins are found in several organs and tissues and are mainly seen in the alveoli present in the lungs, specifically alveolar type II cells. They produce and recycle surfactants. The protein encoded by the gene is pH sensitive. The lower the pH more phosphate is produced, and defects in this gene can cause microlithiasis. It is associated with several human cancers. It was studied in human bladder cancer and was seen to be upregulated after a series of *in vitro* and *in vivo* studies. High expression of SLC34A2 was associated with large size, advanced status, poor growth *in vitro* and decreased suppressed cellular viability, colony formation, and anchorage-independent [52].

1.34. SLIT2- SLIT GUIDANCE LIGAND 2 CHROMOSOME 4; 4p15.31

They belong to the family of secreted glycoproteins, ligands for the Robo family of immunoglobin receptors, providing highly conserved roles in axon guidance, neuron migration, leukocyte migration, and other cell migrations. They are characterized by the N-terminal signal peptide with 4 leucine repeats, 9 EGFR's and C-terminal fragments containing 4 EGFRs and cystine knots. In vitro and *in vivo* demonstrates SLIT2/ROBO1 axis promotes proliferation, inhibits apoptosis, and contributes to Warburg effects in Osteosarcoma cells. SLIT2/ROBO1 axis has a therapeutic approach in OS patients [53].

1.35. SPP1 SECRETED PHOSPHOPROTEIN 1 CHROMOSOME: 4; 4q22.1

The protein encoded by this gene is involved in the attachment of osteoclasts to the bone matrix. The osteoclast vitronectin receptor is found on the cell membrane thus, it is involved in the binding of proteins. They are considered a prognostic marker of ovarian cancer [54] and Gastric cancer [55], which is oncogenic and a target for therapy. The protein is secreted that binds to hydroxyapatite with greater affinity. It is also a cytokine that upregulates the expression of IFN gamma and IL-12. Expression of SPP1 was higher in Epithelial Ovarian Cancer than in normal tissue-cellular proliferation, migration, and invasion. Silencing SPP1 inhibited the pathway β1/FAK/AKT. SPP1 was regulated by miR-181a [54].

1.36. SPRY1 SPROUTY RTK SIGNALLING ANTAGONIST 1 CHROMOSOME: 4; 4q28.1

Sprout proteins are encoded by the SPRY gene that acts as modulators and feedback inhibitors of EGF and FGF. These levels are downregulated in prostate cancer. They are proteins that are evolutionarily conserved modulators of Receptor Tyrosine Kinase signaling. They have an inverse effect on ovarian cancer cell proliferation, migration, invasion, and survival [56].

1.37. TACC3-TRANSFORMING ACIDIC COILED COIL PROTEIN 3 CHROMOSOME: 4;4p16.3

They encode a member of the transforming acidic coiled-coil protein, which is a motor spindle protein that stabilizes the mitotic spindle. This protein also plays a role in the growth and differentiation of certain cancer cells. The dysregulation of these genes is considered important in the development and progression of myeloma and breast and gastric cancer. SNIPER(TACC3) is a method used to degrade target proteins *via* the ubiquitin-proteasome pathway. They are small molecules that target spindle regulatory proteins transforming acidic coiled-coil 3 that induce polyubiquitylation and proteasomal degradation of TACC3, reducing their levels in cells [57].

1.38. TLR1- TOLL-LIKE RECEPTOR 1 CHROMOSOME 4; 4p14

They play a fundamental role in recognizing the pathogen and also activate innate immunity. TLR are highly conserved from Drosophila to Humans, sharing structural and functional similarities. Pathogen Associated Molecular Patterns are expressed in infectious agents and mediate the production of cytokines necessary for effective immunity. They have prognostic value in various adenocarcinoma (PDAC patients), but negative expressions show a poor prognosis [58].

1.39. TET2-TET METHYLCYTOSINE DIOXYGENASE 2 CHROMOSOME 4; 4q24

The protein encoded by this gene catalyzes the conversion of methylcytosine to 5-

hydroxymethylcytosine by the methylcytosine dioxygenase domain found. The protein is involved in myelopoiesis, and defects in this gene have been associated with several myeloproliferative disorders. Two variants of different isoforms have been found for this gene. TET2 is a tumor suppressor substrate of the AMP-activated kinase that phosphorylates TET2 at serine 99, stabilizing the tumor suppressor [59].

1.40. UCHL1- UBIQUITIN C- TERMINAL HYDROLASE L1 CHROMOSOME 4; 4p13

Gene belongs to the peptidase C12 family. The enzyme is a thiol protease that hydrolyses peptide bonds in glycine of ubiquitin. They express in the neurons and cells in the diffuse neuroendocrine system. In cells, damaged or increased proteins are tagged with ubiquitin that serves as signals to move the unneeded proteins into proteasomes that degrade these proteins. UCHL1- HIF1 axis suppresses the formation of metastatic tumors. The association of UCHL1 and HIF1 are also associated with poor prognosis in breast and lung cancers. They are a prognostic marker and a potential therapeutic target as they promote metastasis as a deubiquitinating enzyme for HIF-1 [60].

CONCLUSION

Chromosome 4 has shown various aberrations that have resulted in cancer development. One of the genes from chromosome 4 is PDGFRA which is associated with chronic eosinophilic leukemia. This occurs due to the fusion of the FIP1L1-PDGFRA, which makes the constitutive expression of the PDGFRA gene and allows cellular growth, division and survival. Overexpression of certain genes also supports cancer development, such as AAA2, whose overexpression supports oesophageal squamous cell carcinoma. This list will help the better reach for the ongoing and future research in the field of cancer.

REFERENCES

[1]   Li T, Zhang Y, Guo Y, *et al.* Oncogene ATAD2 promotes cell proliferation, invasion and migration in cervical cancer. Oncol Rep 2015; 33(5): 2337-44.

[2]   Li N, Yu Y, Wang B. Downregulation of AAA-domain-containing protein 2 restrains cancer stem cell properties in esophageal squamous cell carcinoma *via* blockade of the Hedgehog signaling pathway. Am J Physiol Cell Physiol 2020; 319(1): C93-C104.
[http://dx.doi.org/10.1152/ajpcell.00133.2019] [PMID: 31747529]

[3]   Zhao M, Jia W, Jiang WG, *et al.* Adam29 expression in human breast cancer and its effects on breast cancer cells *in vitro.* Anticancer Res 2016; 36(3): 1251-8.
[PMID: 26977022]

[4]   Tamai H, Yamaguchi H, Miyake K, *et al.* Amlexanox downregulates S100A6 to sensitize KMT2A/AFF1-positive acute lymphoblastic leukemia to TNFα treatment. Cancer Res 2017; 77(16): 4426-33.
[http://dx.doi.org/10.1158/0008-5472.CAN-16-2974] [PMID: 28646023]

[5]   Montal R, Andreu-Oller C, Bassaganyas L, *et al.* Molecular portrait of high alpha-fetoprotein in hepatocellular carcinoma: implications for biomarker-driven clinical trials. Br J Cancer 2019; 121(4): 340-3.
[http://dx.doi.org/10.1038/s41416-019-0513-7] [PMID: 31285588]

[6]   Tzartzeva K, Obi J, Rich NE, *et al.* Surveillance Imaging and Alpha Fetoprotein for Early Detection of Hepatocellular Carcinoma in Patients With Cirrhosis: A Meta-analysis. Gastroenterology 2018; 154(6): 1706-1718.e1.
[http://dx.doi.org/10.1053/j.gastro.2018.01.064] [PMID: 29425931]

[7]   Jiang J, Zhao W, Tang Q, Wang B, Li X, Feng Z. Over expression of amphiregulin promoted malignant progression in gastric cancer. Pathol Res Pract 2019; 215(10): 152576.
[http://dx.doi.org/10.1016/j.prp.2019.152576] [PMID: 31466817]

[8]   Li XJ, Ren ZJ, Tang JH, Yu Q. Exosomal MicroRNA MiR-1246 Promotes Cell Proliferation, Invasion and Drug Resistance by Targeting CCNG2 in Breast Cancer. Cell Physiol Biochem 2017; 44(5): 1741-8.
[http://dx.doi.org/10.1159/000485780] [PMID: 29216623]

[9]   Hasegawa S, Eguchi H, Nagano H, *et al.* MicroRNA-1246 expression associated with CCNG2-mediated chemoresistance and stemness in pancreatic cancer. Br J Cancer 2014; 111(8): 1572-80.
[http://dx.doi.org/10.1038/bjc.2014.454] [PMID: 25117811]

[10] Wang S, Zeng Y, Zhou JM, *et al.* MicroRNA-1246 promotes growth and metastasis of colorectal cancer cells involving CCNG2 reduction. Mol Med Rep 2016; 13(1): 273-80.
[http://dx.doi.org/10.3892/mmr.2015.4557] [PMID: 26573378]

[11] Dwivedi S, Rendón-Huerta EP, Ortiz-Navarrete V, *et al.* *et al.* CD38 and Regulation of the Immune Response Cells in Cancer. J Oncol; 2021.

[12] Kiessling S, Beaulieu-Laroche L, Blum ID, *et al.* Enhancing circadian clock function in cancer cells inhibits tumor growth. BMC Biol 2017; 15(1): 13.
[http://dx.doi.org/10.1186/s12915-017-0349-7] [PMID: 28196531]

[13] Jiang W, Zhao S, Jiang X, *et al.* The circadian clock gene Bmal1 acts as a potential anti-oncogene in pancreatic cancer by activating the p53 tumor suppressor pathway. Cancer Lett 2016; 371(2): 314-25.
[http://dx.doi.org/10.1016/j.canlet.2015.12.002] [PMID: 26683776]

[14] Zou A, Lambert D, Yeh H, *et al.* Elevated CXCL1 expression in breast cancer stroma predicts poor prognosis and is inversely associated with expression of TGF-β signaling proteins. BMC Cancer 2014; 14(1): 781.
[http://dx.doi.org/10.1186/1471-2407-14-781] [PMID: 25344051]

[15] Chen MC, Baskaran R, Lee NH, *et al.* CXCL2/CXCR2 axis induces cancer stem cell characteristics in CPT-11-resistant LoVo colon cancer cells *via* Gαi-2 and Gαq/11. J Cell Physiol 2019; 234(7): 11822-34.
[http://dx.doi.org/10.1002/jcp.27891] [PMID: 30552676]

[16] Gui S liang, Teng L chen, Wang S qiu, et al. Overexpression of CXCL3 can enhance the oncogenic potential of prostate cancer. Int Urol Nephrol 2016; 48: 701–709.

[17] Zhang L, Zhang L, Li H, *et al.* CXCL3 contributes to CD133+ CSCs maintenance and forms a positive feedback regulation loop with CD133 in HCC via Erk1/2 phosphorylation. Sci Rep 2016; 6(1): 27426.
[http://dx.doi.org/10.1038/srep27426] [PMID: 27255419]

[18] Hu B, Fan H, Lv X, Chen S, Shao Z. Prognostic significance of CXCL5 expression in cancer patients: a meta-analysis. Cancer Cell Int 2018; 18(1): 68.
[http://dx.doi.org/10.1186/s12935-018-0562-7] [PMID: 29743818]

[19] Romero-Moreno R, Curtis KJ, Coughlin TR, *et al.* The CXCL5/CXCR2 axis is sufficient to promote breast cancer colonization during bone metastasis. Nat Commun 2019; 10(1): 4404.
[http://dx.doi.org/10.1038/s41467-019-12108-6] [PMID: 31562303]

[20]   Ding Q, Lu P, Xia Y, *et al.* CXCL9: evidence and contradictions for its role in tumor progression. Cancer Med 2016; 5(11): 3246-59.
[http://dx.doi.org/10.1002/cam4.934] [PMID: 27726306]

[21]   Newsletter STO, Acir GTO, Digests W, *et al.* Tumor in ltration is governed by CCL5 and 2020.

[22]   Tan S, Wang K, Sun F. *et al* CXCL9 promotes prostate cancer progression through inhibition of cytokines from T cells. Mol Med Rep 2018; 18: 1305-10.

[23]   Puchert M, Obst J, Koch C, Zieger K, Engele J. CXCL11 promotes tumor progression by the biased use of the chemokine receptors CXCR3 and CXCR7. Cytokine 2020; 125: 154809.
[http://dx.doi.org/10.1016/j.cyto.2019.154809] [PMID: 31437604]

[24]   Gao Q, Wang S, Chen X, *et al.* Cancer-cell-secreted CXCL11 promoted CD8$^+$ T cells infiltration through docetaxel-induced-release of HMGB1 in NSCLC. J Immunother Cancer 2019; 7(1): 42.
[http://dx.doi.org/10.1186/s40425-019-0511-6] [PMID: 30744691]

[25]   Hussain M, Adah D, Tariq M, Lu Y, Zhang J, Liu J. CXCL13/CXCR5 signaling axis in cancer. Life Sci 2019; 227: 175-86.
[http://dx.doi.org/10.1016/j.lfs.2019.04.053] [PMID: 31026453]

[26]   Kazanietz MG, Durando M, Cooke M. CXCL13 and its receptor CXCR5 in cancer: Inflammation, immune response, and beyond. Front Endocrinol (Lausanne) 2019; 10: 471.
[http://dx.doi.org/10.3389/fendo.2019.00471] [PMID: 31354634]

[27]   Blevins MA, Huang M, Zhao R. The role of CtBP1 in oncogenic processes & its potential as a therapeutic target. Mol Cancer Ther 2017; 16(6): 981-90.
[http://dx.doi.org/10.1158/1535-7163.MCT-16-0592] [PMID: 28576945]

[28]   Byun JS, Park S, Yi DI, *et al.* Epigenetic re-wiring of breast cancer by pharmacological targeting of C-terminal binding protein. Cell Death Dis 2019; 10(10): 689.
[http://dx.doi.org/10.1038/s41419-019-1892-7] [PMID: 31534138]

[29]   Ding B, Yuan F, Damle PK, Litovchick L, Drapkin R, Grossman SR. CtBP determines ovarian cancer cell fate through repression of death receptors. Cell Death Dis 2020; 11(4): 286.
[http://dx.doi.org/10.1038/s41419-020-2455-7] [PMID: 32332713]

[30]   Smolle E, Pichler M. Non-smoking-associated lung cancer: A distinct entity in terms of tumor biology, patient characteristics and impact of hereditary cancer predisposition. Cancers (Basel) 2019; 11(2): 204.
[http://dx.doi.org/10.3390/cancers11020204] [PMID: 30744199]

[31]   Chen X, Wang X, Wei X, Wang J. EphA5 protein, a potential marker for distinguishing histological grade and prognosis in ovarian serous carcinoma. J Ovarian Res 2016; 9(1): 83.
[http://dx.doi.org/10.1186/s13048-016-0292-1] [PMID: 27887627]

[32]   Smith HR. Oncology letters. Oncol Lett 2015; 9: 1509-14.
[http://dx.doi.org/10.3892/ol.2015.2944] [PMID: 25788991]

[33]   Zhang R, Liu J, Zhang W, Hua L, Qian LT, Zhou SB. EphA5 knockdown enhances the invasion and migration ability of esophageal squamous cell carcinoma *via* epithelial-mesenchymal transition through activating Wnt/β-catenin pathway. Cancer Cell Int 2020; 20(1): 20.
[http://dx.doi.org/10.1186/s12935-020-1101-x] [PMID: 31956298]

[34]   Sunaga N, Kaira K. Epiregulin as a therapeutic target in non-small-cell lung cancer. Lung Cancer (Auckl) 2015; 6: 91-8.
[http://dx.doi.org/10.2147/LCTT.S60427] [PMID: 28210154]

[35]   Wang Y, Jing Y, Ding L, *et al.* Epiregulin reprograms cancer-associated fibroblasts and facilitates oral squamous cell carcinoma invasion *via* JAK2-STAT3 pathway. J Exp Clin Cancer Res 2019; 38(1): 274.
[http://dx.doi.org/10.1186/s13046-019-1277-x] [PMID: 31234944]

[36]   Yumimoto K, Akiyoshi S, Ueo H. *et al* F-box protein FBXW7 inhibits cancer metastasis in a non-cel-
-autonomous manner J Clin Invest 2019; 125: 621-35.

[37]   Lu M, Zhu J, Ling Y, Shi W, Zhang C, Wu H. The lower expression of gonadotropin-releasing
hormone receptor associated with poor prognosis in gastric cancer. Int J Clin Exp Med 2015; 8(8):
13365-70.
[PMID: 26550267]

[38]   Doroszko M, Chrusciel M, Stelmaszewska J, *et al.* GnRH antagonist treatment of malignant
adrenocortical tumors. Endocr Relat Cancer 2019; 26(1): 103-17.
[http://dx.doi.org/10.1530/ERC-17-0399] [PMID: 30400009]

[39]   Zhang L, Lian R, Zhao J, *et al.* IGFBP7 inhibits cell proliferation by suppressing AKT activity and
cell cycle progression in thyroid carcinoma. Cell Biosci 2019; 9: 1-26.

[40]   Rupp C, Scherzer M, Rudisch A, *et al.* IGFBP7, a novel tumor stroma marker, with growth-promoting
effects in colon cancer through a paracrine tumor–stroma interaction. Oncogene 2015; 34(7): 815-25.
[http://dx.doi.org/10.1038/onc.2014.18] [PMID: 24632618]

[41]   Jiang T, Zhou C, Ren S. Role of IL-2 in cancer immunotherapy. OncoImmunology 2016; 5(6):
e1163462.
[http://dx.doi.org/10.1080/2162402X.2016.1163462] [PMID: 27471638]

[42]   Lee SCW, Abdel-Wahab O. Therapeutic targeting of splicing in cancer. Nat Med 2016; 22(9): 976-86.
[http://dx.doi.org/10.1038/nm.4165] [PMID: 27603132]

[43]   Xu D, Pavlidis P, Thamadilok S, *et al.* Recent evolution of the salivary mucin MUC7. Sci Rep 2016;
6(1): 31791.
[http://dx.doi.org/10.1038/srep31791] [PMID: 27558399]

[44]   Lin YL, Wang YL, Fu XL, Li WP, Wang YH, Ma JG. Low expression of protocadherin7 (PCDH7) is
a potential prognostic biomarker for primary non-muscle invasive bladder cancer. Oncotarget 2016;
7(19): 28384-92.
[http://dx.doi.org/10.18632/oncotarget.8635] [PMID: 27070091]

[45]   Xu S, Wu X, Tao Z, *et al.* Effect of aberrantly methylated androgen receptor target gene PCDH7 on
the development of androgen-independent prostate cancer cells. Genes Genomics 2020; 42(3): 299-
307.
[http://dx.doi.org/10.1007/s13258-019-00903-w] [PMID: 31872382]

[46]   Zhu Y, Wang Y, Guan B, *et al.* C-kit and PDGFRA gene mutations in triple negative breast cancer. Int
J Clin Exp Pathol 2014; 7(7): 4280-5.
[PMID: 25120810]

[47]   Onishi H, Ichimiya S, Yanai K, *et al.* RBPJ and MAML3: Potential therapeutic targets for small cell
lung cancer. Anticancer Res 2018; 38(8): 4543-7.
[http://dx.doi.org/10.21873/anticanres.12758] [PMID: 30061220]

[48]   Mi Y, Zhang D, Jiang W, *et al.* miR-181a-5p promotes the progression of gastric cancer *via* RASSF6-
mediated MAPK signalling activation. Cancer Lett 2017; 389: 11-22.
[http://dx.doi.org/10.1016/j.canlet.2016.12.033] [PMID: 28043911]

[49]   Li Y, Gan S, Ren L, *et al.* Multifaceted regulation and functions of replication factor C family in
human cancers. Am J Cancer Res 2018; 8(8): 1343-55.
[PMID: 30210909]

[50]   Prica F, Radon T, Cheng Y, Crnogorac-Jurcevic T. The life and works of S100P - from conception to
cancer. Am J Cancer Res 2016; 6(2): 562-76.
[PMID: 27186425]

[51]   Carneiro P, Moreira AM, Figueiredo J, *et al.* S100P is a molecular determinant of E-cadherin function
in gastric cancer. Cell Commun Signal 2019; 17(1): 155.

[http://dx.doi.org/10.1186/s12964-019-0465-9] [PMID: 31767037]

[52]   Ye W, Chen C, Gao Y, *et al.* Overexpression of SLC34A2 is an independent prognostic indicator in bladder cancer and its depletion suppresses tumor growth *via* decreasing c-Myc expression and transcriptional activity. Cell Death Dis 2017; 8(2): e2581.
[http://dx.doi.org/10.1038/cddis.2017.13] [PMID: 28151475]

[53]   Zhao SJ, Shen YF, Li Q, *et al.* SLIT2/ROBO1 axis contributes to the Warburg effect in osteosarcoma through activation of SRC/ERK/c-MYC/PFKFB2 pathway. Cell Death Dis 2018; 9(3): 390.
[http://dx.doi.org/10.1038/s41419-018-0419-y] [PMID: 29523788]

[54]   zeng B, zhou , Wu H, Xiong Z. SPP1 promotes ovarian cancer progression *via* Integrin β1/FAK/Akt signaling pathway. OncoTargets Ther 2018; 11: 1333-43.
[http://dx.doi.org/10.2147/OTT.S154215] [PMID: 29559792]

[55]   Zhuo C, Li X, Zhuang H, *et al.* Elevated THBS2, COL1A2, and SPP1 Expression Levels as Predictors of Gastric Cancer Prognosis. Cell Physiol Biochem 2016; 40(6): 1316-24.
[http://dx.doi.org/10.1159/000453184] [PMID: 27997896]

[56]   Masoumi-Moghaddam S, Amini A, Wei AQ, Robertson G, Morris DL. Sprouty 1 predicts prognosis in human epithelial ovarian cancer. Am J Cancer Res 2015; 5(4): 1531-41.
[PMID: 26101716]

[57]   Ohoka N, Nagai K, Hattori T, *et al.* Cancer cell death induced by novel small molecules degrading the TACC3 protein *via* the ubiquitin–proteasome pathway. Cell Death Dis 2014; 5(11): e1513-0.
[http://dx.doi.org/10.1038/cddis.2014.471] [PMID: 25375378]

[58]   Lanki M, Seppänen H, Mustonen H, Hagström J, Haglund C. Toll-like receptor 1 predicts favorable prognosis in pancreatic cancer. PLoS One 2019; 14(7): e0219245.
[http://dx.doi.org/10.1371/journal.pone.0219245] [PMID: 31314777]

[59]   Wu D, Hu D, Chen H, *et al.* Glucose-regulated phosphorylation of TET2 by AMPK reveals a pathway linking diabetes to cancer. Nature 2018; 559(7715): 637-41.
[http://dx.doi.org/10.1038/s41586-018-0350-5] [PMID: 30022161]

[60]   Goto Y, Zeng L, Yeom CJ, *et al.* UCHL1 provides diagnostic and antimetastatic strategies due to its deubiquitinating effect on HIF-1α. Nat Commun 2015; 6(1): 6153.
[http://dx.doi.org/10.1038/ncomms7153]

CHAPTER 5

Chromosome 5

Sayooj Madhusoodanan[1], Saurav Panicker[1] and Satish Ramalingam[1,*]

[1] Department of Genetic Engineering, School of Bioengineering, SRM Institute of Science and Technology, Kattankulathur, India

Abstract: Chromosome 5 presents an extensive collection of genes, and includes several cancer-associated ones. The contribution of chromosome 5 in abnormalities is evident through somatic translocations, germline, somatic, and, in some instances, expression of genes. Various syndromes are associated with chromosome 5, such as 5q minus syndrome, leading to the development of acute myeloid leukemia, PDGFRB-associated chronic eosinophilic leukemia contributing to acute myeloid leukemia, and myelodysplastic syndromes. Studies propose that a few genes on chromosome 5 play important roles withinside the increase and department of cells. When chromosome segments are deleted, as in a few instances of AML and MDS, those crucial genes are missing. Without those genes, cells can develop and divide too speedy and in an out-o--control way. Researchers are trying to perceive the genes on chromosome five that might be associated with AML and MDS.

Keywords: Cellular differentiation, Epigenesis, Follicular variants, Hypermethylation, Intercellular communication, Microsatellite instability, Multi-drug resistance, Polymorphism, Signet-ring cancer, Signal transduction, Translocation.

1.1. AACSP1: ACETOACETYL-COA SYNTHETASE PSUEDOGENE 1. CHROMOSOME 5; 5q35.3

AACSP1 is a pseudogene and is reported to regulate genes similarly to LncRNAs in the human genome. In renal cell carcinoma, alterations in this gene are observed, and this was because LncRNAs and pseudogenes are closely related to survival and recurrence, suggesting they can serve as potential prognostic markers and are worth further investigation [1]. AACSP1 is involved in lipid metabolism and serves as a marker for it. In a study on non-small cell lung carcinoma, it was observed that there is a direct correlation between the changes in the concentrations of lipid metabolites with changes in the expression levels of AACSP [2]. In

* **Corresponding author Satish Ramalingam**: Department of Genetic Engineering, School of Bioengineering, SRM Institute of Science and Technology, Kattankulathur, India; E-mail: rsatish76@gmail.com

asbestos-related lung cancer, DNA methylation changes were observed in the DNA methylation regions (DMR) in T and N between the asbestos-exposed and non-exposed cases, and AACSP1 showed lowered asbestos-related hypomethylation in lung tumors with asbestos-exposed cases [3].

1.2. ABLIM3: ACTIN BINDING LIM PROTEIN FAMILY MEMBER 3. CHROMOSOME 5; 5q32

ABLIM3 is the third member of the actin-binding LIM protein subgroup. ABLIM3 expression is highest in the heart, lungs, liver (fetal and adult), brain/-cerebellum, CNS, and spinal cord. The expression profile of the abLIM3 gene supports a suggested role in hepatoma development [4]. The knockdown of ABLIM3 resulted in significant impairment of hepatitis C virus replication in HCV- induced hepatocellular carcinoma [5]. The expression of ABLIM3 mRNA is downregulated for triple-negative breast cancer and adjacent non-tumor tissues [6]. Hyper or hypomethylation of ABLIM3 is observed in connection with thyroid cancer. The mutation of ABLIM3 in Kidney renal clear cell carcinoma may play a key role in kidney cancers. The signal transduction and system processes were enriched and interacted between different cancers, reflecting the standard processes in tumor progression and development [7].

1.3. ACOT12: ACYL-COA THIOESTERASE 12. CHROMOSOME 5; 5q14.1

Acyl-CoA thioesterase 12 (ACOT12) is the major enzyme known to hydrolyze acetyl-CoA's thioester bond in the liver cytosol [8]. In a study, it was observed that there is a close association between increased acetyl-CoA levels and hepatocellular carcinoma (HCC) metastasis. Down-regulation of ACOT12 is correlated with metastasis and poor prognosis of HCC. ACOT12 functionally suppresses HCC metastasis. ACOT12 regulates acetyl-CoA metabolism, and histone acetylation down-regulation of ACOT12 promotes HCC metastasis by epigenetic induction of TWIST2 [9]. ACOT12 is linked with growth and invasion potential.

1.4. ACSL6: ACYL-COA SYNTHETASE LONG-CHAIN FAMILY 6. CHROMOSOME 5; 5q31.1

The ACSL6 gene (Fig. 1), called acyl CoA synthetase 2 (*ACS2*) and fatty acid CoA long chain 6, encodes a long-chain acyl-CoA synthetase. This enzyme is essential in lipid metabolism and cell ATP generation pathways [10]. A study suggests that t(5;12) (q23- 31; p13)/ETV6-ACSL6 gene fusion in chronic leukemia renders cancer cells resistant to treatment using a tyrosine kinase inhibitor [11]. Another study suggests that the expression of ACSL6 was down-regulated and serves as a potential tumor suppressor gene in leukemia. In addition, ACSL6 was decreased in most forms of cancers, except colorectal cancer [12].

ACSL6 is highly expressed in brain tissue. A bioinformatics study in colorectal cancer found that ACSL6 is upregulated compared to healthy tissue. ACSL6 is speculated to support the accumulation of lipid droplets in fatty liver disease, thereby required for the early stages of hepatocellular carcinoma development [13].

1.5. ACTBL2: ACTIN BETA LIKE 2 [HOMO AAPIENS (HUMAN)]. CHROMOSOME 5; 5q11.2

Actin beta-like 2 (ACTBL2) was found to have higher levels in colorectal tumor samples, indicating ACTBL2 association and differential upregulation in colorectal cancer, thereby potentially serving a function in developing markers for colorectal cancer [14]. A study found that increased expression of ACTBL2 was observed in human pancreatic ductal adenocarcinoma [15]. In a survey of human breast cancer cell lines, ACTBL2 was one of the top ten genes to be upregulated [16]. ACTBL2 is a cytoskeletal protein abundantly expressed in vascular smooth muscle cells. ACTBL2 was most strongly associated with epithelial ovarian cancer risk [17]. ACTBL2 is found to differentiate between conventional and follicular variants of papillary thyroid cancer [18].

1.6. ACTBP2: ACTB PSEUDOGENE 2 [HOMO SAPIENS (HUMAN)]. CHROMOSOME 5; 5q14.1

The ACTBP2 locus (Fig. **1**) consisting of AAAG repeats on human chromosome 5 is one of the most polymorphic short tandem repeat systems [19]. ACTBP2 is used as a marker in studying microsatellite instability in cancer cells [20]. In a study on ovarian cancer, the microsatellite instability at the ACTBP2 locus is found in 20% of the cancers [21]. ACTBP2 can be used as a microsatellite repeat marker to assess patients with bladder cancer using a non-invasive technique and thereby can be used as a potential biomarker for bladder cancer patients [22]. Knowing the sensitivity of ACTBP2 in bladder tumors, it was used to detect non-small cell lung cancers (NSCLC), detecting an alteration in primary lung tumors. Hence, markers sensitive to NSCLC may also be used for detecting tumors from other organs [23]. A study detected loss of heterozygosity at the ACTBP2 locus in the plasma of small-cell lung cancer patients [24]. ACTBP2 shows a high rate of microsatellite alterations in small-cell lung carcinoma patients [25].

1.7. ADAM19: ADAM METALLOPEPTIDASE DOMAIN 19. CHROMO-SOME 5; 5q33.3

ADAM19 (Fig. 1) is a member of a disintegrin and metalloproteinases (ADAMs), which are involved in various biological functions, such as fertilization, embryonic development, cell adhesion, cell migration, cell signaling, proteolytic shedding and proteolysis [26, 27]. Dysregulation of many ADAM proteins is observed in regulating growth factor activities and integrin functions, promoting cell growth and invasion in human tumors [28, 29]. ADAM19 is upregulated in human brain tumors, such as astrocytoma and glioblastoma, and is correlated with the invasiveness of glioma [30]. ADAM19 is also overexpressed in cancerous lung cells [31]. Abnormally high expression of ADAM19 is also linked to inflammation and fibrosis of the lung and kidney [32, 33]. Knockdown of ADAM19 inhibited migration and invasion of non-small cell lung carcinoma cells [34]. ADAM19 promotes the invasiveness of colon cancer cells [35]. ADAM19 is a protective factor for human prostate cancer, suggesting that upregulation of ADAM19 expression could be therapeutic in human prostate cancer [36].

1.8. ADAMTS12: ADAM METALLOPEPTIDASE WITH THROMBOS-PONDIN TYPE 1 MOTIF 1. CHROMOSOME 5; 5p13.3-p13.2

ADAMTS12 (Fig. 1) is a complex metalloproteinase whose expression has been detected mainly in some human fetal tissues, carcinomas, and cancer cell lines [37]. The expression of ADAMTS12 in colorectal cancer stroma is essential in inhibiting tumor development, and its expression may be an excellent prognostic marker for colorectal cancer [38]. A study showed that ADAMTS12 confers tumor-protective functions upon cells that produce this proteolytic enzyme [39]. ADAMTS12 gene promoter is hypermethylated in patients with colorectal carcinomas. ADAMTS-12 is a novel anti-tumor protease that can reduce the proliferative properties of tumor cells. ADAMTS-12 might act as a tumor-protective protease in colon cancer and tumors of different origins, such as breast cancer. The dual nature of ADAMTS12 expression was found in colon carcinoma: epigenetic inactivation in epithelial malignant cells and induction in myofibroblasts, suggesting that this metalloprotease could form part of a protective stromal response aimed at limiting tumor progression [39].

1.9. ADAMTS16: ADAM METALLOPEPTIDASE WITH THROMBOSP-ONDIN TYPE 1 MOTIF 16. CHROMOSOME 5; 5p15.32

ADAMTS16 belongs to the family of ADAMTS (a disintegrin and metallo-proteinase domain with thrombospondin motifs), which includes 19 secreted proteinases in man. ADAMTS16 is expressed at high levels in the kidney, adult brain, and ovary. When over-expressed in chondrosarcoma cells, it decreased cell proliferation and migration but not adhesion [40]. IDNA methylation of ADAM-TS16 in colorectal cancer and other epithelial cells was identified in a study ADAMTS16 protein was strongly expressed in goblet cells and colonocytes in control tissue but not in CRC samples [41]. ADAMTS16 transcription is regulated by Wt1 (Wilm's tumor protein), and when knocked down, it reduces branching morphogenesis in cultured embryonic kidneys [42]. ADAMTS16 can be considered a novel gene because of its potential with cancer-specific promoter hypermethylation in colorectal cancer, liver cancer, and squamous cell carcinoma patients, therefore serving as a biomarker for these tumors and may include tumor suppressing properties [41] (Fig. **1**).

1.10. ADRA1B: ADRENO RECEPTOR ALPHA 1B MOTIF 16. CHROMOSOME 5; 5q33.3

ADRA1B; Alpha-1-adrenergic receptors (alpha-1-ARs) are members of the G protein-coupled receptor superfamily. They activate mitogenic responses and regulate the growth and proliferation of many cells. ADRA1B is associated with breast cancer as it was observed to undergo mutations in the replication stage [43]. It has also been noted that ADRA1B's related to gastric cancer. The ADRA1B promoter is frequently methylated in gastric cancer, and the studies suggested that it is an essential tumor-related gene commonly involved in the development and progression of Gastric cancer [44].

1.11. ADRB2: ADRENOCEPTOR BETA 2. CHROMOSOME 5; 5q33.3

ADRB2 (Fig. **1**) encodes for beta-2-androgenic receptors, a member of the G protein-coupled receptor superfamily. Direct association of this gene with the ultimate effectors, the class CL-type calcium channel, is reported. The other inclusion of these receptor channels is the G protein, an adenyl cyclase, cAMP-dependent kinase, and counterbalancing phosphatases.

This assembly of signaling complexes would eventually provide a mechanism that ensures specific and rapid signaling by G protein-coupled receptors. This receptor is also a transcription regulator of the alpha-synuclein gene, and together, both genes are believed to be associated with the risk of Parkinson's disease. This gene is intronless. Different polymorphic forms, point mutations, and downregulation of this gene are associated with nocturnal asthma, obesity, type 2 diabetes, and cardiovascular disease. It has been studied extensively about this gene's properties in cancer progression, where the loss of endothelial ADRB2 leads to the inhibition of angiogenesis through the improvement of endothelial oxidative phosphory-lation. This cross-talk between the nerves and the endothelial metabolism can be targeted for potential anticancer treatment [45]. Activation of ADRB2 contributes to prostate cancer pathophysiology by inhibiting apoptosis [46]. It is also associated with breast cancer by its relation with the HIC1 (Hypermethylated in cancer 1) tumor repressor, which is silenced in many human tumors. It was identified that the early inactivation of HIC1 in breast carcinomas could predispose to stress-induced metastasis through the upregulation of the beta-2-androgenic receptors [47].

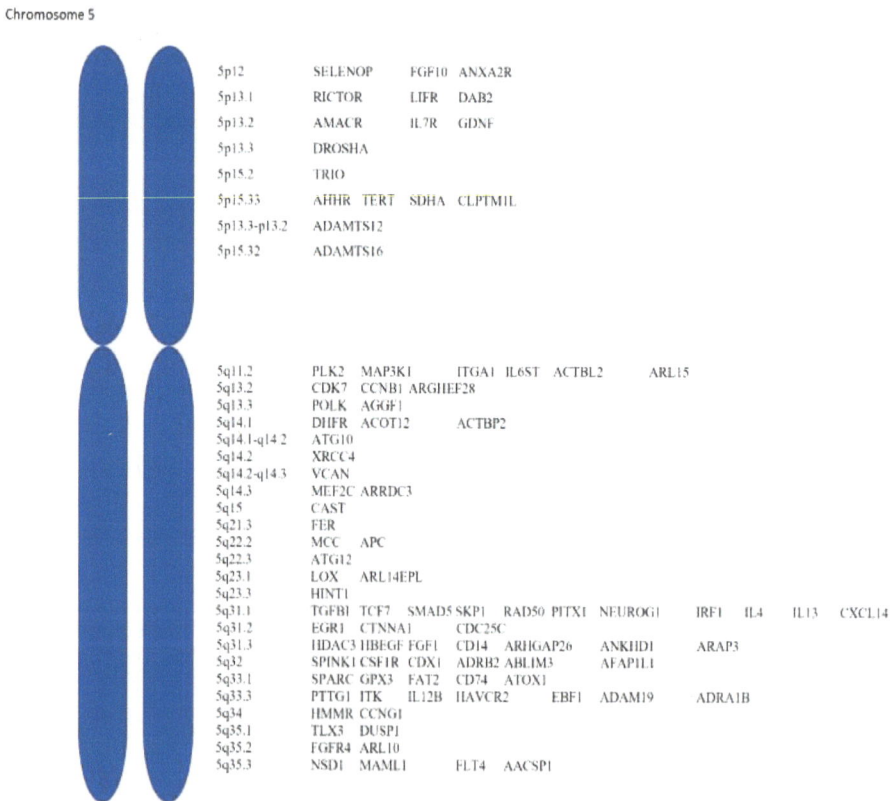

Chromosome 5

Locus	Genes
5p12	SELENOP FGF10 ANXA2R
5p13.1	RICTOR LIFR DAB2
5p13.2	AMACR IL7R GDNF
5p13.3	DROSHA
5p15.2	TRIO
5p15.33	AHHR TERT SDHA CLPTM1L
5p13.3-p13.2	ADAMTS12
5p15.32	ADAMTS16
5q11.2	PLK2 MAP3K1 ITGA1 IL6ST ACTBL2 ARL15
5q13.2	CDK7 CCNB1 ARGHEF28
5q13.3	POLK AGGF1
5q14.1	DHFR ACOT12 ACTBP2
5q14.1-q14.2	ATG10
5q14.2	XRCC4
5q14.2-q14.3	VCAN
5q14.3	MEF2C ARRDC3
5q15	CAST
5q21.3	FER
5q22.2	MCC APC
5q22.3	ATG12
5q23.1	LOX ARL14EPL
5q23.3	HINT1
5q31.1	TGFBI TCF7 SMAD5 SKP1 RAD50 PITX1 NEUROG1 IRF1 IL4 IL13 CXCL14
5q31.2	EGR1 CTNNA1 CDC25C
5q31.3	HDAC3 HBEGF FGF1 CD14 ARHGAP26 ANKHD1 ARAP3
5q32	SPINK1 CSF1R CDX1 ADRB2 ABLIM3 AFAP1L1
5q33.1	SPARC GPX3 FAT2 CD74 ATOX1
5q33.3	PTTG1 ITK IL12B HAVCR2 EBF1 ADAM19 ADRA1B
5q34	HMMR CCNG1
5q35.1	TLX3 DUSP1
5q35.2	FGFR4 ARL10
5q35.3	NSD1 MAML1 FLT4 AACSP1

Fig. (1). This figure displays the loci of the genes from Chromosome 5 whose roles in cancer have been explained in this chapter. Sayooj Madhusoodanan designs this diagram.

1.12. AFAP1L1: ACTIN FILAMENT-ASSOCIATED PROTEIN 1. CHROMOSOME 5; 5q32

AFAP1L1 belongs to the family of actin-filament-associated proteins (AFAP) and is one of the three adapter proteins, the other being AFAP1, and AFAPIL2/-XB130. AFAP1 and AFAPIL2 have already been studied and established to have an oncogenic role. The association with AFAP1L1 is currently being investigated, and there are a few notable connections. AFAP1L1 has been found to promote cell proliferation, acceleration of cell cycle progression, and prevention of cellular apoptosis in lung cancer cells, which suggests that even this member of the AFAP family has an oncogenic role [48]. AFAP1L1 has also been studied in association with spindle cell sarcomas which consists of tumors with different biological features. In this study, AFAP1L1 was identified as a metastatic-predicting marker. When the AFAP1L1 gene knocked down sarcoma cells, it inhibited cell invasion. At the same time, tumor growth was accelerated in AFAP1L1 transduced sarcoma cells [49]. Also, in colorectal cancer, AFAP1L1 plays a role in the progression of modulation of cell shape, motility and biting anoikis [50].

1.13. AFF4: AF4/FMR2 FAMILY MEMBER 4. CHROMOSOME 5; 5q31.1

The AFF4 gene encodes a protein belonging to the family of transcription factors involved in leukemia. It is also a vital component of the SEC (super elongation complex), in which AAF4 act as a scaffold that recruits by utilizing the direct interaction with the ELL proteins and the P- TEFb complex. AFF4 is essential for SEC stability and proper translation by poised RNA polymerase II in metazoans. When the AFF4 gene is knocked down in leukemic cells, it reduces MLL chimera target gene expression, which would justify that AFF4/SEC can be considered a key regulator in the pathogenesis of leukemia. It has been suggested as a biomarker and potential target for therapies for head and neck squamous cell carcinoma (HNSCC). AFF4 was highly expressed in the HNSCC cell lines and tumor tissues. AFF4 promoted migration, proliferation, and invasion of the HNSCC cells. ALDH (Aldehyde dehydrogenase) activity was also enhanced. SOX2 (sex-determining region Y box2) expression changed in parallel with AFF4 expression in response to depletion and overexpression of AFF4 [51]. AFF4 has shown relations in breast cancer progression. It acts as one of the direct targets for modification of methyltransferase-3 (METTL3), a major RNA N6-adenosine methyltransferase, which also has targets like key regulators of NF-κB pathway (IKBKB and RELA) and MYC. In summary, AFF4 is associated with a signal network, AFF4/NF-κB/MYC signaling, which is operated by m6A modification and provides insight into the mechanisms of BCa progression [52].

1.14. AGGF1: ANGIOGENIC FACTOR WITH G-PATCH AND FHA DOMAINS 1. CHROMOSOME 5; 5q13.3

The AGGF1 gene encodes an angiogenic factor that promotes the proliferation of endothelial cells. AGGF1 Promotes angiogenesis and the proliferation of endo-thelial cells. Able to bind to endothelial cells and promote cell proliferation, suggesting that it may act in an autocrine fashion. AGGF1 is important for regulating vascular differentiation and angiogenesis and is also identified as a novel anti-inflammatory factor. When AGGF1 is overexpressed, it represses the expression of pro-inflammatory molecules. Conversely, when AGGF1 was knocked down, it increased the expression of the pro-inflammatory molecules. It was demonstrated that AGGF1 suppresses endothelial activation responses to TNF-α by antagonizing the ERK/NF-κB pathway. This would suggest that AGGF1 is a potential therapeutic candidate for preventing and treating inflammatory diseases [53].

Aberrant expression of AGGF1 is associated with tumor initiation and progression [54]. Expression of AGGF1 was identified to be high in gastric cancer samples; this states that it predicts poor prognosis in gastric cancer patients. It can be used as an independent factor to predict post-operative survival [55]. AGGF1 has also been stated to be critical for autophagy induction and is a novel agent for the treatment of coronary artery disease and myocardial infarction [56]. AGGF1 is also identified as an independent prognostic factor for the patient's disease-free survival (DFS) after surgical resection. Contribute to tumor angiogenesis in Hepatocellular carcinoma, which indicates that AGGF1 may be a potential therapeutic target for anti-angiogenesis treatment for patients with HCC [57].

1.15. AHHR: ARYL-HYDROCARBON RECEPTOR REPRESSOR. CHROMOSOME 5; 5p15.33

AHHR encodes a protein in the aryl hydrocarbon receptor (AhR) signaling cascade. The protein's function is that it mediates Digoxin toxicity and is involved in cell growth and differentiation. AHHR eventually plays a role in inflammation and tumorigenesis [58]. AHHR has been identified to have an expression status that would serve as a potential independent prognostic factor as it plays a sup-pressor gene in primary gastric adenocarcinoma [59]. When AHRR is downre-gulated in human lung cancer cell lines, it confers resistance to apoptotic signals and eventually enhances motility, invasion, and angiogenic potential. At the same time, ectopic expression in tumors decreased anchorage-dependent and independent cell growth and reduced angiogenic potential [60]. A study has also identified a relation with AHHR in breast cancer in which it states to be suppressive on cell growth (MCF-7) by distributing transcriptional and post-post transcriptional actions of estrogen-responsive and cell cycle-related genes [61].

1.16. AMACR: ALPHA-METHYLACYL-COA RACEMASE. CHROMO-SOME 5; 5p13.2

AMACR gene encodes a racemase. The encoded enzyme interconverts pristanoyl-CoA and C27- bile acyl CoA between their (R)- and (S)-stereoisomers. The conversion to the (S)- stereoisomers is necessary for degrading these substrates by peroxisomal beta-oxidation; encoded proteins from this locus localize to both mitochondria and peroxisomes. Mutations in this gene may be associated with adult-onset sensorimotor neuropathy, pigmentary retinopathy, and adrenomyeloneuropathy due to defects in bile acid synthesis. In a study, it was hypothesized that AMACR is overexpressed in the development of cancer, playing a role in providing sufficient energy to the neoplastic cells [62]. There is an increased risk of polymorphism of the AMACR gene in prostate cancer [63]. AMACR is also suggested as a candidate tissue biomarker for prostate cancer [64, 65].

1.17. ANKHD1: ANKYRIN REPEAT AND KH DOMAIN CONTAINING 1. CHROMOSOME 5; 5q31.3

ANKHD1 encodes a protein with multiple ankyrin repeat domains and a single KH domain. The encoded protein is said to have a function that acts as a scaffolding protein and is suggested to be involved in the regulation of caspases, which leads to a play of antiapoptotic role in cell survival. ANKHD1 is highly expressed in cancers, including acute leukemia and Multiple Myeloma. It is also suggested to have a role in cell proliferation and cell cycle progression by regulating the expression of p21 in Multiple myeloma cells. ANKHD1 promotes MM growth by repressing p21, a potent cell cycle regulator [66, 67]. In prostate cancer, ANKHD1 is identified as a novel candidate of the Hippo signaling pathway, a mechanism considered to control tissue growth and organ size, where the core signaling complex is evolutionarily conserved, and also plays a role of tumor suppressor in mammals. Being a novel component of the Hippo signaling pathway, ANKHD1 promotes YAP1 activation and cell cycle progression in prostate cancer cells [68]. As mentioned earlier, ANKHD1 is highly expressed in human acute leukemia cells and potentially regulates multiple cellular functions. ANKHD1 binds to SIVA, which has a vital role in the induction of leukemia cell proliferation and migration *via* the Stathmin 1 pathway, thus suggesting ANKH-D1 could be oncogenic and participate in leukemia cell phenotype [69].

1.18. ANXA2R: ANNEXIN A2 RECEPTOR. CHROMOSOME 5; 5p12

ANXA2R (Annexin A2 Receptor) is a Protein Coding gene. Increased expression of ANXA2 is frequently observed in a broad spectrum of cancer cells, making it a potential cancer biomarker [70]. It is a calcium-dependent phospholipid-binding protein and is found to be expressed in metastatic tumors inclusive of a phenotype of drug resistance and metastasis. Upregulation of ANXA2R might play an important role in modulating the proliferation and invasion of breast cancer cells through many associated downstream target genes [71]. In hepatocellular carcinoma, ANXA2R expression and phosphorylation are upregulated. Over-expression and tyrosine phosphorylation of ANXA2R is suggested to play an important role in the malignant transformation process, leading to Hepatocellular carcinoma [72]. When cancer cells (MCF-7) acquired drug resistance, ANXA2R was enhanced and is said to have a play as an essential role in MDR (Multidrug resistance)- induced tumor invasion [73]. The Association of ANXA2R is linked to tumor cell adhesion, cell proliferation, tumor neovascularization, tumor invasion, and metastasis [74]. ANXA2R has also been identified as a poor prognostic factor for breast cancer and has a novel mechanism to promote breast cancer metastasis [75].

1.19. APC: APC REGULATOR OF WNT SIGNALING PATHWAY/ADENOMATOUS POLYPOSIS COLI. CHROMOSOME 5; 5q22.2

APC Gene codes for the APC protein are important in many cellular processes. APC functions as a tumor suppressor and controls cell division, cell adhesion, and cellular movement. The APC protein accomplishes these tasks mainly through association with other proteins, especially those involved in cell attachment and signaling. One protein with which APC associates is beta-catenin. Beta-catenin helps control the activity (expression) of particular genes and promotes the growth and division (proliferation) of cells and the process by which cells mature to carry out specific functions (differentiation). Beta-catenin also helps cells attach and is important for tissue formation. Association of APC with beta-catenin signals for beta-catenin to be broken down when it is no longer needed. APC gene is usually seen to be mutated in gastric and colorectal cancer, thus suggesting an important role during the carcinogenesis of these cancers [76]. Inactivation of APC plays a role in developing some gastric cancers, particularly well-differentiated adenocarcinomas, and signet-ring cell carcinomas. Results provide evidence that the inactivation of the APC gene plays a significant role in FAP and sporadic tumors of these tissues [77, 78]. It is established that APC mutations sync with other genetic and epigenetic alterations, which add to the extensive genetic heterogeneity of colon cancer [79].

1.20. ARAP3: ARFGAP WITH RHOGAP DOMAIN, ANKYRIN REPEAT, AND PF DOMAINS 3. CHROMOSOME 5; 5q31.3

ARAP3 is responsible for encoding phosphoinositide binding protein ARF-GAP, RHO-GAP, RAS-associating, and pleckstrin homology domains [80]. The ARF-GAP and RHO-GAP domains cooperate in mediating rearrangements in the cell cytoskeleton and cell shape. An unusual expression has been reported in ARAP3 in scirrhous gastric carcinoma cell lines, ARAP3 protein is a substrate of Src family kinases, and it suppresses the peritoneal dissemination of scirrhous gastric carcinoma cell lines [81]. ARAP3 is said to be involved in the regulation of chemotaxis and adhesion-dependent processes in neutrophils [82]. ARAP3 is also significantly upregulated in metastatic breast tumor cells; this expression level might be considered a valuable indicator of breast cancer metastasis. It is also suggested to have an association involving NOTCH4 and CDH5-related signaling pathways [83].

1.21. ARHGEF28: RHO GUANINE NUCLEOTIDE EXCHANGE FACTOR 28. CHROMOSOME 5; 5q13.2

Rgnef (ARHGEF28) is a large protein that canonically functions downstream of integrin receptors to control cell adhesion and RhoA GTPase activity upon cell engagement with matrix proteins [84]. Rgnef is a guanine nucleotide exchange factor that is activated downstream of integrins. It was found that Rgnef protein levels are elevated in late-stage serous ovarian cancer and regulate its progression [85]. ARHGEF28 has been reported to be correlated with migration, invasion, and tumor progression in colon carcinoma and breast cancer cells. ARHGEF28 expression activates the activity of FAK and RhoC, leading to increased migration and invasion in breast cancer [86]. ARHGEF28 was found to be expressed in early- and late-stage oral melanoma [87]. Elevated ArhGEF28 expression promotes colorectal carcinoma invasion and tumor progression *via* interaction with focal adhesion kinase [88].

1.22. ARHGAP26: RHO GTPASE ACTIVATING PROTEIN 26. CHROMOSOME 5; 5q31.3

ARHGAP26 (Rho GTPase Activating Protein 26) is a Protein Coding gene. The protein encoded by this gene is a GTPase-activating protein that binds to focal adhesion kinase and mediates the activity of the GTP-binding proteins RhoA and Cdc42. Among its related pathways is G-protein signaling RhoA regulation pathway and signaling. In gene expression profiling of metastatic brain cancer, it was found that ARGHAP26 is one of the genes which are altered, making cancer cells prone to metastasis. ARGHAP26 associates with CLDN18 to become a recurrent fusion gene CLDN18-ARGHAP26 in gastric cancer, which impairs epithelial barrier properties and wound healing. Its fusion also contributes to GC loss of CLDN18 and gain of ARGHAP26 functions [89]. ARGHAP26 is overexpressed in gastric cancer cells, and its downregulation is said to inhibit cell proliferation and promotion of cell apoptosis [90]. The recurrent fusion CLDN18-ARGHAP26/6 provides evidence of gastric signet-ring cell cancer, highlighting the importance of chemotherapy response [91].

1.23. ARL10: ADP RIBOSYLATION FACTOR LIKE GTPASE 10. CHROMOSOME 5; 5q35.2

ARL10 belongs to the ARF family of GTP-binding proteins, which is known to play an essential role in vesicle biogenesis and intracellular vesicle trafficking [92]. Hsa-miR-1271, located on chromosome 5q35, is an intronic miRNA in the second intron region of the ADP ribosylation factor, like the GTPase 10 (ARL10) gene [93]. The expression and biological significance of miR-1271 on onco-genesis and cancer progression in various malignancies has been reported. MiR-1271 was identified as an upregulated miRNA in patients with head and neck cancers, while it was found to be lower in other tissues and cell lines, such as liver, stomach, ovary, and lung cancer [94 - 96]. ARL10 was down-regulated in endometrial cancer tissues compared to adjacent normal tissues [97]. ARL10 can serve as a marker to predict gastric cancer prognosis.

1.24. ARL14EPL: ADP RIBOSYLATION FACTOR LIKE GTPASE 14 EFFECTOR PROTEIN. CHROMOSOME 5; 5q23.1

ARL14EPL belongs to the ADP ribosylation factor family, which are GTPases, acting as molecular switches by converting guanosine triphosphate (GTP) into guanosine diphosphate (GDP) [98]. A study suggested that ARL14EPL with a combination of genes or independently could indicate a promising and independent prognostic biomarker for lung squamous cell carcinoma (LUSC) patients. ARL14EPL was reported to show a relation to tumorigenesis [99].

1.25. ARL15: ADP RIBOSYLATION FACTOR LIKE GTPASE. CHROMOSOME 5; 5q11.2

ARL15 is expressed in insulin-responsive tissues, including adipose tissue and skeletal muscle (li2014). ARL15 is a tumor suppressor gene and is one of the novel cancer genes [100]. ARL15 is known to regulate the MAPK signaling pathway, cell cycle, metabolism of proteins, and cell-cell communication of cancer cells [101].

ARL15 is found to regulate adiponectin levels, which is dysregulated in cancer [102]. The expression of ARL15 in rheumatoid arthritis synovial fibroblasts shows inflammation and metabolic syndromes through a TNF- independent pathway [103, 104].

1.26. ARRDC3: ARRESTIN DOMAIN CONTAINING 3. CHROMOSOME 5; 5q14.3

Arrestin domain-containing 3 (ARRDC3) overexpression represses cancer cell proliferation, migration, invasion, growth in soft agar, and *in vivo* tumorigenicity, whereas downregulation of ARRCD3 has the opposite effects. The results identify the ARRCD3-ITGβ4 pathway as a new therapeutic target in breast cancer [105]. A study indicates that SIRT2-dependent epigenetic silencing of ARRDC3 is one of the critical events that may contribute to the aggressive nature of basal-like breast cancer cells [106]. Another study suggests that ARRDC3/ITGb4 pathway may play a key role in miR-182-5p's functions in prostate cancer cells [107]. There exists a relationship between ARRDC3 downregulation and aberrant Hippo-Yes-associated protein 1 pathway activation in renal cell carcinoma cells [108]. ARRDC3 could function as a tumor-suppressor gene for cervical cancer and could be involved in cervical cancer development [109].

1.27. ATG10: AUTOPHAGY RELATED 10. CHROMOSOME 5; 5Q14.1-q 14.2

ATG10 is autophagy associated protein-coding gene. Its codes for E2-like enzymes involved in 2 ubiquitin-like modifications are essential for auto-phagosome formation. ATG10 gene, along with the other ATG, is associated with cancer initiation and progression through their mechanisms of autophagy regulation [110]. Most ATG genes are studied extensively, and notable work can be significant. While analyzing single nucleotide polymorphisms in ATGs, ATG10 was identified to have 3 SNPs. In assays, higher expression levels of ATG10 variants elevating showed lesser survival time for lung cancer. Other functional assays have demonstrated ATG10 facilitating lung cancer proliferation and migration, suggesting evidence that variants of ATG10 would be a potential influencer in lung cancer survival through ATG10 regulation [111]. ATG10 in colorectal cancer was found to be upregulated in the tissues, and higher protein expression of ATG10 was associated with tumor lymph node metastasis and invasion. ATG10 was correlated with poor survival, suggesting it is a potential prognostic biomarker [112]. An association was established between ATG10 and Sox2.

Sox2 is a transcription factor in the ting stemness of embryonic stem cells, and induced pluripotent stem cells strongly induced autophagic phenomena, including intracellular vacuole formation and lysosomal activation in colon cancer cells. Sox2 acts as a mediator for ATG10 expression, inhibiting cell proliferation and anchorage-dependent colony growth. While knocking down ATG10 in Sox2 expressing colon cancer cells restored cancer cell properties [113].

1.28. ATG12: AUTOPHAGY RELATED 12. CHROMOSOME 5; 5q22.3

ATG12 is a member of autophagy-related genes, which codes for autophagy-associated proteins. Evidence showed that cancer cells that lack or have reduced ATG12 expression led to undergo oncotic cell death. This led to the finding that inducing costs creating an ATG12 deficiency in solid tumors might be a potential anticancer therapy, preferably to the other conventional options having undesirable outcomes [114]. ATG12, in association with ATG5, is needed as essential for LC3 lipidation and autophagosome formation during macro autophagy. These associations are stable, while free ATG12 was found to be highly unstable and undergo rapid degradation in the proteasomal degradation system, indicating that the accumulation of free ATG12 leads to its contribution towards the proteasome inhibitor-mediated apoptosis. As proteasome inhibitors are used as an anticancer agents through clinical relevance, the ubiquitin-like properties of ATG12 reveal the potential for further studies [115].

1.29. ATOX1: ANTIOXIDANT 1 COPPER CHAPERONE. CHROMOSOME 5; 5q33.1

ATOX1 encodes copper chaperone. Copper chaperones are important in playing a role in copper homeostasis by binding and transporting cytosolic copper to ATPase proteins. The protein is also identified to function as an antioxidant opposing superoxide and hydrogen peroxide., thus suggesting a significant role in cancer carcinogenesis. ATOX1 interacts with the anticancer drug cisplatin, through a study in which cisplatin-induced human melanoma cells contain ATOX1 molecules bound to certain cisplatin derivatives [116]. ATOX1 contributes to cell proliferation through nuclear translocation, DNA binding, and transactivation when copper has activated and ATOX1 functions as a transcription factor [117]. In certain anticancer therapy based on copper ionophores or chelating drugs, it was identified that silencing of the ATOX1 gene would lead to increased susceptibility [118]. In breast cancer migration, evidence suggests that ATOX1 has a role in which ATOX1 accumulates in lamellipodia borders of the migrating cancer cells, and when silenced, it results in migration defects [119].

1.30. CAST: CALPASTATIN. CHROMOSOME 5; 5q15

The CAST gene is encoded by a protein which is a calcium-dependent cysteine protease known as endogenous calpain inhibitor. It is known to be involved in various membrane fusion events; some examples include neural vesicle exocytosis and platelet and red cell aggregation. The protein encoded also has been suggested to affect the expression levels of certain genes, which codes for the structural and regulatory proteins. CAST levels have been evaluated in ovarian cancer in which their levels matched between chemo-sensitive cells and resistant counterparts, suggesting to play a role in ovarian cancer [120]. Initial metastatic dissemination of breast cancer is the other major area where CAST plays a role in regulation [121].

1.31. CCNB1: CYCLIN B1. CHROMOSOME 5; 5q13.2

CCNB1 is responsible for encoding cyclinB1, a regulatory protein involved in mitosis. This protein is essential for the correct control of the G2/M transition phase of the cell. It belongs to the cyclin family, which is highly conserved and is found to be significantly overexpressed in various types of cancer. In ER+ breast cancer patients, it was identified to play a role in the prediction of distant metastasis survival, disease-free survival, recurrence-free survival, and overall survival significantly. Thus, suggesting it to be a potential biomarker for ER+ breast cancer [122]. It has been linked to p53 mutations in enhanced breast cancer, in which it was identified that the delivery of circ-CCNB1 inhibited the function of mutated p53s [123]. In human hepatocellular carcinoma (HCC), it is linked with FOXM1, which promotes the proliferation of the cells by transcriptionally activating CCNB1, which results have suggested that there could be therapeutic potential from FOXM1/CCNB1 axis in HCC [124]. In Human colorectal cancer, CCNB1 and its protein level were upregulated, and evidence suggested a correlation with Chk1expression. Repression of Chk1 decreased CCNB1 protein expression, while downregulation of CCNB1 impaired proliferation. Suppressing CCNB1 caused severe arrest in the G2/M phase; inhibition also led to induced apoptotic death in colorectal cancer cells. These findings suggest that Chk1 activates CCNB1 and lead to oncogenic properties that have a potential role in developing novel therapeutic approach against colorectal cancer [125].

1.32. CCNG1: CYCLIN G1. CHROMOSOME 5; 5q34

CCNG1 is a member of the cyclin family, transcriptional activation of this gene can be induced by tumor protein p53. In high-grade serous CCNG1 play a potential role in the therapeutics due to the molecular mechanism in which the

CCNG1 is regulated by mutant p53, which leads to tumorigenesis and progression by the activation of notch3 expression [126]. CCNG1 is enhanced in cancerous tumors comparatively to its counterparts. MiR-1271 is identified to inhibit ovarian cancer growth by exerting its function by targeting CCNG1 [127]. Similarly, Mir-23b targets CCNG1 by downregulating it through suppression which leads to the inhibition of tumorigenesis and the progression of ovarian cancer [128]. CCNG1 is targeted for studies through its link with cell cycle check control, paving a pathway for therapies [129].

1.33. CD74: CD74 MOLECULE. CHROMOSOME 5; 5q33.1

CD74 encodes the protein that has an association with the class 2 major histocompatibility complex. This protein functions as an important chaperone which helps in regulating the antigen-presenting mechanism for immune response. Furthermore, it also serves the purpose of being a cell surface receptor for cytokine macrophage migration inhibitory factor, which directs the initiation of survival pathways and cell proliferation [130, 131]. Expression of CD74 and MIF were significantly higher in lung cancer and were also identified in other common tumors. In lung cancer, MIF expression is linked to the increased production of angiogenic CXC chemokines [132]. In thyroid cancer, CD74 was found to be overexpressed and associated with the advanced tumor stage [133]. A novel somatic gene fusion of CD74, which is CD74-NRG1, was recognized as a therapeutic opportunity for invasive lung adenocarcinomas [134], and also CD74's several roles throughout the immune system, prominent ones being the association with MIF and cathepsins, promise and potential therapeutic pathway [135].

1.34. CDC25C: CELL DIVISION CYCLE 25. CHROMOSOME 5; 5q31.2

CDC25C is responsible for the encoding of a conserved protein. This protein plays a key role in the regulation of cellular division, the main functions being the suppression of p53-induced growth arrest and facilitating dephosphorylation of cyclin B-bound CDC2 following the triggering of entry towards mitosis. It was identified that the CDC25C undergoes ROS-dependent destruction and hyperphosphorylation by diallyl trisulfide-induced G2-M phase cell cycle arrest in human prostate cancer cells [136]. HSP90 inhibitors were suggested to play a therapeutic role by inhibiting lung cancer cells inducing G2-M arrest by reducing CDC25C levels [137]. CDC25C is impaired when the LZTS1 protein is downregulated or absent, eventually leading to increased susceptibility to spontaneous and carcinogen-induced cancer [138]. CDC25C was identified as one of the factors that, when overexpressed in vulvar squamous cell carcinomas, are suggested to be associated with malignant features and aggressive cancer phenotypes [139]. CDC25C was also linked with prostate cancer playing a role in the progression of cancer, suggesting usefulness in monitoring and predicting the aggressiveness of cancer [140].

1.35. CDK7: CYCLIN-DEPENDENT KINASE 7. CHROMOSOME 5; 5q13.2

CDK7 gene facilitated the coding of a protein that is a member of the cyclin-dependent protein kinase family. It is suggested that CDK7 kinase activity pharmacological modification may serve as an opportunity to identify and treat tumor types that are solely dependent on transcription for maintenance of the oncogenic state [141]. It has been stated to be relevant in triple-negative breast cancer as the TNBC cells are highly dependent on CDK7, in which its activity is critical for the expression of certain genes which are essential factors for TNBC, while the use of CDK7 inhibitors blocks the tumor growth in the patient [142]. Triptolide, a bioactive ingredient having anticancer properties, facilitates CDK-7 mediated degradation of RNA polymerase II, leading to cancer cell death and suggesting a therapeutic property [143].

1.36. CDX1: CAUDAL TYPE HOMEOBOX 1. CHROMOSOME 5; 5q32

CDX1 encodes a DNA-binding protein regulating intestine-specific gene expression and enterocyte differentiation. This gene belongs to the family of the caudal-related homeobox transcription factor gene. In colorectal cancer cell lines, CDX1 is downregulated through the aberrant DNA methylation in the CpG island in the CDX1 promoter [144]. CDX1 is also reported as a key regulator which facilitates differentiation in normal colon and colorectal cancer [145]. Aberrant expression of CDX1 was reported to be correlated with H. pylori infection and studies have suggested that CDX1 in association with CDX2 plays a key role in the progression of Gastric cancer and dysplasia [146]. CDX1 is also stated to be one of the homeobox genes to be dysregulated in colorectal cancer, suggesting the possibility of its association with colorectal cancer development and progression [147]. A study reported that ROS-induced oxidative stress leads to the silencing of CDX1 through epigenetic regulation [148].

1.37. CLPTM1L: CLEFT LIP AND PALATE TRANSMEMBRANE PROTEIN 1-LIKE PROTEIN. CHROMOSOME 5 ; 5p15.33

CLPTM1L is a gene that encodes a membrane protein that causes apoptosis when over-expressed in cisplatin-sensitive cells. Many polymorphisms in this gene facilitating cancer have been reported [149]. One polymorphism, rs2736100, in the TERT-CLPTM1L locus is reported to be significantly associated with the risk of adenocarcinoma of the lung [150]. CLPTM1L also has a common risk variant from the population, a genetic locus that is associated with estrogen receptor-negative breast cancer [151]. TERT-CLPTM1L variants have also been suggested to increase the risk of lung cancer apart from the ones induced by tobacco [152] and are a factor that increases the susceptibility to the development of lung cancer [153].

1.38. CSF1R: COLONY STIMULATING FACTOR 1 RECEPTOR. CHROMOSOME 5; 5q32

CSF1R is responsible for encoding the protein colony-stimulating factor 1 receptor (CSF-1 receptor). In most cell types, these proteins s found in the outer membrane. The association with CSF-1 receptor is that it is involved in stimulating signaling pathways, which is important for various cellular processes, including cell growth, division, maturation, and differentiation. In cancer, CSF1R inhibitors are reported to be a potential for cancer therapy [154]. Usage of CSF1R inhibitor gave good efficacy in prostate cancer and is suggested to undergo a combination therapy with radiotherapy [155]. Using CSF1R inhibitors in macrophage-targeted treatment is suggested to be a promising strategy for controlling the malignant ascites in epithelial ovarian cancer [156]. CSF1R inhibition is one of the important strategies which can be implemented for anticancer therapy and is reported in cervical and mammary tumor growth in which the inhibition of the CSF1R pathway was essential to maintain efficacious macrophage depletion [157].

1.39. CTNNA1: CATENIN ALPHA 1. CHROMOSOME 5; 5q31.2

CTNNA1 gene function in encoding protein. This protein belongs to the family of catenin. The function of this protein is that it is important for adhesion processes by creating a connected network of cadherins located on the plasma membrane to the actin filaments which are present inside the cell [158]. In Advanced myeloid malignancies, the methylation of CTNNA1, inactivation including histone modification, and methylation in the CpG promoter were reported [159]. Similarly, CTNNA1 mutation in hereditary diffuse cancer was also reported [160]. In a study restoring CTNNA1 expression in HL-60 myeloid leukemia cell lines resulted in reduced proliferation and apoptosis [161]. CTNNA1 has also been suggested to be an invasion suppressor gene [162].

1.40. CXCL14: C-X-C MOTIF CHEMOKINE LIGAND 14. CHROMOSO-ME 5; 5q31.1

CXCL14 encodes the proteins which are involved in the immunoregulatory and inflammatory processes and belong to the cytokine family. CXCL14 mRNA is considered to be very common in prostate cancer, and it is also reported that when expressed, it facilitates tumor growth inhibition stating it has tumor suppressive functions [163]. CXCL14 was also reported as one of the susceptible genes for prostate cancer. CXCL14 is upregulated in cancer-associated fibroblasts of human prostate cancer [164]. In lung cancer, CXCL14 is suggested to be an important tumor suppressor gene epigenetically silenced during lung carcinogenesis and a potential biomarker [165]. In pancreatic cancer, CXCL14 was reported to play a major role in pathobiology, suggesting its involvement in cancer invasion regulation [166]. In breast cancer, a novel pathway mediated by CXCL14 promoted breast cancer through mitochondrial dysfunction and ROS imbalance [167].

1.41. DAB2: DAB ADAPTOR PROTEIN 2. CHROMOSOME 5; 5p13.1

DAB2 is a protein-coding gene that codes for a mitogen-responsive phospho-protein. It is normally expressed in ovarian epithelial cells. It has a suggestive tumor suppressor role due to its downregulation or absence in ovarian cancer cell lines. The functionality of the protein is that it binds to the SH3 domains GRB2, adaptor protein coupling with tyrosine kinase receptor, leading to the modulation of growth factor and RAS pathways [168]. Being a tumor suppressor, when expressed, inhibits cancer growth in prostate cancer [169]. Similarly, in lung cancer, DAB2 levels were low, and the studies suggested that miR-93 facilitated the progress of lung cancer cell growth by repressing DAB2 expression [170]. DAB2 interactive protein methylation was identified to be used as a biomarker for the disease stage of malignant lung cancer [171]. DAB2 was also identified to modulate androgen receptor-mediated cell growth in both normal and malignant prostate epithelial cells, which facilitates a potential therapeutic strategy against prostate cancers [172].

1.42. DHFR: DIHYDROFOLATE REDUCTASE. CHROMOSOME 5; 5q14.1

DHFR gene codes for the enzyme Dihydrofolate reductase, which converts dihydrofolate into tetrahydrofolate. This is required for the de novo synthesis of purines, thymidylic acid, and some amino acids. A polymorphism in DHFR, DHFR 19-bp deletion, was identified to affect the transcription of the gene in humans and is associated with breast cancer risk [173, 174]. DHFR is one of the important targets which is taken into account for antifolate and anti-fluoropyrimidine-based chemotherapies [175, 176].

1.43. DROSHA: DROSHA RIBONUCLEASE III. CHROMOSOME 5; 5p13.3

DROSHA gene is responsible for encoding RNase III double-stranded RNA-specific ribonuclease and subunit of the microprocessor protein complex. The functionality is that it catalyzes the initial processing procedure of miRNA synthesis. The absence or lack of this gene would eventually affect the process of miRNA synthesis by reducing it. DROSHA dysregulation was identified in epithelial skin cancer, which suggested that miRNAs involvement in carcinogenesis [177]. DROSHA in association with DICER was found to be downregulated in endometrial cancer [178]. Dysregulation of DROSHA in triple-negative breast cancer and matching lymph node metastases were identified, in which the altered expression may serve as a potential biomarker for disrupted miRNA biogenesis [179]. P53 plays a role regulation of miRNA biogenesis in cancer by interfering with DROSHA, inhibiting the miRNA processing in cancer and facilitating carcinogenesis [180]. DROSHA, in association with DICER has also revealed its role in ovarian cancer patients [181].

1.44. DUSP1: DUAL SPECIFICITY PHOSPHATASE 1. CHROMOSOME 5; 5q35.1

DUSP is responsible for encoding the protein phosphatase, which has dual specificity for tyrosine and threonine. The role is that it dephosphorylates MAPK1/ERL2, which directs its association in various cellular processes and is also responsible for playing a role in human cellular responses to environmental stresses and negative regulation of cellular proliferation. A mechanism was reported that p53 regulates DUSP1; DUSP1 is increased abundantly after oxidative stress in p53 dependent manner and also when apoptosis is triggered [182]. DUSP1 is reported to have an association with gallbladder cancer by its ability to inhibit cell proliferation, metastasis, invasion, and angiogenesis, suggesting the signals associated with being a potential biomarker and therapeutic target for GBC suppression, and lung cancer [183, 184]. It is also considered one of the anti-apoptotic genes which are upregulated under the administration of glucocorticoid in ovarian cancer [185]. In cancer therapy, DUSP1 is suggested to play a role in tumor chemotherapy, immunotherapy, and biotherapy [186]. It's also associated with being a mediator of anti-proliferative and anti-inflammatory actions in breast cancer [187].

1.45. EBF1: EBF TRANSCRIPTION FACTOR 1. CHROMOSOME 5; 5q33.3

EBF1 was identified as a potentially important regulator of breast cancer by studying breast cancer subtypes, through specific methylation and gene expression studies [188]. EBF1 fusion as EBF1-PDGFRB was identified in acute lymphoblastic leukemia occurring within Philadelphia-like ALL subtypes, and positive patients were identified as slow responders to imatinib [189]. In colorectal cancer, overexpression of EBF1-suppressed Ribosome assembly factor PNO1 results in the inhibition of cell proliferation and induction of cell apoptosis through the p53/p21 pathway [190].

1.46. EGR1: EARLY GROWTH RESPONSE 1. CHROMOSOME 5; 5q31.2

EGR1 encodes a protein that is a member that belongs to the EGR family OF C2H2-type zinc-finger proteins. The functionality is that it is a transcriptional regulator since it is a nuclear protein, resulting in the activation of its target genes responsible for differentiation and mitogenesis. EGR1 was reported to promote the growth and survival of prostate cancer and is also responsible for the overexpression of cyclin D2 in tumorigenic prostate cells [191]. EGR1 expression has been linked to tumor suppression which directs cell cycle arrest and apoptosis through regulating tumor suppressive pathways like PTEN, which has suggested that EGR1 expression predicts PTEN levels and survival in non-small-cell lung cancer [192]. EGR1 is can also be considered a major factor for potential prostate cancer therapy [193].

1.47. FAT2: FAT ATYPICAL CADHERIN 2. CHROMOSOME 5; 5q33.1

The FAT2 gene is a human homolog of the Drosophila FAT gene. In drosophila, it encodes a tumor suppressor, which controls the cell proliferation of drosophila development. The protein of this gene in humans mostly functions as a cell adhesion molecule that controls cell proliferation [194]. FAT2 was identified as one of the cell surface markers for lung cancer due to its overexpression in lung cancer cells [195]. FAT2 was also reported as one of the genes which had differential expression between genders showing to play a role in sexual dimorphism in liver cancer [196]. FAT is also recognized as one of the gene families, frequently mutated across various types of human cancers [197].

1.48. FER: FER TYROSINE KINASE. CHROMOSOME 5 ; 5q21.3

The FER gene is responsible for encoding a protein that belongs to the FPS/FES family of non-transmembrane receptor tyrosine kinases. Its function is to regulate cell-cell adhesion and facilitates signaling from the cell surface to the cytoskeleton *via* growth factor receptors. In castrate-resistant prostate cancer, FER is said to contribute to aberrant AR signaling *via* the pSTAT cross-talks during the cancer progression [198]. FER was also suggested to be a promising target for the prevention and inhibition of metastatic breast cancer through its regulation of α6- and β1-integrin-dependent cell adhesion and anoikis resistance [199] and might also serve as a novel drug target in hepatocellular carcinoma cells [200]. In human prostate cancer, FER facilitates cancer cell growth by associating with interleukin-5 activating signal transducer and activator of transcription 3 [201].

1.49. FGF1: FIBROBLAST GROWTH FACTOR 1. CHROMOSOME 5; 5q31

FGF1 is responsible for encoding the protein, which is a member which belongs to the family of Fibroblast growth factor (FGF). The members of these families have properties that involve mitogenic and cell survival activities, involved in the biological process such as embryonic development, cell growth, morphogenesis, tissue repair, tumor growth, and invasion. The functionality of the protein is that it serves as a modifier of endothelial cellular migration and proliferation and as an angiogenic factor. Breast cancer cells generate FGF1 through expression and are suggested to play a role in the proliferation of breast cancer cells both by autocrine and paracrine mechanisms [202]. FGF signaling pathway inhibition might serve as a potential strategy for the treatment of colon cancer as the FGF1 signaling pathway in cancer-associated fibroblasts promotes tumor progression in colon cancer through ERK and MMP-7 [203]. It was reported that FGF1 is a direct downstream target of WNT7A/β- catenin which has a potential therapeutic role in ovarian cancer [204]. The Association of FGF1 isoforms has also been reported in bladder cancer [205].

1.50. FGF10: FIBROBLAST GROWTH FACTOR 10. CHROMOSOME 5; 5p12

FGF10 is responsible for making fibroblast growth factor 10, which is one of the members of the protein family of fibroblast growth factors. Fibroblast growth factors are associated with cellular processes like cell division, growth regulation, maturation, blood vessel formation, healing, and development before birth. Associating it with receptor protein FGF10 triggers various chemical reactions inside the cell, signaling them to undergo the necessary changes. FGF10 was reported to play a role in inducing cell migration and invasion in pancreatic cancer through its interaction with FGFR2 [206]. It is also identified as a candidate gene that is involved in breast cancer [207 - 209]. The FGF10/FGFR1 axis was reported to have potential therapeutic involvement in treating hormone-sensitive or refractory prostate cancer [210]. The differentiation of human stem cells into urothelial cells is stimulated by paracrine signaling of FGF10; it is also suggested to have a lead role in the growth factor of bladder regeneration [211].

1.51. FGFR4: FIBROBLAST GROWTH FACTOR RECEPTOR 4. CHROMOSOME 5; 5q35.2

FGFR4 gene encodes the protein fibroblast growth factor receptor 4, belonging to the family of fibroblast growth factor receptors. FGFR4 Arg388 genotype is recognized as one of the markers for breast cancer progression, involving patients with systemic therapy, and chemotherapy and serves the purpose of indicating therapy resistance [212, 213]. In hepatocellular carcinomas, FGFR4 is specifically targeted by a novel irreversible kinase inhibitor for treatment [214]. FGFR4 plays a role in tumor-stroma interactions when metastases occur in colorectal cancer, as well, FGFR4-associated pathways are preferentially activated in the tumor, suggesting a therapeutic strategy [215].

1.52. FLT4: FMS-RELATED RECEPTOR TYROSINE KINASE 4. CHROMOSOME 5; 5q35.3

FLT4 is responsible for encoding a protein called vascular endothelial growth factor receptor 3 (VEGFR-3), which is important for the regulation of the lymphatic system. FLT4 is considered an important prognostic factor in non-small cell lung cancer [216]. In Angiosarcoma FLT4 gene was suggested to play a role in tumor progression and might have a potential therapeutic strategy for targeting [217]. Invasion and metastasis of many cancer types were reported to be promoted by associations of the VEGF-C/FLT4 axis [218]. Even bladder cancer FLT4 and VEGF-D were suggested to be potential prediction tools and control bladder cancer progression [219]. FLT4 is suggested to be a target for antiangiogenic therapy in breast cancer [220].

1.53. GDNF: GLIAL CELL-DERIVED NEUROTROPHIC FACTOR. CHROMOSOME 5; 5p13.2

GDNF gene is responsible for the production of a ligand belonging to the family of TGF-β superfamily proteins. The function of these ligands is to bind to the TGF-β receptors to result in the activation of SMAD transcription factors and regulate gene expression. GDNF was reported as a key factor that enhances perineural invasion by facilitating GDNF-RET protooncogene signaling [221]. VEGF-VEGFR interaction is supposedly increased by GDNF, which leads to the migration of cells in colon cancer [222]. GDNF signaling through the GDNF receptor enhanced integrin expression, which resulted in a strong influence on the invasion and adhesion of ECM proteins by pancreatic cancer cells [223]. It was also reported that GDNF and RET upregulation might participate in glucose-induced cancer progression [224].

1.54. GPX3: GLUTATHIONE PEROXIDASE 3. CHROMOSOME 5; 5q33.1

GPX3 encodes a protein belonging to the family of glutathione peroxidase, responsible for catalyzing the reduction of organic hydroperoxides and hydrogen peroxide by glutathione resulting in the protection of cells from oxidative stress. In gastric cancer, GPX3 was downregulated, and promoter methylation was identified as the reason for the downregulation [72]. It was suggested that positive ALDH1A3 and negative GPX3 expressions are linked with pathological behaviors and poor prognosis of gall bladder cancer [225]. GPX3 has an immunomodulatory role that limits the development of colitis-associated carcinomas [226]. In relevance to certain studies, GPX3 was said to have tumor suppressor activity stating it to be a tumor suppressor gene [227]. GPX3 levels in the serum of patients having papillary serous ovarian cancer have suggested GPX3 associations in understanding clinical therapeutics, which is beneficial for treatment strategy [228]. It was reported that methylation of GPX3 would have implications for chemotherapy response and clinical outcomes of head and neck cancer patients [229].

1.55. HAVCR2: HEPATITIS A VIRUS CELLULAR RECEPTOR 2. CHROMOSOME 5; 5q33.3

HAVCR2 is responsible for encoding the protein, which is a member that belongs to the immunoglobulin family and TIM family of proteins. It is a cell surface receptor that modulates innate and adaptive immune responses. HAVCR2 was identified as a potentially novel mechanism in regulating the T cells suggesting new pathways for modulating immune checkpoint blockade [230]. It was reported that individuals with HAVCR2 mutations were identified to be highly susceptible to sporadic subcutaneous panniculitis-like T-cell lymphoma [231]. HAVCR2 is suggested to be involved in the pathogenesis of malignant tumors and the progress of many cancer types [232]. HAVCR2 Expression was significantly high in adenocarcinomas[137] and non-small cell lung cancer [233].

1.56. HBEGF: HEPARIN-BINDING EGF-LIKE GROWTH FACTOR. CHROMOSOME 5; 5q31.3

HBEGF is a protein-coding gene that is essential for cardiac valve development, and normal heart function promotes smooth cell proliferation and might have an involvement in macrophage-mediated cell proliferation. This growth factor also mediates its effects through EGFR, ERBB2, and ERBB4. In breast cancer, anti-HBEGF systems were suggested to be a useful treatment method for HBEGF-expressing cells [234]. In breast cancer enhanced tumor invasion which is independent of macrophage signaling was a resultant of short-circuiting the tumor cell/macrophage paracrine invasion loop by expressing HBEGF at high levels [235]. HBEGF is already an established potent inducer of tumor growth and angiogenesis [236]. H. pylori infections increase HBEGF expression levels, suggesting a role of HBEGF in gastric cancer, providing potential targets for therapeutic in H. pylori-induced gastric cancer [237].

1.57. HDAC3: HISTONE DEACETYLASE 3. CHROMOSOME 5; 5q31.3

HDAC3 gene encodes for the protein enzyme histone deacetylase 3, which is responsible for the deacetylation of lysine residues on the N-terminal part of the core histones. It was identified that HDAC3 inhibitors played a potential role in therapeutics by favoring the elimination of the transformed cells by increasing the immunogenicity of epithelial tumors [238]. A novel mechanism in which SOX2 was associated with HDAC3 to suppress microRNA-31 promoting tumor progression in invasive esophageal carcinomas [239]. HDAC3 plays a central role in regulating cellular proliferation and differentiation in colon cancer cells [240]. HDAC3 associates itself with repressing p21, which suggests that the growth inhibitory and apoptotic effects induced by HDAC3 inhibitors are the results of the inhibition of multiple HDAC3 [241]. It is suggested that Epigenetic programming alteration occurs because of HDAC3 overexpression in colon cancer cells which impacts intracellular Wnt signaling [242].

1.58. HINT1: HISTIDINE TRIAD NUCLEOTIDE-BINDING PROTEIN 1. CHROMOSOME 5; 5q23.3

HINT1 gene encodes the protein histidine triad nucleotide-binding protein 1. It is said to have properties to bind to nucleotide molecules and break down nucleotides through hydrolysis *in vitro*. The protein is also said to have involvement in cell apoptosis, blocking the activity of the certain gene and acting as a tumor suppressor. The tumor-suppressing activity of HINT1 was reported in melanoma cells by influencing the formation of non-functional complexes and oncogenic transcription factors [243]. tumor suppression activity in colon cancer was suggested to occur by HINT1 inhibiting the AP-1 activity by binding to the POSH-JNK2 complex [244]. In human hepatoma cells, HINT1 was reported to inhibit β-catenin/TCF3, USF2, and NFκB activity [245]. HINT1 promoter hypermethylation was suggested to play a role in hepatocarcinogenesis [246]. HINT1 expression was found to be low in gastric cancer [247].

1.59. HMMR: HYALURONAN-MEDIATED MOTILITY RECEPTOR. CHROMOSOME 5; 5q34

HMMR encodes a protein receptor that is associated with cell motility, expressed in breast tissue, and forms a complex with BRCA1 and BRCA2, resulting in potential associations in breast cancer risk. HMMR was identified as one of the genes that are novel and important regulators of adipogenesis [248]. HMMR locus is widely associated with a higher risk of breast cancer in humans [249]. HMMR was also reported as a candidate therapeutic target for Glioblastoma stem-like cells and its treatment strategy [250]. A non-coding RNA association HMMR was identified to be considered as a novel prognostic factor in epithelial ovarian cancer [251].

1.60. IL12B: INTERLEUKIN 12B. CHROMOSOME 5 ; 5q33.3

IL12B is responsible for the coding of a subunit belonging to interleukin 12, which is a cytokine that has broad activities by acting on T and natural killer cells. Polymorphism occurring in this gene is widely associated with cervical cancer, which is studied in various populations [252 - 254]. This gene is categorized as a proinflammatory cytokine having pleiotropic effects, having regulatory control over T- lymphocytes and NK responses which are critical for the protection against cancer and other infectious diseases [255]. It was identified that STAT3-dependent expression of NFIL3 plays an important role as a key factor of a negative feedback pathway in myeloid cells that suppresses the proinflammatory responses of IL12B [256].

1.61. IL13: INTERLEUKIN 13. CHROMOSOME 5 ; 5q31.1

IL13 gene codes for a cytokine responsible for immunoregulation which is produced by the activation of Th2 cells. This cytokine is specifically associated with B-cell maturation and differentiation. The functionality of this cytokine is that it upregulates the expression of CD23 and MHC class II and facilitates the promotion of IgE isotype switching to B cell; similarly, it downregulates macrophage activity which results in the inhibition of the production of pro-inflammatory cytokines [257] and chemokines [258, 259]. It was reported that IL13 might be involved in the mediation of CD4+ NKT cells which negatively regulates immunosurveillance in non-regressor tumor in syngeneic colon cancer and lung metastasis was significantly decreased by treatment of IL13 inhibitors in mice [260]. IL13 expression is reported to play a critical role in colon cancer invasion and metastasis, as higher expression levels were reported in later stages of disease progression [261]. IL13 targeting has been reported to play an important role which suggests the killing of primary tumor cells and also prevents cancer metastases, as IL13 is involved in cancer metastasis through the activation of ERK/AP1 [262].

1.62. IL4: INTERLEUKIN 4. CHROMOSOME 5; 5q31.1

IL4 is responsible for the coding of pleiotropic cytokine produced by activated T cells. This particular cytokine acts as a ligand for the interleukin 4 receptor. This receptor binds to IL13, which associates itself with various overlapping functions of this cytokine and IL13. IL4 mediation is reported to be carried out by STAT6, which is a signal transducer and activator of transcription [263]. Human neurological cancer cells are said to express IL4, which was identified as the prime target for the cytotoxic effects of IL4 toxin [264]. IL4 induced through STAT6 has been reported to affect breast cancer through its association with apoptosis and gene expression in breast cancer cells [265], similarly in colon cancer cells [266]. IL4 is an important regulator, which can induce cathepsin protease activity which becomes a critical mediator for promoting cancer growth and invasion [267]. IL4 in association with IL13 is suggested to be one of the targets to approach for cancer therapy [257].

1.63. IL6ST: INTERLEUKIN 6 SIGNAL TRANSDUCER. CHROMOSOME 5; 5q11.2

IL6ST encodes the protein, which is a signal transducer that is used by many cytokines such as interleukin 6 (IL6), ciliary neurotrophic factor (CNTF), leukemia inhibitory factor (LIF), and oncostatin M (OSM). The functionality of this protein is that it is a part of the cytokine receptor complex, while activation of this protein is associated with the binding of cytokines to their receptors. miR-188-5p was identified to have a potential therapeutic potential. In breast cancer, as it was differentially expressed, studies have reported that it facilitates cellular proliferation and migration through IL6ST [268]; IL6ST is also reported to be fundamentally associated with tumor progression and tumor aggressiveness in breast cancer, suggesting it to be a potential therapeutic target [269]. In gastric cancer, PLXNC1 was seen to undergo upregulation associated with poor prognosis and was found to be associated with IL6ST by transcriptional activation of IL6ST to enhance carcinogenesis [270].

1.64. IL7R: INTERLEUKIN 7 RECEPTOR. CHROMOSOME 5; 5p13.2

IL7R is responsible for the coding of the interleukin 7 protein receptor alpha chain. These receptors are embedded in the cell membrane of immune cells. IL7R mutations were reported to associate with the development of diverse types acute leukemias [271]. Bromodomain BET inhibition is a promising therapeutic strategy, which is suggested to be a promising therapeutic strategy, and this achieved by targeting c-MYC and IL7R [272]. Mutation in IL7R promotes cellular transformation and tumor formation as the mutational activation is linked to human T-cell leukemogenesis [273].

1.65. IRF1: INTERFERON REGULATORY FACTOR 1. CHROMOSOME 5; 5q31.1

IRF1 codes for a transcriptional regulator and is a tumor suppressor, which acts as an activator of genes associated with both innate and acquired immune responses. Defects in this gene have been associated with various types of cancer like gastric, myelogenous leukemia, and lung cancer. IRF1 plays a vital role in mediating the mitochondrial apoptotic pathway in IRF1 induced apoptosis in cancer cells through upregulation of PUMA (P53 upregulated modulator of apoptosis) [274]. In human gastric cancer, the loss of IRF1 was found to be critical for development [275]. Identified crosstalk between STAT1, DTX3L, and ARTD-like mono-ADP-ribosyl transferases facilitates proliferation and survival of metastatic prostate cancer by inhibiting IRF1 [276]. IRF1 is also reported to play a central role in influencing different tumor phenotypes [277].

1.66. ITGA1: INTEGRIN SUBUNIT ALPHA 1. CHROMOSOME 5; 5q11.2

ITGA1 is a protein-coding gene that codes for the alpha 1 subunit of integrin receptors [278]. In cancer cells expressing high Grb2, an anticancer property with a therapeutic potential can be promoted by inhibiting ITGA1 and Grb2 while suppressing the ERK phosphorylation [279]. ITGA1 is carried out by MYC, which was identified and reported as a key regulator [280]. MYC, in association with ITGA1, plays a role in colorectal cancers [281]. In pancreatic cancer, ITGA1 is suggested to be a pre-malignant biomarker that facilitates the promotion of therapy resistance and metastatic potential [282]. ITGA1 was also identified as participating in regulating drug resistance in ovarian cancer [283].

1.67. ITK: IL2 INDUCIBLE T CELL KINASE. CHROMOSOME 5; 5q33.3

ITK is responsible for the coding of intracellular tyrosine kinase expressed in T-cells. This protein includes SH2 and SH3 domains, which are common in intra-cellular kinases. The function of this protein is that it is said to have a role in T-cell proliferation and differentiation. ITK inhibitors have been used to treat inflammation, cancer, and autoimmunity [284, 285]. A fusion of ITK as ITK-SYK is suggested as an oncogene that is the cause of T-cell lymphoproliferative disease in mice which mimics the human disease [286].

1.68. LIFR: LIF RECEPTOR SUBUNIT ALPHA. CHROMOSOME 5; 5p13.1

LIFR gene encodes for the protein leukemia inhibitory factor. This receptor protein surrounds the cell membrane allowing ligands to bind. Important for the normal development of and functioning of the autonomous nervous system, blocking the growth of leukemic cells. In colon cancer development, a common inactivation event is a decrease in specific LIFR expression and cancer-specific methylation [287]. In ERα-positive breast cancer cells, LIFR association as PAK4/LIFR axis play a role in breast-to-bone metastasis [288]. LIFR is a novel suppressor gene suggested in hepatocellular carcinoma [289]. In colorectal cancers, IL-8 levels are significantly upregulated by LIFR, resulting in the promotion of tumor angiogenesis [290]. LIFR is also suggested to be a prognostic marker and a metastasis suppressor in breast cancer [291].

1.69. LOX: LYSYL OXIDASE. CHROMOSOME 5; 5q23.1

LOX encodes a protein that is a member of the lysyl oxidase family of proteins. It is suggested to play a role in the post-translational oxidative deamination of peptidyl lysine residues in precursors to fibrous collagen and elastin. LOX is upregulated in human pancreatic cancer and is suggested to play a critical role in cellular proliferation, suggesting LOX inhibitors to be a potential therapeutic approach [292]. LOX/hypoxia axis is suggested to reverse many properties of pancreatic cancer aggravation, and its inhibition is identified to evade metastasis, enhancing drug efficacy [293]. LOX has been reported to play a role in cancer cell invasion in breast cancer [294]. LOX association involves regulating tumor progression, invasion, and metastasis [295]. LOX family have been reported both to upregulate and downregulated in stromal and tumor cells in various cancer types [296].

1.70. MAML1: MASTERMIND-LIKE TRANSCRIPTIONAL COACTIVATOR 1. CHROMOSOME 5; 5q35.3

The MAML1 gene is the human homolog of the drosophila protein mastermind, which plays a role in the notch signaling pathway associated with cell fate determination [297]. It was suggested that MAML1 is a part of the transcriptional networks that regulateg the EGR1 target genes during nephrogenesis, and is reported to have associations with the development of renal cancer [298]. In esophageal cancer, MAML1 is utilized for targeted therapy by eliminating CD44+ cancer stem cells *via* the inhibiby inhibiting NOTCH pathway [299]. Apart from NOTCH regulation, MAML1 acts as a coactivator for p53 [300, 301]. In cervical cancer cell lines, it was reported that the regulation of cell viability is carried out by MAML1 through the NFκB pathway [302]. MAML1 is suggested to be a molecular marker of advanced tumors helping to determine the characteristics and aggressiveness in Esophageal squamous cell carcinoma [303].

1.71. MAP3K1: MITOGEN-ACTIVATED PROTEIN KINASE KINASE KINASE 1. CHROMOSOME 5; 5q11.2

MAP3K1 is responsible for encoding the protein which functions to regulate signaling pathways controlling various biological processes. MAP3K1 is reported to be having genetic variants which facilitate susceptibility to breast cancer [304]. In breast cancer, MAP3K puts forth an important oncogenic property in developing breast cancer cells which suggest that targeting MAP3K1 through artificial miRNA is a potential therapeutic strategy [305]. MAP3K1 was found to have mutations in Langerhans cell histiocytosis [306]. MAP3K mutations are frequent in breast, prostate, and colon cancer, and they can be linked as a potential drug target with the combination of MEK inhibitors [306].

1.72. MCC: MCC REGULATOR OF WNT SIGNALING PATHWAY. CHROMOSOME 5; 5q22.2

MCC is a potential colorectal tumor suppressor gene and is suggested to negatively regulate the cell cycle progression. Abnormalities in the MCC gene are also associated with gastric cancer [307]. Polymorphism of the MCC gene is also reported to be associated with Human small-cell lung cancer [308]. MCC has also been linked to playing a role in breast cancer [309].

1.73. MEF2C: MYOCYTE ENHANCER FACTOR 2C. CHROMOSOME 5; 5q14.3

MEF2C gene instructs to encode the protein, which is a member of the MADS-box transcription enhancer factor 2 (MEF2) family. Deregulation of MEF2C expression was reported to accelerate myeloid leukemia [310]. MEF2C is identified as an oncogene in T-lineage acute lymphoblastic leukemia, a malignancy of thymocytes [311]. MEF2C functions as a regulator of cell proliferation [312]. MEF2C inhibition has been suggested to have a therapeutic potential in hepatic cancer [313].

1.74. MTRR: 5-METHYLTETRAHYDROFOLATE-HOMOCYSTEINE METHYLTRANSFERASE REDUCTASE. CHROMOSOME 5; 5q15.31

MTRR gene encodes for the protein enzyme methionine synthase reductase. This protein plays an important role in the proper functioning of methionine synthase, which is a protein that helps in processing amino acids. MTRR polymorphisms have been identified and reported to be susceptible to sporadic colon cancer [314], breast cancer [315 - 317], and pancreatic cancer [318]. Associations of polymorphic variants have also been identified in prostate [319] and colorectal cancers [320, 321].

1.75. NEUROG1: NEUROGENIN 1. CHROMOSOME 5 ; 5q14.3

NEUROG1 is a protein-coding gene that acts as a transcriptional regulator and is suggested to be involved in the initiation of neuronal differentiation. NEUROG1 is reported to play a role in medulloblastomas [322]. NEUROG1 methylation is frequent in patients with colorectal cancers [323].

1.76. NSD1: NUCLEAR RECEPTOR BINDING SET DOMAIN PROTEIN 1. CHROMOSOME 5; 5q35.3

The NSD1 gene is responsible for the coding of a protein functioning as a histone methyltransferase which is an enzyme having the ability to modify histones. Frameshift mutations of NSD1 have been reported in colorectal cancer [324]. NSD1 inhibitors are associated with epigenetic therapy of cancers [325]. NSD1 is suggested to play a role in tumorigenesis [326]. NSD1 mutations have been identified to have an important role in skin cancer. The inactivation of NSD1 has resulted in causing epigenetic deregulation across cancer sites and suggests associations with immunotherapy [327].

1.77. PITX1: PAIRED LIKE HOMEODOMAIN 1. CHROMOSOME 5; 5q35.3

PITX1 gene encodes for the protein, which plays an important role in the development of lower limbs, primarily found in developing legs and feet. Also identified in the developing pituitary gland, suggesting it plays a role in the development of the gland and tissues derived from the branchial arch. In non-small cell lung cancer, a miRNA was identified for the progression and cell proliferation of cancer by downregulating PITX1 [328]. PITX1 is reported to have the ability to suppress tumorigenicity by downregulation of RAS activity [329]. PITX1 is also suggested to be one of the genes which are involved in Barrett's-associated adenocarcinoma [330]. In gastric cancer, a miRNA identified to promote cell malignancy achieves the effect through PITX1 downregulation [331]. PITX1 has been associated with breast cancer as an ERα transcriptional target, which functions as a repressor to coordinate and target specific ERα mediated transcriptional activity in the cancer cells [332]. PITX1 is also responsible for the direct transcriptional targeting of p53 [333].

1.78. PDGFRB: PLATELET-DERIVED GROWTH FACTOR RECEPTOR BETA. CHROMOSOME 5; 5q32

PDGFRB gene encodes platelet-derived growth factor receptor beta, which is a member belonging to the family of proteins named receptor tyrosine kinases. The protein is found in the cell membrane of certain cell types in which the platelet-derived growth factor binds to the receptor activating other proteins inside the cells. PDGFRB expression is reported to be induced in cancer stem cell properties of gastric cancer. PDGFRB is deregulated in non-small cell lung cancer [334]. gain of function point mutations in PDGFRB was identified in patients with familial infantile myofibramatosis [335]. P53 regulates PDGFRB receptor-mediated signaling to drive pancreatic cancer metastasis [336]. In esophageal cancer, SATB1 plays an oncogenic role by upregulating PDGFRB [337].

1.79. PLK2: POLO-LIKE KINASE 2. CHROMOSOME 5; 5q11.2

PLK2 is a protein-coding gene in which the protein belongs to the family of serine/threonine protein kinases, playing a role in normal cellular division. PLK2 is associated with tuberculosis sclerosis complex proteins which affect affecting, tumor growth, and chemosensitivity under hypoxic conditions [338]. PLK2 is a target for p53 and has been reported to be lost in colorectal carcinomas [339]. PLK2 is suggested to be an important representative as an independent prognostic marker, regulating tumor growth and apoptosis in colorectal cancer, suggesting PLK2 as a potential target [340]. PLK2 inhibitors provide potential therapeutic strategies [341].

1.80. POLK: DNA POLYMERASE KAPPA. CHROMOSOME 5; 5q13.3

POLK gene instructs to code for a protein that is a member belonging to the DNA polymerase type-Y family of proteins [342]. The protein is a special DNA polymerase that catalyzes translesion DNA synthesis, allowing DNA replication in the presence of DNA lesions. POLK polymorphism influences the susceptibility toward breast cancer [343]. POLK is associated with p53 as loss of p53 function led to the upregulation of POLK in human lung cancer [344]. POLK core somatic mutations were reported in prostate cancer which alters translesion DNA synthesis [345].

1.81. PTTG1: PTTG1 REGULATOR OF SISTER CHROMATID SEPARATION, SECURING. CHROMOSOME 5; 5q33.3

PTTG1 gene codes for the homolog of yeast securing proteins. The function of this protein is that it prevents separins from promoting sister chromatid separation. It was found that PTTG1 negatively regulates the ability of p53 to induce apoptosis in hepatoma cell lines where PTTG1 is overexpressed [346]. In prostate cancer cells, SMAD3 is inhibited by PTTG1, facilitating the advancement of the proliferation of the cells [347]. A miRNA (Mir-186) is modulated by PTTG1, which results in promoting the migration and invasion of human non-small cell lung cancer cells [348]. PTTG1 is identified as a prognostic factor that acts as an oncogene in colorectal cancers. Experiments proved that PTTG1 knockdown facilitated the inhibition of colorectal cancer growth and metastasis [349]. PTTG1 is reported to promote malignancy by facilitating epithelial to mesenchymal transition by activation of AKT, suggesting PTTG1 is a potential target for therapy in breast cancer [350, 351].

1.82. PRLR: PROLACTIN RECEPTOR. CHROMOSOME 5; 5p13.2

PRLR gene is responsible for providing instructions to code for anterior pituitary hormone prolactin, which is a member belonging to the type I cytokine receptor family. Prolactin has a pathogenic role in human breast cancer in which the mediation is carried out by PRLR [352]. PRLR is one important gene that is studied under breast cancer type as it plays a major important role and strategizing therapies through PRLR targeting [353 - 355]. The Association of PRLR has also been linked to Prostate cancer [356].

1.83. RAD50: RAD50 DOUBLE STRAND BREAK REPAIR PROTEIN. CHROMOSOME 5; 5q31.1

RAD5O encodes a protein involved in double-strand break repair. The protein is said to form a complex with MRE11 and NSB1; through binding to DNA, it facilitates numerous enzymatic activities required for the nonhomologous joining of DNA. It is also involved in cell cycle checkpoint activation, telomere maintenance and meiotic recombination. In breast cancer, RAD50 is one of the identified genes associated with breast cancer risk and is also said to be associated with ovarian cancer [357 - 361].

1.84. RICTOR: RPTOR INDEPENDENT COMPANION OF MTOR COMPLEX 2. CHROMOSOME 5 ; 5p13.1

RICTOR is associated as a part of a protein complex that integrates nutrient and growth factor-derived signals resulting in the regulation of cell growth. RICTOR has been stated to play a role in cancer onset and progression [362]. RICTOR forms a complex with mTOR, phosphorylates, and activates Akt. RICTOR is said to have a role in the accumulation of cyclin E and c-myc in colorectal cancer cells [363]. Promoting Akt regulation is one of the important steps RICTOR is associated with, which is achieved through the regulation of ILK [364]. RICTOR contributes a central role in oral cancer; a tumor suppressive miRNA was identified to target RICTOR, which facilitates inhibition of AKT phosphorylation in oral cancer [365]. It is suggested that sustained Akt activation while mTOR inhibition counteracts the anticancer efficacy of mTOR inhibitors [366]. In breast cancer, RICTOR is reported to be an important mediator of chemotaxis and metastasis [367].

1.85. RACK1: RECEPTOR FOR ACTIVATED C KINASE 1. CHROMOSOME 5; 5q35.3

The RACK1 gene is a protein-coding gene that is related to pathways like ERK signaling and TNF signaling. In chronic pancreatitis and pancreatic cancer, RACK1 supposedly plays a role through the expression patterns of Protein Kinase

C Isoenzymes [368]. Overexpression of RACK1 was reported in colon cancer [369]. In Squamous cell lung cancer cells, RACK1 facilitates growth and migration by forming a complex with FGFR1 and PKM2 [370].

1.86. SPRY4: SPROUTY RTK SIGNALING ANTAGONIST 4. CHROMOSOME 5; 5q31.3

SPRY4 gene gives instructions to code a protein member belonging to the family of cysteine and proline-rich proteins; this protein acts as an inhibitor of the receptor-transduced mitogen-activated protein kinases (MAPK) signaling pathway. SPRY4 is suggested to be a potential tumor suppressor in prostate cancer, having negative regulation of fibroblast growth signaling factor [371].

SPRY4 is considered to be the molecular switch for MAPK signaling [372]. SPRY4 associates itself with the Urokinase plasminogen activator by its degradation leading to the inhibition of uPAR-mediated cell adhesion and proliferation [373]. Rhabdomyosarcoma tumors carrying mutated RAS genes were identified to regress through the silencing of SPRY [374, 375].

1.87. SDHA: SUCCINATE DEHYDROGENASE COMPLEX FLAVOPROTEIN SUBUNIT A. CHROMOSOME 5 ; 5p15.33

SDHA encodes for making one of the four subunits of succinate dehydrogenase enzyme. This enzyme plays a role in the mitochondria and is linked to important pathways in energy conversion, the Krebs cycle, and oxidative phosphorylation. SDHA is suggested to contribute a role in hereditary pheochromocytoma and paraganglioma [376]. A mutation in SDHA was reported under pituitary adenoma [377]. SDHA mutations are also associated with neuroblastoma tumorigenesis [378]. SDHA loss is found in gastrointestinal tumors suggesting SDHA mutations [379, 380]. SDHA loss was also observed in breast cancer [381].

1.88. SELENOP: SELENOPROTEIN P. CHROMOSOME 5 ; 5p12

SELENOP is responsible for giving instructions to code for the protein selenoprotein, which is predominantly expressed in the liver and secreted into the plasma. SELENOP contributes a role in indicating an interactive role with the selenium status in prostate cancer [382 - 384]. In colorectal cancers, altered expression of SELENOP is considered to serve as a marker of functional Selenium status and colorectal adenoma to cancer progression [385]. SELENOP polymorphism is identified to be one of the causes of the selenium levels in human breast carcinoma tissues [386].

1.89. SKP1: S-PHASE KINASE-ASSOCIATED PROTEIN 1. CHROMO-SOME 5; 5q31.1

SKP1 gene codes for a unit of SCF complexes that plays a role in various cellular processes and physiological dysfunctions in cancer biology. SKP1 is the central regulator of the SCF complex [387]. SKP1 associated with the SCF has been suggested for an SCF-based knockout system which plays as a tool to target abnormal proteins that effects growth and transformation [388]. SKP has been reported to play a role in skin cancer [389].

1.90. SMAD5: SMAD FAMILY MEMBER 5. CHROMOSOME 5; 5q31.1

SMAD5 is involved in encoding the protein which associates with the transforming growth factor beta signaling pathway resulting in inhibition of the proliferation of hematopoietic progenitor cells. SMAD5 is associated with TGFβ signaling. A miRNA (miRNA-155) directly targets SMAD5, linking to the TGFβ pathway and lymphomagenesis [390]. SMAD5 is suggested to be a tumor suppressor candidate in the human leukemia cell line [391]. SMAD5, in association with the BMP4 signal transduction pathway, can activate hematopoietic differentiation, which is impaired in anemia manifestations in secondary myelodysplasias and Acute myeloid leukemia patients having SMAD5 haploinsufficiency [392]. SMAD5 is recognized as a candidate myeloid tumor suppressor [393]. SMADs are identified to be critical for the development of ovaries and testis when disrupted, leading to malignant transformation [394]. SMAD5 overexpression was reported in the hepatocellular carcinoma cell line (Hep-40) [395]. SMAD5, in association with SMAD1, functions together to govern BMP target gene expression in the early mammalian embryo [396].

1.91. SPARC: SECRETED PROTEIN ACIDIC AND CYSTEINE-RICH. CHROMOSOME 5; 5q33.1

SPARC gene is involved in providing instructions to code for cysteine-rich acidic matric protein which is required for the collagen in the bone to become calcified, and is also involved in extracellular matrix synthesis and facilitating cellular shape changes. Upregulation of SPARC has been stated to be a poor prognostic factor in head and neck cancer. SPARC helps albumin accumulation in the tumor [397]. SPARC is associated with adipogenesis as it modulates interactions between cells and extracellular matrix and proved to have an anticancer role [398]. Host SPARC was reported to normalize the microenvironment of ovarian cancer malignant sites by achieving the repression of VEGF -the integrin MMP axis [399]. SPARC has also been stated to be associated with and responsible for cancer progression [400]. In ovarian cancer cells, SPARC induced apoptosis [401]. In cancer cells, gamma-linolenic acid is the key regulator of SPARC secretion [402].

1.92. SPINK1: SERINE PEPTIDASE INHIBITOR KAZAL TYPE 1. CHROMOSOME 5; 5q32

SPINK1 gene encodes a trypsin inhibitor secreted in the pancreatic acinar cells into pancreatic juice. The function of this protein is suggested to be the prevention of trypsin-catalyzed premature activation of zymogens within the pancreas and the pancreatic duct. High expression of SPINK1 was first reported in ovarian cancer and later has been seen in many cancer types [403]. In prostate cancer, SPINK1 is targeted as a strategy for a therapeutic role [404]. Polymorphisms in SPINK1 have been reported in both sporadic and familial pancreatic types [405]. Metallothionein expression is downregulated by SPINK1which leads to the contribution of SPINK1 in promoting the progression of colorectal cancer [406]. SPINK1 inhibition may increase the risk of pancreatitis and is suggested to be a potential biomarker for cancer therapy [407]. SPINK1 is widely studied in prostate cancer studies [404, 408-410].

1.93. TCF7: TRANSCRIPTION FACTOR 7. CHROMOSOME 5; 5q31.1

TCF7 gene is responsible for encoding a member belonging to the T-cell factor/lymphoid enhancer binding factor family or known as the High mobility group box transcriptional activators. TCF7 long noncoding RNA is suggested to be a potential novel diagnostic biomarker and a therapeutic target for colorectal cancer treatment [411]. TCF7 is also suggested to be a prognostic factor for gastric cancer [412]. A miRNA was identified to regulate TCF7/WNT signaling, which led to the inhibition of bone metastasis in prostate cancer activated by RAS [413]. In human osteosarcoma, upregulation of microRNA-192 targeted TCF7, inhibiting cell growth and invasion and leading to cell apoptosis [414].

1.94. TERT: TELOMERASE REVERSE TRANSCRIPTASE. CHROMO-SOME 5 ; 5p15.33

TERT is responsible for making one of the components required for forming the enzyme telomerase. TERT-CLPTM1L locus sequence variants were identified to be associated with various types of cancer [415] TERT locus is categorized as a general cancer susceptible locus [416]. TERT promoter mutations have been reported in certain cancer types [417]. TERT variants are also associated with testicular germ cell cancer [418]. In cancer, the GABP transcription factor is said to have a selective binding property and activated mutant TERT promoter [419]. In urothelial cancer, TERT promoter mutations and telomerase reactivation have been reported [420].

1.95. TGFB1: TRANSFORMING GROWTH FACTOR BETA-INDUCED. CHROMOSOME 5; 5q31.1

TGFB1 gene encodes transforming growth factor beta-1; it facilitates chemical signaling that regulates various cellular activities, which includes proliferation, differentiation, motility, and apoptosis. TGFB1 polymorphisms have been repor ted in breast cancer and are said to be associated with higher risk [421, 422]. Similarly, TGFB1 polymorphism was reported in gastric cancer [423, 424]. TGFB1 was identified to play a role in advanced-stage prostate cancer, where the identified variant affected the expression of TGFβ1 [425]. TGFB1 is suggested to be one of the genes to be a potential target for prostate cancer and benign prostatic hyperplasia [426].

1.96. TLX3: T CELL LEUKEMIA HOMEOBOX 3. CHROMOSOME 5; 5q35.1

TLX3 gene encodes an orphan homeobox protein which then encodes a DNA-binding nuclear transcription factor. TLX3 methylation is considered a potential novel biomarker for cisplatin resistance, to have a therapeutic strategy to counteract the resistance in bladder cancer [427]. TLX3 locus has been reported as a target for studies related to T-cell acute lymphoblastic leukemia [428]. The t(5;14)(q35;q32) chromosomal translocation is one of the important associations in T-cell acute lymphoblastic leukemia [429 - 433].

1.97. TRIO: TRIO RHO GUANINE NUCLEOTIDE EXCHANGE FACTOR. CHROMOSOME 5; 5p15.2

TRIO gene is responsible for encoding a large protein that functions as a GDP to GTP exchange factor. The function of these proteins is that facilitates the reorganization of the actin cytoskeleton, playing a role in cell migration and growth. TRIO expression is high in breast tumors and frequent in those with poor prognoses [434]. TRIO plays a role in cell migration of breast cancer, where CDH1 recruits TRIO to the plasma membrane to activate RAS. This novel signaling mechanism contributes to cellular migration [435]. In urinary bladder cancer, TRIO is associated with tumor growth and tumor cell proliferation [436].

It is also suggested to have a role in the invasion and metastasis of colorectal cancer [437].

1.98. VCAN: VERSICAN. CHROMOSOME 5; 5q14.2-q14.3

VCAN gene encodes for the protein Versican, a proteoglycan. It has several sugar molecules attached to it; this protein is found in the extracellular matrix of various tissues and organs. The function of this protein is to associate itself with other proteins and molecules to ensure extracellular matrix stability. VCAN is differentially expressed in gastric cancer and is reported as a potential prognostic biomarker [438]. VCAN functions in ECM regulating tumor cell behavior, essential for cancer-associated fibroblast function to inhibit cancer growth [439]. In advanced-stage serous ovarian cancer, VCAN was found to be upregulated [440]. It is also a suggested prognostic biomarker for disease recurrence in colon cancer [441].

1.99.   XRCC4:   X-RAY   REPAIR   CROSS-COMPLEMENTING   4. CHROMOSOME 5; 5q14.2

XCCR4 encodes a protein that functions with DNA ligase IV, DNA-dependent protein kinase. The function of the protein is that it plays a part in both nonhomologous ends joining and the completion of V(D)J recombination. XCC-R4 polymorphism has been reported in bladder cancer populations [442, 443]. A polymorphism variant of XCCR4 was reported to contribute to colorectal carcinogenesis [443]. Other polymorphisms of this gene are reported to be associated with oral cancer [444, 445], urothelial bladder cancer [446] and breast cancer.

CONCLUSION

The chapter has defined several genes associated with chromosome 5. The insights from the chapter indicate that cancer types such as lung, breast and prostate cancers are very important as genes are associated with chromosome 5. Important studies have been targeted in chromosome 5 to identify genes targeting Acute Myeloid Leukemia and Myelodysplastic syndromes. Relative association of genes in sarcomas and melanomas have also been indicated in the chapter giving a concise indication of the contribution of chromosome 5 in cancer genetics.

REFERENCES

[1]   Chen B, Wang C, Zhang J, *et al.* New insights into long noncoding RNAs and pseudogenes in prognosis of renal cell carcinoma Cancer Cell Int 2018; 18: 1-12.

[2]   M S, N Z, KA, B, *et al.* Metabolic shifts induced by fatty acid synthase inhibitor orlistat in non- small cell lung carcinoma cells provide novel pharmacodynamic biomarkers for positron emission tomography and magnetic resonance spectroscopy Mol imaging Biol 2013; 15: 136-47.

[3]   Kettunen E, Hernandez-Vargas H, Cros MP, *et al.* Asbestos-associated genome-wide DNA methylation changes in lung cancer. Int J Cancer 2017; 141(10): 2014-29.
        [http://dx.doi.org/10.1002/ijc.30897] [PMID: 28722770]

[4]   Krupp M, Weinmann A, Galle PR, Teufel A. Actin binding LIM protein 3 (abLIM3). Int J Mol Med 2006; 17(1): 129-33.
        [PMID: 16328021]

[5]   Song Q, Zhao C, Ou S, *et al.* Co-expression analysis of differentially expressed genes in hepatitis C virus-induced hepatocellular carcinoma. Mol Med Rep 2015; 11(1): 21-8.
        [http://dx.doi.org/10.3892/mmr.2014.2695] [PMID: 25339452]

[6]   Shen X, Xie B, Ma Z, *et al.* Identification of novel long non-coding RNAs in triple-negative breast cancer. Oncotarget 2015; 6(25): 21730-9.
        [http://dx.doi.org/10.18632/oncotarget.4419] [PMID: 26078338]

[7]   Wang Y, Liu Z, Lian B, Liu L, Xie L. Integrative Analysis of Dysfunctional Modules Driven by Genomic Alterations at System Level Across 11 Cancer Types. Comb Chem High Throughput Screen 2019; 21(10): 771-83.
        [http://dx.doi.org/10.2174/1386207322666190122110726] [PMID: 30666908]

[8]   Horibata Y, Ando H, Itoh M, Sugimoto H. Enzymatic and transcriptional regulation of the cytoplasmic acetyl-CoA hydrolase ACOT12. J Lipid Res 2013; 54(8): 2049-59.
        [http://dx.doi.org/10.1194/jlr.M030163] [PMID: 23709691]

[9]   Lu M, Zhu WW, Wang X, *et al.* ACOT12-Dependent Alteration of Acetyl-CoA Drives Hepatocellular Carcinoma Metastasis by Epigenetic Induction of Epithelial-Mesenchymal Transition. Cell Metab 2019; 29(4): 886-900.e5.
        [http://dx.doi.org/10.1016/j.cmet.2018.12.019] [PMID: 30661930]

[10]   Chen X, Wang X, Hossain S, *et al.* Haplotypes spanning SPEC2, PDZ-GEF2 and ACSL6 genes are associated with schizophrenia. Hum Mol Genet 2006; 15(22): 3329-42.
        [http://dx.doi.org/10.1093/hmg/ddl409] [PMID: 17030554]

[11]   Su RJ, Jonas BA, Welborn J, Gregg JP, Chen M. Chronic eosinophilic leukemia, NOS with t(5;12)(q31;p13)/ETV6-ACSL6 gene fusion: A novel variant of myeloid proliferative neoplasm with eosinophilia. Hum Pathol (N Y) 2016; 5: 6-9.
        [http://dx.doi.org/10.1016/j.ehpc.2015.10.001] [PMID: 27458550]

[12]   Chen WC, Wang CY, Hung YH, Weng TY, Yen MC, Lai MD. Systematic Analysis of Gene Expression Alterations and Clinical Outcomes for Long-Chain Acyl-Coenzyme A Synthetase Family in Cancer. PLoS One 2016; 11(5): e0155660.
        [http://dx.doi.org/10.1371/journal.pone.0155660] [PMID: 27171439]

[13]   Rossi Sebastiano M, Konstantinidou G. Targeting long chain acyl-CoA synthetases for cancer therapy. Int J Mol Sci. 2019; 20(15): 3624.
        [http://dx.doi.org/10.3390/ijms20153624]

[14]   Ghazanfar S, Fatima I, Aslam M, *et al.* Identification of actin beta-like 2 (ACTBL2) as novel, upregulated protein in colorectal cancer. J Proteomics 2017; 152: 33-40.
        [http://dx.doi.org/10.1016/j.jprot.2016.10.011] [PMID: 27989943]

[15]   Kuwae Y, Kakehashi A, Wakasa K, *et al.* Paraneoplastic Ma Antigen–Like 1 as a Potential Prognostic Biomarker in Human Pancreatic Ductal Adenocarcinoma. Pancreas 2015; 44(1): 106-15.
        [http://dx.doi.org/10.1097/MPA.0000000000000220] [PMID: 25251443]

[16]   Wang B, Zhao H, Zhao L, *et al.* Up-regulation of OLR1 expression by TBC1D3 through activation of TNFα/NF-κB pathway promotes the migration of human breast cancer cells. Cancer Lett 2017; 408:

60-70.
[http://dx.doi.org/10.1016/j.canlet.2017.08.021] [PMID: 28844714]

[17]   Permuth JB, Pirie A, Ann Chen Y, *et al.* Exome genotyping arrays to identify rare and low frequency variants associated with epithelial ovarian cancer risk. Hum Mol Genet 2016; 25(16): 3600-12.
[http://dx.doi.org/10.1093/hmg/ddw196] [PMID: 27378695]

[18]   Stokowy T, Gawel D, Wojtas B. Differences in miRNA and mRNA profile of papillary thyroid cancer variants. Int J Endocrinol. 2016; 2016: 1427042.
[http://dx.doi.org/10.1155/2016/1427042]

[19]   Katsuyama Y, Inoko H, Imanishi T, Mizuki N, Gojobori T, Ota M. Genetic relationships among Japanese, northern Han, Hui, Uygur, Kazakh, Greek, Saudi Arabian, and Italian populations based on allelic frequencies at four VNTR (D1S80, D4S43, COL2A1, D17S5) and one STR (ACTBP2) loci. Hum Hered 1998; 48(3): 126-37.
[http://dx.doi.org/10.1159/000022793] [PMID: 9618060]

[20]   Awadalla A, Harraz AM, Abol-Enein H, *et al.* Prognostic influence of microsatellite alterations of muscle-invasive bladder cancer treated with radical cystectomy. Urol Oncol Semin Orig Investig 2021; 17.
[http://dx.doi.org/10.1016/j.urolonc.2021.08.020] [PMID: 34538725]

[21]   Mullokandov M, Cass I, Achary PM, Klinger HP. Assignment of ACTBP8 (alias ACTBP2) within or close to human chromosome band 6q13 using a radiation hybrid panel. Cytogenet Genome Res 1997; 78(1): 46-7.
[http://dx.doi.org/10.1159/000134624] [PMID: 9345905]

[22]   Zekri ARN, Khaled HM, Mohammed MB, *et al.* Microsatellite instability profiling in Egyptian bladder cancer patients: A pilot study. Curr Probl Cancer 2019; 43(6): 100472.
[http://dx.doi.org/10.1016/j.currproblcancer.2019.03.002] [PMID: 30929752]

[23]   Xu L, Chow J, Bonacum J, Eisenberger C, *et al.* Microsatellite instability at AAAG repeat sequences in respiratory tract cancers. Int J Cancer. 2001; 91(2): 200-4.

[24]   Kozulic M, Chen XQ, Bonilla F, Silva J. Loss of heterozygosity at the ACTBP2 locus in lung cancer detected on Elchrom precast Spreadex gels. Ann N Y Acad Sci 2000; 906(1): 83-6.
[http://dx.doi.org/10.1111/j.1749-6632.2000.tb06595.x] [PMID: 10818601]

[25]   Gonzalez R, Silva JM, Sanchez A, *et al.* Microsatellite alterations and TP53 mutations in plasma DNA of small-cell lung cancer patients: Follow-up study and prognostic significance. Ann Oncol 2000; 11(9): 1097-104.
[http://dx.doi.org/10.1023/A:1008305412635] [PMID: 11061602]

[26]   Edwards D, Handsley M, Pennington C. The ADAM metalloproteinases. Mol Aspects Med 2008; 29(5): 258-89.
[http://dx.doi.org/10.1016/j.mam.2008.08.001] [PMID: 18762209]

[27]   Wolfsberg TG, Primakoff P, Myles DG, White JM. ADAM, a novel family of membrane proteins containing A Disintegrin And Metalloprotease domain: multipotential functions in cell-cell and cell-matrix interactions. J Cell Biol 1995; 131(2): 275-8.
[http://dx.doi.org/10.1083/jcb.131.2.275] [PMID: 7593158]

[28]   Duffy MJ, McKiernan E, O'Donovan N, McGowan PM. Role of ADAMs in cancer formation and progression. Clin Cancer Res 2009; 15(4): 1140-4.
[http://dx.doi.org/10.1158/1078-0432.CCR-08-1585] [PMID: 19228719]

[29]   Mochizuki S, Okada Y. ADAMs in cancer cell proliferation and progression. Cancer Sci 2007; 98(5): 621-8.
[http://dx.doi.org/10.1111/j.1349-7006.2007.00434.x] [PMID: 17355265]

[30]   Wildeboer D, Naus S, Sang Q-XA, Bartsch JW, Pagenstecher A. Metalloproteinase disintegrins ADAM8 and ADAM19 are highly regulated in human primary brain tumors and their expression

levels and activities are associated with invasiveness. J Neuropathol Exp Neurol 2006; 65(5): 516-27.
[http://dx.doi.org/10.1097/01.jnen.0000229240.51490.d3] [PMID: 16772875]

[31]   A D, DS P, JA N, *et al.* Expression of ADAMs ('a disintegrin and metalloprotease') in the human lung. Virchows Arch. 2009; 454: 441–449.

[32]   Keating DT, Sadlier DM, Patricelli A, *et al.* Microarray identifies ADAM family members as key responders to TGF-β1 in alveolar epithelial cells. Respir Res 2006; 7(1): 114.
[http://dx.doi.org/10.1186/1465-9921-7-114] [PMID: 16948840]

[33]   Melenhorst WBWH, van den Heuvel MC, Timmer A, *et al.* ADAM19 expression in human nephrogenesis and renal disease: Associations with clinical and structural deterioration. Kidney Int 2006; 70(7): 1269-78.
[http://dx.doi.org/10.1038/sj.ki.5001753] [PMID: 16900093]

[34]   Shan N, Shen L, Wang J, He D, Duan C. MiR-153 inhibits migration and invasion of human non-small-cell lung cancer by targeting ADAM19. Biochem Biophys Res Commun 2015; 456(1): 385-91.
[http://dx.doi.org/10.1016/j.bbrc.2014.11.093] [PMID: 25475731]

[35]   Zhang Q, Yu L, Qin D, *et al.* Role of microRNA-30c targeting ADAM19 in colorectal cancer. PLoS One 2015; 10(3): e0120698.
[http://dx.doi.org/10.1371/journal.pone.0120698] [PMID: 25799050]

[36]   Hoyne G, Rudnicka C, Sang QX, *et al.* Genetic and cellular studies highlight that A Disintegrin and Metalloproteinase 19 is a protective biomarker in human prostate cancer. BMC cancer. 2016 Dec;16:1-2.

[37]   Cal S, Argüelles JM, Fernández PL, López-Otín C. Identification, characterization, and intracellular processing of ADAM-TS12, a novel human disintegrin with a complex structural organization involving multiple thrombospondin-1 repeats. J Biol Chem 2001; 276(21): 17932-40.
[http://dx.doi.org/10.1074/jbc.M100534200] [PMID: 11279086]

[38]   Wang D, Zhu T, Zhang FB, He C. Expression of ADAMTS12 in colorectal cancer-associated stroma prevents cancer development and is a good prognostic indicator of colorectal cancer. Dig Dis Sci 2011; 56(11): 3281-7.
[http://dx.doi.org/10.1007/s10620-011-1723-x] [PMID: 21559743]

[39]   Llamazares M, Obaya AJ, Moncada-Pazos A, *et al.* The ADAMTS12 metalloproteinase exhibits anti-tumorigenic properties through modulation of the Ras-dependent ERK signalling pathway. J Cell Sci 2007; 120(20): 3544-52.
[http://dx.doi.org/10.1242/jcs.005751] [PMID: 17895370]

[40]   Surridge AK, Rodgers UR, Swingler TE, *et al.* Characterization and regulation of ADAMTS-16. Matrix Biol 2009; 28(7): 416-24.
[http://dx.doi.org/10.1016/j.matbio.2009.07.001] [PMID: 19635554]

[41]   Kordowski F, Kolarova J, Schafmayer C, *et al.* Aberrant DNA methylation of ADAMTS16 in colorectal and other epithelial cancers. BMC Cancer. 2018; 18: 1–10.

[42]   Jacobi CLJ, Rudigier LJ, Scholz H, Kirschner KM. Transcriptional regulation by the Wilms tumor protein, Wt1, suggests a role of the metalloproteinase Adamts16 in murine genitourinary development. J Biol Chem 2013; 288(26): 18811-24.
[http://dx.doi.org/10.1074/jbc.M113.464644] [PMID: 23661704]

[43]   Zhang Y, Cai Q, Shu XO, *et al.* Whole-Exome Sequencing Identifies Novel Somatic Mutations in Chinese Breast Cancer Patients. J Mol Genet Med 2015; 9(4): 25.
[http://dx.doi.org/10.4172/1747-0862.1000183] [PMID: 26870154]

[44]   Noda H, Miyaji Y, Nakanishi A, Konishi F, Miki Y. Frequent reduced expression of alpha-1--adrenergic receptor caused by aberrant promoter methylation in gastric cancers. Br J Cancer 2007; 96(2): 383-90.
[http://dx.doi.org/10.1038/sj.bjc.6603555] [PMID: 17242706]

[45] Lehrer S, Rheinstein PH. The ADRB1 (Adrenoceptor Beta 1) and ADRB2 genes significantly co-express with commonly mutated genes in prostate cancer. Discov Med 2020; 30(161): 163-71.
[PMID: 33593484]

[46] Kulik G. ADRB2-targeting therapies for prostate cancer. Cancers. 2019; 11(3): 358.
[http://dx.doi.org/10.3390/cancers11030358]

[47] Boulay G, Malaquin N, Loison I, *et al.* Loss of Hypermethylated in Cancer 1 (HIC1) in breast cancer cells contributes to stress-induced migration and invasion through ?-2 adrenergic receptor (ADRB2) misregulation. JBiolChem; 287, https://hsrc.himmelfarb.gwu.edu/smhs_peds_facpubs/5573 (2012, accessed 25 September 2021).

[48] Wang M, Han X, Sun W, Li X, Jing G, Zhang X. Actin Filament-Associated Protein 1-Like 1 Mediates Proliferation and Survival in Non-Small Cell Lung Cancer Cells. Med Sci Monit 2018; 24: 215-24.
[http://dx.doi.org/10.12659/MSM.905900] [PMID: 29323101]

[49] Furu M, Kajita Y, Nagayama S, *et al.* Identification of AFAP1L1 as a prognostic marker for spindle cell sarcomas. Oncogene. 2011; 30(38): 4015-25.

[50] Takahashi R, Nagayama S, Furu M, *et al.* AFAP 1L1, a novel associating partner with vinculin, modulates cellular morphology and motility, and promotes the progression of colorectal cancers. Cancer Med 2014; 3(4): 759-74.
[http://dx.doi.org/10.1002/cam4.237] [PMID: 24723436]

[51] Deng P, Wang J, Zhang X, *et al.* AFF4 promotes tumorigenesis and tumor-initiation capacity of head and neck squamous cell carcinoma cells by regulating SOX2. Carcinogenesis 2018; 39(7): 937-47.
[http://dx.doi.org/10.1093/carcin/bgy046] [PMID: 29741610]

[52] Cheng M, Sheng L, Gao Q, *et al.* The m⁶A methyltransferase METTL3 promotes bladder cancer progression *via* AFF4/NF-κB/MYC signaling network. Oncogene 2019; 38(19): 3667-80.
[http://dx.doi.org/10.1038/s41388-019-0683-z] [PMID: 30659266]

[53] Hu FY, Wu C, Li Y, *et al.* AGGF1 is a novel anti-inflammatory factor associated with TNF-α-induced endothelial activation. Cell Signal 2013; 25(8): 1645-53.
[http://dx.doi.org/10.1016/j.cellsig.2013.04.007] [PMID: 23628701]

[54] Wang W, Li GY, Zhu JY, *et al.* Overexpression of AGGF1 is correlated with angiogenesis and poor prognosis of hepatocellular carcinoma. Med Oncol. 2015; 32(4): 131.

[55] Yao HH, Wang BJ, Wu Y, Huang Q. High Expression of Angiogenic Factor with G-Patch and FHA Domain1 (AGGF1) Predicts Poor Prognosis in Gastric Cancer. Med Sci Monit 2017; 23: 1286-94.
[http://dx.doi.org/10.12659/MSM.903248] [PMID: 28289272]

[56] Lu Q, Yao Y, Hu Z, *et al.* Angiogenic Factor AGGF1 Activates Autophagy with an Essential Role in Therapeutic Angiogenesis for Heart Disease. PLoS Biol 2016; 14(8): e1002529.
[http://dx.doi.org/10.1371/journal.pbio.1002529] [PMID: 27513923]

[57] Tu J, Ying X, Zhang D, *et al.* High expression of angiogenic factor AGGF1 is an independent prognostic factor for hepatocellular carcinoma. Oncotarget 2017; 8(67): 111623-30.
[http://dx.doi.org/10.18632/oncotarget.22880] [PMID: 29340079]

[58] Vogel CFA, Haarmann-Stemmann T. The aryl hydrocarbon receptor repressor – More than a simple feedback inhibitor of AhR signaling: Clues for its role in inflammation and cancer. Curr Opin Toxicol 2017; 2: 109-19.
[http://dx.doi.org/10.1016/j.cotox.2017.02.004] [PMID: 28971163]

[59] Li Y fang, Wang D dan, Zhao B wei, *et al.* Poor prognosis of gastric adenocarcinoma with decreased expression of ahrr. PLoS One; 2012, 7.
[http://dx.doi.org/10.1371/journal.pone.0043555]

[60] Zudaire E, Cuesta N, Murty V, *et al.* The aryl hydrocarbon receptor repressor is a putative tumor

suppressor gene in multiple human cancers. J Clin Invest 2008; 118(2): 640-50.
[http://dx.doi.org/10.1172/JCI30024] [PMID: 18172554]

[61]　Kanno Y, Takane Y, Izawa T, Nakahama T, Inouye Y. The inhibitory effect of aryl hydrocarbon receptor repressor (AhRR) on the growth of human breast cancer MCF-7 cells. Biol Pharm Bull 2006; 29(6): 1254-7.
[http://dx.doi.org/10.1248/bpb.29.1254] [PMID: 16755028]

[62]　Kuefer R, Varambally S, Zhou M, *et al.* alpha-Methylacyl-CoA racemase: expression levels of this novel cancer biomarker depend on tumor differentiation. Am J Pathol 2002; 161(3): 841-8.
[http://dx.doi.org/10.1016/S0002-9440(10)64244-7] [PMID: 12213712]

[63]　Thornburg T, Turner AR, Chen YQ, Vitolins M, Chang B, Xu J. Phytanic acid, AMACR and prostate cancer risk. Future Oncol 2006; 2(2): 213-23.
[http://dx.doi.org/10.2217/14796694.2.2.213] [PMID: 16563090]

[64]　Jiang Z. BA W, XJ Y. Alpha-methylacyl coenzyme A racemase as a marker for prostate cancer. JAMA 2002; 287(23): 3080-a-1.
[http://dx.doi.org/10.1001/jama.287.23.3080-a]

[65]　Luo J, Zha S, Gage WR, *et al.* Alpha-methylacyl-CoA racemase: a new molecular marker for prostate cancer. Cancer Res 2002; 62(8): 2220-6.
[PMID: 11956072]

[66]　A D, AS D, JA M-N, *et al.* ANKHD1 regulates cell cycle progression and proliferation in multiple myeloma cells. FEBS Lett 2012; 586: 4311–4318.

[67]　A D, JA M-N, P F, *et al.* ANKHD1 represses p21 (WAF1/CIP1) promoter and promotes multiple myeloma cell growth. Eur J Cancer 2015; 51: 252–259.

[68]　Machado-Neto JA, Lazarini M, Favaro P, *et al.* ANKHD1, a novel component of the Hippo signaling pathway, promotes YAP1 activation and cell cycle progression in prostate cancer cells. Exp Cell Res 2014; 324(2): 137-45.
[http://dx.doi.org/10.1016/j.yexcr.2014.04.004] [PMID: 24726915]

[69]　Machado-Neto JA, Lazarini M, Favaro P, *et al.* ANKHD1 silencing inhibits Stathmin 1 activity, cell proliferation and migration of leukemia cells. Biochim Biophys Acta Mol Cell Res 2015; 1853(3): 583-93.
[http://dx.doi.org/10.1016/j.bbamcr.2014.12.012] [PMID: 25523139]

[70]　Wang CY, Lin CF. Annexin A2: its molecular regulation and cellular expression in cancer development. Dis Markers 2014; 2014: 1-10.
[http://dx.doi.org/10.1155/2014/308976] [PMID: 24591759]

[71]　Wu B, Zhang F, Yu M, *et al.* Up-regulation of *Anxa2* gene promotes proliferation and invasion of breast cancer MCF -7 cells. Cell Prolif 2012; 45(3): 189-98.
[http://dx.doi.org/10.1111/j.1365-2184.2012.00820.x] [PMID: 22452352]

[72]　Kondo T, Oka T, Sato H, *et al.* Accumulation of aberrant CpG hypermethylation by Helicobacter pylori infection promotes development and progression of gastric MALT lymphoma. Int J Oncol 2009; 35(3): 547-57.
[PMID: 19639175]

[73]　Zhang F, Zhang L, Zhang B, *et al.* Anxa2 plays a critical role in enhanced invasiveness of the multidrug resistant human breast cancer cells. J Proteome Res 2009; 8(11): 5041-7.
[http://dx.doi.org/10.1021/pr900461c] [PMID: 19764771]

[74]　Xu XH, Pan W, Kang LH, Feng H, Song YQ. Association of annexin A2 with cancer development (Review). Oncol Rep 2015; 33(5): 2121-8.
[http://dx.doi.org/10.3892/or.2015.3837] [PMID: 25760910]

[75]　Wang T, Yuan J, Zhang J, *et al.* Anxa2 binds to STAT3 and promotes epithelial to mesenchymal transition in breast cancer cells. Oncotarget 2015; 6(31): 30975-92.

[http://dx.doi.org/10.18632/oncotarget.5199] [PMID: 26307676]

[76] Horii A, Nakatsuru S, Miyoshi Y, *et al.* The APC Gene, Responsible for Familial Adenomatous Polyposis, Is Mutated in Human Gastric Cancer. Cancer Res; 52.

[77] Nakatsuru S, Yanagisawa A, Ichii S, *et al.* Somatic mutation of the *APC* gene in gastric cancer: frequent mutations in very well differentiated adenocarcinoma and signet-ring cell carcinoma. Hum Mol Genet 1992; 1(8): 559-63.
[http://dx.doi.org/10.1093/hmg/1.8.559] [PMID: 1338691]

[78] Nagase H, Nakamura Y. Mutations of theAPC adenomatous polyposis coli) gene. Hum Mutat 1993; 2(6): 425-34.
[http://dx.doi.org/10.1002/humu.1380020602] [PMID: 8111410]

[79] Samowitz WS, Slattery ML, Sweeney C, Herrick J, Wolff RK, Albertsen H. APC mutations and other genetic and epigenetic changes in colon cancer. Mol Cancer Res 2007; 5(2): 165-70.
[http://dx.doi.org/10.1158/1541-7786.MCR-06-0398] [PMID: 17293392]

[80] Krugmann S, Anderson KE, Ridley SH, *et al.* Identification of ARAP3, a novel PI3K effector regulating both Arf and Rho GTPases, by selective capture on phosphoinositide affinity matrices. Mol Cell 2002; 9(1): 95-108.
[http://dx.doi.org/10.1016/S1097-2765(02)00434-3] [PMID: 11804589]

[81] Groden J, Joslyn G, Samowitz W, *et al.* Response of Colon Cancer Cell Lines to the Introduction of APC, a Colon-specific Tumor Suppressor Gene. Cancer Res; 55.

[82] Gambardella L, Anderson KE, Nussbaum C, *et al.* The GTPase-activating protein ARAP3 regulates chemotaxis and adhesion-dependent processes in neutrophils. Blood 2011; 118(4): 1087-98.
[http://dx.doi.org/10.1182/blood-2010-10-312959] [PMID: 21490342]

[83] J-J Han, B-R Du, C-H Zhang. Bioinformatic analysis of prognostic value of ARAP3 in breast cancer and the associated signaling pathways - PubMed. Eur Rev Med Pharmacol Sci; 21(10), https://pubmed.ncbi.nlm.nih.gov/28617548/ (2017, accessed 28 September 2021).

[84] Miller NLG, Kleinschmidt EG, Schlaepfer DD. RhoGEFs in cell motility: novel links between Rgnef and focal adhesion kinase. Curr Mol Med 2014; 14(2): 221-34.
[http://dx.doi.org/10.2174/1566524014666140128110339] [PMID: 24467206]

[85] Kleinschmidt EG, Miller NLG, Ozmadenci D, *et al.* Rgnef promotes ovarian tumor progression and confers protection from oxidative stress. Oncogene 2019; 38(36): 6323-37.
[http://dx.doi.org/10.1038/s41388-019-0881-8] [PMID: 31308489]

[86] Zhang HD, Jiang LH, Hou JC, *et al.* Circular RNA hsa_circ_0072995 promotes breast cancer cell migration and invasion through sponge for miR-30c-2-3p. Epigenomics 2018; 10(9): 1229-42.
[http://dx.doi.org/10.2217/epi-2018-0002] [PMID: 30182731]

[87] Cook DR, Rossman KL, Der CJ. Rho guanine nucleotide exchange factors: regulators of Rho GTPase activity in development and disease. Oncogene 2014; 33(31): 4021-35.
[http://dx.doi.org/10.1038/onc.2013.362] [PMID: 24037532]

[88] Pisamai S, Roytrakul S, Phaonakrop N, Jaresitthikunchai J, Suriyaphol G. Proteomic analysis of canine oral tumor tissues using MALDI-TOF mass spectrometry and in-gel digestion coupled with mass spectrometry (GeLC MS/MS) approaches. PLoS One 2018; 13(7): e0200619.
[http://dx.doi.org/10.1371/journal.pone.0200619] [PMID: 30001383]

[89] Yao F, Kausalya JP, Sia YY, *et al.* Recurrent Fusion Genes in Gastric Cancer: CLDN18-ARHGAP26 Induces Loss of Epithelial Integrity. Cell Rep 2015; 12(2): 272-85.
[http://dx.doi.org/10.1016/j.celrep.2015.06.020] [PMID: 26146084]

[90] Bessissow T, Chao C-Y, Lemieux C, *et al.* Maladaptive coping, low self-efficacy and disease activity are associated with poorer patient-reported outcomes in inflammatory bowel disease. Saudi J Gastroenterol 2019; 25(3): 159-66.
[http://dx.doi.org/10.4103/sjg.SJG_566_18] [PMID: 30900609]

[91]   Shu Y, Zhang W, Hou Q, *et al.* Prognostic significance of frequent CLDN18-ARHGAP26/6 fusion in gastric signet-ring cell cancer. Nat Commun 2018; 9(1): 2447.
       [http://dx.doi.org/10.1038/s41467-018-04907-0]

[92]   Yang WM, Min KH, Lee W. MiR-1271 upregulated by saturated fatty acid palmitate provokes impaired insulin signaling by repressing INSR and IRS-1 expression in HepG2 cells. Biochem Biophys Res Commun 2016; 478(4): 1786-91.
       [http://dx.doi.org/10.1016/j.bbrc.2016.09.029] [PMID: 27613089]

[93]   Yang M, Shan X, Zhou X, *et al.* miR-1271 regulates cisplatin resistance of human gastric cancer cell lines by targeting IGF1R, IRS1, mTOR, and BCL2. Anticancer Agents Med Chem 2014; 14(6): 884-91.
       [http://dx.doi.org/10.2174/1871520614666140528161318] [PMID: 24875127]

[94]   Nurul-Syakima AM, Yoke-Kqueen C, Sabariah AR, Shiran MS, Singh A, Learn-Han L. Differential microRNA expression and identification of putative miRNA targets and pathways in head and neck cancers. Int J Mol Med 2011; 28(3): 327-36.
       [PMID: 21637912]

[95]   Maurel M, Jalvy S, Ladeiro Y, *et al.* A functional screening identifies five micrornas controlling glypican-3: role of mir-1271 down-regulation in hepatocellular carcinoma. Hepatology 2013; 57(1): 195-204.
       [http://dx.doi.org/10.1002/hep.25994] [PMID: 22865282]

[96]   Xiang XJ, Deng J, Liu YW, *et al.* MiR-1271 Inhibits Cell Proliferation, Invasion and EMT in Gastric Cancer by Targeting FOXQ1. Cell Physiol Biochem 2015; 36(4): 1382-94.
       [http://dx.doi.org/10.1159/000430304] [PMID: 26159618]

[97]   Zhang J, Zhang Q, Sun C, Huang Y, Zhang J, Wang Q. Clinical relevance of ARF/ARL family genes and oncogenic function of ARL4C in endometrial cancer. Biomed Pharmacother 2020; 125: 110000.
       [http://dx.doi.org/10.1016/j.biopha.2020.110000] [PMID: 32070877]

[98]   Gillingham AK, Munro S. The small G proteins of the Arf family and their regulators. Annu Rev Cell Dev Biol 2007; 23(1): 579-611.
       [http://dx.doi.org/10.1146/annurev.cellbio.23.090506.123209] [PMID: 17506703]

[99]   Wang Z, Wang Z, Niu X, *et al.* Identification of seven-gene signature for prediction of lung squamous cell carcinoma. OncoTargets Ther 2019; 12: 5979-88.
       [http://dx.doi.org/10.2147/OTT.S198998] [PMID: 31440059]

[100] Uren AG, Kool J, Matentzoglu K, *et al.* Large-scale mutagenesis in p19(ARF)- and p53-deficient mice identifies cancer genes and their collaborative networks. Cell 2008; 133(4): 727-41.
       [http://dx.doi.org/10.1016/j.cell.2008.03.021] [PMID: 18485879]

[101] Cilek EE, Ozturk H, Gur Dedeoglu B. Construction of miRNA-miRNA networks revealing the complexity of miRNA-mediated mechanisms in trastuzumab treated breast cancer cell lines. PLoS One 2017; 12(10): e0185558.
       [http://dx.doi.org/10.1371/journal.pone.0185558]

[102] Scaglione KM, Basrur V, Ashraf NS, *et al.* The ubiquitin-conjugating enzyme (E2) Ube2w ubiquitinates the N terminus of substrates. J Biol Chem 2013; 288(26): 18784-8.
       [http://dx.doi.org/10.1074/jbc.C113.477596] [PMID: 23696636]

[103] Kashyap S, Kumar U, Pandey AK, *et al.* Functional characterisation of ADP ribosylation factor-like protein 15 in rheumatoid arthritis synovial fibroblasts. Clin Exp Rheumatol 2018; 36(4): 581-8.
       [PMID: 29465355]

[104] Li Y, Yang Y, Yao Y, *et al.* Association study of ARL15 and CDH13 with T2DM in a Han Chinese population. Int J Med Sci 2014; 11(5): 522-7.
       [http://dx.doi.org/10.7150/ijms.8206] [PMID: 24688318]

[105] Draheim KM, Chen H-B, Tao Q, Moore N, Roche M, Lyle S. ARRDC3 suppresses breast cancer

progression by negatively regulating integrin β4. Oncogene 2010; 29(36): 5032-47.
[http://dx.doi.org/10.1038/onc.2010.250] [PMID: 20603614]

[106]   Soung YH, Pruitt K, Chung J. Epigenetic silencing of ARRDC3 expression in basal-like breast cancer cells. Sci Rep 2014; 4(1): 3846.
[http://dx.doi.org/10.1038/srep03846]

[107]   Yao J, Xu C, Fang Z, *et al.* Androgen receptor regulated microRNA miR-182-5p promotes prostate cancer progression by targeting the ARRDC3/ITGB4 pathway. Biochem Biophys Res Commun 2016; 474(1): 213-9.
[http://dx.doi.org/10.1016/j.bbrc.2016.04.107] [PMID: 27109471]

[108]   Xiao J, Shi Q, Li W, *et al.* ARRDC1 and ARRDC3 act as tumor suppressors in renal cell carcinoma by facilitating YAP1 degradation. Am J Cancer Res 2018; 8(1): 132-43.
[PMID: 29416926]

[109]   Takeuchi F, Kukimoto I, Li Z, *et al.* Genome-wide association study of cervical cancer suggests a role for *ARRDC3* gene in human papillomavirus infection. Hum Mol Genet 2019; 28(2): 341-8.
[http://dx.doi.org/10.1093/hmg/ddy390] [PMID: 30412241]

[110]   Liang C, Jung JU. Autophagy genes as tumor suppressors. Curr Opin Cell Biol 2010; 22(2): 226-33.
[http://dx.doi.org/10.1016/j.ceb.2009.11.003] [PMID: 19945837]

[111]   Xie K, Liang C, Li Q, *et al.* Role of *ATG* 10 expression quantitative trait loci in non-small cell lung cancer survival. Int J Cancer 2016; 139(7): 1564-73.
[http://dx.doi.org/10.1002/ijc.30205] [PMID: 27225307]

[112]   Burada F, Nicoli ER, Ciurea ME, Uscatu DC, Ioana M, Gheonea DI. Autophagy in colorectal cancer: An important switch from physiology to pathology. World J Gastrointest Oncol 2015; 7(11): 271-84.
[http://dx.doi.org/10.4251/wjgo.v7.i11.271] [PMID: 26600927]

[113]   Cho YY, Kim DJ, Lee HS, *et al.* Autophagy and cellular senescence mediated by Sox2 suppress malignancy of cancer cells. PLoS One 2013; 8(2): e57172.
[http://dx.doi.org/10.1371/journal.pone.0057172] [PMID: 23451179]

[114]   Liu H, He Z, Germič N, *et al.* ATG12 deficiency leads to tumor cell oncosis owing to diminished mitochondrial biogenesis and reduced cellular bioenergetics. Cell Death Differ 2019 276 2019; 27: 1965–1980.

[115]   M H, AK H, E G, *et al.* Ubiquitination and proteasomal degradation of ATG12 regulates its proapoptotic activity. Autophagy 2014; 10: 2269–2278.

[116]   Palm-Espling M, Lundin C, Björn E, Naredi P, Wittung- Stafshede P. Interaction between the anticancer drug Cisplatin and the copper chaperone Atox1 in human melanoma cells. Protein Pept Lett 2013; 21(1): 63-8.
[http://dx.doi.org/10.2174/09298665113209990036] [PMID: 23988033]

[117]   Itoh S, Kim HW, Nakagawa O, *et al.* Novel role of antioxidant-1 (Atox1) as a copper-dependent transcription factor involved in cell proliferation. J Biol Chem 2008; 283(14): 9157-67.
[http://dx.doi.org/10.1074/jbc.M709463200] [PMID: 18245776]

[118]   Barresi V, Spampinato G, Musso N, Trovato Salinaro A, Rizzarelli E, Condorelli DF. ATOX1 gene silencing increases susceptibility to anticancer therapy based on copper ionophores or chelating drugs. J Inorg Biochem 2016; 156: 145-52.
[http://dx.doi.org/10.1016/j.jinorgbio.2016.01.002] [PMID: 26784148]

[119]   Blockhuys S, Wittung-Stafshede P. Copper chaperone Atox1 plays role in breast cancer cell migration. Biochem Biophys Res Commun 2017; 483(1): 301-4.
[http://dx.doi.org/10.1016/j.bbrc.2016.12.148] [PMID: 28027931]

[120]   Zhang S, Deen S, Storr SJ, *et al.* Calpain system protein expression and activity in ovarian cancer. J Cancer Res Clin Oncol 2019; 145(2): 345-61.
[http://dx.doi.org/10.1007/s00432-018-2794-2] [PMID: 30448882]

[121] Storr SJ, Mohammed RAA, Woolston CM, *et al.* Calpastatin is associated with lymphovascular invasion in breast cancer. Breast 2011; 20(5): 413-8.
[http://dx.doi.org/10.1016/j.breast.2011.04.002] [PMID: 21531560]

[122] Ding K, Li W, Zou Z, Zou X, Wang C. CCNB1 is a prognostic biomarker for ER+ breast cancer. Med Hypotheses 2014; 83(3): 359-64.
[http://dx.doi.org/10.1016/j.mehy.2014.06.013] [PMID: 25044212]

[123] Fang L, Du WW, Lyu J, *et al.* Enhanced breast cancer progression by mutant p53 is inhibited by the circular RNA circ-Ccnb1. Cell Death Differ 2018; 25(12): 2195-208.
[http://dx.doi.org/10.1038/s41418-018-0115-6] [PMID: 29795334]

[124] Chai N, Xie H, Yin J, *et al.* FOXM1 promotes proliferation in human hepatocellular carcinoma cells by transcriptional activation of CCNB1. Biochem Biophys Res Commun 2018; 500(4): 924-9.
[http://dx.doi.org/10.1016/j.bbrc.2018.04.201] [PMID: 29705704]

[125] Fang Y, Yu H, Liang X, Xu J, Cai X. Chk1-induced CCNB1 overexpression promotes cell proliferation and tumor growth in human colorectal cancer. Cancer Biol Ther 2014; 15(9): 1268-79.
[http://dx.doi.org/10.4161/cbt.29691] [PMID: 24971465]

[126] Xu Y, Zhang Q, Miao C, *et al.* CCNG1 (Cyclin G1) regulation by mutant-P53 *via* induction of Notch3 expression promotes high-grade serous ovarian cancer (HGSOC) tumorigenesis and progression. Cancer Med 2019; 8(1): 351-62.
[http://dx.doi.org/10.1002/cam4.1812] [PMID: 30565428]

[127] Liu X, Ma L, Rao Q, *et al.* MiR-1271 Inhibits Ovarian Cancer Growth by Targeting Cyclin G1. Med Sci Monit 2015; 21: 3152-8.
[http://dx.doi.org/10.12659/MSM.895562] [PMID: 26477861]

[128] Yan J, Jiang J, Meng X-N, *et al.* MiR-23b targets cyclin G1 and suppresses ovarian cancer tumorigenesis and progression. J Exp Clin Cancer Res 2016 351 2016; 35: 1–10.

[129] A A-S, SP C, FL H, *et al.* Exploiting Oncogenic Drivers along the CCNG1 Pathway for Cancer Therapy and Gene Therapy. Mol Ther oncolytics 2018; 11: 122–126.

[130] Schröder B. The multifaceted roles of the invariant chain CD74 — More than just a chaperone. Biochim Biophys Acta Mol Cell Res 2016; 1863(6): 1269-81.
[http://dx.doi.org/10.1016/j.bbamcr.2016.03.026] [PMID: 27033518]

[131] Beswick EJ, Reyes VE. CD74 in antigen presentation, inflammation, and cancers of the gastrointestinal tract. World J Gastroenterol 2009; 15(23): 2855-61.
[http://dx.doi.org/10.3748/wjg.15.2855] [PMID: 19533806]

[132] McClelland M, Zhao L, Carskadon S, Arenberg D. Expression of CD74, the receptor for macrophage migration inhibitory factor, in non-small cell lung cancer. Am J Pathol 2009; 174(2): 638-46.
[http://dx.doi.org/10.2353/ajpath.2009.080463] [PMID: 19131591]

[133] Cheng SP, Liu CL, Chen MJ, *et al.* CD74 expression and its therapeutic potential in thyroid carcinoma. Endocr Relat Cancer 2015; 22(2): 179-90.
[http://dx.doi.org/10.1530/ERC-14-0269] [PMID: 25600560]

[134] Fernandez-Cuesta L, Plenker D, Osada H, *et al.* CD74-NRG1 fusions in lung adenocarcinoma. Cancer Discov 2014; 4(4): 415-22.
[http://dx.doi.org/10.1158/2159-8290.CD-13-0633] [PMID: 24469108]

[135] Borghese F, Clanchy FIL. CD74: an emerging opportunity as a therapeutic target in cancer and autoimmune disease. Expert Opin Ther Targets 2011; 15(3): 237-51.
[http://dx.doi.org/10.1517/14728222.2011.550879] [PMID: 21208136]

[136] Xiao D, Herman-Antosiewicz A, Antosiewicz J, *et al.* Diallyl trisulfide-induced G2–M phase cell cycle arrest in human prostate cancer cells is caused by reactive oxygen species-dependent destruction and hyperphosphorylation of Cdc25C. Oncogene 2005 2441 2005; 24: 6256–6268.

[137] M S, N S, A S, *et al.* Hsp90 inhibitors cause G2/M arrest associated with the reduction of Cdc25C and Cdc2 in lung cancer cell lines. J Cancer Res Clin Oncol 2006; 132: 150–158.

[138] Vecchione A, Baldassarre G, Ishii H, *et al.* Fez1/Lzts1 absence impairs Cdk1/Cdc25C interaction during mitosis and predisposes mice to cancer development. Cancer Cell 2007; 11(3): 275-89.
[http://dx.doi.org/10.1016/j.ccr.2007.01.014] [PMID: 17349584]

[139] Wang Z, Trope CG, Førenes VA, Suo Z, Nesland JM, Holm R. Overexpression of CDC25B, CDC25C and phospho-CDC25C (Ser216) in vulvar squamous cell carcinomas are associated with malignant features and aggressive cancer phenotypes. BMC Cancer 2010; 10(1): 233.
[http://dx.doi.org/10.1186/1471-2407-10-233] [PMID: 20500813]

[140] Ozen M, Ittmann M. Increased expression and activity of CDC25C phosphatase and an alternatively spliced variant in prostate cancer. Clin Cancer Res 2005; 11(13): 4701-6.
[http://dx.doi.org/10.1158/1078-0432.CCR-04-2551] [PMID: 16000564]

[141] Kwiatkowski N, Zhang T, Rahl PB, *et al.* Targeting transcription regulation in cancer with a covalent CDK7 inhibitor. Nat 2014 5117511 2014; 511: 616–620.

[142] Wang Y, Zhang T, Kwiatkowski N, *et al.* CDK7-dependent transcriptional addiction in triple-negative breast cancer. Cell 2015; 163(1): 174-86.
[http://dx.doi.org/10.1016/j.cell.2015.08.063] [PMID: 26406377]

[143] Manzo SG, Zhou ZL, Wang YQ, *et al.* Natural product triptolide mediates cancer cell death by triggering CDK7-dependent degradation of RNA polymerase II. Cancer Res 2012; 72(20): 5363-73.
[http://dx.doi.org/10.1158/0008-5472.CAN-12-1006] [PMID: 22926559]

[144] Suh ER, Ha CS, Rankin EB, Toyota M, Traber PG. DNA methylation down-regulates CDX1 gene expression in colorectal cancer cell lines. J Biol Chem 2002; 277(39): 35795-800.
[http://dx.doi.org/10.1074/jbc.M205567200] [PMID: 12124393]

[145] Jones MF, Hara T, Francis P, *et al.* The CDX1–microRNA-215 axis regulates colorectal cancer stem cell differentiation. Proc Natl Acad Sci USA 2015; 112(13): E1550-8.
[http://dx.doi.org/10.1073/pnas.1503370112] [PMID: 25775580]

[146] Kang JM, Lee BH, Kim N, *et al.* CDX1 and CDX2 expression in intestinal metaplasia, dysplasia and gastric cancer. J Korean Med Sci 2011; 26(5): 647-53.
[http://dx.doi.org/10.3346/jkms.2011.26.5.647] [PMID: 21532856]

[147] Vider BZ, Zimber A, Chastre E, *et al.* Deregulated expression of homeobox-containing genes, HOXB6, B8, C8, C9, and Cdx-1, in human colon cancer cell lines. Biochem Biophys Res Commun 2000; 272(2): 513-8.
[http://dx.doi.org/10.1006/bbrc.2000.2804] [PMID: 10833444]

[148] Zhang R, Kang KA, Kim KC, *et al.* Oxidative stress causes epigenetic alteration of CDX1 expression in colorectal cancer cells. Gene 2013; 524(2): 214-9.
[http://dx.doi.org/10.1016/j.gene.2013.04.024] [PMID: 23618814]

[149] Rafnar T, Sulem P, Stacey SN, *et al.* Sequence variants at the TERT-CLPTM1L locus associate with many cancer types. Nat Genet 2009; 41(2): 221-7.
[http://dx.doi.org/10.1038/ng.296] [PMID: 19151717]

[150] Lan Q, Cawthon R, Gao Y, *et al.* Longer telomere length in peripheral white blood cells is associated with risk of lung cancer and the rs2736100 (CLPTM1L-TERT) polymorphism in a prospective cohort study among women in China. PLoS One 2013; 8(3): e59230.
[http://dx.doi.org/10.1371/journal.pone.0059230] [PMID: 23555636]

[151] Haiman CA, Chen GK, Vachon CM, *et al.* A common variant at the TERT-CLPTM1L locus is associated with estrogen receptor–negative breast cancer. Nat Genet 2011; 43(12): 1210-4.
[http://dx.doi.org/10.1038/ng.985] [PMID: 22037553]

[152] Wang Y, Broderick P, Matakidou A, Eisen T, Houlston RS. Role of 5p15.33 (TERT-CLPTM1L),

6p21.33 and 15q25.1 (CHRNA5-CHRNA3) variation and lung cancer risk in never-smokers. Carcinogenesis 2010; 31(2): 234-8.
[http://dx.doi.org/10.1093/carcin/bgp287] [PMID: 19955392]

[153] Zienolddiny S, Skaug V, Landvik NE, *et al.* The TERT-CLPTM1L lung cancer susceptibility variant associates with higher DNA adduct formation in the lung. Carcinogenesis 2009; 30(8): 1368-71.
[http://dx.doi.org/10.1093/carcin/bgp131] [PMID: 19465454]

[154] Cannarile MA, Weisser M, Jacob W, Jegg AM, Ries CH, Rüttinger D. Colony-stimulating factor 1 receptor (CSF1R) inhibitors in cancer therapy. J Immunother Cancer 2017; 5(1): 53.
[http://dx.doi.org/10.1186/s40425-017-0257-y] [PMID: 28716061]

[155] Xu J, Escamilla J, Mok S, *et al.* CSF1R signaling blockade stanches tumor-infiltrating myeloid cells and improves the efficacy of radiotherapy in prostate cancer. Cancer Res 2013; 73(9): 2782-94.
[http://dx.doi.org/10.1158/0008-5472.CAN-12-3981] [PMID: 23418320]

[156] Moughon DL, He H, Schokrpur S, *et al.* Macrophage Blockade Using CSF1R Inhibitors Reverses the Vascular Leakage Underlying Malignant Ascites in Late-Stage Epithelial Ovarian Cancer. Cancer Res 2015; 75(22): 4742-52.
[http://dx.doi.org/10.1158/0008-5472.CAN-14-3373] [PMID: 26471360]

[157] Strachan DC, Ruffell B, Oei Y, *et al.* CSF1R inhibition delays cervical and mammary tumor growth in murine models by attenuating the turnover of tumor-associated macrophages and enhancing infiltration by CD8 + T cells. OncoImmunology 2013; 2(12): e26968-8.
[http://dx.doi.org/10.4161/onci.26968] [PMID: 24498562]

[158] Furukawa Y, Nakatsuru S, Nagafuchi A, *et al.* Structure, expression and chromosome assignment of the human catenin (cadherin-associated protein) alpha 1 gene (CTNNA1). Cytogenet Genome Res 1994; 65(1-2): 74-8.
[http://dx.doi.org/10.1159/000133603] [PMID: 8404069]

[159] Ye Y, McDevitt MA, Guo M, *et al.* Progressive chromatin repression and promoter methylation of CTNNA1 associated with advanced myeloid malignancies. Cancer Res 2009; 69(21): 8482-90.
[http://dx.doi.org/10.1158/0008-5472.CAN-09-1153] [PMID: 19826047]

[160] Majewski IJ, Kluijt I, Cats A, *et al.* An α-E-catenin (*CTNNA1*) mutation in hereditary diffuse gastric cancer. J Pathol 2013; 229(4): 621-9.
[http://dx.doi.org/10.1002/path.4152] [PMID: 23208944]

[161] Liu TX, Becker MW, Jelinek J, *et al.* Chromosome 5q deletion and epigenetic suppression of the gene encoding α-catenin (CTNNA1) in myeloid cell transformation. Nat Med 2007; 13(1): 78-83.
[http://dx.doi.org/10.1038/nm1512] [PMID: 17159988]

[162] Vermeulen SJ, Nollet F, Teugels E, *et al.* The αE-catenin gene (CTNNA1) acts as an invasion-suppressor gene in human colon cancer cells. Oncogene 1999 184 1999; 18: 905–915.

[163] Williams KA, Lee M, Hu Y, *et al.* A systems genetics approach identifies CXCL14, ITGAX, and LPCAT2 as novel aggressive prostate cancer susceptibility genes. PLoS Genet 2014; 10(11): e1004809.
[http://dx.doi.org/10.1371/journal.pgen.1004809] [PMID: 25411967]

[164] Augsten M, Hägglöf C, Olsson E, *et al.* CXCL14 is an autocrine growth factor for fibroblasts and acts as a multi-modal stimulator of prostate tumor growth. Proc Natl Acad Sci USA 2009; 106(9): 3414-9.
[http://dx.doi.org/10.1073/pnas.0813144106] [PMID: 19218429]

[165] Tessema M, Klinge DM, Yingling CM, Do K, Van Neste L, Belinsky SA. Re-expression of CXCL14, a common target for epigenetic silencing in lung cancer, induces tumor necrosis. Oncogene 2010; 29(37): 5159-70.
[http://dx.doi.org/10.1038/onc.2010.255] [PMID: 20562917]

[166] Wente MN, Mayer C, Gaida MM, *et al.* CXCL14 expression and potential function in pancreatic cancer. Cancer Lett 2008; 259(2): 209-17.

[http://dx.doi.org/10.1016/j.canlet.2007.10.021] [PMID: 18054154]

[167] Pelicano H, Lu W, Zhou Y, *et al.* Mitochondrial dysfunction and reactive oxygen species imbalance promote breast cancer cell motility through a CXCL14-mediated mechanism. Cancer Res 2009; 69(6): 2375-83.
[http://dx.doi.org/10.1158/0008-5472.CAN-08-3359] [PMID: 19276362]

[168] Wang Z, Tseng CP, Pong RC, *et al.* The mechanism of growth-inhibitory effect of DOC-2/DAB2 in prostate cancer. Characterization of a novel GTPase-activating protein associated with N-terminal domain of DOC-2/DAB2. J Biol Chem 2002; 277(15): 12622-31.
[http://dx.doi.org/10.1074/jbc.M110568200] [PMID: 11812785]

[169] Zhou J, Scholes J, Hsieh JT. Characterization of a novel negative regulator (DOC-2/DAB2) of c-Src in normal prostatic epithelium and cancer. J Biol Chem 2003; 278(9): 6936-41.
[http://dx.doi.org/10.1074/jbc.M210628200] [PMID: 12473651]

[170] Du L, Zhao Z, Ma X, *et al.* miR-93-directed downregulation of DAB2 defines a novel oncogenic pathway in lung cancer. Oncogene 2014; 33(34): 4307-15.
[http://dx.doi.org/10.1038/onc.2013.381] [PMID: 24037530]

[171] Yano M, Toyooka S, Tsukuda K, *et al.* Aberrant promoter methylation of human DAB2 interactive protein(hDAB2IP) gene in lung cancers. Int J Cancer 2005; 113(1): 59-66.
[http://dx.doi.org/10.1002/ijc.20531] [PMID: 15386433]

[172] Zhoul J, Hernandez G, Tu SW, Huang CL, Tseng CP, Hsieh JT. The role of DOC-2/DAB2 in modulating androgen receptor-mediated cell growth *via* the nongenomic c-Src-mediated pathway in normal prostatic epithelium and cancer. Cancer Res 2005; 65(21): 9906-13.
[http://dx.doi.org/10.1158/0008-5472.CAN-05-1481] [PMID: 16267015]

[173] Xu X, Gammon MD, Wetmur JG, *et al.* A functional 19-base pair deletion polymorphism of dihydrofolate reductase (DHFR) and risk of breast cancer in multivitamin users. Am J Clin Nutr 2007; 85(4): 1098-102.
[http://dx.doi.org/10.1093/ajcn/85.4.1098] [PMID: 17413111]

[174] Eskandari-Nasab E, Hashemi M, Rezaei H, *et al.* Evaluation of UDP-glucuronosyltransferase 2B17 (UGT2B17) and dihydrofolate reductase (DHFR) genes deletion and the expression level of NGX6 mRNA in breast cancer. Mol Biol Reports 2012 3912 2012; 39: 10531–10539.

[175] Song B, Wang Y, Titmus MA, *et al.* Molecular mechanism of chemoresistance by miR-215 in osteosarcoma and colon cancer cells. Mol Cancer 2010; 9(1): 96.
[http://dx.doi.org/10.1186/1476-4598-9-96] [PMID: 20433742]

[176] J Neradil, G Pavlasova, R Veselska. New mechanisms for an old drug; DHFR- and non-DHFR-mediated effects of methotrexate in cancer cells - PubMed. Klin Onkol; 2:2S87-92, https: //pubmed .ncbi.nlm.nih.gov/23581023/ (2012, accessed 28 September 2021).

[177] M S, T G, M S, *et al.* Expression levels of the microRNA processing enzymes Drosha and dicer in epithelial skin cancer. Cancer Invest 2010; 28: 649–653.

[178] Torres A, Torres K, Paszkowski T, *et al.* Major regulators of microRNAs biogenesis Dicer and Drosha are down-regulated in endometrial cancer. Tumour Biol 2011; 32(4): 769-76.
[http://dx.doi.org/10.1007/s13277-011-0179-0] [PMID: 21559780]

[179] Avery-Kiejda KA, Braye SG, Forbes JF, Scott RJ. The expression of Dicer and Drosha in matched normal tissues, tumours and lymph node metastases in triple negative breast cancer. BMC Cancer 2014; 14(1): 253.
[http://dx.doi.org/10.1186/1471-2407-14-253] [PMID: 24725360]

[180] A G, E F, F G, *et al.* Dysregulation of microRNA biogenesis in cancer: the impact of mutant p53 on Drosha complex activity. J Exp Clin Cancer Res; 35.
[http://dx.doi.org/10.1186/s13046-016-0319-x]

[181] Cho SH, Ko JJ, Kim JO, *et al.* 3'-UTR Polymorphisms in the MiRNA Machinery Genes DROSHA,

DICER1, RAN, and XPO5 Are Associated with Colorectal Cancer Risk in a Korean Population. PLoS One 2015; 10(7): e0131125.
[http://dx.doi.org/10.1371/journal.pone.0131125] [PMID: 26147304]

[182] Liu YX, Wang J, Guo J, Wu J, Lieberman HB, Yin Y. DUSP1 is controlled by p53 during the cellular response to oxidative stress. Mol Cancer Res 2008; 6(4): 624-33.
[http://dx.doi.org/10.1158/1541-7786.MCR-07-2019] [PMID: 18403641]

[183] Shen J, Zhou S, Shi L, *et al.* DUSP1 inhibits cell proliferation, metastasis and invasion and angiogenesis in gallbladder cancer. Oncotarget 2017; 8(7): 12133-44.
[http://dx.doi.org/10.18632/oncotarget.14815] [PMID: 28129656]

[184] Moncho-Amor V, Ibañez de Cáceres I, Bandres E, *et al.* DUSP1/MKP1 promotes angiogenesis, invasion and metastasis in non-small-cell lung cancer. Oncogene 2011; 30(6): 668-78.
[http://dx.doi.org/10.1038/onc.2010.449] [PMID: 20890299]

[185] Melhem A, Yamada SD, Fleming GF, *et al.* Administration of glucocorticoids to ovarian cancer patients is associated with expression of the anti-apoptotic genes SGK1 and MKP1/DUSP1 in ovarian tissues. Clin Cancer Res 2009; 15(9): 3196-204.
[http://dx.doi.org/10.1158/1078-0432.CCR-08-2131] [PMID: 19383827]

[186] Shen J, Zhang Y, Yu H, *et al.* Role of DUSP1/MKP1 in tumorigenesis, tumor progression and therapy. Cancer Med 2016; 5(8): 2061-8.
[http://dx.doi.org/10.1002/cam4.772] [PMID: 27227569]

[187] Chen CC, Hardy DB, Mendelson CR. Progesterone receptor inhibits proliferation of human breast cancer cells *via* induction of MAPK phosphatase 1 (MKP-1/DUSP1). J Biol Chem 2011; 286(50): 43091-102.
[http://dx.doi.org/10.1074/jbc.M111.295865] [PMID: 22020934]

[188] Fernandez-Jimenez N, Sklias A, Ecsedi S, *et al.* Lowly methylated region analysis identifies EBF1 as a potential epigenetic modifier in breast cancer. Epigenetics 2017; 12(11): 964-72.
[http://dx.doi.org/10.1080/15592294.2017.1373919] [PMID: 29099283]

[189] Schwab C, Ryan SL, Chilton L, *et al.* EBF1-PDGFRB fusion in pediatric B-cell precursor acute lymphoblastic leukemia (BCP-ALL): genetic profile and clinical implications. Blood 2016; 127(18): 2214-8.
[http://dx.doi.org/10.1182/blood-2015-09-670166] [PMID: 26872634]

[190] Shen A, Chen Y, Liu L, *et al.* EBF1-Mediated Upregulation of Ribosome Assembly Factor PNO1 Contributes to Cancer Progression by Negatively Regulating the p53 Signaling Pathway. Cancer Res 2019; 79(9): 2257-70.
[http://dx.doi.org/10.1158/0008-5472.CAN-18-3238] [PMID: 30862720]

[191] Virolle T, Krones-Herzig A, Baron V, De Gregorio G, Adamson ED, Mercola D. Egr1 promotes growth and survival of prostate cancer cells. Identification of novel Egr1 target genes. J Biol Chem 2003; 278(14): 11802-10.
[http://dx.doi.org/10.1074/jbc.M210279200] [PMID: 12556466]

[192] Ferraro B, Bepler G, Sharma S, Cantor A, Haura EB. EGR1 predicts PTEN and survival in patients with non-small-cell lung cancer. J Clin Oncol 2005; 23(9): 1921-6.
[http://dx.doi.org/10.1200/JCO.2005.08.127] [PMID: 15774784]

[193] Gitenay D, Baron VT. Is EGR1 a potential target for prostate cancer therapy? Future Oncol 2009; 5(7): 993-1003.
[http://dx.doi.org/10.2217/fon.09.67] [PMID: 19792968]

[194] Katoh M. Function and cancer genomics of FAT family genes. Int J Oncol 2012; 41(6): 1913-8.
[http://dx.doi.org/10.3892/ijo.2012.1669] [PMID: 23076869]

[195] Cohen AS, Khalil FK, Welsh EA, *et al.* Cell-surface marker discovery for lung cancer. Oncotarget 2017; 8(69): 113373-402.

[http://dx.doi.org/10.18632/oncotarget.23009] [PMID: 29371917]

[196] Li Y, Kang K, Krahn JM, *et al.* A comprehensive genomic pan-cancer classification using The Cancer Genome Atlas gene expression data. BMC Genomics 2017; 18(1): 508-8.
[http://dx.doi.org/10.1186/s12864-017-3906-0] [PMID: 28673244]

[197] Morris LGT, Ramaswami D, Chan TA. The FAT epidemic: A gene family frequently mutated across multiple human cancer types. Cell Cycle 2013; 12(7): 1011-2.
[http://dx.doi.org/10.4161/cc.24305] [PMID: 23493187]

[198] Rocha J, Zouanat FZ, Zoubeidi A, *et al.* The Fer tyrosine kinase acts as a downstream interleukin-6 effector of androgen receptor activation in prostate cancer. Mol Cell Endocrinol 2013; 381(1-2): 140-9.
[http://dx.doi.org/10.1016/j.mce.2013.07.017] [PMID: 23906537]

[199] Ivanova IA, Vermeulen JF, Ercan C, *et al.* FER kinase promotes breast cancer metastasis by regulating α6- and β1-integrin-dependent cell adhesion and anoikis resistance. Oncogene 2013 3250 2013; 32: 5582–5592.

[200] Li H, Ren Z, Kang X, *et al.* Identification of tyrosine-phosphorylated proteins associated with metastasis and functional analysis of FER in human hepatocellular carcinoma cells. BMC Cancer 2009; 9(1): 366-6.
[http://dx.doi.org/10.1186/1471-2407-9-366] [PMID: 19835603]

[201] Zoubeidi A, Rocha J, Zouanat FZ, *et al.* The Fer tyrosine kinase cooperates with interleukin-6 to activate signal transducer and activator of transcription 3 and promote human prostate cancer cell growth. Mol Cancer Res 2009; 7(1): 142-55.
[http://dx.doi.org/10.1158/1541-7786.MCR-08-0117] [PMID: 19147545]

[202] Yoshimura N, Sano H, Hashiramoto A, *et al.* The expression and localization of fibroblast growth factor-1 (FGF-1) and FGF receptor-1 (FGFR-1) in human breast cancer. Clin Immunol Immunopathol 1998; 89(1): 28-34.
[http://dx.doi.org/10.1006/clin.1998.4551] [PMID: 9756721]

[203] Bai YP, Shang K, Chen H, *et al.* FGF -1/-3/ FGFR 4 signaling in cancer-associated fibroblasts promotes tumor progression in colon cancer through Erk and MMP -7. Cancer Sci 2015; 106(10): 1278-87.
[http://dx.doi.org/10.1111/cas.12745] [PMID: 26183471]

[204] King ML, Lindberg ME, Stodden GR, *et al.* WNT7A/β-catenin signaling induces FGF1 and influences sensitivity to niclosamide in ovarian cancer. Oncogene 2015; 34(26): 3452-62.
[http://dx.doi.org/10.1038/onc.2014.277] [PMID: 25174399]

[205] Tomlinson DC, Knowles MA. Altered splicing of FGFR1 is associated with high tumor grade and stage and leads to increased sensitivity to FGF1 in bladder cancer. Am J Pathol 2010; 177(5): 2379-86.
[http://dx.doi.org/10.2353/ajpath.2010.100354] [PMID: 20889570]

[206] Nomura S, Yoshitomi H, Takano S, *et al.* FGF10/FGFR2 signal induces cell migration and invasion in pancreatic cancer. Br J Cancer 2008; 99(2): 305-13.
[http://dx.doi.org/10.1038/sj.bjc.6604473] [PMID: 18594526]

[207] Ghoussaini M, French JD, Michailidou K, *et al.* Evidence that the 5p12 Variant rs10941679 Confers Susceptibility to Estrogen-Receptor-Positive Breast Cancer through FGF10 and MRPS30 Regulation. Am J Hum Genet 2016; 99(4): 903-11.
[http://dx.doi.org/10.1016/j.ajhg.2016.07.017] [PMID: 27640304]

[208] Huijts PE, van Dongen M, de Goeij MC, *et al.* Allele-specific regulation of FGFR2 expression is cell type-dependent and may increase breast cancer risk through a paracrine stimulus involving FGF10. Breast Cancer Res 2011 134 2011; 13: 1–12.

[209] A A, GH R, E A, *et al.* FGF10: Type III Epithelial Mesenchymal Transition and Invasion in Breast Cancer Cell Lines. J Cancer 2014; 5: 537–547.

[210] Memarzadeh S, Xin L, Mulholland DJ, *et al.* Enhanced paracrine FGF10 expression promotes formation of multifocal prostate adenocarcinoma and an increase in epithelial androgen receptor. Cancer Cell 2007; 12(6): 572-85.
[http://dx.doi.org/10.1016/j.ccr.2007.11.002] [PMID: 18068633]

[211] Chung SS, Koh CJ. Bladder cancer cell in co-culture induces human stem cell differentiation to urothelial cells through paracrine FGF10 signaling. *In Vitro* Cell Dev Biol Anim 2013; 49(10): 746-51.
[http://dx.doi.org/10.1007/s11626-013-9662-9] [PMID: 23949743]

[212] Thussbas C, Nahrig J, Streit S, *et al.* FGFR4 Arg388 allele is associated with resistance to adjuvant therapy in primary breast cancer. J Clin Oncol 2006; 24(23): 3747-55.
[http://dx.doi.org/10.1200/JCO.2005.04.8587] [PMID: 16822847]

[213] Bange J, Prechtl D, Cheburkin Y, *et al.* Cancer Progression and Tumor Cell Motility Are Associated with the FGFR4 Arg388 Allele. Cancer Res; 62.

[214] M H, C M, M S, *et al.* First Selective Small Molecule Inhibitor of FGFR4 for the Treatment of Hepatocellular Carcinomas with an Activated FGFR4 Signaling Pathway. Cancer Discov 2015; 5: 424–437.

[215] Liu R, Li J, Xie K, *et al.* Molecular and Cellular Pathobiology FGFR4 Promotes Stroma-Induced Epithelial-to-Mesenchymal Transition in Colorectal Cancer 2013.
[http://dx.doi.org/10.1158/0008-5472.CAN-12-4718]

[216] Chen F, Takenaka K, Ogawa E, *et al.* Flt-4-positive endothelial cell density and its clinical significance in non-small cell lung cancer. Clin Cancer Res 2004; 10(24): 8548-53.
[http://dx.doi.org/10.1158/1078-0432.CCR-04-0950] [PMID: 15623638]

[217] Türkmen S, Riehn M, Klopocki E, Molkentin M, Reinhardt R, Burmeister T. A BACH2-BCL2L1 fusion gene resulting from a t(6;20)(q15;q11.2) chromosomal translocation in the lymphoma cell line BLUE-1. Genes Chromosomes Cancer 2011; 50(6): 389-96.
[http://dx.doi.org/10.1002/gcc.20863] [PMID: 21412927]

[218] Su JL, Yang PC, Shih JY, *et al.* The VEGF-C/Flt-4 axis promotes invasion and metastasis of cancer cells. Cancer Cell 2006; 9(3): 209-23.
[http://dx.doi.org/10.1016/j.ccr.2006.02.018] [PMID: 16530705]

[219] Herrmann E, Eltze E, Bierer S, *et al.* VEGF-C, VEGF-D and Flt-4 in transitional bladder cancer: relationships to clinicopathological parameters and long-term survival. Anticancer Res 2007; 27(5A): 3127-33.
[PMID: 17970053]

[220] Nakamura Y, Yasuoka H, Tsujimoto M, *et al.* Flt-4-Positive Vessel Density Correlates with Vascular Endothelial Growth Factor-D Expression, Nodal Status, and Prognosis in Breast Cancer.

[221] He S, Chen CH, Chernichenko N, *et al.* GFRα1 released by nerves enhances cancer cell perineural invasion through GDNF-RET signaling. Proc Natl Acad Sci USA 2014; 111(19): E2008-17.
[http://dx.doi.org/10.1073/pnas.1402944111] [PMID: 24778213]

[222] Huang SM, Chen TS, Chiu CM, *et al.* GDNF increases cell motility in human colon cancer through VEGF–VEGFR1 interaction. Endocr Relat Cancer 2014; 21(1): 73-84.
[http://dx.doi.org/10.1530/ERC-13-0351] [PMID: 24165321]

[223] Funahashi H, Okada Y, Sawai H, *et al.* The role of glial cell line-derived neurotrophic factor (GDNF) and integrins for invasion and metastasis in human pancreatic cancer cells. J Surg Oncol 2005; 91(1): 77-83.
[http://dx.doi.org/10.1002/jso.20277] [PMID: 15999351]

[224] Liu H, Ma Q, Li J. High glucose promotes cell proliferation and enhances GDNF and RET expression in pancreatic cancer cells. Mol Cell Biochem 2010 3471 2010; 347: 95–101.

[225] Yang Z, Yang L, Zou Q, *et al.* Positive ALDH1A3 and negative GPX3 expressions are biomarkers for

poor prognosis of gallbladder cancer. Dis Markers 2013; 35(3): 163-72.
[http://dx.doi.org/10.1155/2013/187043] [PMID: 24167362]

[226]   Barrett CW, Ning W, Chen X, *et al.* Tumor suppressor function of the plasma glutathione peroxidase gpx3 in colitis-associated carcinoma. Cancer Res 2013; 73(3): 1245-55.
[http://dx.doi.org/10.1158/0008-5472.CAN-12-3150] [PMID: 23221387]

[227]   Yu YP, Yu G, Tseng G, *et al.* Glutathione peroxidase 3, deleted or methylated in prostate cancer, suppresses prostate cancer growth and metastasis. Cancer Res 2007; 67(17): 8043-50.
[http://dx.doi.org/10.1158/0008-5472.CAN-07-0648] [PMID: 17804715]

[228]   Agnani D, Camacho-Vanegas O, Camacho C, *et al.* Decreased levels of serum glutathione peroxidase 3 are associated with papillary serous ovarian cancer and disease progression. J Ovarian Res 2011 41 2011; 4: 1–8.

[229]   Chen B, Rao X, House MG, Nephew KP, Cullen KJ, Guo Z. GPx3 promoter hypermethylation is a frequent event in human cancer and is associated with tumorigenesis and chemotherapy response. Cancer Lett 2011; 309(1): 37-45.
[http://dx.doi.org/10.1016/j.canlet.2011.05.013] [PMID: 21684681]

[230]   McGuire MH, Herbrich SM, Dasari SK, *et al.* Pan-cancer genomic analysis links 3'UTR DNA methylation with increased gene expression in T cells. EBioMedicine 2019; 43: 127-37.
[http://dx.doi.org/10.1016/j.ebiom.2019.04.045] [PMID: 31056473]

[231]   Polprasert C, Takeuchi Y, Kakiuchi N, *et al.* Frequent germline mutations of *HAVCR2* in sporadic subcutaneous panniculitis-like T-cell lymphoma. Blood Adv 2019; 3(4): 588-95.
[http://dx.doi.org/10.1182/bloodadvances.2018028340] [PMID: 30792187]

[232]   F P, F C, Z Z, *et al.* Functional variants of TIM-3/HAVCR2 3'UTR in lymphoblastoid cell lines. Futur Sci OA; 2018, 4.
[http://dx.doi.org/10.4155/fsoa-2017-0121]

[233]   Lisberg A, Mckenna R, Dering J, *et al.* P2.01-078 Frequent High TIM-3 (HAVCR2) Expression in Resected NSCLC Specimens, Most Notably in Adenocarcinoma Histology. Epub ahead of print 2017.
[http://dx.doi.org/10.1016/j.jtho.2016.11.1130]

[234]   Nishikawa K, Asai T, Shigematsu H, *et al.* Development of anti-HB-EGF immunoliposomes for the treatment of breast cancer. J Control Release 2012; 160(2): 274-80.
[http://dx.doi.org/10.1016/j.jconrel.2011.10.010] [PMID: 22020380]

[235]   Zhou ZN, Sharma VP, Beaty BT, *et al.* Autocrine HBEGF expression promotes breast cancer intravasation, metastasis and macrophage-independent invasion *in vivo.* Oncogene 2014; 33(29): 3784-93.
[http://dx.doi.org/10.1038/onc.2013.363] [PMID: 24013225]

[236]   Ongusaha PP, Kwak JC, Zwible AJ, *et al.* HB-EGF is a potent inducer of tumor growth and angiogenesis. Cancer Res 2004; 64(15): 5283-90.
[http://dx.doi.org/10.1158/0008-5472.CAN-04-0925] [PMID: 15289334]

[237]   Yin Y, Grabowska AM, Clarke PA, *et al.* Helicobacter pylori potentiates epithelial:mesenchymal transition in gastric cancer: links to soluble HB-EGF, gastrin and matrix metalloproteinase-7. Gut 2010; 59(8): 1037-45.
[http://dx.doi.org/10.1136/gut.2009.199794] [PMID: 20584780]

[238]   A L-S, AR F, E S, *et al.* HDAC3 represses the expression of NKG2D ligands ULBPs in epithelial tumour cells: potential implications for the immunosurveillance of cancer. Oncogene 2009; 28: 2370–2382.

[239]   Koumangoye RB, Andl T, Taubenslag KJ, *et al.* SOX4 interacts with EZH2 and HDAC3 to suppress microRNA-31 in invasive esophageal cancer cells. Mol Cancer 2015; 14(1): 24-4.
[http://dx.doi.org/10.1186/s12943-014-0284-y] [PMID: 25644061]

[240]   Ren H, Tang L. HDAC3-mediated lncRNA-LOC101928316 contributes to cisplatin resistance in

gastric cancer *via* activating the PI3K-Akt-mTOR pathway. Neoplasma 2021; 68(5): 1043-51.
[http://dx.doi.org/10.4149/neo_2021_210317N356]

[241] Wilson AJ, Byun DS, Popova N, *et al.* Histone deacetylase 3 (HDAC3) and other class I HDACs regulate colon cell maturation and p21 expression and are deregulated in human colon cancer. J Biol Chem 2006; 281(19): 13548-58.
[http://dx.doi.org/10.1074/jbc.M510023200] [PMID: 16533812]

[242] Godman CA, Joshi R, Tierney BR, *et al.* HDAC3 impacts multiple oncogenic pathways in colon cancer cells with effects on Wnt and vitamin D signaling. Cancer Biol Ther 2008; 7(10): 1570-80.
[http://dx.doi.org/10.4161/cbt.7.10.6561] [PMID: 18769117]

[243] Genovese G, Ghosh P, Li H, *et al.* The tumor suppressor HINT1 regulates MITF and β-catenin transcriptional activity in melanoma cells. Cell Cycle 2012; 11(11): 2206-15.
[http://dx.doi.org/10.4161/cc.20765] [PMID: 22647378]

[244] Wang L, Zhang Y, Li H, Xu Z, Santella RM, Weinstein IB. Hint1 inhibits growth and activator protein-1 activity in human colon cancer cells. Cancer Res 2007; 67(10): 4700-8.
[http://dx.doi.org/10.1158/0008-5472.CAN-06-4645] [PMID: 17510397]

[245] Wang L, Li H, Zhang Y, Santella RM, Weinstein IB. HINT1 inhibits β-catenin/TCF4, USF2 and NFκB activity in human hepatoma cells. Int J Cancer 2009; 124(7): 1526-34.
[http://dx.doi.org/10.1002/ijc.24072] [PMID: 19089909]

[246] Zhang YJ, Li H, Wu HC, *et al.* Silencing of Hint1, a novel tumor suppressor gene, by promoter hypermethylation in hepatocellular carcinoma. Cancer Lett 2009; 275(2): 277-84.
[http://dx.doi.org/10.1016/j.canlet.2008.10.042] [PMID: 19081673]

[247] Huang H, Wei X, Su X, *et al.* Clinical significance of expression of Hint1 and potential epigenetic mechanism in gastric cancer. Int J Oncol 2011; 38(6): 1557-64.
[PMID: 21468541]

[248] Liu XF, Bera TK, Kahue C, *et al.* ANKRD26 and its interacting partners TRIO, GPS2, HMMR and DIPA regulate adipogenesis in 3T3-L1 cells. PLoS One 2012; 7(5): e38130-0.
[http://dx.doi.org/10.1371/journal.pone.0038130] [PMID: 22666460]

[249] Pujana MA, Han J-DJ, Starita LM, *et al.* Network modeling links breast cancer susceptibility and centrosome dysfunction. Nat Genet 2007 3911 2007; 39: 1338–1349.

[250] Tilghman J, Wu H, Sang Y, *et al.* HMMR maintains the stemness and tumorigenicity of glioblastoma stem-like cells. Cancer Res 2014; 74(11): 3168-79.
[http://dx.doi.org/10.1158/0008-5472.CAN-13-2103] [PMID: 24710409]

[251] Chu ZP, Dai J, Jia LG, *et al.* Increased expression of long noncoding RNA HMMR-AS1 in epithelial ovarian cancer: an independent prognostic factor. Eur Rev Med Pharmacol Sci 2018; 22(23): 8145-50.
[PMID: 30556852]

[252] Han SS, Cho EY, Lee TS, *et al.* Interleukin-12 p40 gene (IL12B) polymorphisms and the risk of cervical caner in Korean women. Eur J Obstet Gynecol Reprod Biol 2008; 140(1): 71-5.
[http://dx.doi.org/10.1016/j.ejogrb.2008.02.007] [PMID: 18367309]

[253] Chen X, Han S, Wang S, *et al.* Interactions of IL-12A and IL-12B polymorphisms on the risk of cervical cancer in Chinese women. Clin Cancer Res 2009; 15(1): 400-5.
[http://dx.doi.org/10.1158/1078-0432.CCR-08-1829] [PMID: 19118071]

[254] A R, A M, A S, *et al.* Contribution of IL12A and IL12B polymorphisms to the risk of cervical cancer. Pathol Oncol Res 2012; 18: 997–1002.

[255] Morahan G, Kaur G, Singh M, *et al.* Association of variants in the *IL12B* gene with leprosy and tuberculosis. Tissue Antigens 2007; 69 (Suppl. 1): 234-6.
[http://dx.doi.org/10.1111/j.1399-0039.2006.773_3.x] [PMID: 17445208]

[256] Smith AM, Qualls JE, O'Brien K, *et al.* A distal enhancer in Il12b is the target of transcriptional

repression by the STAT3 pathway and requires the basic leucine zipper (B-ZIP) protein NFIL3. J Biol Chem 2011; 286(26): 23582-90.
[http://dx.doi.org/10.1074/jbc.M111.249235] [PMID: 21566115]

[257]   A S, P L, BH J, *et al.* Targeting of IL-4 and IL-13 receptors for cancer therapy. Cytokine 2015; 75: 79–88.

[258]   Hallett MA, Venmar KT, Fingleton B. Cytokine stimulation of epithelial cancer cells: the similar and divergent functions of IL-4 and IL-13. Cancer Res 2012; 72(24): 6338-43.
[http://dx.doi.org/10.1158/0008-5472.CAN-12-3544] [PMID: 23222300]

[259]   Murata T, Obiri NI, Debinski W, Puri RK. Structure of IL-13 receptor: analysis of subunit composition in cancer and immune cells. Biochem Biophys Res Commun 1997; 238(1): 90-4.
[http://dx.doi.org/10.1006/bbrc.1997.7248] [PMID: 9299458]

[260]   Park JM, Terabe M, van den Broeke LT, Donaldson DD, Berzofsky JA. Unmasking immuno-surveillance against a syngeneic colon cancer by elimination of CD4+ NKT regulatory cells and IL-13. Int J Cancer 2005; 114(1): 80-7.
[http://dx.doi.org/10.1002/ijc.20669] [PMID: 15523692]

[261]   Barderas R, Bartolomé RA, Fernandez-Aceñero MJ, Torres S, Casal JI. High expression of IL-13 receptor α2 in colorectal cancer is associated with invasion, liver metastasis, and poor prognosis. Cancer Res 2012; 72(11): 2780-90.
[http://dx.doi.org/10.1158/0008-5472.CAN-11-4090] [PMID: 22505647]

[262]   Fujisawa T, Joshi BH, Puri RK. IL-13 regulates cancer invasion and metastasis through IL-13Rα2 *via* ERK/AP-1 pathway in mouse model of human ovarian cancer. Int J Cancer 2012; 131(2): 344-56.
[http://dx.doi.org/10.1002/ijc.26366] [PMID: 21858811]

[263]   Puri RK, Siegel JP. Interleukin-4 and cancer therapy. Cancer Invest 1993; 11(4): 473-86.
[http://dx.doi.org/10.3109/07357909309018879] [PMID: 8324651]

[264]   Puri RK, Leland P, Kreitman RJ, Pastan I. Human neurological cancer cells express interleukin-4 (IL-4) receptors which are targets for the toxic effects of IL4-pseudomonas exotoxin chimeric protein. Int J Cancer 1994; 58(4): 574-81.
[http://dx.doi.org/10.1002/ijc.2910580421] [PMID: 8056454]

[265]   Zhang WJ, Li BH, Yang XZ, *et al.* IL-4-induced Stat6 activities affect apoptosis and gene expression in breast cancer cells. Cytokine 2008; 42(1): 39-47.
[http://dx.doi.org/10.1016/j.cyto.2008.01.016] [PMID: 18342537]

[266]   Li BH, Yang XZ, Li PD, *et al.* IL-4/Stat6 activities correlate with apoptosis and metastasis in colon cancer cells. Biochem Biophys Res Commun 2008; 369(2): 554-60.
[http://dx.doi.org/10.1016/j.bbrc.2008.02.052] [PMID: 18294957]

[267]   Gocheva V, Wang HW, Gadea BB, *et al.* IL-4 induces cathepsin protease activity in tumor-associated macrophages to promote cancer growth and invasion. Genes Dev 2010; 24(3): 241-55.
[http://dx.doi.org/10.1101/gad.1874010] [PMID: 20080943]

[268]   Wang M, Zhang H, Yang F, *et al.* miR-188-5p suppresses cellular proliferation and migration *via* IL6ST: A potential noninvasive diagnostic biomarker for breast cancer. J Cell Physiol 2020; 235(5): 4890-901.
[http://dx.doi.org/10.1002/jcp.29367] [PMID: 31650530]

[269]   Pietro L, Bottcher-Luiz F, Velloso LA, *et al.* Expression of interleukin-6 (IL-6), signal transducer and activator of transcription-3 (STAT-3) and telomerase in choriocarcinomas. Surg Exp Pathol 2020 31 2020; 3: 1–8.

[270]   Chen J, Liu H, Chen J, Sun B, Wu J, Du C. PLXNC1 Enhances Carcinogenesis Through Transcriptional Activation of IL6ST in Gastric Cancer. Front Oncol 2020; 10: 33.
[http://dx.doi.org/10.3389/fonc.2020.00033] [PMID: 32117710]

[271]   Kim MS, Chung NG, Kim MS, Yoo NJ, Lee SH. Somatic mutation of IL7R exon 6 in acute leukemias

and solid cancers. Hum Pathol 2013; 44(4): 551-5.
[http://dx.doi.org/10.1016/j.humpath.2012.06.017] [PMID: 23069254]

[272] Ott CJ, Kopp N, Bird L, *et al.* BET bromodomain inhibition targets both c-Myc and IL7R in high-risk acute lymphoblastic leukemia. Blood 2012; 120(14): 2843-52.
[http://dx.doi.org/10.1182/blood-2012-02-413021] [PMID: 22904298]

[273] Zenatti PP, Ribeiro D, Li W, *et al.* Oncogenic IL7R gain-of-function mutations in childhood T-cell acute lymphoblastic leukemia. Nat Genet 2011; 43(10): 932-9.
[http://dx.doi.org/10.1038/ng.924] [PMID: 21892159]

[274] Gao J, Senthil M, Ren B, *et al.* IRF-1 transcriptionally upregulates PUMA, which mediates the mitochondrial apoptotic pathway in IRF-1-induced apoptosis in cancer cells. Cell Death Differ 2010; 17(4): 699-709.
[http://dx.doi.org/10.1038/cdd.2009.156] [PMID: 19851330]

[275] H Nozawa, E Oda, S Ueda, *et al.* Functionally inactivating point mutation in the tumor-suppressor IRF-1 gene identified in human gastric cancer - PubMed, https://pubmed.ncbi.nlm.nih.gov/9679752/ (1998, accessed 28 September 2021).

[276] Bachmann SB, Frommel SC, Camicia R, Winkler HC, Santoro R, Hassa PO. DTX3L and ARTD9 inhibit IRF1 expression and mediate in cooperation with ARTD8 survival and proliferation of metastatic prostate cancer cells. Mol Cancer 2014; 13(1): 125-5.
[http://dx.doi.org/10.1186/1476-4598-13-125] [PMID: 24886089]

[277] Murtas D, Maric D, De Giorgi V, *et al.* IRF-1 responsiveness to IFN-γ predicts different cancer immune phenotypes. Br J Cancer 2013 1091 2013; 109: 76–82.

[278] Boudjadi S, Beaulieu JF. ITGA1 (integrin, alpha 1). Atlas Genet Cytogenet Oncol Haematol 2017; (9):
[http://dx.doi.org/10.4267/2042/62325]

[279] Qingxia Ma, Jingyi Song, Hailong Ma, *et al.* Synergistic anticancer effect of Grb2 and ITGA1 on cancer cells highly expressing Grb2 through suppressing ERK phosphorylation - PubMed. 2019; 182–189.

[280] Boudjadi S, Carrier JC, Groulx J-F, *et al.* Integrin α1β1 expression is controlled by c-MYC in colorectal cancer cells. Oncogene 2016 3513 2015; 35: 1671–1678.

[281] Boudjadi S, Beaulieu JF. MYC and integrins interplay in colorectal cancer. Oncoscience 2016; 3(2): 50-1.
[http://dx.doi.org/10.18632/oncoscience.293] [PMID: 27014720]

[282] Gharibi A, La Kim S, Molnar J, *et al.* ITGA1 is a pre-malignant biomarker that promotes therapy resistance and metastatic potential in pancreatic cancer. Sci Reports 2017 71 2017; 7: 1–14.

[283] Wei L, Yin F, Zhang W, *et al.* Original Article ITGA1 and cell adhesion-mediated drug resistance in ovarian cancer. Int J Clin Exp Pathol 2017; 10: 5522-9.

[284] Vargas L, Hamasy A, Nore BF, Smith CI. Inhibitors of BTK and ITK: state of the new drugs for cancer, autoimmunity and inflammatory diseases. Scand J Immunol 2013; 78(2): 130-9.
[http://dx.doi.org/10.1111/sji.12069] [PMID: 23672610]

[285] Sagiv-Barfi I, Kohrt HEK, Czerwinski DK, Ng PP, Chang BY, Levy R. Therapeutic antitumor immunity by checkpoint blockade is enhanced by ibrutinib, an inhibitor of both BTK and ITK. Proc Natl Acad Sci USA 2015; 112(9): E966-72.
[http://dx.doi.org/10.1073/pnas.1500712112] [PMID: 25730880]

[286] Dierks C, Adrian F, Fisch P, *et al.* The ITK-SYK fusion oncogene induces a T-cell lymphoproliferative disease in mice mimicking human disease. Cancer Res 2010; 70(15): 6193-204.
[http://dx.doi.org/10.1158/0008-5472.CAN-08-3719] [PMID: 20670954]

[287] Cho YG, Chang X, Park IS, *et al.* Promoter methylation of leukemia inhibitory factor receptor gene in colorectal carcinoma. Int J Oncol 2011; 39(2): 337-44.

[PMID: 21617854]

[288] Li Y, Zhang H, Zhao Y, *et al.* A mandatory role of nuclear PAK4-LIFR axis in breast-to-bone metastasis of ERα-positive breast cancer cells. Oncogene 2019; 38(6): 808-21.
[http://dx.doi.org/10.1038/s41388-018-0456-0] [PMID: 30177834]

[289] Okamura Y, Nomoto S, Kanda M, *et al.* Leukemia inhibitory factor receptor (LIFR) is detected as a novel suppressor gene of hepatocellular carcinoma using double-combination array. Cancer Lett 2010; 289(2): 170-7.
[http://dx.doi.org/10.1016/j.canlet.2009.08.013] [PMID: 19733004]

[290] Wu H, Cheng X, Jing X, *et al.* LIFR promotes tumor angiogenesis by up-regulating IL-8 levels in colorectal cancer. Biochim Biophys Acta Mol Basis Dis 2018; 1864(9): 2769-84.
[http://dx.doi.org/10.1016/j.bbadis.2018.05.004] [PMID: 29751081]

[291] Chen D, Sun Y, Wei Y, *et al.* LIFR is a breast cancer metastasis suppressor upstream of the Hippo-YAP pathway and a prognostic marker. Nat Med 2012; 18(10): 1511-7.
[http://dx.doi.org/10.1038/nm.2940] [PMID: 23001183]

[292] Ding XZ, Iversen P, Cluck MW, Knezetic JA, Adrian TE. Lipoxygenase inhibitors abolish proliferation of human pancreatic cancer cells. Biochem Biophys Res Commun 1999; 261(1): 218-23.
[http://dx.doi.org/10.1006/bbrc.1999.1012] [PMID: 10405349]

[293] Miller BW, Morton JP, Pinese M, *et al.* Targeting the LOX / hypoxia axis reverses many of the features that make pancreatic cancer deadly: inhibition of LOX abrogates metastasis and enhances drug efficacy. EMBO Mol Med 2015; 7(8): 1063-76.
[http://dx.doi.org/10.15252/emmm.201404827] [PMID: 26077591]

[294] Kirschmann DA, Seftor EA, Fong SFT, *et al.* A molecular role for lysyl oxidase in breast cancer invasion. Cancer Res 2002; 62(15): 4478-83.
[PMID: 12154058]

[295] Payne SL, Hendrix MJC, Kirschmann DA. Paradoxical roles for lysyl oxidases in cancer—A prospect. J Cell Biochem 2007; 101(6): 1338-54.
[http://dx.doi.org/10.1002/jcb.21371] [PMID: 17471532]

[296] Barker HE, Cox TR, Erler JT. The rationale for targeting the LOX family in cancer. Nat Rev Cancer 2012; 12(8): 540-52.
[http://dx.doi.org/10.1038/nrc3319] [PMID: 22810810]

[297] Wu L, Aster JC, Blacklow SC, *et al.* MAML1, a human homologue of Drosophila Mastermind, is a transcriptional co-activator for NOTCH receptors. Nat Genet 2000 264 2000; 26: 484–489.

[298] Hansson ML, Behmer S, Ceder R, *et al.* MAML1 acts cooperatively with EGR1 to activate EGR1-regulated promoters: implications for nephrogenesis and the development of renal cancer. PLoS One 2012; 7(9): e46001.
[http://dx.doi.org/10.1371/journal.pone.0046001] [PMID: 23029358]

[299] Moghbeli M, Mosannen Mozaffari H, Memar B, *et al.* Role of MAML1 in targeted therapy against the esophageal cancer stem cells. J Transl Med 2019 171 2019; 17: 1–12.

[300] Zhao Y, Katzman RB, Delmolino LM, *et al.* The notch regulator MAML1 interacts with p53 and functions as a coactivator. J Biol Chem 2007; 282(16): 11969-81.
[http://dx.doi.org/10.1074/jbc.M608974200] [PMID: 17317671]

[301] Yun J, Espinoza I, Pannuti A, *et al.* p53 Modulates Notch Signaling in MCF-7 Breast Cancer Cells by Associating With the Notch Transcriptional Complex *via* MAML1. J Cell Physiol 2015; 230(12): 3115-27.
[http://dx.doi.org/10.1002/jcp.25052] [PMID: 26033683]

[302] Kuncharin Y, Sangphech N, Kueanjinda P, Bhattarakosol P, Palaga T. MAML1 regulates cell viability *via* the NF-κB pathway in cervical cancer cell lines. Exp Cell Res 2011; 317(13): 1830-40.
[http://dx.doi.org/10.1016/j.yexcr.2011.05.005] [PMID: 21640102]

[303] Forghanifard MM, Moaven O, Farshchian M, *et al.* Expression analysis elucidates the roles of MAML1 and Twist1 in esophageal squamous cell carcinoma aggressiveness and metastasis. Ann Surg Oncol 2012; 19(3): 743-9.
[http://dx.doi.org/10.1245/s10434-011-2074-8] [PMID: 22006371]

[304] Jara L, Gonzalez-Hormazabal P, Cerceño K, *et al.* Genetic variants in FGFR2 and MAP3K1 are associated with the risk of familial and early-onset breast cancer in a South-American population. Breast Cancer Res Treat 2013; 137(2): 559-69.
[http://dx.doi.org/10.1007/s10549-012-2359-z] [PMID: 23225170]

[305] Liu C, Wang S, Zhu S, *et al.* MAP3K1-targeting therapeutic artificial miRNA suppresses the growth and invasion of breast cancer *in vivo* and *in vitro*. Springerplus 2016; 5(1): 11-1.
[http://dx.doi.org/10.1186/s40064-015-1597-z] [PMID: 26759750]

[306] Xue Z, Vis DJ, Bruna A, *et al.* MAP3K1 and MAP2K4 mutations are associated with sensitivity to MEK inhibitors in multiple cancer models. Cell Res 2018; 28(7): 719-29.
[http://dx.doi.org/10.1038/s41422-018-0044-4] [PMID: 29795445]

[307] Achille A, Baron A, Zamboni G, Di Pace C, Orlandini S, Scarpa A. Chromosome 5 allelic losses are early events in tumours of the papilla of Vater and occur at sites similar to those of gastric cancer. Br J Cancer 1998; 78(12): 1653-60.
[http://dx.doi.org/10.1038/bjc.1998.738] [PMID: 9862579]

[308] D'Amico D, Carbone DP, Johnson BE, Meltzer SJ, Minna JS. Polymorphic sites within the MCC and APC loci reveal very frequent loss of heterozygosity in human small cell lung cancer. Lung Cancer 1993; 8(5-6): 337.
[http://dx.doi.org/10.1016/0169-5002(93)90534-5]

[309] Thompson A, Morris R, Wallace M, *et al.* Allele loss from 5q21 (APC/MCC) and 18q21 (DCC) and DCC mRNA expression in breast cancer. Br J Cancer 1993 681 1993; 68: 64–68.

[310] Du Y, Spence SE, Jenkins NA, Copeland NG. Cooperating cancer-gene identification through oncogenic-retrovirus–induced insertional mutagenesis. Blood 2005; 106(7): 2498-505.
[http://dx.doi.org/10.1182/blood-2004-12-4840] [PMID: 15961513]

[311] Homminga I, Pieters R, Langerak AW, *et al.* Integrated transcript and genome analyses reveal NKX2-1 and MEF2C as potential oncogenes in T cell acute lymphoblastic leukemia. Cancer Cell 2011; 19(4): 484-97.
[http://dx.doi.org/10.1016/j.ccr.2011.02.008] [PMID: 21481790]

[312] Badodi S, Baruffaldi F, Ganassi M, Battini R, Molinari S. Phosphorylation-dependent degradation of MEF2C contributes to regulate G2/M transition. Cell Cycle 2015; 14(10): 1517-28.
[http://dx.doi.org/10.1080/15384101.2015.1026519] [PMID: 25789873]

[313] Zhang H, Liu W, Wang Z, *et al.* MEF2C promotes gefitinib resistance in hepatic cancer cells through regulating MIG6 transcription. Tumori 2018; 104(3): 221-31.
[http://dx.doi.org/10.1177/0300891618765555] [PMID: 29714661]

[314] Zhao Y, Zhou H, Ma K, *et al.* Abnormal methylation of seven genes and their associations with clinical characteristics in early stage non-small cell lung cancer. Oncol Lett 2013; 5(4): 1211-8.
[http://dx.doi.org/10.3892/ol.2013.1161] [PMID: 23599765]

[315] Weiner AS, Boyarskikh UA, Voronina EN, *et al.* Polymorphisms in the folate-metabolizing genes MTR, MTRR, and CBS and breast cancer risk. Cancer Epidemiol 2012; 36(2): e95-e100.
[http://dx.doi.org/10.1016/j.canep.2011.11.010] [PMID: 22236648]

[316] Shrubsole MJ, Gao YT, Cai Q, *et al.* MTR and MTRR polymorphisms, dietary intake, and breast cancer risk. Cancer Epidemiol Biomarkers Prev 2006; 15(3): 586-8.
[http://dx.doi.org/10.1158/1055-9965.EPI-05-0576] [PMID: 16537721]

[317] Hu J, Zhou G-W, Wang N, *et al.* MTRR A66G polymorphism and breast cancer risk: a meta- analysis. Breast Cancer Res Treat 2010 1243 2010; 124: 779–784.

[318]   Ohnami S, Sato Y, Yoshimura K, *et al.* His595Tyr polymorphism in the methionine synthase reductase (MTRR) gene is associated with pancreatic cancer risk. Gastroenterology 2008; 135(2): 477-488.e3.
[http://dx.doi.org/10.1053/j.gastro.2008.04.016] [PMID: 18515090]

[319]   López-Cortés A, Jaramillo-Koupermann G, Muñoz MJ, *et al.* Genetic polymorphisms in MTHFR (C677T, A1298C), MTR (A2756G) and MTRR (A66G) genes associated with pathological characteristics of prostate cancer in the Ecuadorian population. Am J Med Sci 2013; 346(6): 447-54.
[http://dx.doi.org/10.1097/MAJ.0b013e3182882578] [PMID: 23459165]

[320]   Wettergren Y, Odin E, Carlsson G, Gustavsson B. MTHFR, MTR, and MTRR polymorphisms in relation to p16INK4A hypermethylation in mucosa of patients with colorectal cancer. Mol Med 2010; 16(9-10): 425-32.
[http://dx.doi.org/10.2119/molmed.2009.00156] [PMID: 20549016]

[321]   Pardini B, Kumar R, Naccarati A, *et al.* 5-Fluorouracil-based chemotherapy for colorectal cancer and MTHFR/MTRR genotypes. Br J Clin Pharmacol 2011; 72(1): 162-3.
[http://dx.doi.org/10.1111/j.1365-2125.2010.03892.x] [PMID: 21204909]

[322]   Salsano E, Croci L, Maderna E, *et al.* Expression of the neurogenic basic helix-loop-helix transcription factor NEUROG1 identifies a subgroup of medulloblastomas not expressing ATOH1. Neuro-oncol 2007; 9(3): 298-307.
[http://dx.doi.org/10.1215/15228517-2007-014] [PMID: 17522332]

[323]   A H, K R, P S, *et al.* Methylation of NEUROG1 in serum is a sensitive marker for the detection of early colorectal cancer. Am J Gastroenterol 2011; 106: 1110–1118.

[324]   Jo YS, Kim MS, Yoo NJ, Lee SH. NSD1 encoding a histone methyltransferase exhibits frameshift mutations in colorectal cancers. Pathology 2016; 48(3): 284-6.
[http://dx.doi.org/10.1016/j.pathol.2016.01.002] [PMID: 27020509]

[325]   Morishita M, di Luccio E. Structural insights into the regulation and the recognition of histone marks by the SET domain of NSD1. Biochem Biophys Res Commun 2011; 412(2): 214-9.
[http://dx.doi.org/10.1016/j.bbrc.2011.07.061] [PMID: 21806967]

[326]   Morishita M, di Luccio E. Cancers and the NSD family of histone lysine methyltransferases. Biochim Biophys Acta 2011; 1816(2): 158-63.
[PMID: 21664949]

[327]   Quintana RM, Dupuy AJ, Bravo A, *et al.* A transposon-based analysis of gene mutations related to skin cancer development. J Invest Dermatol 2013; 133(1): 239-48.
[http://dx.doi.org/10.1038/jid.2012.245] [PMID: 22832494]

[328]   Jiang W, He Y, Shi Y, *et al.* MicroRNA-1204 promotes cell proliferation by regulating PITX1 in non-small-cell lung cancer. Cell Biol Int 2019; 43(3): 253-64.
[PMID: 30549141]

[329]   Kolfschoten IGM, van Leeuwen B, Berns K, *et al.* A genetic screen identifies PITX1 as a suppressor of RAS activity and tumorigenicity. Cell 2005; 121(6): 849-58.
[http://dx.doi.org/10.1016/j.cell.2005.04.017] [PMID: 15960973]

[330]   Lord RVN, Brabender J, Wickramasinghe K, *et al.* Increased CDX2 and decreased PITX1 homeobox gene expression in Barrett's esophagus and Barrett's-associated adenocarcinoma. Surgery 2005; 138(5): 924-31.
[http://dx.doi.org/10.1016/j.surg.2005.05.007] [PMID: 16291394]

[331]   Qiao F, Gong P, Song Y, *et al.* Downregulated PITX1 Modulated by MiR-19a-3p Promotes Cell Malignancy and Predicts a Poor Prognosis of Gastric Cancer by Affecting Transcriptionally Activated PDCD5. Cell Physiol Biochem 2018; 46(6): 2215-31.
[http://dx.doi.org/10.1159/000489590] [PMID: 29734189]

[332]   Stender JD, Stossi F, Funk CC, Charn TH, Barnett DH, Katzenellenbogen BS. The estrogen-regulated

transcription factor PITX1 coordinates gene-specific regulation by estrogen receptor-alpha in breast cancer cells. Mol Endocrinol 2011; 25(10): 1699-709.
[http://dx.doi.org/10.1210/me.2011-0102] [PMID: 21868451]

[333] Liu DX, Lobie PE. Transcriptional activation of p53 by Pitx1. Cell Death Differ 2007; 14(11): 1893-907.
[http://dx.doi.org/10.1038/sj.cdd.4402209] [PMID: 17762884]

[334] Negri T, Casieri P, Miselli F, *et al.* Evidence for PDGFRA, PDGFRB and KIT deregulation in an NSCLC patient. Br J Cancer 2007; 96(1): 180-1.
[http://dx.doi.org/10.1038/sj.bjc.6603542] [PMID: 17213828]

[335] Arts FA, Chand D, Pecquet C, *et al.* PDGFRB mutants found in patients with familial infantile myofibromatosis or overgrowth syndrome are oncogenic and sensitive to imatinib. Oncogene 2016; 35(25): 3239-48.
[http://dx.doi.org/10.1038/onc.2015.383] [PMID: 26455322]

[336] Weissmueller S, Manchado E, Saborowski M, *et al.* Mutant p53 drives pancreatic cancer metastasis through cell-autonomous PDGF receptor β signaling. Cell 2014; 157(2): 382-94.
[http://dx.doi.org/10.1016/j.cell.2014.01.066] [PMID: 24725405]

[337] Song G, Liu K, Yang X, *et al.* SATB1 plays an oncogenic role in esophageal cancer by up-regulation of FN1 and PDGFRB. Oncotarget 2017; 8(11): 17771-84.
[http://dx.doi.org/10.18632/oncotarget.14849] [PMID: 28147311]

[338] Matthew EM, Hart LS, Astrinidis A, *et al.* The p53 target Plk2 interacts with TSC proteins impacting mTOR signaling, tumor growth, and chemosensitivity under hypoxic conditions. Cell Cycle 2009; 8(24): 4168-75.
[http://dx.doi.org/10.4161/cc.8.24.10800] [PMID: 20054236]

[339] Matthew EM, Yang Z, Peri S, *et al.* Plk2 Loss Commonly Occurs in Colorectal Carcinomas but not Adenomas: Relationship to mTOR Signaling. Neoplasia 2018; 20(3): 244-55.
[http://dx.doi.org/10.1016/j.neo.2018.01.004] [PMID: 29448085]

[340] Ou B, Zhao J, Guan S, *et al.* Plk2 promotes tumor growth and inhibits apoptosis by targeting Fbxw7/Cyclin E in colorectal cancer. Cancer Lett 2016; 380(2): 457-66.
[http://dx.doi.org/10.1016/j.canlet.2016.07.004] [PMID: 27423313]

[341] Strebhardt K. Multifaceted polo-like kinases: drug targets and antitargets for cancer therapy. Nat Rev Drug Discov 2010 98 2010; 9: 643–660.

[342] Makridakis NM, Reichardt JKV. JK R. Translesion DNA polymerases and cancer. Front Genet 2012; 3.
[http://dx.doi.org/10.3389/fgene.2012.00174]

[343] Dai Z-J, Liu X-H, Ma Y-F, *et al.* Association Between Single Nucleotide Polymorphisms in DNA Polymerase Kappa Gene and Breast Cancer Risk in Chinese Han Population. Medicine (Baltimore) 2016; 95(2): e2466.
[http://dx.doi.org/10.1097/MD.0000000000002466]

[344] Wang Y, Seimiya M, Kawamura K, *et al.* Elevated expression of DNA polymerase κ in human lung cancer is associated with p53 inactivation: Negative regulation of POLK promoter activity by p53. Int J Oncol 2004; 25(1): 161-5.
[http://dx.doi.org/10.3892/ijo.2013.2170] [PMID: 15202001]

[345] Yadav S, Mukhopadhyay S, Anbalagan M, Makridakis N. Somatic Mutations in Catalytic Core of *POLK* Reported in Prostate Cancer Alter Translesion DNA Synthesis. Hum Mutat 2015; 36(9): 873-80.
[http://dx.doi.org/10.1002/humu.22820] [PMID: 26046662]

[346] Jung C-R, Yoo J, Jang YJ, *et al.* Adenovirus-mediated transfer of siRNA against PTTG1 inhibits liver cancer cell growth *in vitro* and *in vivo*. Hepatology 2006; 43(5): 1042-52.

[http://dx.doi.org/10.1002/hep.21137] [PMID: 16628636]

[347] Huang S, Liao Q, Li L, *et al.* PTTG1 inhibits SMAD3 in prostate cancer cells to promote their proliferation. Tumor Biol 2014 357 2014; 35: 6265–6270.

[348] Li H, Yin C, Zhang B, *et al.* PTTG1 promotes migration and invasion of human non-small cell lung cancer cells and is modulated by miR-186. Carcinogenesis 2013; 34(9): 2145-55.
[http://dx.doi.org/10.1093/carcin/bgt158] [PMID: 23671127]

[349] Ren Q, Jin B. The clinical value and biological function of PTTG1 in colorectal cancer. Biomed Pharmacother 2017; 89: 108-15.
[http://dx.doi.org/10.1016/j.biopha.2017.01.115] [PMID: 28219049]

[350] Yoon CH, Kim MJ, Lee H, *et al.* PTTG1 oncogene promotes tumor malignancy *via* epithelial to mesenchymal transition and expansion of cancer stem cell population. J Biol Chem 2012; 287(23): 19516-27.
[http://dx.doi.org/10.1074/jbc.M111.337428] [PMID: 22511756]

[351] Ghayad SE, Vendrell JA, Bieche I, *et al.* Identification of TACC1, NOV, and PTTG1 as new candidate genes associated with endocrine therapy resistance in breast cancer. J Mol Endocrinol 2009; 42(2): 87-103.
[http://dx.doi.org/10.1677/JME-08-0076] [PMID: 18984771]

[352] Li Y, Clevenger CV, Minkovsky N, *et al.* Stabilization of prolactin receptor in breast cancer cells. Oncogene 2006; 25(13): 1896-902.
[http://dx.doi.org/10.1038/sj.onc.1209214] [PMID: 16278670]

[353] Clevenger CV, Gadd SL, Zheng J. New mechanisms for PRLr action in breast cancer. Trends Endocrinol Metab 2009; 20(5): 223-9.
[http://dx.doi.org/10.1016/j.tem.2009.03.001] [PMID: 19535262]

[354] Galsgaard ED, Rasmussen BB, Folkesson CG, *et al.* Re-evaluation of the prolactin receptor expression in human breast cancer. J Endocrinol 2009; 201(1): 115-28.
[http://dx.doi.org/10.1677/JOE-08-0479] [PMID: 19153125]

[355] Swaminathan G, Varghese B, Fuchs SY. Regulation of prolactin receptor levels and activity in breast cancer. J Mammary Gland Biol Neoplasia 2008; 13(1): 81-91.
[http://dx.doi.org/10.1007/s10911-008-9068-6] [PMID: 18204982]

[356] O'Sullivan CC, Bates SE. Targeting Prolactin Receptor (PRLR) Signaling in PRLR-Positive Breast and Prostate Cancer. Oncologist 2016; 21(5): 523-6.
[http://dx.doi.org/10.1634/theoncologist.2016-0108] [PMID: 27107001]

[357] Bartkova J, Tommiska J, Oplustilova L, *et al.* Aberrations of the MRE11-RAD50-NBS1 DNA damage sensor complex in human breast cancer: *MRE11* as a candidate familial cancer-predisposing gene. Mol Oncol 2008; 2(4): 296-316.
[http://dx.doi.org/10.1016/j.molonc.2008.09.007] [PMID: 19383352]

[358] Hsu HM, Wang HC, Chen ST, Hsu GC, Shen CY, Yu JC. Breast cancer risk is associated with the genes encoding the DNA double-strand break repair Mre11/Rad50/Nbs1 complex. Cancer Epidemiol Biomarkers Prev 2007; 16(10): 2024-32.
[http://dx.doi.org/10.1158/1055-9965.EPI-07-0116] [PMID: 17932350]

[359] Damiola F, Pertesi M, Oliver J, *et al.* Rare key functional domain missense substitutions in MRE11A, RAD50, and NBNcontribute to breast cancer susceptibility: results from a Breast Cancer Family Registry case-control mutation-screening study. Breast Cancer Res 2014; 16(3): R58.
[http://dx.doi.org/10.1186/bcr3669] [PMID: 24894818]

[360] Heikkinen K, Rapakko K, Karppinen SM, *et al.* RAD50 and NBS1 are breast cancer susceptibility genes associated with genomic instability. Carcinogenesis 2005; 27(8): 1593-9.
[http://dx.doi.org/10.1093/carcin/bgi360] [PMID: 16474176]

[361] Tommiska J, Seal S, Renwick A, *et al.* Evaluation ofRAD50 in familial breast cancer predisposition.

Int J Cancer 2006; 118(11): 2911-6.
[http://dx.doi.org/10.1002/ijc.21738] [PMID: 16385572]

[362] Gkountakos A, Pilotto S, Mafficini A, *et al.* Unmasking the impact of Rictor in cancer: novel insights of mTORC2 complex. Carcinogenesis 2018; 39(8): 971-80.
[http://dx.doi.org/10.1093/carcin/bgy086] [PMID: 29955840]

[363] Guo Z, Zhou Y, Evers BM, Wang Q. Rictor regulates FBXW7-dependent c-Myc and cyclin E degradation in colorectal cancer cells. Biochem Biophys Res Commun 2012; 418(2): 426-32.
[http://dx.doi.org/10.1016/j.bbrc.2012.01.054] [PMID: 22285861]

[364] McDonald PC, Oloumi A, Mills J, *et al.* Rictor and integrin-linked kinase interact and regulate Akt phosphorylation and cancer cell survival. Cancer Res 2008; 68(6): 1618-24.
[http://dx.doi.org/10.1158/0008-5472.CAN-07-5869] [PMID: 18339839]

[365] Uesugi A, Kozaki K, Tsuruta T, *et al.* The tumor suppressive microRNA miR-218 targets the mTOR component Rictor and inhibits AKT phosphorylation in oral cancer. Cancer Res 2011; 71(17): 5765-78.
[http://dx.doi.org/10.1158/0008-5472.CAN-11-0368] [PMID: 21795477]

[366] Wang X, Yue P, Kim YA, Fu H, Khuri FR, Sun SY. Enhancing mammalian target of rapamycin (mTOR)-targeted cancer therapy by preventing mTOR/raptor inhibition-initiated, mTOR/rictor-independent Akt activation. Cancer Res 2008; 68(18): 7409-18.
[http://dx.doi.org/10.1158/0008-5472.CAN-08-1522] [PMID: 18794129]

[367] Zhang F, Zhang X, Li M, *et al.* mTOR complex component Rictor interacts with PKCzeta and regulates cancer cell metastasis. Cancer Res 2010; 70(22): 9360-70.
[http://dx.doi.org/10.1158/0008-5472.CAN-10-0207] [PMID: 20978191]

[368] Foster, MD, PhD, DSc, FRCPath CS, Dodson A, Neoptolemos, MA, MD, FRCS JP, *et al.* Expression Patterns of Protein Kinase C Isoenzymes Are Characteristically Modulated in Chronic Pancreatitis and Pancreatic Cancer. Am J Clin Pathol 2003; 119: 0–0.

[369] Saito A, Fujii G, Sato Y, *et al.* Detection of genes expressed in primary colon cancers by *in situ* hybridisation: overexpression of RACK 1. Mol Pathol 2002; 55(1): 34-9.
[http://dx.doi.org/10.1136/mp.55.1.34] [PMID: 11836445]

[370] Fan Y, Si W, Ji W, *et al.* Rack1 mediates Src binding to drug transporter P-glycoprotein and modulates its activity through regulating Caveolin-1 phosphorylation in breast cancer cells. Cell Death Dis 2019; 10(6): 394-4.
[http://dx.doi.org/10.1038/s41419-019-1633-y] [PMID: 31113938]

[371] Darimipourain M, Wang S, Ittmann M, Kwabi-Addo B. Transcriptional and post-transcriptional regulation of Sprouty1, a receptor tyrosine kinase inhibitor in prostate cancer. Prostate Cancer Prostatic Dis 2011; 14(4): 279-85.
[http://dx.doi.org/10.1038/pcan.2011.33] [PMID: 21826097]

[372] Fritzsche S, Kenzelmann M, Hoffmann MJ, *et al.* Concomitant down-regulation of SPRY1 and SPRY2 in prostate carcinoma. Endocr Relat Cancer 2006; 13(3): 839-49.
[http://dx.doi.org/10.1677/erc.1.01190] [PMID: 16954433]

[373] Zou M, Baitei EY, Al-Rijjal RA, *et al.* KRAS-mediated oncogenic transformation of thyroid follicular cells requires long-term TSH stimulation and is regulated by SPRY1. Lab Invest 2015; 95(11): 1269-77.
[http://dx.doi.org/10.1038/labinvest.2015.90] [PMID: 26146959]

[374] Liu X, Lan Y, Zhang D, Wang K, Wang Y, Hua ZC. SPRY1 promotes the degradation of uPAR and inhibits uPAR-mediated cell adhesion and proliferation. Am J Cancer Res 2014; 4(6): 683-97.
[PMID: 25520860]

[375] Schaaf G, Hamdi M, Zwijnenburg D, *et al.* Silencing of SPRY1 triggers complete regression of rhabdomyosarcoma tumors carrying a mutated RAS gene. Cancer Res 2010; 70(2): 762-71.

[http://dx.doi.org/10.1158/0008-5472.CAN-09-2532] [PMID: 20068162]

[376] Bausch B, Schiavi F, Ni Y, *et al.* Clinical Characterization of the Pheochromocytoma and Paraganglioma Susceptibility Genes *SDHA*, *TMEM127*, *MAX*, and *SDHAF2* for Gene-Informed Prevention. JAMA Oncol 2017; 3(9): 1204-12.
[http://dx.doi.org/10.1001/jamaoncol.2017.0223] [PMID: 28384794]

[377] Dwight T, Mann K, Benn DE, *et al.* Familial SDHA mutation associated with pituitary adenoma and pheochromocytoma/paraganglioma. J Clin Endocrinol Metab 2013; 98(6): E1103-8.
[http://dx.doi.org/10.1210/jc.2013-1400] [PMID: 23633203]

[378] Dubard Gault M, Mandelker D, DeLair D, *et al.* Germline *SDHA* mutations in children and adults with cancer. Molecular Case Studies 2018; 4(4): a002584.
[http://dx.doi.org/10.1101/mcs.a002584] [PMID: 30068732]

[379] Wagner AJ, Remillard SP, Zhang YX, Doyle LA, George S, Hornick JL. Loss of expression of SDHA predicts SDHA mutations in gastrointestinal stromal tumors. Mod Pathol 2013; 26(2): 289-94.
[http://dx.doi.org/10.1038/modpathol.2012.153] [PMID: 22955521]

[380] A I, CL C, YS S, *et al.* SDHA loss of function mutations in a subset of young adult wild-type gastrointestinal stromal tumors. BMC Cancer; 2012, 12.
[http://dx.doi.org/10.1186/1471-2407-12-408]

[381] Kim S, Kim DH, Jung WH, Koo JS. Succinate dehydrogenase expression in breast cancer. Springerplus 2013; 2(1): 299.
[http://dx.doi.org/10.1186/2193-1801-2-299] [PMID: 23888270]

[382] Ekoue DN, Ansong E, Liu L, *et al.* Correlations of SELENOF and SELENOP genotypes with serum selenium levels and prostate cancer. Prostate 2018; 78(4): 279-88.
[http://dx.doi.org/10.1002/pros.23471] [PMID: 29314169]

[383] Donadio JLS, Liu L, Freeman VL, Ekoue DN, Diamond AM, Bermano G. Interaction of NKX3.1 and SELENOP genotype with prostate cancer recurrence. Prostate 2019; 79(5): 462-7.
[http://dx.doi.org/10.1002/pros.23752] [PMID: 30582190]

[384] Diamond AM. Selenoproteins of the Human Prostate: Unusual Properties and Role in Cancer Etiology. Biol Trace Elem Res 2019; 192(1): 51-9.
[http://dx.doi.org/10.1007/s12011-019-01809-0] [PMID: 31300958]

[385] Hughes D, Kunická T, Schomburg L, Liška V, Swan N, Souček P. Expression of Selenoprotein Genes and Association with Selenium Status in Colorectal Adenoma and Colorectal Cancer. Nutrients 2018; 10(11): 1812.
[http://dx.doi.org/10.3390/nu10111812] [PMID: 30469315]

[386] Ekoue DN, Zaichick S, Valyi-Nagy K, *et al.* Selenium levels in human breast carcinoma tissue are associated with a common polymorphism in the gene for SELENOP (Selenoprotein P). J Trace Elem Med Biol 2017; 39: 227-33.
[http://dx.doi.org/10.1016/j.jtemb.2016.11.003] [PMID: 27908419]

[387] M H, Y L, YQ L, *et al.* Skp1: Implications in cancer and SCF-oriented anti-cancer drug discovery. Pharmacol Res 2016; 111: 34–42.

[388] Su Y, Ishikawa S, Kojima M, Liu B. Eradication of pathogenic β-catenin by Skp1/Cullin/F box ubiquitination machinery. Proc Natl Acad Sci USA 2003; 100(22): 12729-34.
[http://dx.doi.org/10.1073/pnas.2133261100] [PMID: 14563921]

[389] Xie CM, Wei W, Sun Y. Role of SKP1-CUL1-F-box-protein (SCF) E3 ubiquitin ligases in skin cancer. J Genet Genomics 2013; 40(3): 97-106.
[http://dx.doi.org/10.1016/j.jgg.2013.02.001] [PMID: 23522382]

[390] Rai D, Kim SW, McKeller MR, Dahia PLM, Aguiar RCT. Targeting of SMAD5 links microRNA-155 to the TGF-β pathway and lymphomagenesis. Proc Natl Acad Sci USA 2010; 107(7): 3111-6.
[http://dx.doi.org/10.1073/pnas.0910667107] [PMID: 20133617]

[391] Zavadil J, Březinová J, Svoboda P, Zemanová Z, Michalová K. Smad5, a tumor suppressor candidate at 5q31.1, is hemizygously lost and not mutated in the retained allele in human leukemia cell line HL60. Leukemia 1997; 11(8): 1187-92.
[http://dx.doi.org/10.1038/sj.leu.2400750] [PMID: 9264367]

[392] Fuchs O, Simakova O, Klener P, *et al.* Inhibition of Smad5 in human hematopoietic progenitors blocks erythroid differentiation induced by BMP4. Blood Cells Mol Dis 2002; 28(2): 221-33.
[http://dx.doi.org/10.1006/bcmd.2002.0487] [PMID: 12064918]

[393] 1997. Hejlik DP, Kottickal LV, Liang H, *et al.* Localization of SMAD5 and its evaluation as a candidate myeloid tumor suppressor. Cancer research. 1997; 57(17): 3779-83.

[394] Pangas SA, Li X, Umans L, *et al.* Conditional deletion of Smad1 and Smad5 in somatic cells of male and female gonads leads to metastatic tumor development in mice. Mol Cell Biol 2008; 28(1): 248-57.
[http://dx.doi.org/10.1128/MCB.01404-07] [PMID: 17967875]

[395] Zimonjic DB, Durkin ME, Keck-Waggoner CL, Park SW, Thorgeirsson SS, Popescu NC. SMAD5 gene expression, rearrangements, copy number, and amplification at fragile site FRA5C in human hepatocellular carcinoma. Neoplasia 2003; 5(5): 390-6.
[http://dx.doi.org/10.1016/S1476-5586(03)80041-6] [PMID: 14670176]

[396] Arnold SJ, Maretto S, Islam A, Bikoff EK, Robertson EJ. Dose-dependent Smad1, Smad5 and Smad8 signaling in the early mouse embryo. Dev Biol 2006; 296(1): 104-18.
[http://dx.doi.org/10.1016/j.ydbio.2006.04.442] [PMID: 16765933]

[397] Desai N, Trieu V, Damascelli B, Soon-Shiong P. SPARC Expression Correlates with tumor Response to Albumin-Bound Paclitaxel in Head and Neck Cancer Patients. Transl Oncol 2009; 2(2): 59-64.
[http://dx.doi.org/10.1593/tlo.09109] [PMID: 19412420]

[398] Nagaraju GPC, Sharma D. Anti-cancer role of SPARC, an inhibitor of adipogenesis. Cancer Treat Rev 2011; 37(7): 559-66.
[http://dx.doi.org/10.1016/j.ctrv.2010.12.001] [PMID: 21237573]

[399] Said N, Socha MJ, Olearczyk JJ, Elmarakby AA, Imig JD, Motamed K. Normalization of the ovarian cancer microenvironment by SPARC. Mol Cancer Res 2007; 5(10): 1015-30.
[http://dx.doi.org/10.1158/1541-7786.MCR-07-0001] [PMID: 17951402]

[400] Tai IT, Tang MJ. SPARC in cancer biology: Its role in cancer progression and potential for therapy. Drug Resist Updat 2008; 11(6): 231-46.
[http://dx.doi.org/10.1016/j.drup.2008.08.005] [PMID: 18849185]

[401] Yiu GK, Chan WY, Ng SW, *et al.* SPARC (secreted protein acidic and rich in cysteine) induces apoptosis in ovarian cancer cells. Am J Pathol 2001; 159(2): 609-22.
[http://dx.doi.org/10.1016/S0002-9440(10)61732-4] [PMID: 11485919]

[402] Watkins G, Martin TA, Bryce R, Mansel RE, Jiang WG. γ-Linolenic acid regulates the expression and secretion of SPARC in human cancer cells. Prostaglandins Leukot Essent Fatty Acids 2005; 72(4): 273-8.
[http://dx.doi.org/10.1016/j.plefa.2004.12.004] [PMID: 15763439]

[403] Stenman UH. Role of the tumor-associated trypsin inhibitor SPINK1 in cancer development. Asian J Androl 2011; 13(4): 628-9.
[http://dx.doi.org/10.1038/aja.2011.45] [PMID: 21602832]

[404] Ateeq B, Tomlins SA, Laxman B, *et al.* Therapeutic targeting of SPINK1-positive prostate cancer. Sci Transl Med 2011; 3(72): 72ra17.
[http://dx.doi.org/10.1126/scitranslmed.3001498] [PMID: 21368222]

[405] Matsubayashi H, Fukushima N, Sato N, *et al.* Polymorphisms of SPINK1 N34S and CFTR in patients with sporadic and familial pancreatic cancer. Cancer Biol Ther 2003; 2(6): 650-3.
[http://dx.doi.org/10.4161/cbt.2.6.530] [PMID: 14688470]

[406] Tiwari R, Pandey SK, Goel S, *et al.* SPINK1 promotes colorectal cancer progression by downregulating Metallothioneins expression. Oncogenesis 2015; 4(8): e162.
[http://dx.doi.org/10.1038/oncsis.2015.23] [PMID: 26258891]

[407] Räsänen K, Itkonen O, Koistinen H, Stenman UH. Emerging Roles of SPINK1 in Cancer. Clin Chem 2016; 62(3): 449-57.
[http://dx.doi.org/10.1373/clinchem.2015.241513] [PMID: 26656134]

[408] Bismar TA, Yoshimoto M, Duan Q, Liu S, Sircar K, Squire JA. Interactions and relationships of PTEN, ERG, SPINK1 and AR in castration-resistant prostate cancer. Histopathology 2012; 60(4): 645-52.
[http://dx.doi.org/10.1111/j.1365-2559.2011.04116.x] [PMID: 22260502]

[409] Tomlins SA, Rhodes DR, Yu J, *et al.* The role of SPINK1 in ETS rearrangement-negative prostate cancers. Cancer Cell 2008; 13(6): 519-28.
[http://dx.doi.org/10.1016/j.ccr.2008.04.016] [PMID: 18538735]

[410] Flavin R, Pettersson A, Hendrickson WK, *et al.* SPINK1 protein expression and prostate cancer progression. Clin Cancer Res 2014; 20(18): 4904-11.
[http://dx.doi.org/10.1158/1078-0432.CCR-13-1341] [PMID: 24687926]

[411] Jin FS, Wang HM, Song XY. Long non-coding RNA TCF7 predicts the progression and facilitates the growth and metastasis of colorectal cancer. Mol Med Rep 2018; 17(5): 6902-8.
[http://dx.doi.org/10.3892/mmr.2018.8708] [PMID: 29532890]

[412] Xu X, Liu Z, Tian F, Xu J, Chen Y. Clinical Significance of Transcription Factor 7 (TCF7) as a Prognostic Factor in Gastric Cancer. Med Sci Monit 2019; 25: 3957-63.
[http://dx.doi.org/10.12659/MSM.913913] [PMID: 31133633]

[413] Chen WY, Liu SY, Chang YS, *et al.* MicroRNA-34a regulates WNT/TCF7 signaling and inhibits bone metastasis in Ras-activated prostate cancer. Oncotarget 2015; 6(1): 441-57.
[http://dx.doi.org/10.18632/oncotarget.2690] [PMID: 25436980]

[414] Wang Y, Zhang S, Xu Y, *et al.* Upregulation of miR-192 inhibits cell growth and invasion and induces cell apoptosis by targeting TCF7 in human osteosarcoma. Tumor Biol 2016 3711 2016; 37: 15211–15220.

[415] Heidenreich B, Rachakonda PS, Hemminki K, Kumar R. TERT promoter mutations in cancer development. Curr Opin Genet Dev 2014; 24: 30-7.
[http://dx.doi.org/10.1016/j.gde.2013.11.005] [PMID: 24657534]

[416] Johnatty SE, Beesley J, Chen X, *et al.* Evaluation of candidate stromal epithelial cross-talk genes identifies association between risk of serous ovarian cancer and TERT, a cancer susceptibility "hot-spot". PLoS Genet 2010; 6(7): e1001016.
[http://dx.doi.org/10.1371/journal.pgen.1001016] [PMID: 20628624]

[417] Huang FW, Bielski CM, Rinne ML, *et al.* TERT promoter mutations and monoallelic activation of TERT in cancer. 2015, 4.
[http://dx.doi.org/10.1038/oncsis.2015.39]

[418] Turnbull C, Rapley EA, Seal S, *et al.* Variants near DMRT1, TERT and ATF7IP are associated with testicular germ cell cancer. Nat Genet 2010; 42(7): 604-7.
[http://dx.doi.org/10.1038/ng.607] [PMID: 20543847]

[419] Bell RJA, Rube HT, Kreig A, *et al.* The transcription factor GABP selectively binds and activates the mutant TERT promoter in cancer. Science 2015; 348(6238): 1036-9.
[http://dx.doi.org/10.1126/science.aab0015] [PMID: 25977370]

[420] Borah S, Xi L, Zaug AJ, *et al. TERT* promoter mutations and telomerase reactivation in urothelial cancer. Science 2015; 347(6225): 1006-10.
[http://dx.doi.org/10.1126/science.1260200] [PMID: 25722414]

[421] Andreassen CN, Alsner J, Overgaard J, *et al.* TGFB1 polymorphisms are associated with risk of late normal tissue complications in the breast after radiotherapy for early breast cancer. Radiother Oncol 2005; 75(1): 18-21.
[http://dx.doi.org/10.1016/j.radonc.2004.12.012] [PMID: 15878096]

[422] Cox DG, Penney K, Guo Q, Hankinson SE, Hunter DJ. TGFB1 and TGFBR1 polymorphisms and breast cancer risk in the Nurses' Health Study. BMC Cancer 2007; 7(1): 175.
[http://dx.doi.org/10.1186/1471-2407-7-175] [PMID: 17848193]

[423] Guan X, Zhao H, Niu J, Tan D, Ajani JA, Wei Q. Polymorphisms of TGFB1 and VEGF genes and survival of patients with gastric cancer. J Exp Clin Cancer Res 2009; 28(1): 94-4.
[http://dx.doi.org/10.1186/1756-9966-28-94] [PMID: 19566948]

[424] Jin G, Wang L, Chen W, *et al.* Variant alleles ofTGFB1 andTGFBR2 are associated with a decreased risk of gastric cancer in a Chinese population. Int J Cancer 2007; 120(6): 1330-5.
[http://dx.doi.org/10.1002/ijc.22443] [PMID: 17187359]

[425] A E-T, JM C, J Y, *et al.* A gain of function TGFB1 polymorphism may be associated with late stage prostate cancer. Cancer Epidemiol Biomarkers Prev 2004; 13: 759–764.

[426] Soulitzis N, Karyotis I, Delakas D, Spandidos D. Expression analysis of peptide growth factors VEGF, FGF2, TGFB1, EGF and IGF1 in prostate cancer and benign prostatic hyperplasia. Int J Oncol 2006; 29(2): 305-14.
[http://dx.doi.org/10.3892/ijo.29.2.305] [PMID: 16820871]

[427] Tada Y, Yokomizo A, Shiota M, Tsunoda T, Plass C, Naito S. Aberrant DNA methylation of T-cell leukemia, homeobox 3 modulates cisplatin sensitivity in bladder cancer. Int J Oncol 2011; 39(3): 727-33.
[PMID: 21617853]

[428] Su XY, Busson M, Della Valle V, *et al.* Various types of rearrangements targetTLX3 locus in T-cell acute lymphoblastic leukemia. Genes Chromosomes Cancer 2004; 41(3): 243-9.
[http://dx.doi.org/10.1002/gcc.20088] [PMID: 15334547]

[429] Su XY, Della-Valle V, Andre-Schmutz I, *et al.* HOX11L2/TLX3 is transcriptionally activated through T-cell regulatory elements downstream of BCL11B as a result of the t(5;14)(q35;q32). Blood 2006; 108(13): 4198-201.
[http://dx.doi.org/10.1182/blood-2006-07-032953] [PMID: 16926283]

[430] Gottardo NG, Jacoby PA, Sather HN, *et al.* Significance of HOX11L2/TLX3 expression in children with T-cell acute lymphoblastic leukemia treated on Children's Cancer Group protocols. Leuk 2005 199 2005; 19: 1705–1708.

[431] Ballerini P, Landman-Parker J, Cayuela JM, *et al.* Impact of genotype on survival of children with T-cell acute lymphoblastic leukemia treated according to the French protocol FRALLE-93: the effect of TLX3/HOX11L2 gene expression on outcome. Haematologica 2008; 93(11): 1658-65.
[http://dx.doi.org/10.3324/haematol.13291] [PMID: 18835836]

[432] Borghini S, Vargiolu M, Di Duca M, Ravazzolo R, Ceccherini I. Nuclear factor Y drives basal transcription of the human TLX3, a gene overexpressed in T-cell acute lymphocytic leukemia. Mol Cancer Res 2006; 4(9): 635-43.
[http://dx.doi.org/10.1158/1541-7786.MCR-05-0250] [PMID: 16966433]

[433] Van Vlierberghe P, Homminga I, Zuurbier L, *et al.* Cooperative genetic defects in TLX3 rearranged pediatric T-ALL. Leukemia 2008; 22(4): 762-70.
[http://dx.doi.org/10.1038/sj.leu.2405082] [PMID: 18185524]

[434] Lane J, Martin TA, Mansel RE, Jiang WG. The expression and prognostic value of the guanine nucleotide exchange factors (GEFs) Trio, Vav1 and TIAM-1 in human breast cancer. Int Semin Surg Oncol 2008; 5(1): 23.
[http://dx.doi.org/10.1186/1477-7800-5-23] [PMID: 18925966]

[435] Li Y, Guo Z, Chen H, *et al.* HOXC8-Dependent Cadherin 11 Expression Facilitates Breast Cancer Cell Migration through Trio and Rac. Genes Cancer 2011; 2(9): 880-8.
[http://dx.doi.org/10.1177/1947601911433129] [PMID: 22593800]

[436] Zheng M, Simon R, Mirlacher M, *et al.* TRIO amplification and abundant mRNA expression is associated with invasive tumor growth and rapid tumor cell proliferation in urinary bladder cancer. Am J Pathol 2004; 165(1): 63-9.
[http://dx.doi.org/10.1016/S0002-9440(10)63275-0] [PMID: 15215162]

[437] Sonoshita M, Itatani Y, Kakizaki F, *et al.* Promotion of colorectal cancer invasion and metastasis through activation of NOTCH-DAB1-ABL-RHOGEF protein TRIO. Cancer Discov 2015; 5(2): 198-211.
[http://dx.doi.org/10.1158/2159-8290.CD-14-0595] [PMID: 25432929]

[438] Jiang K, Liu H, Xie D, Xiao Q. Differentially expressed genes *ASPN, COL1A1, FN1, VCAN* and *MUC5AC* are potential prognostic biomarkers for gastric cancer. Oncol Lett 2019; 17(3): 3191-202.
[http://dx.doi.org/10.3892/ol.2019.9952] [PMID: 30867749]

[439] Fanhchaksai K, Okada F, Nagai N, *et al.* Host stromal versican is essential for cancer-associated fibroblast function to inhibit cancer growth. Int J Cancer 2016; 138(3): 630-41.
[http://dx.doi.org/10.1002/ijc.29804] [PMID: 26270355]

[440] Ghosh S, Albitar L, LeBaron R, *et al.* Up-regulation of stromal versican expression in advanced stage serous ovarian cancer. Gynecol Oncol 2010; 119(1): 114-20.
[http://dx.doi.org/10.1016/j.ygyno.2010.05.029] [PMID: 20619446]

[441] Zahid S, Branham K, Schlegel D, *et al.* Retinal dystrophy gene atlas. Cham: Springer International Publishing; 2018.

[442] Chiu CF, Wang CH, Wang CL, *et al.* A novel single nucleotide polymorphism in XRCC4 gene is associated with gastric cancer susceptibility in Taiwan. Ann Surg Oncol 2008; 15(2): 514-8.
[http://dx.doi.org/10.1245/s10434-007-9674-3] [PMID: 17987338]

[443] Da-Tian Bau, Mei-Due Yang, Yung-An Tsou, *et al.* Colorectal cancer and genetic polymorphism of DNA double-strand break repair gene XRCC4 in Taiwan - PubMed. Anticancer Res; 30(7):2727- 30., https://pubmed.ncbi.nlm.nih.gov/20683005/ (2010, accessed 28 September 2021).

[444] Yen CY, Liu SY, Chen CH, *et al.* Combinational polymorphisms of four DNA repair genes XRCC1, XRCC2, XRCC3, and XRCC4 and their association with oral cancer in Taiwan. J Oral Pathol Med 2008; 37(5): 271-7.
[http://dx.doi.org/10.1111/j.1600-0714.2007.00608.x] [PMID: 18410587]

[445] Hsien-Chang Tseng, Ming-Hsui Tsai, Chang-Fang Chiu, *et al.* Association of XRCC4 codon 247 polymorphism with oral cancer susceptibility in Taiwan - PubMed. Anticancer Res; 28(3A):1687- 91, https://pubmed.ncbi.nlm.nih.gov/18630527/ (2008, accessed 28 September 2021).

[446] Mittal RD, Gangwar R, Mandal RK, *et al.* Gene variants of XRCC4 and XRCC3 and their association with risk for urothelial bladder cancer. Mol Biol Reports 2011 392 2011; 39: 1667– 1675.

CHAPTER 6

Chromosome 6

Shivani Singh[1], Saurav Panicker[1] and **Satish Ramalingam[1,*]**

[1] Department of Genetic Engineering, School of Bioengineering, SRM Institute of Science and Technology, Kattankulathur, India

Abstract: Chromosome 6 is among the 23 pairs of chromosomes in humans and it spans about 170 million base pairs. Several cancer genes have been identified to have a role in cancer development. Cancer is also a genetic disease caused due to changes in the genes that control cell function, such as cell division and cell growth. Most of these cancer genes either act as tumor suppressors or possess an oncogenic potential. Oncogenes like ROS1, MYB, HMGA1, *etc.*, induce tumorigenesis by playing a role in DNA repair, replication, transcriptional regulation, and mRNA splicing. When these genes are highly expressed, they result in the transformation of normal cells to malignant cells; on the other side, tumor suppressor genes like IGF2R, AIM1, IRF4, *etc.*, reduce tumorigenicity and invasive potential. Thus, reduced expression of these genes due to loss of heterozygosity, deletion or any epigenetic modifications can induce tumor formation. Also, some genes can either suppress or induce tumor formation given the cellular location and condition, such as CCN2, TNF, *etc.* Along with these, different types of structural abnormalities can be observed on chromosome 6, such as chromosomal translocation, deletion, duplication, and inversion. These abnormalities on both p and q arms have been known to contribute to the growth and spread of cancer by impacting the expression of cancer genes. Aberrant expression of the genes can also be influenced by fusions, missense mutations, non-missense mutations, silent mutations, frame-shift deletions, and insertion at the molecular level. Some genes can maintain stem-cell-like properties by regulating the expression of cell surface markers like Oct4, Nanog, Sox4, *etc.* This chapter explains important cancer genes, genetic mutations, and gene variations that can influence the risk of having cancer and induces cancer formation.

Keywords: A Cancer stem cell, Chromosome 6, Chromosomal translocation, Deletion, Oncogenes, Tumor suppressor genes.

---

* **Corresponding author Satish Ramalingam**: Department of Genetic Engineering, School of Bioengineering, SRM Institute of Science and Technology, Kattankulathur, India; E-mail: rsatish76@gmail.com

Satish Ramalingam (Ed.)

1.1. GENE- AFDN; AF-6; AFADIN, ADHERENS JUNCTION FORMAT-ION FACTOR LOCATION: 6p27

AFDN gene (Fig. **1**) encodes a multi-domain protein that plays a key role in the organization of epithelial structures of the embryonic ectoderm and is also involved in the signaling and organization of cell junctions during embryogenesis. Aberrant expression of the *AFDN* gene has been shown to induce epithelial-to-mesenchymal [EMT] transition leading to cell migration, invasion, and proliferation in cancer, such as breast cancer, colon cancer, and pancreatic cancer.

Low expression of *AFDN* has been associated with many types of tumors, such as osteosarcoma, breast cancer, and gastric cancer.

1.1.1. The Disease of Relevance

- *AFDN* gene is involved in chromosomal translocation [6, 11][q27;q23] in the case of acute myeloid leukemia [AML] by forming a fusion partner with the acute lymphoblastic leukemia [*ALL-1*] gene. This self-association of the protein afadin activates the oncogenic potential of the MLL-afadin fusion protein. Maintaining the expression on *MLL-AFDN* [*AF6*] driven oncogenic gene expression requires the continuous activity of the histone-methyltransferase DOT1L [1, 2].
- In breast cancer, phosphorylation of afadin by the Akt signaling pathway at Ser1718 promotes the relocalization of afadin from the adherens junction to the nucleus, which further results in breast epithelial cell migration. This relocalization can also occur due to the presence of wild-type or Ser1718Asp mutant afadin that is nuclear restricted and also enhances cell migration. Increased metastatic relapse in breast carcinoma is associated with afadin low expression [3, 4].
- Silencing of *AFDN* expression is known to reactivate the ERK signaling pathway, and this interaction promotes the metastasis phenotype in osteo-sarcoma cells by stably expressing claudin-2 [*CLDN2*]. Reduced expression of *CLDN2* and *AFDN* are found to participate in pulmonary metastasis of OS and thus can be used as a potential molecular marker for the diagnosis of OS and can also help to determine the prognosis [5].
- Downregulation of long non-coding RNA [lncRNA] MLLT4-AS1 is signi-ficantly associated with lymph node metastasis, distant metastasis, and a shorter disease-free interval in Gastric Cancer. Thus in this cancer, it acts as a tumor suppresser gene, and down-regulation of *MLLT4-AS1* is a potential marker of a poor prognosis. Few studies have shown that infection with *H.pylori* can reduce the expression of afadin, leading to cell migration [6, 7].
- In colon cancer, *AFDN* or afadin physically interacts with Cystic fibrosis

transmembrane conductance regulator [*CFTR*] at a cell to cell contacts, so knockdown of *CFTR* results in reduced stability of afadin protein and enhanced malignancies [8].

- Reduced expression of *AFDN* induces transcription of Snail, which is an EMT inducer, thus promoting *tumorigenesis* in human pancreatic adenocarcinoma [9].
- Loss of *AFDN* expression results in myometrial invasion and high histological grade in patients with `uterine corpus endometrial carcinoma. It is known to induce chemoresistance to cisplatin and so can be used as a marker of chemo-resistance to cisplatin [10].

1.2. GENE- DEK; DEK PROTO-ONCOGENE LOCATION: 6p22.3

DEK gene (Fig. 1) codes for nuclear protein, and its expression has been linked to numerous cancer occurring through multiple mechanisms. It is involved in DNA repair, replication, transcriptional regulation, and mRNA splicing, so any changes in the gene expression can lead to tumorigenesis. *DEK* overexpression has been reported in several malignancies like leukemia, melanoma, hepatocellular carcinoma, malignant brain tumors, uterine cervical cancer, lung cancer, glioblastoma, urinary bladder cancer, ovarian cancer, and most sarcoma cell carcinoma. The resequence project of the cancer genome has shown a heterozygous missense mutation [K348N] of *DEK* in the case of renal tumors.

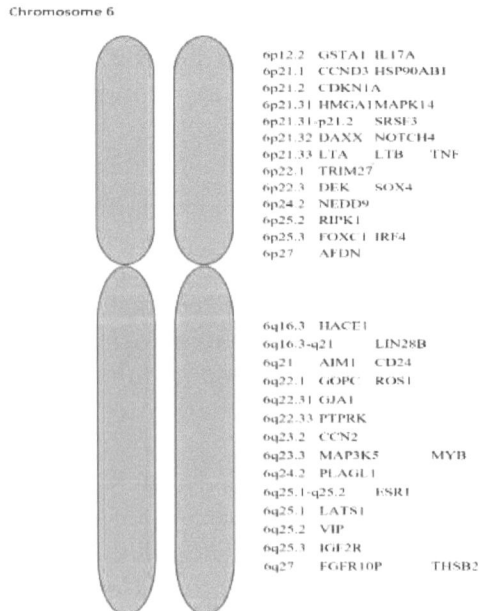

Fig. (1). This figure displays the loci of the genes from Chromosome 6 whose roles in cancer have been explained in this chapter. Sayooj Madhusoodanan designed this diagram.

1.2.1. The Disease of Relevance

- Frequently gained chromosomal regions of 6p in retinoblastoma are represented as isochromosome I [6p], and patients with this unbalanced rearrangement have four copies of the entire 6p genomic region. The oncogenes *DEK* along with E2F3, which are 2.1 megabases apart at band 6p22.3, are overexpressed in retinoblastoma [11, 12].
- Copy number increases at 6p22 have also led to aggressive tumor formation in bladder cancer just like retinoblastoma tumors. *DEK* overexpression is also involved in superficial bladder cancers which is known to be a result of an increase in gene copy number or amplification, and this gene can be used to differentiate superficial from invasive tumors [13].
- *DEK* forms a fusion partner with *NUP214 [CAN]* by undergoing recurrent chromosomal translocation t[6, 9][p23;q34] and forms a DEK-CAN fusion protein in AML and myelodysplasia [MDS]. This rare translocation involves a fusion of the 5' part of the *DEK* gene at 6p22.3 and the 3' part of the *NUP214* gene at 9p34 [14].
- *DEK* overexpression has been associated with malignancy in most squamous cell carcinomas [SCC] including squamous epithelium of the uterine cervix, lung, esophagus, and other tissues. DEK protein can be upregulated in both Human papillomavirus HPV-positive and negative cervical cancer cells, precancerous lesions, and human head and neck sarcoma cell carcinoma [HNSCC]. A *DEK-AFF2* fusion has been currently discovered in patients diagnosed with middle ear and temporal bone non-keratinizing/basaloid SCC [15].
- *DEK* is highly expressed in a higher percentage of tumor cells from high-grade primary invasive ductal carcinomas compared with benign tissue and low-grade carcinomas in breast cancer and helps in maintaining the breast cancer stem cell-like population. *DEK* and *RON* [Recepteur d'Origine Nantaise] together are known to promote breast cancer and contribute to relapse and metastasis through alterations in β-catenin signaling [16].
- CUGBP Elav-like family member 1 [*CELF1*] is known to initiate cutaneous melanoma, having *DEK* as a signal amplifier, and this positive correlation between DEK mRNA expression and CELF1 has also been reported in other tumor types such as diffuse large B cell lymphoma, thyroid carcinoma or prostate adenocarcinoma [17].

1.3. GENE: ROS1, ROS PROTO-ONCOGENE 1, RECEPTOR TYROSINE KINASE LOCATION: 6q22.1

ROS1 is a proto-oncogene (Fig. **1**), coding for a receptor tyrosine kinase of the insulin receptor family, and is highly expressed in a variety of tumor cell lines.

Overexpression of the *ROS1* gene has been associated with brain and lung cancers, breast fibroadenomas, liver, colon, and kidney cancers, chemically induced stomach cancer, and myelomonocytic leukemia. *ROS1* rearrangements and somatic chromosomal fusions have been detected in several malignancies, including inflammatory myofibroblastic tumor, cholangiocarcinoma, ovarian cancer, gastric cancer, colorectal cancer, angiosarcoma, spitzoid melanoma, and non-small cell lung carcinoma [NSCLC]. Chromosomal rearrangements occur at the kinase domain of *ROS1,* which leads to constitutive activation of *ROS1* signaling, accompanied by phosphorylation of SHP-2 and downstream signaling pathways such as MEK/ERK, JAK/STAT or PI3K/AKT. Any sudden change in any on these signaling pathways by *ROS1* fusions result in malignancies. Several *ROS1* fusion partner genes have been reported in lung cancer, including cluster of differentiation 74 [*CD74*], solute carrier family 34 members 2 gene [*SLC34A2*], tropomyosin 3 gene [*TMP3*], syndecan 4 gene [*SDC4*], ezrin gene [*EZR*], leucine-rich repeats and immunoglobulin-like domains 3 gene [*LRIG3*], KDEL endoplasmic reticulum protein retention receptor 2 gene [*KDELR2*], coiled-coil domain containing 6 gene [*CCDC6*], LIM domain and actin-binding 1 gene [*LIMA1*], moesin gene [*MSN*], tumor protein D52 like 1 gene [*TPD52L1*], transmembrane protein 106B gene [*TMEM106B*], clathrin heavy chain gene [*CLTC*] and *FIG* gene. *CD74-ROS1* is the most common fusion in *ROS1*-rearranged NSCLC, and all ROS1 fusions retain their entire kinase domain [18].

1.3.1. The Disease of Relevance

• Much *ROS1* fusion and translocational genes have been detected as an oncogenic driver in primary NSCLC. One of the most common *ROS1* fusion found is *CD74- ROS1* which has been detected in NSCLC tumors as well as in adenocarcinoma. This fusion protein is formed due to chromosomal translocation that fused the 5' region of *CD74* to the 3' region of *ROS1*. The same pattern is observed in *SLC342A-ROS1* fusion in HCC78 cell lines. Within this chimeric protein, *ROS1* is fused with its partner at exons 32, 34, 35, or 36 on the gene. This kind of fusion allows for maintaining the ROS1 kinase domain and its kinase activity. *ROS1* kinase activity is activated by the dimerization of the *ROS1* fusion, which is mediated by the N-terminal fusion partner, followed by stimulation of downstream signaling that results in enhanced cell growth. Another *ROS1* fusion found is *SDC4-ROS1,* and there exist two forms: a long form in which *SDC4* is fused to *ROS1* at exon 32 and a short form in which *SDC4* is fused to *ROS1* at exon 34. Apart from all these ROS1 fusion proteins, other novel *ROS*1 fusion partners detected are *FIG, TPM3, SDC4, EZR,* and *LRIG3*. Some studies have shown that overexpression in a small fraction of NSCLC tumors has resulted in hypo-methylation in the *ROS1* promoter region, but the molecular mechanism is yet to be studied. Approximately 1-2% of NSCLC patients have been detected with tumors driven by *ROS1* fusion [19 - 22].

- The first *ROS1* fusion was discovered in glioblastoma. This fusion involves chromosomal interstitial deletion of 240 kilobases on 6q21 resulting in the formation of FIG-ROS1 fusion protein where the 3, a region of the *ROS1,* is fused to the 5' region of the glioblastoma gene [*FIG*]. Short and long isoforms of FIG-ROS1 have been detected as an oncogenic driver in cholangio-carcinoma. In some cases, *ROS1* undergoes chromosomal translocation t[6, 12][q21;q24.3] and forms a fusion gene between the 5' region of *ZCCH8* and the 3' region of *ROS1* represented as ZCCH8-ROS1 fusion. This rearrangement is considered to be a key potential driver in a subset of Glioblastoma. A *CEP85L-ROS1* rearrangement has also been reported in an adult glioblastoma [19, 23].
- *SLC34A2-ROS1* fusion has been detected in gastric cancer other than NSCLC [24].
- In smoldering multiple myeloma, the *ROS1* fusion gene was detected and results in the activation of the MEK/ERK pathway through phosphorylation of Ras [25, 26].
- Enhancer of zeste homolog 2 [EZH2], a histone-lysine N-methyltransferase enzyme, mediated changes in the epigenome of oral squamous cell carcinoma [OSCC] enhances expressions of *ROS1* and its target genes. These epigenetic changes confer greater invasiveness and plasticity to cope with the tumor microenvironment [27].
- *TGF-ROS1* and fibronectin-1 *FN1-ROS1* fusions have been detected in infantile inflammatory myofibroblastic tumors involving the liver and lung, respectively [28].

1.4. GENE: CCND3, CYCLIN D3 LOCATION: 6p21.1

CCND3 gene codes for G1/S specific cyclin D3 protein that functions in the regulation of CDK kinases in the cell cycle. Cyclin D3 is critical for cell growth, proliferation, and cancer development and is also involved in the phosphorylation of tumor suppressor protein Rb. Fusions, missense mutations, nonsense mutations, silent mutations, frame-shift deletions, and insertions are the mechanism involved in aberrant expression of *CCND3* and is observed in cancers such as endometrial cancer, skin cancer, and stomach cancer. Amplification in the *CCND3* gene is observed in breast invasive ductal carcinoma, lung adenocarcinoma, osteosar-coma, colon adenocarcinoma, and adenocarcinoma of the gastro-oesophageal junction, and mutation is observed in lung adenocarcinoma, endometrial endo-metrioid adenocarcinoma, colon adenocarcinoma, diffuse large B-cell lymphoma, and breast invasive ductal carcinoma. Mutant *CCND3* isoforms are known to have shorter half-lives than the wild type. *CCND3* has a carcinogenic potential and is considered a biomarker in many cancer types and is directly targeted by various miRNAs for cancer therapy.

1.4.1. The Disease of Relevance:

- Chromosomal rearrangement involving the cryptic insertion of Immunoglobulin kappa locus *[IGK]* enhancer in chromosome 2 and Immunoglobulin lambda locus [*IGL*] enhancer in chromosome 22 near 3' of the *CCND3* gene has been reported in Mantle Cell Lymphoma [MCL], and this rearrangement resulted in *CCND3* overexpression. *CCND3/IGH* translocation has also been in low-grade B-cell lymphoma, splenic lymphoma, and aggressive B-cell lymphomas [29].
- Initially, *CCND3* translocation involving t[6, 14][p21.1;q32.3] was observed in Non-Hodgkin Lymphoma. In splenic lymphoma, missense mutations affecting the PEST domain [proline, glutamic acid, serine, and threonine] resulted in overexpression of *CCND3* [30].
- *CCND3* has been confirmed to acquire multiple nonsenses and frameshift mutations that remove up to 41 amino acids from the cyclin D3 carboxy-terminus in Burkitt Lymphoma. Like MCL, frequent missense mutations are known to affect threonine residue at 283, proline at 284, and isoleucine at 290; and at each position, multiple amino acid substitutions have been known to occur, and most of them were heterozygous [31].
- In Lymphoma, mutations like cytosine duplication at C811 result in protein elongating frameshift, and amino acid substitution, including T869G and C58-0T, are positively associated with an advanced stage of the disease, supporting pro-proliferative and cell cycle driving role [32].
- One of the most recurrent translocations observed in multiple myeloma is t[6, 14][p21:32] involving *CCND3* and *IGH*, and this rearrangement leads to dere-gulated expression of the *CCND3* gene [33].
- In colorectal cancer, many researchers have identified a gain in 6p as a metastasis-specific change, and this led to further detection of high-level amplification of *CCND3* [6p21.1]. *CCND3* expression is up-regulated in the development of hepatic metastasis and is associated with vascular invasion, liver metastasis, and reduced disease-specific survival [34, 35].

1.5. GENE: CCN2, CELLULAR COMMUNICATION NETWORK FACTOR 2, CTGF LOCATION: 6q23.2

CCN2, commonly known as *CTGF,* is a multifunctional signaling modulator that is involved in a variety of biological or pathological processes. It has been identified as an oncogene in many types of human cancer and plays a different role in different types of cancer, and also serves as a prognostic marker in many types of human cancer. *CCN2/CTGF* overexpression is associated with tumorigenesis and poor prognosis in prostate cancer, glioblastoma growth, breast cancer, adult acute lymphoblastic leukemia, breast cancer-induced bone metastasis, pancreatic cancer, liver cancer, melanoma, papillary thyroid carcinoma, esophageal squamous cell carcinoma, gastric cancer, and cervical tumors. Contrarily, it is known to inhibit the invasion and metastasis of cancer cells in colorectal cancer, non-small cell lung carcinoma, ovarian cancer, and oral squamous cell carcinoma. Its overexpression is also associated with chemo-resistance in glioma, breast cancer, osteosarcoma, and thyroid cancer [36, 37].

1.5.1. The Disease of Relevance:

- *CCN2* expression differs from benign thyroid tumors to thyroid carcinomas, and its expression can accelerate tumor growth and inhibits cell apoptosis. *CCN2* expression is upregulated in thyroid carcinoma compared to benign thyroid; this suggests that it plays a role in thyroid malignancy [36].
- *CCN2* is overexpressed in a subset of Wilms tumors and its expression is activated in early tumorigenesis and gradually decreases with tumor progression [38].
- Vascular cell adhesion molecule [VCAM]-1 is upregulated in osteosarcoma and this upregulation along with *CCN2* influences osteosarcoma development. In some cases, *CCN2* is known to promote osteosarcoma migration and metastasis through the upregulation of matrix metalloproteinase [MMP]-2 and MMP-3 [39].
- *CCN2* promotes angiogenesis in breast cancer. The C-terminal domain of *CCN2* has a binding site for integrin $\alpha v \beta 3$. Activation of kinases such as ILK and MAPK results in the activation of the integrin $\alpha v \beta 3$, and this interaction enhances the cell motility leading to the formation of aggressive breast cancer phenotype [39].
- *CCN2* acts as a tumor suppressor in nasopharyngeal carcinoma [NPC], so the loss of *CCN2* expression induces the stage of initiation and precancerous lesion in NPC [40].
- In gastric cancer, *CCN2* is the key downstream effector for the oncogene *YAP1* and together they exhibit a positive correlation in primary tumors. It plays an oncogenic role by down-regulating E-cadherin expression through activation of the NF-κB pathway, also enhances the expression of cyclin D1/MMP-2/MMP-9 and lastly, induces EMT transition, which is a hallmark of *tumorigenesis* [41].

1.6. GENE: GOPC, GOLGI-ASSOCIATED PDZ, AND COILED-COIL MOTIF-CONTAINING PROTEIN, FIG LOCATION: 6q22.1

GOPC, initially known as *FIG*, undergoes chromosomal rearrangement involving intrachromosomal deletion resulting in the formation of a *FIG-ROS1* fusion protein. The fusion gene results from 240 kilobases interstitial deletion on 6q21, which fuses the first seven exons of the *GOPC* gene to the last nine exons of the *ROS1* gene. FIG-ROS1 fusion proteins have been reported in anaplastic astrocytoma, glioblastoma, ovarian serous tumor, cholangiocarcinoma, NSCLC, and acral lentiginous melanoma.

1.6.1. The Disease of R Elevance:

- One of the reasons for glial brain tumors is the formation of a ROS1-GOPC fusion protein. Most tumors with this fusion arise in midline brain structures, often the thalamus and basal ganglia. This del [6][q22;q22] and the resulting rearrangement produces a constitutively active tyrosine kinase fusion product that has been demonstrated to be sufficient to produce neoplastic transformation and tumor development. ROS1-GOPC fusion results in shorter overall survival in patients with glioblastoma [42, 43].
- In Lung adenocarcinoma, ROS1-GOPC fusion has been known to help in acquiring resistance to osimertinib and responding to crizotinib combined treatments with osimertininb [44].
- In colorectal cancer, knockdown or loss of *GOPC* has been reported to increase activation of the mitogen-activated protein kinase [MAPK] and extracellular signal-regulated kinase [Erk] ½ pathway. These two pathways are involved in regulating cell differentiation, proliferation, survival and migration. Venous invasion significantly increases in the low *GOPC* tissue as well as the proportion of cancer recurrence [45].

1.7. GENE: MAP3K5, MITOGEN-ACTIVATED PROTEIN KINASE KINASE KINASE 5 LOCATION: 6q23.3

MAP3K5 belonging to the MAPK family has a significant role in biological mechanisms like stress and cytokine-induced apoptosis. Overexpression of *MAP3K5* regulates reactive oxygen species [ROS]-induced JNK and p38 signaling pathways leading to differentially regulated apoptosis. *MAP3K5* is upregulated in many cancers, such as Hepatitis C [HCV] associated hepatocellular carcinoma [HCC].

1.7.1. The Disease of Relevance:

• Somatic non-synonymous mutations have been found in the protein-coding regions of the *MAP3K5* gene in case of metastatic melanoma. The position of the mutations and the loss of heterozygosity [LOH] of the *MAP3K5* gene indicates reduced kinase activity, such as in the *MAP3K5* I780F variant, which affects the packing of helices in the kinase domain. Homozygous deletion in *MAP3K5* results in increased tumor initiation. Other somatic mutations in *MAP3K5* known to be involved are arginine to a cytosine substitution at 256 [8R256C], and cytosine to thymine substitution at 766 [C766T]. Somatic mutation *MAP3K5* [R256C] can help cancer cells to evade cell death induced by *MAP3K5*-dependent stress by suppressing its pro-apoptotic activity [46, 47].

• It has been revealed that oxidative stress contributes to the pathogenesis of prostate cancer. Since mitochondria are known to be a major source of ROS, any changes in mitochondrial bioenergetics can induce *MAP3K5* over-expression, further favoring malignant progression [48].

1.8. GENE: FOXC1, FORKHEAD BOX C1 LOCATION: 6p25.3

FOXC1 regulates the expression of genes involved in embryogenesis, differentiation, and angiogenesis; any mutation in *FOXC1* can result in developmental anomalies. *FOXC1* regulates the Epithelial-Mesenchymal transition [EMT], and its overexpression is associated with metastasis and poor survival in several cancer types, such as hepatocellular carcinoma [HCC], pancreatic ductal adenocarcinoma, lymphoma, lung cancer, oral cancer, melanoma, cervical cancer, breast cancer, and gastric cancer. In cervical cancers and melanoma, *FOXC1* promotes tumor development through PI3K/AKT signaling pathway. Some studies have revealed that *FOXC1* can regulate cancer stem cell [CSC] like properties through activation of smoothened independent Hedgehog signaling [49, 50].

1.8.1. The Disease of Relevance:

• *FOXC1* expression in basal-like breast cancers [BLBC], enhances cell invasion, proliferation, metastasis, and EMT and is also associated with poor overall survival. Overexpression of *FOXC1* in BLBC cells increases CSC-like properties and the process by which it is achieved is through regulation of non-canonical Smoothened [SMO]-Independent Hedgehog [Hh] signaling. *FOXC1* regulates and maintains breast tumorigenesis by activating the NF-κB signaling pathway. It is also known to promote tumor growth by upregulating Matrix metalloproteinase- 7 [MMP7] expression in cancer cells. *FOXC1* overexpression has been revealed to play a role in shorter brain metastasis-free survival and better bone metastasis-free survival [51, 52].

- In HCC, overexpression of *FOXC1* has been observed to aggravate malignancy by promoting EMT and MIV generation. It transactivates genes important for angiogenesis and metastasis, *CXCR2* and *CCL2*, through the IL-8-regulated PI2K/Akt/HIF-α inflammatory signaling pathway. In some cases, it has been found to promote tumor growth through the upregulation of *NEDD9* gene expression [51].

- *FOXC1* is highly expressed in colorectal cancers [CRCs], and it has an important role in tumor development. For any type of invasive cancer, glycolysis is the primary feature of metabolic signature; *FOXC1* enhances glycolysis in CRCs by targeting *FBP1,* which is a gluconeogenesis regulatory enzyme. It regulates *FBP1* expression by directly binding to the FBP1 promoter region and thus weakens the promoter activity of the gene*;* as a result, *FBP1* expression is downregulated in CRCs. In some CRC cases, *FOXC1* promotes metastasis by upregulating the expression of MMP10, SOX4, and SOX3. Also, the positive relationship between p38 and FOXC1 has been considered a contributor to CRC metastasis [53, 54].

- Overexpression of *FOXC1* leads to cancer metastasis in non-small cell lung carcinoma [NSCLC]. It induces and maintains CSC-like properties in NSCLC by regulating the expression of cell surface markers for cancer stem cell-like CD133. The Wnt/β-catenin pathway, which is important for regulating CSC-like properties, is also regulated by *FOXC1*, and its knockdown can result in a reduction of β- catenin mRNA levels as well as total and nuclear β-catenin protein levels. *Oct4,NANOG, SOX2,* and *ABCG2,* which are the downstream target genes of beta-catenin and important for maintaining CSC-like properties, are also regulated by *FOXC1* [55].

- Overexpression of *FOXC1* has been observed during the development of both Hodgkin's lymphoma [HL] and non-Hodgkin's lymphoma [NHL], and it has contributed to *tumorigenesis* either through differentiation and apoptosis or migration and invasion. In the HL case, *FOXC1* regulates the expression of NKL homeobox gene, *i.e., MSX1,* which is important in B-cell development, in conjugation with shuttle-protein encoding gene *IPO7* inhibits the B-cell specific factor involved in differentiation and apoptosis, and the NOTCH signaling pathway, ZHX2. In NHL cases, a positive relationship has been observed between *FOXC1* and CARD11-Jun pathway, wherein overexpression of *FOXC1* resulted in elevated Jun protein levels, which led to increased occurrence of migration and invasion of solid tumors [51].

- In pancreatic cancer, *FOXC1* is the transcription factor that is regulated by growth factor IGF-1R and the expression of both genes is independent, thus indicating strong positive feedback regulation between *IGF-1R* and *FOXC1*. As a downstream signaling molecule of IGF-1R, it is known to have the same effect as IGF-1R on cancer cells. It activates the translation of genes having a role in processes such as proliferation, cell survival, metastasis, and angiogenesis through IGF-1R signaling. *FOXC1* expression increases as the pancreatic tumor advance. *FOXC1* promotes tumor growth and increases survival potential by regulating the PI3K/AKT and ERK signaling pathways. *FOXC1* expression level also regulates the expression level of important EMT markers such as Zeb, β-Catenin, Notch-2, Snail, Slug, N-cadherin, and Vimentin in cancer cells. *FOXC1* has an active role in angiogenesis, and so it enhances the invasiveness or the aggressiveness of the pancreatic cancer cells by increasing the levels of angiogenic markers VEGFR2 and delta-like ligand-protein 4 [DLL4] [56].

1.9. GENE: FGFR1OP, FGFR1 ONCOGENE PARTNER LOCATION: 6q27

FGFR1OP is a centrosomal protein that plays a major role in cell polarization and ciliogenesis. Aberrant expression of *FGFR1OP* can induce centrosome abnormalities and tumor development through the induction of chromosome instability. Overexpression of *FGFR1OP* has been found in most bladder cancer, cervical cancer, prostate cancer, renal cell carcinoma, and osteosarcoma.

1.9.1. The Disease of Relevance:

- *FGFR1OP* gene undergoes chromosomal translocation t[6, 10][q27;q11] with *RET* gene and forms a chimeric protein called FGFR1OP-RET in a patient affected by primary myelofibrosis case with secondary acute myeloid leukemia [AML]. Sequencing has shown that exon 11 of *FGFR1OP* fuses in-frame to the 3' portion of exon 11 of *RET* and forms the fusion gene. This fusion protein confers anchorage-independent growth in cancer cells and has oncogenic potential. In FGFR1OP-RET fusion protein, the LISH domain on *FGFR1OP* results in continuous activation of RET tyrosine kinase. FGFR1OP-RET fusion protein exhibits oncogenic activity mostly due to the constitutive dimerization and activation of its kinase domain [57].
- In myeloproliferative disorders with lymphoma and myeloid hyperplasia, the *FGFR1OP* gene is involved in translocation with *FGFR1*, t[6, 8][q27;q12], and forms FGFR1OP-FGFR1 fusion protein, regulates the *tumorigenesis* [58].
- *FGFR1OP* variants involved in the *tumorigenesis* are rs151606 and rs12212247 and of this, rs15606 is associated with a high risk of lung cancer. Also, overexpression of *FGFR1OP* has been reported in most of the primary non-small cell lung carcinoma [NSCLC], and it induces a highly malignant phenotype of lung cancer cells [59, 60].

1.10. GENE: IGF2R, INSULIN-LIKE GROWTH FACTOR 2 RECEPTOR LOCATION: 6q25.3

One of the main functions of *IGF2R* is the degradation of insulin-like growth factor 2 [*IGF2*], so any alteration in its expression results in *IGF2*-induced proliferation and reduces susceptibility to tumor necrosis factor-induced apoptosis. *IGF2R* usually acts as a tumor suppressor in many types of cancer, but in some cancers, such as cervical cancers and glioblastoma, it acts as an oncogene. Loss of heterozygosity [LOH] at 6q26-27, where this gene resides and reduction in protein expression has been observed in many malignant tumors such as breast cancer, ovarian cancer, melanoma, lymphoma, renal cell carcinoma, hepatocellular carcinoma [HCC], lung cancer, colorectal cancer, hemangioma, and androgen insensitive prostate cancer. Some studies have found the 3' UTR *IGF2R-A2/B2* variant to be involved in increased tumor growth and advanced stages in the case of non-small cell lung carcinoma [NSCLC] [61 - 63].

1.10.1. The Disease of Relevance

- Association between *IGF2R* c.901C>G allele and esophageal gastric cardia adenocarcinoma is observed mostly in white males with a history of cigarette smoking and none or irregular use of NSAIDs [64].
- *IGF2R* act as a tumor suppressor gene by reducing the tumorigenicity and invasive potential of HCC. LOH at the *IGF2R* locus is considered to be an early event in HCC. Many types of mutations in *IGF2R* have been considered to induce *tumorigenesis*. Point mutations such as Gly1449Val, Gly1464Glu, Cys1262Ser, Asp1268Asn, Met1625Leu, Pro1444Ser, Ser1628Phe, Gly1315-Gln, His1878Gln, and Thr1650Ile; and frame-shift mutations induced by "G" deletion in poly[G]8 repeats present in exon 28 has been reported to be involved in HCC exhibiting LOH [62, 65].
- LOH at the *IGF2R* locus has been observed in invasive ductal carcinomas and ductal carcinoma in situ. Later two mutations, one in exon 31 [Gln144His] and the other in exon 40 [Thr2379Pro], were reported in case of ductal carcinoma in situ. *IGF2R* is overexpressed in high-grade ductal carcinoma in situ, whereas its expression is decreased in invasive ductal carcinomas [62].
- Two-point mutations in *IGF2R* that is Gly1296Arg and Gly1564Arg, have been associated with lung adenocarcinoma. In the first mutation, glycine in coding triplet GGT changes into CGT; whereas in the second mutation, glycine in coding triplet, GGG changes into CGG [62].
- Unlike other cancers, *IGF2R* is upregulated in cervical cancer and has prognoses. In the absence of *IGF2R*, cervical cells undergo caspase-mediated and cell viability is decreased, and also vulnerability to cisplatin is increased. *IGF2R* plays an oncogenic role through the transportation of M6P-tagged cargo

in cervical cancer and can be used as a predictive biomarker for prognostic classification [66].

1.11. GENE: AIM1, ABSENT IN MELANOMA, CRYBG1 LOCATION: 6q21

AIM1 is an important regulator of actin cytoskeletal dynamics. It is mainly known for its role in malignant melanoma as a tumor suppressor. *AIM1* hypermethylation has been associated with human melanoma and prostate cancers. Its methylation has also been associated with nasopharyngeal carcinoma and primary tumor invasion of bladder cancer.

1.11.1. The Disease of Relevance:

- *AIM1* is localized within the putative tumor suppressor gene region for human melanoma, and alteration in *AIM1* gene expression has been observed in malignant melanoma. Promoter hypermethylation of *AIM1* along with LINE-1 hypomethylation together increases tumor progression in melanoma. Deletion of 6q21 and methylation of *AIM1* results in decreased expression, and as well as promoter hypermethylation of *AIM1* has been reported to downregulate the expression in natural killer-cell malignancies [67, 68].
- *AIM1* expression is strongly associated with the regulation of the actin cytoskeleton, and it acts as a tumor suppressor by suppressing cytoskeletal remodeling and invasive properties in the case of benign prostate epithelial cells. Depletion in *AIM1* expression promotes cell migration and invasion, cytoskeletal remodeling, and anchorage-independent growth in prostate epithelial cells and also results in increased metastatic dissemination. Reduced expression or deletion of *AIM1* can dissociate *AIM1* from the actin cytoskeleton in advanced prostate cancers. In some cases of prostate cancers, *AIM1* acts as an oncogene as a result of promoter hypermethylation. *AIM1* is highly expressed in primary prostate cancers [69, 70].

1.12. GENE: HACE1, HECT DOMAIN, AND ANKYRIN REPEAT-CONTAINING E3 UBIQUITIN-PROTEIN LIGASE 1 LOCATION: 6q16.3

HACE1 protein as a potential tumor suppressor has been described in the pathophysiology of several tumors. Reduced expression of *HACE1* as a result of a loss of heterozygosity [LOH] at the *HACE1* locus or epigenetic inactivation due to methylation in the *HACE1* gene has been associated with tumors such as natural killer/T-cell lymphomas of the nasal type, B-cell non-Hodgkin's ladlymphomas, childhood acute lymphoblastic leukemia, osteosarcoma, prostate cancers, pancreatic tumors, gastric carcinomas, ovarian carcinomas, cervical adenocarcinomas, aggressive breast cancer, Wilms tumor, lung adenocarcinoma, angiosarcoma, and advanced neuroblastoma.

1.12.1. The Disease of Relevance:

- Reduction in *HACE1* expression levels and LOH has been described in osteosarcoma. *HACE1* reduces reactive oxygen species [ROS] generation by targeting *RAC1* at RAC1-dependent NADPH oxidases to inhibit superoxide production. So HACE1 loss in osteosarcoma cells had elevated levels of active *RAC1*, which further led to an increased level of ROS [71].
- A de novo balanced translocation t[5, 6][q21;q21] involving *HACE1* has been reported in the case of bilateral Wilms tumor, and this rearrangement shortens *HACE1*, which led to its inactivation in cancer tissues. Two somatic translocations involving *HACE1*, t[2, 6][q35;q21] and t[6, 15][q21;q21], have been reported in Wilms tumor. In the case of somatic translocation, the breakpoint was found to be 50kb upstream of *HACE1*, and thus resulted in reduced expression of *HACE1*. There are few cases of Wilms tumor, wherein somatic heterozygous interstitial 6q21 deletion comprising 7.3 Mb of *HACE1* has been reported. Hypermethylation of CpG island in the promoter region, that is upstream of *HACE1* has been associated with reduced expression in tumor cells [72].
- *HACE1* displayed pro-tumoral functions in melanoma cells and it is known to favor cell adhesion, migration, and lung colonization in melanoma [73].

1.13. GENE: RIPK1, RECEPTOR-INTERACTING SERINE/THREONINE KINASE 1 LOCATION: 6p25.2

RIPK1 is a member of the receptor-interacting protein [RIP] family of serine/threonine protein kinases. It plays a dual role in the cell such as cell death and pro-survival signaling and overexpression of RIPK1 have been observed in melanoma, lung cancers, glioblastoma, hepatocellular carcinoma [HCC], and pancreatic ductal adenocarcinoma.

1.13.1. The Disease of Relevance:

- *RIPK1* expression is reduced as a consequence of epigenetic modification caused by promoter methylation in head and neck squamous cell carcinoma [HNSCC] cells. This downregulation of *RIPK1* allows tumor cells to escape anoikis which is a form of programmed cell death wherein cells detach from the surrounding extracellular matrix and thus contribute to tumorigenesis [74].
- In higher grades of human glioblastoma, the *RIPK1* gene is overexpressed, and

this overexpression results in the downregulation of tumor suppressor p53 and thus favors the development of the tumor [75].

- Elevated *RIPK1* level, along with adenosine deaminase, has been associated with malignant breast tumors. *RIPK1* promotes breast cancer metastasis *via* the NF-kB signaling pathway [76].

- Increased level of *RIPK1* has been positively correlated with cell proliferation in colon adenocarcinoma. In colorectal cells, RIPK1 protein targets mitochondrial Ca^{2+} uniporter [MCU]; this interaction enhances mitochondrial Ca^{2+} uptake and energy metabolism, which as a result, mediate RIPK1-dependent cell proliferation. In some cases, *RIPK1* recruits the essential modulator NFκB to the TNFR1 complex and undergoes ubiquitination, thus playing a role in cell proliferation [77].

- In HCC, reduced expression of *RIPK1* inhibits a *TRAF2*- and caspase-8-dependent apoptosis checkpoint and thus promotes tumorigenesis in HCC. *TRAF2* is also known to inhibit necroptosis [78].

1.14. GENE: THSB2, THROMBOSPONDIN 2 LOCATION: 6q27

THBS2 is a matricellular glycoprotein that plays multiple roles including bone growth, cell adhesion, extracellular matrix modeling, inflammatory responses, development, and pathological angiogenesis. THBS2 protein acts as a potential inhibitor of angiogenesis, mitogenesis, and the formation of focal adhesion in endothelial cells. Reduced *THBS2* expression is associated with poor prognoses in gastric cancer, prostate cancer, colon cancer, endometrial carcinoma, non-small cell lung carcinoma [NSCLC], and pancreatic cancer. It is highly expressed in cancers such as renal cancer, ovarian cancer, oral cavity squamous cell carcinoma, gastric cancer, lung carcinoma, and hepatocellular carcinoma [HCC] [79].

1.14.1. The Disease of Relevance:

- *THBS2* expression is reduced in malignant ovarian cancers and alteration in the expression is mostly observed in the early stages. Whereas in late-stage tumors, THBS2 mRNA has been detected indicating its association with an aggressive phenotype. Epigenetic inactivation of *THBS2* by promoter hypermethylation participates in the angiogenesis of malignant ovarian tumors through *THBS2* downregulation [80].

- In Myxoid liposarcomas [MLS], highly expressed miR-135b suppresses the expression of *THBS2* and results in increased levels of MMP2 in the extracellular matrix. However, there are few cases found wherein patients with MLS displayed a high expression level of *THBS2* even in the presence of miR-135b, and the reason for this contradiction would be single nucleotide mutations, deletions, and insertion at miRNA target sites [81].

- *THBS2* is overexpressed in gastric cancer and is known to exhibit anti-angiogenic function. Highly expressed *THBS2* plays a critical role in the ECM-receptor interaction pathway, focal adhesion pathway, and TGF-β signaling during gastric *tumorigenesis* and it is used as a potential predictor of good gastric cancer prognosis. It influences the proteolysis of tumor cytoplasm, thus contributing to the activation and expression of certain proteins in the PI3K/Akt signaling pathway [82, 83].

- *THBS2* expression is significantly regulated by miR-221-3p in cervical cancer tissues. Deletion or reduced *THBS2* expression contributes to cervical cancer progression and is associated with poor prognosis. The inhibitory role of *THBS2* in tumors involves multiple interactions with cell surface receptors [LRP, CD36, CD47, and numerous integrins], ECM components, growth factors [TGF-β, FGF2], enzymes [MMPs, elastase], and calcium-binding in cancer cells [84].

- *THBS2* expression is upregulated and increased expression is associated with poor overall survival in colorectal cancers. *THBS2* expression promotes tumor growth and is also associated with lymphatic invasion, and distant metastasis clinical stage. In a few studies, *THBS2* has displayed hypomethylation in both colorectal adenocarcinoma and CRC-adjacent normal tissues [85].

1.15. GENE: PTPRK, PROTEIN TYROSINE PHOSPHATASE RECEPTOR TYPE K LOCATION: 6q22.33

PTPRK is a putative tumor suppressor gene located within a region on chromosome 6 [6q22.2-q22.3]. PTPRK are signaling molecules that regulate a variety of cellular processes, including cell growth, differentiation, mitotic cycle, and oncogenic transformation. *PTPRK* gene expression is reduced in certain malignancies such as sporadic endocrine pancreatic tumors, juvenile intestinal carcinoma, breast cancer, ovarian carcinoma, melanoma, lung cancers, leukemia, and non-Hodgkin lymphoma [NHL]. Knockdown of *PTPRK* resulted in increased cell proliferation, adhesion, and invasion. Dysregulation or loss of heterozygosity [LOH] mutation within *PTPRK* increases the susceptibility to intestinal lesions, including intraepithelial neoplasia, adenoma, adenocarcinoma, nasal-type NK/T-cell lymphoma [NKTCL], glioblastoma, colon cancer metastasis, primary central nervous system lymphomas [PCNSL] and primary ocular lymphoma. Epigenetic silencing of *PTPRK* has been reported in certain blood malignancies and acute lymphoblastic leukemia [ALL]. Increased expression of *PTPRK* is associated with cancers like breast and prostate cancer tissues. *PTPRK* can weaken or downregulate the activation of various signaling pathways involving tyrosine phosphorylation of cellular proteins through the removal of their phosphate groups [86].

1.15.1. The Disease of Relevance:

- A chromosomal rearrangement involving PTPRK–RSPO3 fusions has been reported in serrated adenomas. This genetic alteration activates the Wnt pathway; this function distinguishes them from other serrated polys, as well as ROPO3 regulates stem cell-like function in PTPRK-RSPO3 fusion-positive tumors [87].
- Depletion or silencing of *PTPRK* gene expression leads to phosphorylation of CD133, which is a stem cell marker and enhances the pro-oncogenic Akt –Bad pathway resulting in an aggressive form of colon cancer. In some colon cancer cases, *PTPRK* suppresses the pro-oncogenic EGF/EGFR signaling pathway through EGFR dephosphorylation, which further activates Akt phosphorylation leading to malignant colon cancer [88].
- In non-small cell lung carcinoma [NSCLC] cells, elevated miR-126b directly targets the *PTPRK* gene and downregulates its expression, this interaction increases the migratory and invasive properties in the tumor. Decreased level of *PTPRK* mRNA has been reported in NKTCL cells and is associated with poor prognosis. In NKTCL, *PTPRK* negatively regulates signal transducer and activator of transcription 3 [STAT3] activation, which is a vital pro-oncogenic transcription factor involved in many cancers and thus contributes to NKTCL pathogenesis [89].
- Both *PTPRK* mRNA and protein levels are upregulated in prostate cancer tissues. *PTPRK* promotes the development of tumors by regulating and maintaining a balance between the cell cycle; and necrosis and apoptosis. *PTPRK* in prostate cancer cells downregulates apoptosis by suppressing the JNK pathway and whereas knockdown of *PTPRK* increases expressions of caspase-3 and -8, responsible for cell death [90].

1.16. GENE: HSP90AB1; HEAT SHOCK PROTEIN 90 ALPHA FAMILY CLASS B MEMBER 1 LOCATION: 6p21.1

HSP90AB1 gene encodes a member of the heat shock protein 90 family and is involved in signal transduction, protein folding and degradation, and morphological evolution. It has a significant role in the regulation of tumorigenesis, such as overexpression of *HSP90AB1* promotes angiogenesis, metastasis, and differentiation. It has been implicated to have an oncogenic role in hepatocellular carcinoma [HCC], lung cancer, laryngeal carcinoma, breast cancer, non-small cell lung cancer [NSCLC], prostate cancer, and multiple myeloma. It has been shown that *HSP90AB1* stabilizes Cdc25A and increases its expression levels; this interaction further promotes cell cycle activation in cancers like pancreatic carcinoma cells. Similarly, it promotes leukemia cell proliferation by preventing the auto-ubiquitination and degradation of c-IAP1, which is a member of the [inhibitor of apoptosis protein] IAP family.

HSP90AB1 in certain cancers is known to be methylated by the histone methyl-transferase *SMYD2* and it plays a critical role 30 in human *tumorigenesis*. *HSP90AB1* and *SMYD2* interact through the C-terminal region of *HSP90AB1* 31 and the SET domain of *SMYD2*. Lysines 531 and 574 of *HSP90AB1* are known to be methylated and these sites are important for the dimerization and chaperone complex formation of *HSP90AB1*. Furthermore, methylated *HSP90AB1* accelerated the proliferation of cancer cells [91].

1.16.1. The Disease of Relevance:

- *HSP90AB1* expression is upregulated in gastric cancer cells, which is associated with aggressive stages. Increased *HSP90AB1* stabilizes [Low-density lipoprotein receptor-related protein 5] LRP5 by inhibiting the ubiquitin degradation of LRP5 to promote EMT *via* activating the AKT and Wnt/β-catenin signaling pathways. Thus *HSP90AB1* protein is important to promote the invasion and migration of gastric cancer tumorigenesis [92].
- A chromosomal rearrangement involving EEF1A1-HSP90AB1 in-frame fusion has been reported in a few colorectal cancer cells. *EEF1A1* in fusion protein plays an important role in tumor pathophysiology and contributes to cell growth, cell cycle regulation, and maintenance of cell survival. On the other hand, the *HSP90AB1* gene is involved in signal transduction, protein folding, degradation, and morphological evolution [93].
- HSP90AB1 protein is highly expressed in NSCLC and is responsible for the pathological type of lung cancer. In lung adenocarcinoma, *HSP90AB1* is highly expressed as a result of the high mutation rate of EGFR, which is a substrate protein of HSP90AB1 and is associated with poor prognosis. However, the expression rate of *HSP90AB1* is high in lung adenocarcinoma when compared to squamous cell carcinoma. *HSP90AB1* is generally identified as a significant prognostic factor in NSCLC patients with a smoking history but not in those without a smoking history. Although increased mRNA level of HSP90AB1 has been revealed to be a significant prognostic factor in NSCLC patients with no smoking history but not in those with a smoking history [94, 95].
- Constitutively expressed heat shock factor *HSP90AB1* is epigenetically regulated by [ubiquitin-specific protease 22] USP22 in human breast and colorectal cancer cells. High *HSP90AB1* expression in both tumor cells is associated with poor prognosis. *HSP90AB1* level was reduced as a consequence of USP22 loss, effectively reducing tumor growth [96].

1.17. GENE: IRF4, INTERFERON REGULATORY FACTOR 4 LOCAT-ION: 6p25.3

IRF4 is a potential candidate transcription factor, which is highly expressed in B cells and plasma cells and has an essential role in controlling B cell to plasma cell differentiation and immunoglobulin class switching. *IRF4* binds to the *MYC* promoter region and enhances *MYC* expression, which is a proto-oncogene, favoring the formation of the tumor. *IRF4* is highly expressed in multiple myeloma, and lymphoid malignancies and is considered a prognostic marker for various hematological malignancies. *IRF4* acts as a tumor suppressor in human neoplasias, and its expression is reduced in cancers like pre-B-cell leukemias, c-Myc–induced malignancies, myeloid leukemia, and acute myeloid leukemia.

1.17.1. The Disease of Relevance:

- *IRF4* is highly expressed in almost all myeloma cells and knockdown of *IRF4* induces apoptosis in myeloma cells, thus it acts as an oncogene in case of myeloma. A chromosomal translocation involving *IRF4* t[6, 14][p25;q32] has been observed in multiple myeloma, which results in overexpression or activation of *IRF4* in tumor cells. In some multiple myeloma tissues, histone demethylase KDM3A activates the expression of *IRF4*, so KDM3A is considered an important epigenetic regulator [97].
- One of the translocation partners identified for *IGH* [14q32] in primary plasma cell leukemia is *IRF4* [6p23-25]. The IRF4-IgH fusion protein is formed as a result of either t[6, 14] or IgH insertion into the *IRF4* locus. This chromosomal rearrangement t[6, 14] has been reported in mature B-cell malignancies, such as diffuse large B-cell lymphoma, splenic marginal zone lymphoma, and mantle cell lymphoma [98].
- *IRF4* is highly expressed in Epstein-Barr virus-transformed cells, multiple myeloma and human T cell leukemia virus 1 [HTLV1]- infected cells and associated T cell lymphoma and it has the potential to induce tumor growth. Expression of *IRF4* is associated with poor survival of NSCLC patients. *IRF4* acts as a tumor promoter by activating the Notch-Akt signaling pathway in many types of cancer cells and is known to promote cell survival [99].
- *IRF4* is frequently downregulated as a consequence of DNA methylation in gastric cancer cells [100].
- SNP in the *IRF4* gene has been associated with chronic lymphocytic leukemia [CLL]. It acts as a tumor suppressor in CLL, so the reduction in its expression enhances CLL disease progression. Reduced *IRF4* level is associated with severe downregulation of genes involved in T-cell activation, also including genes involved in antigen presentation and T-cell costimulation, this interaction enhances the CLL malignancies. CD4-specific *IRF4* deletion is associated with immune defects and T-cell exhaustion; on the other hand, CD8-specific *IRF4*

deletion contributed to the establishment of chronic infections because of abrogated effector T-cell differentiation. Missense somatic substitution has been observed in exon 2 after sequencing of *IRF4* coding exons in CLL cells. The substitution comprising of leucine → arginine [L116R–M1] is located in the DNA-binding domain of the gene, and another substitution comprising of leucine → proline [L116P–M2] has been reported to affect the same base in CLL [101, 102].

1.18. GENE: VIP, VASOACTIVE INTESTINAL PEPTIDE LOCATION: 6q25.2

VIP gene is a neuropeptide, which can act as autocrine or paracrine growth factors in tumor cells. It has carcinogenic potential and can induce tumor formation in human cancers such as breast cancer, lung cancer, pancreatic carcinoma, prostate cancer, and in various CNS tumors like gliomas, and astrocytomas. Further, the *VIP* gene can also exhibit an inhibitory effect on tumor growth in cancers such as retinoblastoma and renal cell carcinoma. Their biological actions are mediated by G-protein-coupled receptors [GPCR] such as VPAC1 and VPAC2, which are members of class II/class-B secretin-like receptors.

VPAC1 receptors are overexpressed in epithelial neoplasms such as bladder, breast, colon, liver, lung, pancreatic, prostate, thyroid, and uterus- cancer. *VPAC2* receptors are present in gastric leiomyomas; thyroid, gastric/pancreatic adenocarcinomas; lung tumors, various sarcomas, and neuroendocrine tumors. It is well known that excessive *VIPR* signaling, which arises from receptor overexpression and autocrine stimulation by *VIP*, is a hallmark for a range of tumors. Since in most of the tumors, *VIPRs* are overexpressed, so when VIP binds to these VIPRs, it activates them, leading to an interaction with a stimulatory guanine nucleotide-binding protein [Gs] and ultimately resulting in the stimulation of adenylate cyclase [103].

1.18.1. The Disease of Relevance:

- VIP receptors are present in the majority of lung carcinoma cells. It has been shown that VIP through GPCR stimulates tumor growth by transactivating the epidermal growth factor [EGFR], which requires phospholipase-c and stimulates matrix-metalloproteinases [MMPs], Src-kinases, TGF-α release and generates oxygen-free-radical in the cancer cell [104].
- VIP receptors or effector systems, including VPAC1 and VPC2, are highly expressed in human breast carcinoma and promote breast *tumorigenesis* by increasing cell proliferation. Many studies have shown that *VIP* activates adenylate cyclase, which further increases vascular endothelial growth factor [VEGF] expression and secretion, and stimulates tumor growth. It is also known

to stimulate the transactivation of both EGFR and the related receptor, human epidermal growth factor receptor 2 [HER2/Neu], in breast cancer cell lines [104].

- VIP receptors, predominantly VPAC1, are highly expressed in prostate cancer cells. It acts as a cytokine in the early metastatic stages of prostate cancer. *VIP* stimulates cAMP generation increases transactivation of HER2/Neu as well as transactivates androgen receptor *via* a PK-ERK mechanism and also increases the expression and secretion of c-Fos, VEGF, and COX-2. It has a carcinogenic potential and can induce malignancy in normal human prostate epithelial cells as a consequence of stimulation of MMP2, MMP9, and cyclin D1; which further decreases E-cadherin-mediated cell-to-cell adhesion and increases cell motility and cell proliferation. In some prostate cancer cells, it can induce tumor formation by stimulating cell proliferation and invasiveness *via* an NF-kB mechanism, which further increases expression of cyclin D1, MMP-2, and MMP-9 and also angiogenic factors like VEGF and COX-2 [104].

- *VIP* receptor is highly expressed in colon adenocarcinoma. In colon cancer where *VPAC1* is highly expressed, increased translocation of activated EGFR to the cell's cytoplasm has been observed. In some cancer cells, VPAC receptors increase cAMP, alter cellular calcium, and activate chloride-activated CA^{2+} channels, which further stimulates ornithine decarboxylase activity and finally stimulates tumor growth [104].

- VPAC1 and VPAC2 receptors are expressed in various human gliomas such as astrocytomas, ependymomas, and oligodendrogliomas. In some gliomas, activation of *VIP* receptors inhibits cell migration but does not have an effect on cell proliferation and is found to be mediated by inhibition of AKT signaling. In childhood, primitive neuroectodermal tumors such as medulloblastomas and expression of both VPAC1 and VPAC2 mRNA have been reported [104].

- VPAC1 receptor is majorly expressed in neuroblastoma cells when compared to the VPAC2 receptor. In tumor cells, *VIP* gene transcription and c-Fos expression are stimulated by pituitary adenylate cyclase-activating polypeptide [PACAP], which also activates phospholipase-c. It is also known to induce tumor formation by activating adenylate cyclase [104].

- *VIP* receptors are frequently expressed in pancreatic ductal cancers and expression of VIP increases cAMP and c-fos mRNA, which results in enhanced proliferation [104].

- *VIP* and its receptor VPAC1 are highly expressed in human primary gastric cancer tissues. Activation of VPAC1 leads to increased *VIP* expression, which is generally attenuated by Ca^{2+} chelation. It is also known to promote tumor formation *via* the VPAC1/TRPV4/Ca^{2+} signaling cascade, which activates *VIP* expression and secretion *via* cAMP-response element-binding protein [CREB] [105].

1.19. GENE: HMGA1, HIGH MOBILITY GROUP AT-HOOK 1 LOCATION: 6p21.31

HMGA1 gene is an oncogene that is highly expressed in cancer cells and is known to play a crucial role in tumorigenesis. It is overexpressed in epithelial cancers such as breast, lung, colorectal and uterine cancer; and also in mesenchymal tumors such as liposarcoma, glioblastoma, fibrosarcoma, leiomyoma, and osteosarcoma. It contributes to metastatic progression by encoding a chromatin-associated protein that primarily binds to the minor groove of AT-rich regions in double-stranded DNA. Its overexpression is associated with poor outcomes, distant metastasis, and advanced tumor stage in several human cancers [106].

1.19.1. The Disease of Relevance:

- In pituitary tumors, it is known to promote the growth hormone prolactin and leads to the formation of prolactinomas by inducing the expression of IL-2 and IL-15 proteins. In some studies, *HMGA1* pseudogenes *HMGA1P6* and *HMGA1P7* are found to act as competitive endogenous decoys for *HMGA1* and therefore contribute to pituitary tumorigenesis by increasing the level of *HMGA1*. It has been found that transcription factor Sp1 interacts with *E2F1* to promote *HMGA1* expression and thus facilitates tumor development. MicroRNAs like miR-34b, miR-326, miR-432, miR-548c-3p, miR-570, and miR-603 are known to target *HMGA1* and result in overexpression in pituitary tumorigenesis [106].
- In blastoma including glioblastomas, medulloblastomas, retinoblastomas, and neuroblastoma, *HMGA1* is associated with malignant progression, histological grade, and time to recurrence as well as with glioblastoma stem cells [GSCs]. In cancer cells, it promotes the maintenance of GSCs by encouraging the transcription of SOX2. During hypoxic stress, *IGF2BP2* and *DHX9* genes bind to each other and promote *HMGA1*-mediated modulation of GSC responses. In medulloblastomas, *HMGA1* expression has been associated with tumorigenesis by promoting cdc25A expression or inhibiting *CRMP1* expression and in neuroblastoma, it facilitates tumorigenesis by increasing the expression of the transcription factor N-Myc [106].
- In thyroid cancer, HMGA1 is overexpressed and thus is used as a diagnostic marker to differentiate between nodular thyroid and thyroid cancer. Its expression results in the suppression of p53 and *HAND1* in thyroid tissue, and it induces the TGF-β1 and S100A13 pathways in tumor cells. *HMGA1* pseudogenes *HMGA1P6* and *HMGA1P7* also function in promoting thyroid malignant progression [106].
- In non-small cell lung cancer [NSCLC], *HMGA1* expression causes an increase

in miR-222 level and simultaneously increases the p-Akt levels by suppressing *PPP2R2A*; by this, it facilitates the progression of NSCLC and can be used as a diagnostic marker [106].

- In breast cancer, *HMGA1* is associated with the histological grade, clinical stage, tumor size, lymph node metastasis, and distant metastasis. In a cancer cell, *HMGA1* pseudogene *HMGA1P7* competitively binds to endogenous RNA and thereby promotes cancer progression. In some cases, it promotes tumorigenesis by promoting miR-181b and inhibiting *CBX7* expression. In basal-like breast cancer and triple-negative breast cancer, *HMGA1* has been seen to promote the transformation of tumor cells into breast stem cells and maintain stemness. It can also promote tumor formation by activating *YAP* through cyclin E2 [*CCNE2*], thereby promoting nuclear localization and basal-like breast cancer progression. In MCF-7 breast cancer cells, *HMGA1* has been known to increase the activity of the Ras/ERK signaling pathway to promote tumor progression [106].

- *HMGA1* is overexpressed in gastric, colorectal, liver, pancreatic cancer, and cholangiocarcinoma. In gastric cancer, it is known to increase the expression of the Wnt/β-catenin pathway, while in colorectal cancer [CRC], its expression is associated with advanced tumors and lymph node metastasis and in some CRC cases, it is known to regulate Wnt/β signaling to promote tumorigenesis. *HMGA1* is shown to have a negative expression in hepatocellular carcinoma [HCC], whereas different degrees of positive expression is also observed in intrahepatic cholangiocarcinoma and metastatic adenocarcinoma [106].

- *HMGA1* expression is prominently increased in pancreatic intraepithelial neoplasia, therefore it is used as a potential diagnostic molecular marker in intra-ductal papillary mucinous tumors and pancreatic duct cell carcinomas. *HMGA1* transcription induces the expression of cyclooxygenase 2 [*COX-2*], or it can also regulate the insulin receptor to increase cyclin D1 translation and later promotes malignant progression [106].

- *HMGA1* is overly expressed in reproductive system cancers such as prostate, ovarian, uterine, cervical, and endometrial cancer, therefore, considered a useful diagnostic marker. In prostate cancer, its expression is positively correlated with malignant properties. In ovarian cancer, its overexpression can elevate spheroid-forming cancer stem cells by increasing stemness-related gene expressions such as *ALDH, SOX2, ABCB1, ABCG2,* and *KLF4*. In uterine cancer, *HMGA1* directly binds to the *COX-2* promoter and facilitates angiogenesis and tumor invasion. *HMGA1* is also known to regulate MMP-2 to induce cervical cancer positively [106].

1.20. GENE: MYB, MYB PROTO-ONCOGENE LOCATION: 6q23.3

MYB gene plays an important role in the regulation of hematopoiesis and acts as an oncogene in many human cancers. Aberrant expression of the gene or rearrangement, such as translocation involving the gene, has been associated with leukemias and lymphomas. *MYB* target genes that can be linked to oncogenicity are divided into those that are connected to proliferation, such as *MYC, CCNA1* [cyclin A1], *CCNB1, CCNE1,* and *KIT*; survival, including BCL2 [B-cell lymphoma 2], HSPA5 [heat shock protein A5; also known as GRP78] and HSP70; or differentiation, such as GATA3. *MYB* is highly expressed in immature, proliferating epithelial, endothelial, and hematopoietic cells and is downregulated as cells become more differentiated. *MYB* is overexpressed in human breast tumors, colorectal cancer, melanoma, pancreatic cancer, and oesophageal cancer.

1.20.1. The Disease of Relevance:

- Overexpression of the *MYB* gene has been associated with a human breast tumor, and its expression is correlated with estrogen receptor [ER] positivity. Its expression is regulated by transcriptional attenuation, mostly occurring within a region between 1.4 kbp and 2.2 kbp from the start of intron 1, which includes the SL–poly[dT] motif. As *MYB* is an effector of estrogen/ ER signaling, estrogen directly acts to relieve attenuation due to sequences within the first intron and results in enhanced expression of *MYB*. Amplification of the *MYB* gene has been described to be correlated to *BRCA1* mutation in breast cancer cells [107, 108].
- Oncogenic alteration in *MYB* expression, particularly in myeloid cells has been associated with leukemogenesis. It plays a crucial role in the continuous proliferation of acute myeloid leukemia [ALL] and chronic myeloid leukemia [CML] cells and also enhances their viability. Recently rearrangement such as translocation or duplication involving *MYB* has been reported in a subset of T-cell acute lymphoblastic leukemia [T-ALL] cells. *MYB* duplication in T-ALL is mediated somatically by homologous recombination between Alu-elements flanking the *MYB* locus. In T-ALL cells, *MYB* undergoes translocation t[6, 7][q23;q34], and in this rearrangement, *MYB* and TCRB [T-cell receptor β] are juxta-posed on the derivative chromosome 6, leading to activation of *MYB* expression, defining a new T-ALL cell [108, 109].
- Overexpression of the *MYB* gene has been described in colorectal cancers. Frequent mutation in the transcriptional attenuation region, including the sequences present in the first intron, is known to regulate transcriptional elongation of *MYB*; hyper-mutation of the poly-T tract and the stem-loop motif is associated with colorectal cancer [108].
- Downregulation of *MYB* expression is known to promote tumorigenesis and tumor progression in gastric cancer tissues and its expression is positively correlated with the prognosis of gastric cancer [110].
- *MYB* gene undergoes chromosomal translocation t[6, 9][q22–23;p23–24] in adenoid cystic carcinomas [ACC]. This translocation involves a fusion of exon

14 of the *MYB* gene to exon 8c or 9 of the *NFIB* gene and results in the formation of fusion protein, including *MYB* and *NFIB* genes. The MYB-NFIB fusion protein retains the DNA-binding and transactivation domains of wild-type MYB and is therefore expected to activate MYB target genes [109].

1.21. GENE: TNF, TUMOR NECROSIS FACTOR, TNF-ALPHA LOCATION: 6p21.33

The *TNF* gene encodes a proinflammatory cytokine that belongs to the TNF superfamily. It regulates a wide spectrum of biological processes, including cell proliferation, differentiation, apoptosis, metabolism, and coagulation. It has been involved in inflammatory-associated tumor development. *TNF-alpha* has biphasic effects it can induce tumor cell apoptosis at high doses while it can promote tumor invasion and metastasis with long-term administration of low doses. TNF protein stimulates the expression of angiogenic factors and promotes tumor angiogenesis. *TNF* is highly expressed in various malignant tumors such as chronic lymphocytic leukemia, Barrett's adenocarcinoma, and prostate, breast, and cervical cancers.

Many SNPs have also been found in the *TNF* gene, which can cause cancer. Individuals carrying an AA/GA genotype at *TNF*-308 have higher *TNF* expression levels and increased cancer risk, including non-Hodgkin's lymphoma, hepatocellular carcinoma [HCC], gastric cancer, invasive cervical cancer, ulcerative colitis-associated colorectal cancer, and non-small cell lung cancer [NSCLC]. Another SNP *TNF*-857T allele is found to be associated with an increased risk of B-cell lymphoma [111]. *TNF* may promote tumor development *via* inducing secretory leukocyte protease inhibitor [SLPI], platelet-type 12-lipoxygenase [p12LOX], or activation-induced cytidine deaminase [AID]. It has been observed that *TNF* promotes tumorigenesis by inducing gene mutations and DNA instability by upregulating reactive oxygen species [ROS] production in the cells.

1.21.1. The Disease of Relevance:

• In head and neck cancer [HNC] patients, the AA haplotype of -308G/A has been associated with increased aggressiveness, worse prognosis, and short overall survival. In some HNC case, the occurrence of either CC genotype or C allele positivity is found to be unfavorable prognostic factors and patients with CC phenotype has a higher risk of early death compared to CT and TT haplotypes [112].
• In hepatic *tumorigenesis*, *TNF* promotes tumor progression by inducing NFkB-regulated anti-apoptotic proteins in hepatocytes during the pre-neoplastic phase

by driving oval cell proliferation [113].

- *TNF* upregulates the expression of angiogenic factors, including interleukin [IL]-8 and vascular endothelial growth factor [VEGF] in glioma cells. *TNF* also enhances the invasiveness of tumor cells by stimulating matrix metalloproteases [MMP-2, -3, -9, -12] [111].

- *TNF* gene has been known to stimulate tumor angiogenesis and is involved in the progression of prostate cancer from androgen-dependent to castrate-resistant prostate cancer. It also facilitates EMT and may contribute to aberrant regulation of eicosanoid pathways which results in enhanced proliferation and reduced apoptosis [114].

- In breast cancer, *TNF-α* activates the MAPK/ERK pathway, which further upregulates matrix metallopeptidase [MMP]-9, CD26, and fibroblast activation protein [FAP]-α levels and results in enhanced tumor cell invasion and metastasis in cancer tissues. Also, increased levels of lectin-like oxidized-low-density lipoprotein [oxLDL] receptor-1 [LOX-1] by *TNF* in an endothelial cell can promote the adhesion and trans-endothelial migration of cancer cells [111, 115].

- *TNF-α* in cancer cells is known to promote lymphangiogenesis and lymphatic metastasis in gallbladder carcinoma by activating the ERK1/2 or the activator protein-1/ [VEGF]-D pathway [115].

- Low concentrations of TNF protein upregulate trophoblast cell surface antigen 2 [TROP-2] protein levels in colon cancer tissues, this way, it promotes tumor cell migration and invasion. Its expression can also induce tumor cells to metastasize to the lungs *via* the ERK signaling pathway [115].

- In ovarian carcinoma, *TNF-α* enhances the metastatic potential of cancer cells by activating the JNK signaling pathway and modulating CD44 levels. Also, in some cases, *TNF* secretion is known to stimulate a constitutive network consisting of cytokines, chemokines, and angiogenic factors such as interleukin [IL]-8 and VEGF, which promote colonization of the peritoneum and neovascularization for developing tumor deposits [111].

1.22. GENE: SRSF3, SERINE AND ARGININE-RICH SPLICING FACTOR 3 LOCATION: 6p21.31-p21.2

SRSF3 protein belongs to the serine/arginine [SR]-rich family of pre-mRNA splicing factors, which constitute part of the spliceosome. *SRSF3* is a proto-oncogene and is highly expressed in several high-grade cancers such as breast tumors, oral cancer, lymphatic metastasis, ovarian, cervical, lung, stomach, colorectal, bladder, skin, thyroid, liver, and kidney cancer. The expression of the splicing factor *SRSF3* is triggered by oncogenic signaling pathways, such as the Wnt signaling pathway that drives the formation of several cancers.

1.22.1. The Disease of Relevance:

- *SRSF3* overexpression has been associated with tumor progression and a poor prognosis in breast cancer. It plays a central role in regulating the production of different splice variants within the HER2 transcript. The switch in splicing from the p100 isoform, which is an inhibitor of tumor cell proliferation and oncogene signaling to the highly tumorigenic Δ16HER2, increases malignant transformation [116].

- TAR DNA-binding protein, also named "TARDBP" [TDP43], and SRSF3 together form a splicing-regulatory complex and are known to regulate alternative splicing [AS] in triple-negative breast cancer [TNBC]. This complex co-regulate the splicing switch from the oncogenic Δ12PAR3 isoform to the PAR3-FL isoform as a downstream splicing event. Overexpression of *SRSF3* is associated with shorter survival time and poorer prognosis [117].

- *SRSF3* is overexpressed in oral squamous cell carcinoma cells [OSCC], and it regulates the expression of N-cadherin through the twist-independent pathway and promotes tumor metastasis. Elevated levels of heterogeneous nuclear ribonucleoprotein [hnRNP] L are reported to enhance relative levels of SRSF3 transcripts in OSCC cells through alternative splicing [AS]- coupled nonsense-mediated decay [NMD] mechanism. The interaction between polypyrimidine tract binding proteins [PTBPs] and the CU element within *SRSF3* exon 4′ is known to impair *SRSF3*-mediated auto-regulation, which establishes a feed-forward pathway to enhance the expression of SRSF3 in OSCC further [118, 119].

- Upregulation of *SRSF3* has been observed in colorectal cancer and imbalanced upregulation reprogrammes the splicing profiles of caspase-2 and pyruvate kinase muscle genes, which results in anti-apoptosis and aerobic glycolysis of cancer cells. SRSF3 is one of the splicing factors of the pyruvate kinase M [*PKM*] gene, and it binds specifically to exonic splicing enhancer [ESE] on *PKM* exon 10. This interaction activates the inclusion of exon 10 of the *PKM* gene to promote the expression of the oncogenic *PKM2* isoform, thus facilitating aerobic analysis and tumor formation. Expression of *SRSF3* is also stimulated by the oncogenic Wnt signaling pathway and its protein levels correlate with the extent of β- catenin/TCF4 signaling in the cancer cell. Expression profiles of *SRSF3* and /RNA binding protein 4 [RBM4] in colorectal carcinoma tissues activates the activity of the MAP4K4 protein through reprogramming the splicing profiles of MAP4K4, which is partially related to the EMT phenomenon and downstream JNK signaling. Upregulated expression of *SRSF3* with a concomitant decrease in the RBM4 protein constitutes a regulatory mechanism for *tumorigenesis*-related splicing events in colorectal cancer [118].

- In hepatocellular carcinoma, AS of kruppel-like factor 6 [*KLF6*] tumor promotes cell proliferation through *SRSF1* mediated AS of KLF6. Also, *SRSF3* loss results in aberrant splicing of genes involved in glucose and lipid metabolisms such as *HNF1α*, *ERN1*, *HMGCS1*, *DHCR7,* and *SCAP;* as a result, it leads to impaired morphological and functional differentiation of hepatocytes [120].

1.23. GENE: CD24, CD24 ZMOLECULE LOCATION: 6q21

CD24 protein function is associated with cell adhesion, proliferation, growth, invasion, metastases, and apoptosis inhibition of tumor cells. Its overexpression results in aggressive tumor formation in various malignant tumors, including B-cell lymphomas, gliomas, non-small cell lung, hepatocellular, uterine, ovarian, breast, prostate, bladder, and pancreatic carcinomas, and salivary gland cancer. The significance of *CD24* expression depends on the tumor type and its cellular localization. Cytoplasmic overexpression of the *CD24* gene has been described as a prognostic marker in prostate, colorectal, bladder, and breast cancers as well as in non-small cell lung carcinomas [NSCLCs]. *CD24* is significantly the most upregulated CSC marker, and its overexpression is associated with lymph node metastasis and poor prognosis. It has been described as one of the important cancer stem cell [CSCs] markers in ovarian, colorectal, and pancreatic cancers as well as in nasopharyngeal carcinoma.

Various mechanisms have been described through which *CD24* expression regulates tumorigenesis: firstly, the *CD24* gene encodes for a glycogen-integrated membrane protein, and this protein binds to P-selectin. As P-selectin is expressed on endothelial cells, so this interaction facilitates endothelial migration and invasion. Second, *CD24* maintains cell stemness by activating signaling factors such as Src kinases. It promotes tumor invasion and metastasis *via* activation of STAT3 transcription factor and some integrins, also, it downregulates tumor suppressor *TFP1-2* [Tissue Factor Pathway Inhibitor 2]. Activated Src promotes the STAT3 signaling pathway through its phosphorylation at tyrosine 705. Once activated, STAT3 transcripts enhance the expression of survivin, matrix metalloproteinase-7 [MMP-7], OPG and STC-1, and Cyclin D1. *CD24* also activates α3β1 and α4β1 integrins in the cancer cell. The activated integrins promote tumor invasion and metastasis by enhancing cell adhesion to an extracellular component such as fibronectin, collagens I and IV, and laminin [121].

1.23.1. The Disease of Relevance:

- In colon cancer, N-acetylglucosaminyltransferase V [GnT-V] modifies the Wnt signaling receptors such as FZD-7 and promotes *CD24* expressing colon CSCs compartment and tumor progression. *CD24* can activate the Wnt signaling pathway, so any heavy and variable glycosylation of *CD24* due to the action of

GnT- V in the cells can accelerate cancer metastasis. The association between CD24 and MAPK [mitogen-activated protein kinase] pathway proteins such as p-ERK 1/2, JNK, and p38 MAPK has been observed in colorectal cancer. Overexpression of *CD24* induces cell proliferation due to increased activity of ERK1/2, p38 MAPK Raf-1, and the upstream ERK1/2 activator. The expression of *CD24* also correlates with the signaling protein epidermal growth factor receptor [EGFR], which is overexpressed in many types of cancer cells [122].

- In gastric cancer, expression levels of *CD24* and *EGFR* are known to be positively correlated. Expression of *CD24* regulates the function and expression of *EGFR* by the activation of RhoA, a GTPase protein of the Rho family; once activated, RhoA maintains *EGFR* expression and reduces its endocytosis. *CD24* indirectly upregulates *EGFR* through the reduction of internalization and degradation of EGFR protein. Thus reduction of EGFR endocytosis prolongs ERK activation and promotes the proliferation, survival, and motility of cells [122].

- In prostate cancer, CD24 mRNA is significantly increased according to stages and is associated with positive lymph node metastasis. Also, the positive correlation between *CD24* expression and the Wnt signaling pathway facilitates tumor invasiveness and bone metastasis [123].

- In nasopharyngeal carcinoma [NPC] cells, upregulation of *CD24* triggers the expression of stem cell genes such as *Sox2*, *Oct4*, *Nanog,* and *Bmi*-1 with Wnt/β- catenin signal activation [123].

- *CD24* gene is expressed 59% in the cytoplasm and 84% in the membrane in case of invasive ovarian carcinomas. *CD24* exhibits its oncogenic function and maintains the cancer cell stemness through activation of Src kinase, which enhances STAT3 phosphorylation and also the expression of its target genes such as *cyclin-D1*, *Nanog,* and c-*myc*. Also, in tumor cells, *CD24* expression promotes EMT phenotype, which is accompanied by overexpression of Twist1, Snail, and Vimentin and downregulation of E-cadherin [121].

- CD24 mRNA overexpression in breast carcinomas is strongly correlated with *CD24* gene amplification, which is further correlated with the expression of genes important for tumor growth and metastasis, such as *CCL18*, *HDAC2,* and *DSC2*. *CD24* exhibit oncogenic activity through its regulation of the Src/STAT3 pathway. *CD24* amplification is considered the most impactful genetic alteration for the prognosis of *BRCA* [124].

1.24. GENE: VEGFA, VASCULAR ENDOTHELIAL GROWTH FACTOR A LOCATION: 6p21.1

VEGFA is a pro-angiogenic factor that induces the proliferation and migration of vascular endothelial cells and is essential for both physiological and pathological angiogenesis. *VEGFA* prevents apoptosis through the PI3-kinase/Akt pathway and it also induces expression of the anti-apoptotic proteins such as Bcl-2 and A1 in endothelial cells. Upregulation of *VEGFA* expression has been correlated with tumor stage and progression in many tumors, such as renal cell carcinomas, and ovarian cancer, and is associated with poor prognosis. Oncogenic mutations or amplification of Ras or mutations in the Wnt signaling pathway can lead to the upregulation of *VEGFA*. It is also known to stimulate stem-like cells in skin and breast cancer tissues and also in glioblastoma.

Hypoxia resulting from inhibition of angiogenesis upregulates *VEGFA* expression, contributing to aggressive disease recurrence and angiogenic therapy failure. Hypoxia stimulates hypoxia-inducible factor [HIF]- 1α-dependent *VEGFA* induction which may stimulate the aggressive hypoxia-tolerant, chemoresistant cancer stem cell [CSC] to metastatic niches.

1.24.1. The Disease of Relevance:

- In ovarian cancer, *VEGF-A* produced works through VEGF receptor 2 [VEGFR2] and stimulates activation of Src kinases which results in increased CSC. Expression of *VEGF-A* induced due to hypoxia can also result in the expansion of stem-like cancer cells. Hypoxia can permit *VEGF-A* to stimulate Src kinases and induce DNA methyltransferase [DNMT]3A above basal levels to maintain cancer cell stemness, which further leads to hyper-methylation and silencing of *miR-128-2*, and also increases expression of Bmi1 to expand CSC. This Bmi1 upregulation due to *VEGF-A* leads to enhanced expression of CSC markers such as cMyc, KLF4, and Sox2 [125].
- In breast cancer, *SOX2* expression induced by *VEGFA* results in *VEGFA*-mediated *SNAI2* induction. A putative metastasis suppressor, miR-452, is significantly downregulated as a result of the increased level of *VEGFA*. Therefore, the prognostic value of high VEGFA levels is increased by the sequential addition of high *SOX2, SNAI2,* and decreased miR-452 expression. Thus *VEGFA* stimulated EMT and CSC expansion *via SOX2* induction [126].
- In renal cell carcinoma, inactivation of mutation in the *von Hippel-Landau [VHL]* tumor suppressor gene results in high transcription of the HIF-target genes under normoxic conditions, which further results in higher expression of *VEGFA* in tumor cells [127].

1.25. GENE: LTA, LYMPHOTOXIN A LOCATION: 6p21.33

LTA protein is a cytokine produced by lymphocytes that belong to the TNF family. *LTA* signaling plays an important role in anti-tumor surveillance *via* the maturation and recruitment of NK cells. Many genetic polymorphisms in this gene have been associated with the risk of developing various types of cancer and the rate of survival according to different ethnic groups. The *LTA* gene is multifunctional because it can promote growth and cell adhesion and can also potentially favor the growth of certain tumors. The risk of cancer and the rate of survival among patients with *LTA* polymorphisms differ according to the cancer type.

1.25.1. The Disease of Relevance:

- In the *LTA* gene, *NcoI* restriction fragment length polymorphism [A252G], the 252G allele results in increased LTA mRNA and protein levels. In elderly Japanese men, *LTA* SNP C804A *LTA* [rs1041981] is known to be associated with a lower presence of cancer, particularly lung cancer. Both these polymorphisms in regards to cancer survival rates and risk of developing cancer have been reported in various types of cancers such as lung, stomach, colorectal, breast, cervix, endometrium, and bladder cancers, also in cancers like leukemia, lymphoma, and myeloma. The high bioactive allele is associated with the risk of developing cancers of the lung, colon, or rectum, non-Hodgkin lymphoma [NHL], and myeloma, whereas the low bioactive allele is associated with the risk of developing cervical and endometrial cancer [128].
- A positive correlation between the *LTA* RS909253GA genotype and gastric cancer has been observed in the Asian population [129].
- The four *LTA* polymorphisms as rs1041981:Thr26Asn; rs2239704; rs2229094: Cys13Arg; rs746868 positively correlated with a potential risk factor for cancer development. One of the functional polymorphisms, rs909253 is associated with gastric and breast cancers in Asians. All four SNPs are known to be present in high linkage disequilibrium [LD] with rs909253 polymorphism, inconsistent results of the four SNPs and cancer risk have been observed for different cancers in Asian, North American, and European populations. *LTA* polymorphisms like rs2239704 and rs2229094 are associated with a high risk of hematological malignancy and adenocarcinoma. *LTA* rs2009658 is an intronic SNP, which is located near the UTR at the 5′ ends of the *LTA* gene and is known to be associated with a high risk of breast cancer among Caucasian women aged 45–64 years [130].
- *LTA* polymorphism A252G is found to be associated with the DLBCL and follicular lymphoma, where the AG haplotype compared to the GA haplotype is associated with the risk of developing lymphoma. *LTA* 252A>G is in LD with TNF –308G>A, and a haplotype analysis could not separate the effects of risk for these 2 variants. Strong inverse associations for *LTA* C-91A SNP were observed in the case of chronic lymphocytic leukemia [CLL]/ small lymphocytic lymphoma [SLL] and follicular lymphomas. Also, a strong haplotype asso-

ciation, including the C-G-C-A-G haplotype compared to the A-A-C-G-G haplotype was observed in the case of CLL/SLL and follicular lymphoma. Thus, SNP and haplotype analysis suggests that TNF G-308A, LTA C-91A, or LTA A252G, plays a role in the etiology of NHL [131, 132].

1.26. GENE: LIN28B, LIN-28 HOMOLOG B LOCATION: 6q16.3-q21

LIN28B gene acts as an oncogene by promoting malignant transformation, including metastasis, regulating inflammation, and maintaining cancer stem cells [CSCs]. Its overexpression in primary tumors is linked to activation of the PI3-kinase/AKT pathway *via* the repression of the let-7 family of microRNAs and derepression of let-7 targets, which facilitates cellular transformation. It is overexpressed in hepatocellular carcinomas [HCC], non-small cell lung cancers [NSCLC], breast cancers, ovarian cancers and melanoma, lymphoma, and neuroblastoma. *LIN28B* in many cancers is considered the more relevant homolog in *tumorigenesis*. It also plays essential role in the formation of CSCs and contributes to tumor aggressiveness and metastasis.

1.26.1. The Disease of Relevance:

- In colon cancer, *LIN28B* expression induces pluripotency when expressed in somatic fibroblasts in conjunction with *OCT4, SOX2*, and *KLF4. LIN28B* expression is upregulated as the consequence of adenomatous polyposis coli [APC] mutations, which further results in sustained β-catenin stabilization and upregulation of the Wnt pathway targets such as the oncogenic transcription factor *c-myc*. Its overexpression is associated with reduced patient survival and increased probability of tumor recurrence. The colonic stem cell markers *LGR5* and *PROM1* are also upregulated in response to increased expression of *LIN28B*. In Wilm's tumor, the c-myc binding site on the LIN28B promoter is frequently demethylated [133, 134].
- Both the LIN28B protein and mRNA are highly expressed in ovarian cancer. The elevated level of *LIN28B* is significantly associated with the risk of disease progression and death in cancer patients. Also, the *LIN28B* polymorphism rs12194974 [G>A] in the promoter region, has been known to influence susceptibility to ovarian cancer [135].
- *LIN28B* is one of the Cancer-testis [CT] genes that are highly expressed in lung adenocarcinoma and is known to drive the development and metastasis of lung adenocarcinoma. Activation of *LIN28B* can promote the proliferation and metastasis of tumor cells and can also influence the cell cycle, DNA damage repair, and genome instability. *LIN28B-AS1*, a let-7-independent Cis-regulator of LIN28B, alters the stability of LIN28B mRNA by directly interacting with

another CT protein IGF2BP1 but not with LIN28B and this together constitutes a novel regulation network. As a result, *LIN28B* is identified as an "epi-driver" of lung adenocarcinoma [136].

- In pancreatic cancer, loss of *SIRT6* results in hyperacetylation of H3K9 and H3K5 at the promoter region of *LIN28B*; this leads to reactivation of *LIN28B* in tumor cells. As a result, a more permissive chromatin state is created that allows the *Myc* transcription factor to drive its expression and thus promote an aggressive form of pancreatic cancer. Reactivation of *LIN28B* also upregulates the expression of oncofetal RNA binding proteins like Igf2bp1 and Igf2bp3, which have been associated with poorly differentiated pancreatic cancer. Expression of Igf2bps increases progressively with tumor stage and high levels of Igf2bps correlate with increased metastasis and extremely poor survival outcome. Pancreatic stellate cells [PSCs] can enhance the CSCs-like phenotypes in pancreatic cancer cells through the induction of *ABCG2, Nestin,* and *LIN28* [134, 137].

- In prostate cancer, the CSCs acquire EMT phenotype *via* stimulation of SOX2, NANOG, OCT, LIN28B, or NOTCH1 expression [134].

1.27. GENE: LTB, LYMPHOTOXIN BETA LOCATION: 6p21.33

LTB protein is a type II membrane protein of the TNF family. LTB is an inducer of the inflammatory response system and is involved in the normal development of lymphoid tissue. *LTB* is highly expressed in breast, oropharynx, tonsil cancers, and hepatocellular carcinoma.

1.27.1. The Disease of Relevance:

- A three-gene set, *LTB,* together with *IL7* and *CXCL13*, are found to be upregulated in human oral cancer-associated tertiary lymphoid structures [TLSs]. These genes are known to regulate the recirculation of lymphocytes and dendritic cells homing into lymphoid structures and thus exert essential roles in the development and maintenance of TLSs [138].

- In high endothelial venules [HEVs] high breast cancer, *LTA* and *LTB* both are highly expressed, and dendritic cells [DCs] are the major producers of the membrane-associated LTB [LTA1B2] within the breast tumor micro-environment. Therefore, DCS is known to contribute to the formation of HEVs in breast tumors through LTB protein production [139].

- *LTB*/*LTBR* promotes activation of the alternative NIK-IKKa-RELB/NF-κB2 pathway, to enhance MET-mediated cell migration in Head and neck squamous cell carcinoma [HNSCC]. *LTBR* is overexpressed in the larynx or oral cavity HNSCC whereas *LTB* is overexpressed in oropharynx and tonsil cancers. So overexpression of *LTB* promotes HNSCC migration and metastasis to local lymph nodes [140].

1.28. GENE: LATS1, LARGE TUMOR SUPPRESSOR KINASE 1 LOCATION: 6q25.1

LATS1 protein is a putative serine/threonine kinase of the AGC kinase family. *LATS1* plays a role as a tumor suppressor, and its down-regulation has been observed in many several human cancers. Loss of *LATS1* results in the development of soft-tissue derived tumors such as sarcomas and astrocytomas, ovarian stromal cell tumors, breast and cervical cancers, and head and neck squamous cell carcinoma [HNSCC]. It is involved in tumor development by either inducing apoptosis or negatively regulating cell proliferation, genetic stability, cell migration, and metastasis. *LATS1* is identified as a central player of the tumor suppressor pathway Hippo signaling pathway in *Drosophila*. Tumor suppressors Mst 1/2, a mammalian homolog of the *Drosophila* Hippo pathway, phosphorylates and activates *LATS1* and its homolog *LATS2*, which subsequently phosphorylates and inhibits oncogene *YAP* and *TAZ* by preventing them from translocating to the nucleus. E3 ubiquitin ligase Itch, a member of the NEDD4-like ubiquitin ligase family, negatively regulates *LATS1* gene expression [141]. Loss of heterozygosity [LOH] at this locus has been reported in ovarian, cervical, and breast cancers [142].

1.28.1. The Disease of Relevance:

- In breast cancer, *WWP1* [WW domain containing E3 ubiquitin-protein ligase 1] regulates tumor cell proliferation by downregulating *LATS1*. *WWP1* down-regulates *LATS1* tumor suppressor activity through ubiquitination and degradation in cancer tissues. Aberrant methylation of the promoter region of LATS1 has been found in breast cancers [141].
- Loss of *LATS1* activity due to hypermethylation of CpG islands in the promoter region has decreased expression of *LATS1* in colorectal, breast, and ovarian cancers and soft-tissue sarcomas [143].

1.29. GENE: IL17A, INTERLEUKIN 17A LOCATION: 6p12.2

IL17A protein is a pro-inflammatory cytokine produced by activated T cells. This cytokine regulates the activities of NF-kB and mitogen-activated protein kinases. This cytokine can stimulate the expression of *IL6* and *cyclooxygenase-2 [PTGS2/COX-2]*, as well as enhance nitric oxide production [NO]. Association between T helper 17 [Th17] cells and the *IL17A* gene has been found in various human tumors. Overexpression of *IL17A* in tumor cells promotes angiogenesis, cell proliferation, and invasiveness and inhibits apoptosis in several human cancers, including prostate, breast, ovarian, colorectal, and gastric cancer.

1.29.1. The Disease of Relevance:

- *IL17A* has a pro-angiogenic role in the occurrence of lung adenocarcinoma. Overexpression of IL17A upregulates the expression of CXCL1, CXCL5, CXCL6, and CXCL8, which further promotes tumor-associated angiogenesis and may favor the secretion of VEGF [144].
- *IL17A* is highly expressed in breast cancer cells and is associated with poor prognosis. The tumor cells and tumor-associated fibroblasts secrete factors and generate a pro-inflammatory cytokine environment that leads to the recruitment of Th17 cells, a distinct lineage of CD4+ effector cells, in the tumor micro-environment. *IL17A activates the ERK kinases in breast cancer cells and promotes cell proliferation, invasion,* and resistance to chemotherapy [145].
- *IL17A* polymorphism G197A [rs2275913 G > A] is associated with suscep-tibility to gastric *tumorigenesis,* and ulcerative colitis. *IL17A* rs2275913 AA homozygote is associated with an increased risk of developing intestinal and diffuse types of gastric cancer [146].
- Overexpression of *IL17A* in non-small cell lung cancer [NSCLC] induces the production of, angiogenic factor *CXCL8*, which is involved in the tumor-associated angiogenic activity of NSCLC [147].
- *IL17A* stimulates activation of all three MAPK genes, *i.e., ERK, p38*, and *JNK*; downstream transcription factors AP-1 and p65 NFKB, and andotesc *IL8* secretion in gastric cancer cells. It directly induces tumor cell proliferation, suppresses apopgastric cancer cell apoptosis, promotes cell invasion, and reduces expression of pro-tumor factors IL6 and MMP13, thereby participating in protumor activities [148].

1.30.   GENE 30: SOX4, SRY-BOX TRANSCRIPTION FACTOR 4 LOCATION: 6p22.3

Overexpression of *SOX4* is associated with poor prognosis and is considered a pan-cancer prognostic marker. Overexpression of the *SOX4* gene as a conse-quence of amplificati, ovarian, bladderian cancers, bladder cancers [BLCA], triple-negative breast cancers [TNBC], and metastatic prostate cancer. *SOX4* mRNA is overexpressed in leukemias, melanomas, glioblastomas, medullo-blastomas, and prostate, bladder, lung, and breast cancers. *SOX4* plays a crucial role in tumor development and progression *via* various mechanisms: [i] directly regulating the expression, transcription, and/or epigenetic reprogramming of numerous genes involved in EMT like enhancer of *zeste homolog 2 [EZH2], E-cadherin [CDH1], N-cadherin [CDH2], vimentin [VIM]* and *TGFB*; [ii] targeting gene networks involved in miRNA processing and posttranscriptional regulation; [iii] enhancing proliferative signals in tumors and activating the signal transduction phosphatidylinositol-3 kinase [PI3K]/Akt pathway by targeting growth factor receptors such as epidermal growth factor receptor [EGFR] and fibroblast growth factor receptor-like 1 [FGFRL1], and insulin-like growth factor 2 receptor [IGF2R]; [iv] interacting with and activating developmental pathways like the Wnt, Notch, and Hedgehog pathways; and [v] inhibiting differentiation through the repression of transcription factors and induction of homeobox [HOX] gene expression [149].

1.30.1. The Disease of Relevance:

- In breast cancer, *SOX4* promotes tumorigenesis by inducing the transcription of the EMT regulators like *Snail, ZEB*, and *TWIST* through intermediate protein or epigenetic modifications. Ectopic expression of *SOX4* causes increases in the expression of a transmembrane protein, TMEM2, which can mediate metastatic migration and invasion of cancer cells. Likewise, androgen receptor negatively induced lncRNA [ARNILA] acts as a competing endogenous RNA [ceRNA] for miR204 to upregulate *SOX4* expression; as a result, stimulating EMT and promoting invasion and metastasis in TNBC. Its expression also regulates TGFβ-mediated induction of a subset of SMAD3/SOX4-co-bound genes that regulate migration and extracellular matrix-associated processes in claudin-low breast cancer cells [150].
- In lung cancer, *SOX4* exhibits oncogenic properties by essentially increasing the transforming ability of the weakly oncogenic RHOA-Q63 L mutation. It also promotes cell proliferation through Krüppel-like factor 5 [KLF5]-mediated tumorigenesis [150].
- In myeloid leukemias, *SOX4* promotes tumorigenesis by cooperating with myocyte-specific enhancer factor 2C [Mef2c] and cAMP response element-binding [CREB] protein. *SOX4* is overexpressed due to the inactivation of the transcription factor CCAAT/enhancer-binding proteins [C/EBPα]. It leads to the development of leukemia with a distinct acute myeloid leukemia [AML] leukemia-initiating cells [LICs] phenotype. In acute lymphoblastic leukemia [ALL], *SOX4* activates PI3K/AKT and MAPK signaling in ALL cells [150].
- In prostate cancer, *SOX4* expression stimulates anchorage-independent growth of prostate epithelial cells. Removal of *SOX4* reduces activation of both AKT and β- catenin, resulting in an attenuated invasive phenotype, and arresting cancer progression at the high-grade prostatic intraepithelial neoplasia [HGPIN] precancerous stage. *SOX4* expression induced by phosphatase and tensin homolog due to the consequence of the activation of PI3K-AKT-mTOR signaling, suggests a positive feedback loop between *SOX4* and PI3K-AK--mTOR activity. In prostate cancer, 282 high-confidence direct *SOX4* target genes including *DICER, EGFR, FOXA1, NKX3*-1, and plenty of regulators of pivotal cancer signaling networks of differentiation, cell survival, and apoptosis

including the Wnt [*e.g.*, FZD4, FZD5, FZD8] and PI3K pathways [*e.g.*, PIK3R1, PIK3R4] are identified. *SOX4* may play a crucial role at the intersection of PI3K and Wnt signaling in metastatic prostate cancer [150].

- *SOX4* regulates the transcriptional activity of p53 and results in the inhibition of p53- mediated apoptosis in hepatocellular carcinoma [HCC]. STAT3 signaling induces the expression of lncRNA HOXD-AS1, thereby inhibiting miR-130a-3p-mediated SOX4 repression and enhancing metastasis [150].
- In pancreatic cancer, SOX4 induces tumorigenesis by cooperating with *KLF5* which prevents *SOX4*-induced apoptosis [150].

1.31. GENE: ESR1; ESTROGEN RECEPTOR 1, ER LOCATION: 6q25.1-q 25.2

ESR1 gene encodes an estrogen receptor, a ligand-activated transcription factor composed of several essential domains important for hormone binding, DNA binding, and transcription activation. The ER-ligand complex is essential in various physiological and pathological processes such as tumorigenesis and tumor progression. Estrogen receptors are associated with breast cancer and endometrial cancer, and downregulation of *ESR1* expression has been associated with cancers such as prostate, breast, lung, colorectal, and hematopoietic cancers.

1.31.1. The Disease of Relevance:

- Two in-frame *ESR1* fusions that are ESR1-e6>DAB2 and ESR1-e6>GYG1, are identified in metastatic ER⁺ breast cancer. These fusion genes are known to follow the same pattern that is, *ESR1* exon 6 in-frame fusions with 3′ partners provided by inter-chromosomal translocation [151].
- A functional SNP rs2295190 is a known missense SNP located 19kb downstream of *ESR1* in the COOH terminus region of *SYNE1*, and its G to T change results in a conservative amino acid substitution from leucine to methionine. The T allele of this SNP has been correlated with increased invasive ovarian cancer risk. Another SNP associated with breast cancer risk is rs2046210, which is located nearly 296 kb away from SNP [rs2295190] and is not in LD with SNP rs2295190 [152].
- Several *ESR1* gene polymorphisms such as *ESR1* PvuII [rs2234693 T>C], XbaI [rs9340799 A>G] and T594T [rs2228480 G>A] polymorphisms and have been reported to be significantly associated with the development of cancer. These SNPs play an important role in tumorigenesis, development, and prognosis of cancers such as colorectal, prostate, breast, and endometrial cancer. PvuII [T>C] has been associated with an increased risk of hepatocellular carcinoma [HCC] and prostate cancer. XbaI [A>G] has been associated with increased cancer of prostate cancer. T594T [G>A] has a significant association with cancer risk in

Asian populations [153].

- DNA Methylation of CpG island in the promoter region and its first exon has been reported in breast, prostate, lung, and colorectum cancers. Reduction in the levels of *ESR1* due to promoter methylation by the action on *ESR1* negative regulator *EZH2* has been known to increase invasiveness in cervical cancer [154].

- Loss or down-regulation of *ESR1* expression due to methylation of *ESR1* promoter has been associated with prostate cancer and ESR1 methylation increases significantly with age, and methylation spreads predominantly along the CpG island during aging [155].

- Overexpression of the *ESR1* gene as a consequence of amplification and copy number is found in ER+ breast cancers. *ESR1* amplifications are present in the early stage and are known to drive cancer progression in breast cancers such as precancerous ductal and lobular carcinoma *in situ* [DCIS and LCIS]. Amino acid substitution of tyrosine at position 537 to serine [Y537N] within the ligand-binding domain [LBD] of ESR1 and aspartate at position 538 to glutamate [D538G], has been identified in metastatic breast cancer. These point mutations result in constitutive hormone-independent transcriptional activation of *ESR1* and enhance cell proliferation. Expression of two ESR1 fusion transcripts involving the first two non-coding exons of *ESR1* fused to various C-termini sequences from the coiled-coil domain containing 170 genes, *i.e.*, *CCDC170* [ESR1-e2>CCDC170] and another fusion containing the first 6 exons of *ESR1* fused to *AKAP12, i.e.*, [ESR1- e6>AKAP12] in breast tumors results in enhanced growth. The translocation produced as a result of the in-frame *ESR1* fusion gene consisting of exons 1-6 of *ESR1* [ESR1-e6] and the C-terminus of the Hippo pathway co-activator gene, *YAP1* [ESR1-e6>YAP1] and another fusion gene involving the protocadherin 11 X-linked gene, *PCDH11X* [ESR1-e6>PCDH11X] have been found in patients with endocrine refractory and metastatic ER+ breast cancer. Upregulation of both fusion genes induces cell motility and increases lung metastatic frequency, thus enhancing EMT. Additional in-frame *ESR1* translocations with diverse partner genes, including ESR1-e6>DAB2, ESR1-e6>GYG1, and ESR1-e6>SOX9 have been identified, and among these ESR1-e6>DAB2 and ESR1-e6>GYG1 fusions can drive hormone-independent activation [156].

1.32. Gene: CDKN1A, Cyclin Dependent Kinase Inhibitor 1A, P21 Location: 6p21.2

CDKN1A, also known as *p21,* encodes for a potent cyclin-dependent kinase [Cdk] inhibitor [CKI] and functions as a regulator of cell cycle progression at the G1 phase, ensuring genomic stability. Its expression is mainly transcriptionally controlled by the tumor suppressor protein p53, through which this protein mediates the p53- dependent cell cycle G1 phase arrest in response to a variety of stress stimuli. It acts either as a tumor suppressor or as an oncogene, depending largely on the cellular context, its subcellular localization, and posttranslational modifications [157, 158]. Low concentrations of *CDKN1A* are known to promote proliferation through the assembly and activation of cyclin D/Cdk4 or Cdk6 complexes in cancer cells. Its oncogenic potential is correlated to its cytoplasmic localization, promoting cell cycle progression, favoring cell migration, and inhibiting cell apoptosis also, upregulated expression of *p21/CDKN1A* leads to escaping from senescent cell arrest. It plays a key role in the differentiation of several normal or malignant cells and tissues; however, its impact depends on the cell type and the stage of differentiation. Its overexpression leading to its oncogenic activity, is found in a variety of human cancers, including breast cancer, renal cell carcinoma, testicular cancer, hepatocellular carcinoma, multiple myeloma, gliomas, prostate cancer, cervical carcinoma, ovarian cancer, acute myeloid cancer, oesophageal squamous cell carcinoma, and soft tissue sarcomas [157].

1.32.1. The Disease of Relevance:

• The presence of mutant p53 or repression of *p21 via* long non-coding RNA [lncRNA] small nucleolar RNA host gene 20 [*SNHG20*] in non-small lung cell cancer [NSCLC] results in increased cell invasiveness. Cytoplasmic *p21* promotes cell migration and invasion in gastric cancer. Epigenetic silencing has been reported in NSCLC, prostate cancer, cholangiocarcinoma, high-grade breast cancer, and acute lymphoblastic leukemia [ALL]. Various *p21* SNPs have been observed to influence the risk of developing oesophageal, colorectal, and estrogen-related cancer and are also associated with a higher risk of secondary primary malignancies in head and neck carcinoma [HNC] [157].

• In gastric cancer, lncRNA HOXA-AS2 promotes cancer cells proliferation by epigenetically silencing *CDKN1A* expression and lncRNA PANDAR decreases *CDKN1A* gene transcription by competitively binding to the p53 protein, acting as a p53-response element decoy [159, 160].

• In colorectal cancer, lncRNA CRNDE [Colorectal Neoplasia Differentially Expressed] promotes cell proliferation, mediated by the regulation of *DUSP5* and *CDKN1A* expression by binding to EZH2 [159].

• *CDKN1A* has been identified as a direct target of miR-93, and so upregulation of miR-93 enhances cell proliferation, and migration, inhibits apoptosis and increases drug resistance *via* regulating *CDKN1A* expression in nasopharyngeal carcinoma, hepatocellular carcinoma [HCC], colorectal carcinoma and osteo-sarcoma as well as cervical cancer [161].

• Upregulation of miR-96 may contribute to aggressive malignancy partly through suppressing CDKN1A protein expression in bladder cancer cells [162].

1.33. GENE: TRIM27. TRIPARTITE MOT6IF CONTAINING 27 LOCATION: 6p22.1

TRIM27 acts as an oncogene in various human cancers, including ovarian cancer, endometrial cancer, breast cancer, colon cancer, lung cancer, colitis-associated cancer, salivary gland intraductal carcinoma, uterus cancer, and prostate cancer. It plays an important role in promoting anticancer drug resistance in specific tumors. [163] *TRIM27* gene is also known to be involved in oncogenic rearrangements with the *RET* proto-oncogene. It is a multifunctional protein involved in cell proliferation, transcriptional repression, negative regulation of NF-κB activation, apoptosis, and innate immune response [164] and could act as a potential prognostic indicator in some cancers.

1.31.1. The Disease of Relevance:

- *TRIM27* expression is upregulated and can predict deeper invasion, increased lymph node metastasis, high tumor stage, and increased distant metastasis in colorectal carcinoma [CRC] cells. Knockdown of *TRIM27* has resulted in cell cycle arrest and apoptosis by upregulating the expression of p-p38 and downregulating the expression of p-AKT in ovarian cancer, impaired cancer cell migration and invasion with concomitant decreases in levels of integrin b1 and a2 in endometrial cancer. In lung cancer, *TRIM27* has been known to be involved in mutated EFGR signaling [163].
- *TRIM27* is upregulated in esophageal carcinoma [ESCC] tissues and acts as a pro-proliferation factor. Overexpression of *TRIM27* in ESCC cells promotes tumorigenesis by enhancing cell proliferation and inhibiting cell apoptosis. *TRIM27* inhibits apoptosis of ESCC cells *via* enhancing the ubiquitination of PTEN, which subsequently promotes the activity of the PI3/AKT signaling pathway in ESCC cells [165].
- Overexpression of *TRIM27* in breast carcinomas has been associated with epidermal growth factor receptor II [ERBB2] protein expression and ERBB2 gene amplification in breast cancer cells. *TRIM27* is highly expressed in ovarian serous carcinoma cells [OSCC], and high expression is significantly related to the International Federation of Obstetrics and Gynecology [FIGO] stage of ovarian serous carcinoma patients [166].
- *TRIM27* is highly expressed in lung cancer and is known to play an important role in cancer prognosis. RET rearrangements are known to be involved in non-small cell lung carcinoma [NSCLC]. DNA methylation at the CpG site, cg05293407, located at the 200 kb transcription start site region of *TRIM27,* results in upregulated gene expression in tumor tissues and is considered an

exclusive biomarker of early-stage lung squamous cell carcinoma [LSCC] prognosis [167].

1.34. GENE: PLAGL1; PLAG1 LIKE ZINC FINGER 1 LOCATION: 6q24.2

PLAGL1 is considered a tumor suppressor gene because it shares its activity with p53 and controls cell cycle progression by regulating *p21* expression. Down-regulation of *PLAGL1* due to loss of heterozygosity [LOH] at the *PLAGL1* locus or hypermethylation of the P1 promoter of the *PLAGL1* gene is frequently observed in pheochromocytoma, ovarian cancer, breast cancer, prostate cancer, colon cancer, gastric cancer, pituitary adenomas like non-functioning pituitary adenomas, hepatocellular carcinoma [HCC], hemangioblastoma, head and neck squamous cell carcinoma [HNSCC], diffused large B-cell lymphoma and basal cell carcinoma [168 - 170]. Molecular mechanisms through which it contributes to tumorigenesis revealed that functional alterations are more frequent than structural alterations [168].

1.34.1. The Disease of Relevance:

- *PLAGL1* is involved in the pathology of Beckwith-Wiedemann Syndrome [BWS], and patients with BWS are susceptible to developing cancer, mostly hepatoblastoma and Wilms' tumor [168].
- In HCC, low and steady levels of PLAGL1 protein promote cell proliferation *via* regulating the transcription of the *PRARy* gene [169].
- *PLAGL1* is also found to have an oncogenic function in some cancers, such as clear cell renal cell carcinoma [ccRCC], and embryonal cancer, where the expression of *PLAGL1* is up-regulated. The increased PLAGL1 protein level in ccRCC tissue is positively correlated with the presence of distant metastases and worse patient outcomes and can serve as a potential prognostic marker [171].
- The mechanism behind the reduced level of *PLAG1* in colorectal cancer could be either transcriptional silencing regulated by epigenetic processes such as methylation of CpG islands and histone deacetylation or downregulation *via* EGFR, which is known to promote tumor growth. It has also been observed that the protein encoded by the *PLAGL1* gene may act as a regulator of nuclear receptor activity, including the glucocorticoid receptor, whose expression in colorectal cancer correlated with the expression of cell cycle-related molecules, such as Rb protein and p16 [170].
- In diffuse B-cell lymphoma [DLBCL], loss or de novo methylation of the active, paternal allele leads to downregulation of *PLAGL1* expression in tumor cells, also the de novo hypermethylation or hypomethylation at the CpG island of the gene suggests an epigenetic modification of the promoter occurs in DLBCL [172].

1.35. GENE: NOTCH4; NOTCH RECEPTOR 4 LOCATION: 6p21.32

Notch4, a family member of the Notch signaling pathway, has important roles in cellular developmental pathways, including proliferation, differentiation, and apoptosis. Overexpression of *Notch4* has been observed in various types of cancer, including colon, breast, pancreatic, cervical, prostate cancer, gastric cancer, large-cell and Hodgkin lymphomas, renal carcinoma, adenoid cystic carcinoma, and lung cancer. Notch4, also known as EMT-trigger, induces metastasis in breast cancer, prostate cancer, melanoma cells, and head and neck squamous cell carcinoma [HNSCC].

1.35.1. The Disease of Relevance:

- The *NOTCH4* expression is significantly upregulated in colorectal cancer tissues and is associated with advanced N stage, distant metastases, and the presence of lymphovascular invasion and thus can be used as a potential new biomarker [173].
- *Notch4* expression is highly expressed in invasive ductal carcinoma, invasive lobular carcinoma, Her-2-overexpressing breast cancer, and triple-negative breast cancer [TNBC]. Aberrant mutations in the *Notch4* gene may inhibit the differentiation of mammary stem cells and enhance mammary epithelial cell proliferation, thus leading to the occurrence of breast cancer. *Notch4* expression is inversely associated with prognostic factors such as small tumor size, less lymph node involvement, and positive p53 expression. Overexpression of *Notch4* induces EMT by decreasing the level of E-cadherin [174].
- *Notch-4* is highly expressed in prostate cancer cells and can affect invasion and metastasis by regulating the expression of EMT markers such as E-cadherin, vimentin, and N-cadherin and by also regulating NF-κB pathway activity [175].
- In HNSCC, the Notch4-Hey1 pathway is specifically upregulated and induces EMT by decreasing E-cadherin expression and increasing *vimentin, fibronectin, TWIST1*, and *SOX2* expression. *NOTCH4* is also associated with proliferation, chemo-resistance, apoptosis inhibition, and cell-cycle alteration in HNSCC [176].
- Overexpression of the Notch4 signaling pathway may promote the initiation and progression of gastric tumor cells partly by inducing Wnt1/β-catenin signaling and by upregulating c-Myc and cyclin D1 expressions in gastric tumor cells. *Notch4* and Wnt1/β-catenin activation result in a decreased level of E-cadherin [177].

1.36. GENE: NEDD9; NEURAL PRECURSOR CELL EXPRESSED, DEVELOPMENTALLY DOWN-REGULATED 9 LOCATION: 6p24.2

NEDD9 protein is a non-catalytic scaffolding protein and has been reported to have a role in cancer metastasis. Its function is to assemble various complexes involving oncogenic kinases, including focal adhesion kinase [FAK], ABL, SRC, Aurora-A [AURKA], and others, and this is how it regulates the magnitude and duration of cell signaling cascades that are important for tumorigenesis and metastases. So any alteration in the *NEDD9* expression can predict poor outcomes, metastatic potential, and resistance to chemotherapy. Many studies have stated that neither overexpression nor gene loss of *NEDD9* induces tumorigenesis in the absence of other driver lesions. *NEDD9* overexpression, as an oncogenic signaling abnormality, has been observed in several cancers, including breast, lung, colon, liver, pancreatic, ovarian, prostate, cervical, and kidney cancer, gastrointestinal stromal tumors, melanoma, glioblastoma, neuroblastoma. Activation of chemokine receptors causes *NEDD9* phosphorylation by ABL and ABL2 kinases. Ligation of beta-integrin signaling causes NEDD9 tyrosine phosphorylation by FAK and by the FAK-related kinase RAFTK, and subsequently phosphorylation by SRC kinases. Ligation of either β1 integrin or the B-cell receptor promotes interaction of phosphorylated NEDD9 with an SH2- domain-containing adaptor protein CRKL [cellular regulator of kinase like], commonly deregulated in human malignancies and associated with tumor progression [178].

1.36.1. Disease if Relevance:

• Overexpression of *NEDD9* promotes the development, progression, and metastasis of breast cancer through various mechanisms that include activating proteins of the focal adhesion complex, *i.e.*, FAK and SRC, mediating effects of TGFβ, increasing the expression and activity of matrix metalloproteases [MMPs], regulating trafficking and enzymatic recovery of MMPs and integrins, increasing the synthesis of the tumor-associated glycocalyx, and downregulating E-cadherin. It can induce EMT by increasing EMT-inducing transcription factors expressions such as *SNAIL* and *SLUG*, which further binds and repress the E-cadherin promoter. Also, in some tumor cells, *NEDD9* induces EMT through SRC to promote the removal of E-cadherin [178, 179].

• *NEDD9* is upregulated in LKB1 [tumor suppressor gene]-deficient lung cancer cells. LKB1 negatively regulates the transcription of *NEDD9* by promoting cytosolic translocation of the NEDD9 transcriptional co-activator *CRTC1* from the nucleus. It induces EMT by regulating EMT markers or *via* FAK activation [178].

• *NEDD9* overexpression has been associated with metastatic potential in melanoma. The gain of chromosome 6p, containing the *NEDD9* gene, is frequently observed in metastatic melanomas, but not in primary melanomas. Elevated expression of *NEDD9* activates FAK to promote cell invasion and metastasis. Also, it has been observed that *NEDD9* forms complexes with DOCK3 and regulates the activation of Rac, and promote the mesenchymal-type movement of melanoma cells [178].

- Expression of *NEDD9* in colorectal cancer mediates hypoxia-induced migration of cancer cells. In some colorectal cancer, inflammatory mediator prostaglandin E has been known to induce overexpression of *NEDD9* and subsequent cell proliferation, cell cycle progression, and tumor growth, which are mediated by an activating interaction of *NEDD9* with the mitotic kinase AURKA. Also, NEDD9 has been considered a novel Wnt signaling target in colorectal cancer [178 - 180].
- In hepatocellular carcinoma [HCC] cells, *forkhead box C1 [FOXC1]* regulates the overexpression of *NEDD9* and induces EMT and cell migration, thus promoting metastases. In prostate cancer cells, stable overexpression of *NEDD9* promotes metastases by inducing TGFβ signaling [178, 179].
- *NEDD9* is overexpressed in cervical cancer cells and promotes cell migration and invasions, mostly *via* regulating tyrosine dephosphorylation of FAK and SRC and the expression of EMT-associated protein E-cadherin [179].
- In gastric cancer, *NEDD9* is overexpressed, and its expression is known to be induced by hypoxia in cancer cells. Hypoxia results in increased expression of *NEDD9,* and that further increases its interaction with MICAL1 [Cas L 1]. MICAL1 is regulated by *NEDD9,* which facilitates hypoxia-induced gastric cancer cell migration *via* a Rac1-dependent manner. Also, *NEDD9* expression is positively correlated with the expression of EMT marker proteins such as vimentin and Zeb and negatively correlated to E-cadherin [180].

1.37. GENE: MAPK14; MITOGEN ACTIVATED PROTEIN KINASE 14; P38 LOCATION: 6p21.31

MAPK14 [also known as p38α] is involved in a wide variety of cellular processes such as proliferation, differentiation, transcription regulation, and development. *MAPK14* is highly expressed in several human cancers, such as breast cancer, ovarian serous adenocarcinoma, and gastric cancer can promote tumorigenesis. However, *MAPK14* is known to play a dual role it can promote the occurrence and progression of breast cancer by activating its downstream target genes, and can also act as a tumor suppressor in some malignancies, such as liver, colon, and lung cancer [181]. Therefore, the effect of MAPK14 activity seems to depend on cell-specific differences [182]. Phosphorylated MAPK14 [P-MAPK14, Thr180, and Tyr182] has been observed to stimulate the progression or recurrence of lung, pancreatic, and colon cancers.

1.37.1. The Disease of Relevance:

- Phosphorylated MAPK14 and cell division cycle 25B [CDC25B] are highly expressed in clear cell renal cell carcinoma [ccRCC]. *MAPK14* promotes tumor cell proliferation and migration in cancer cells probably by influencing the expression stability of the CDC25B protein [181].

- In lung cancer, *MAPK14* acts as a tumor suppressor gene, and so inactivation of *MAPK14* results in immature and hyper-proliferative lung epithelium [182].

- In triple-negative breast cancer [TNBC], TGF-β induces *MAPK14*, which further phosphorylates nuclear receptor 4A1 [NR4A1], resulting in nuclear export of the receptor. This interaction results in the induction of EMT and induction of β- catenin in TNBC cells [183]. *MAPK14* is highly expressed in breast cancer and is associated with poor prognosis, lymph node metastasis, and tamoxifen resistance in breast cancer patients [184].

- The *MAPK14* SNP rs851023 is significantly associated with prostate cancer risk. In men, compared to two copies of allele A, the presence of one or two copies of allele G is associated with decreased risks of overall prostate cancer [185].

- Downregulation of *MAPK14* promotes colon tumor progression by increasing proliferation. Reducing mucus-producing goblet cells affect epithelial barrier function by affecting the tight junction assembly and thus makes it more susceptible to colitis-associated colon tumorigenesis [184].

- Enhanced levels of phosphorylated MAPK14 have been observed in high-grade human pancreatic cancers and are correlated with reduced expression of the [dual-specificity [Thr/Tyr] phosphatases] *DUSP1*. Also, reduced levels of *MAPK14* are inversely associated with relapse probability in colorectal tumor patients. Increased levels of MAPK14 phosphorylation have been reported in lung tumors, indicating its role in tumorigenesis [184].

1.38. GENE: GSTA1; GLUTATHIONE S-TRANSFERASE ALPHA 1 LOCATION: 6p12.2

GSTA1 has been shown to have both stimulatory and inhibitory effects on tumorigenesis. *GSTA1* gene is expressed in most cells at moderate levels and has been shown to possess both GST and glutathione peroxidase activity protecting against oxidative stress. *GSTA1* is overexpressed in various cancers such as colon cancer, lung cancer, bladder cancer, gastric cancer, breast cancer, and clear cell renal cell carcinoma.

1.38.1. The Disease of Relevance:

- In the Japanese population, polymorphism in *GSTA1* in the 5′-regulatory region of the gene involving the substitution of C to T at −69 nucleotides is known to reduce the expression of the *GSTA1* gene and is associated with increased risk of hepatocellular carcinoma and oral cancer [186].
- *GSTA1* is highly expressed in lung cancer and is known to enhance tumor cell proliferation. It promotes lung cancer cell invasion and adhesion and also mediates the effect of nicotine on lung cancer cell metastasis by promoting EMT [187].
- The genetic polymorphism of *GSTA1* is denoted by two alleles, *GSTA1*A* and *GSTA1*B*. These alleles differ in their promoter regions based on three linked single nucleotide substitutions at positions −567, −69, and −52. Specifically, the − 52 substitutions are known to increase promoter activity in *GSTA1*A*, thus making it more highly expressed. These *GSTA1* polymorphisms have been associated with colorectal, prostate, breast, and bladder cancer. The *GSTA1* BB genotype is associated with an increased risk for colorectal cancer in Caucasians [188, 189].
- In hepatocellular carcinoma [HCC], the *GSTA1* gene acts as a tumor suppressor and controls cell proliferation and metastasis. It suppresses tumorigenesis by regulating Liver kinase B1 [LKB1]/ an upstream gene of adenylate-activated protein kinase [AMPK]/mTOR directly or indirectly in HCC tissues [190].
- Expression of GSTA1 mRNA is down-regulated in HCC tissues and is considered a marker of advanced and highly aggressive cancers. *GSTA1* SNP rs3957357C>T has been reported to be a functional SNP that affects the transcriptional activity of its gene in the liver and is correlated to the risk of HCC occurrence among European individuals. Patients with two copies of T alleles are associated with reduced transcriptional activity, resulting in low expression of *GSTA1* in hepatic tissues, thereby increasing the risk of occurrence of developing HCC. *GSTA1* SNP rs3957357T is also found to be associated with a higher risk of developing several malignant cancers, such as colorectal, and breast cancer [191].
- Genetic polymorphism in *GSTA1* involving the substitution of C to T at -69 in the promoter region of the GSTA1 gene results in decreased expression in oral cancer tissues. Patients with at least 1 variant G allele are considered to have a higher susceptibility to oral cancer, whereas the presence of the T allele may prevent tumor size progression of oral cancer in the Taiwanese population. T allele of *GSTA1* results in decreased expression of *GSTA1*, and thus inhibits the proliferation effect of the gene and decreases the development of tumor cell proliferation in oral cancer [192].

39. GENE: GJA1; GAP JUNCTION PROTEIN ALPHA 1, CONNEXIN 43 [CX43] LOCATION: 6q22.31

GJA1 protein is a component of gap junctions, which provide direct intercellular communication between polarized epithelial cells and are subject to down-regulation with loss of polarity during EMT. *GJA1* is involved in critical cellular processes, including cell migration and cell cycle regulation during EMT. Reduced levels of *GJA1* have been reported in lung cancer, mammary carcinoma, endometrial adenocarcinoma, and colon cancer and the role of *GJA1* in breast cancer has been controversial. It is generally considered a tumor suppressor and is demonstrated with downregulation of *GJA1* expression or aberrant localization and phosphorylation in tumor tissues. In some studies, its metastatic role in later stages of breast cancer progression has been reported and is known to mediate the interaction between tumor and endothelial cells to facilitate adhesion and extravasation at secondary sites [193]. *GJA1* expression is highly expressed in prostate cancer and is used as a potential marker of prostate cancer cell metastasis [194].

1.39.1. The Disease of Relevance:

- *GJA1* expression is often downregulated in several human cancer, such as mammary carcinoma, endometrial adenocarcinoma, and lung cancer. This downregulation is probably due to promoter hypermethylation, but the same has not been found in colorectal cancer instead, it was suggested that the silencing of the gene could be mediated by another mechanism through estrogen activation [195].
- Reduced levels of GJA1 mRNA in aggressive basal-like and Her2e tumor subtypes and increased level of lymph node metastasis has been observed. Hence dysregulation of *GJA1* can either increase or decrease its expression so it can be suggested that the role of *GJA1* depends on the molecular context of different breast cancer subtypes. GJA1 mRNA expression also depends on the tumor grades; as the grade increases, the GJA1 mRNA expression decreases like most basal and Her2e tumors that express a low level of GJA1 mRNA are of grade 3, whereas luminal tumors are a grade of 1 and 2 thus some of them overexpresses *GJA1*. Also, low levels of amplification and deletions at the position where *GJA1* is located have been observed in a few cases, mostly in Her2e and basal subtypes [193].
- Downregulation of *GJA1* expression, mostly due to epigenetic silencing, has been reported in lung cancer. It also has the potential to reverse several neoplastic characteristics and can reduce the expression of human lungs CSC markers such as *Nanog, Oct4,* and *Sox2* [196].
- *GJA1* is highly expressed in gastric cancer and is associated with poor OS in patients, mostly in those that are Her2 positive. It may facilitate tumor

proliferation and migration. The abnormal expression of *GJA1* encoded Cx43 can induce lymph node metastasis and peritoneal metastasis of gastric cancer *via* Cx43-mediated heterocellular gap-junctional intercellular communication [197].

1.40. GENE: DAXX, DEATH DOMAIN-ASSOCIATED PROTEIN LOCATION: 6p21.32

DAXX gene can function as a tumor suppressor or as an oncogene, depending on cell type and context. It can exert an anti-apoptotic activity in unstressed primary cells, and act as a pro-apoptotic factor in tumor cells or transformed cells exposed to various types of stress. DAXX proteins interact with a wide variety of proteins such as apoptosis antigen Fas, centromere protein C, and transcription factor erythroblastosis virus E26 oncogene homolog. When in the nucleus, the protein functions as a potent transcription repressor that binds to sumoylated transcription factors. Overexpression of *DAXX* has been observed in cancers such as breast, prostate, ovarian, gastric, kidney, and colon cancers, and oral squamous cell carcinoma.

1.40.1. The Disease of Relevance

- In ovarian cancer, *DAXX* is highly expressed and is known to act as a potential regulator of cell proliferation, metastasis, and drug resistance. It is actively involved in DNA damage responses through its associations with promyelocytic leukemia nuclear bodies [PML-NBs]. It is known to promote DNA repair to protect cancer cells from DNA damage-induced cell death [198].
- *DAXX* is upregulated in glioblastoma cells and acts as an oncogene. It was studied that in PTEN-null glioblastoma [GBM] cells, *DAXX* antagonizes PTEN-mediated repression of oncogenes and their expression levels are inversely correlated [198, 199].
- *DAXX* expression is elevated in prostate cancer tissues and its expression is associated with metastasis. Strong *DAXX* expression is associated with both *TMPRSS2/ERG* gene rearrangement and *ERG* expression. In cancer cells, increased expression of *DAXX* interferes with nuclear localization of tumor suppressor PTEN *via* USP7-mediated PTEN deubiquitination, thus resulting in nuclear exclusion, and this is how it exhibits oncogenic function [198].
- Expression of *DAXX* is reduced in pancreatic neuroendocrine tumors [PanNETs], as a consequence of somatic *DAXX* mutations or its loss. *DAXX* loss is associated with tumor stage, metastasis, and decreased survival. This mutation leads to impairment of the heterochromatic state of telomeres, with reduced levels of histone variant H3.3. Loss of function mutation of *DAXX* has been associated with the formation of abnormal telomeres due to alternative lengthening of telomeres [ALT] independent of telomerase activity. *DAXX*

mutations frequently occur in PanNETs in the regions encoding the folded 4HB and HBD domains, thus indicating that the loss of *DAXX's* H3.3 chaperone function may lead to abnormal chromatin structures, epigenetic dysregulation, and chromosome instability [198, 199].

- In Hürthle cell carcinoma, recurrent mutations involving frameshift and nonsense mutations have been observed [198].
- In kidney cancer, *DAXX* mRNA levels in tumor cells have been reported to be increased. Speckle-Type Poz Protein [SPOP] causes degradation of *DAXX* and thus plays a role in kidney tumorigenesis [198].
- In osteosarcoma, a chromosome translocation involving an in-frame fusion of *DAXX* with *KIFC3* has been observed. The fusion product fails to maintain telomere by suppressing ALT [198].
- In lung cancer, hypoxia-induced activation of hypoxia-inducible factor [HIF]-1α inhibits *DAXX* expression, resulting in increased invasion and metastasis to the lungs. Therefore, *DAXX* expression is significantly higher in lung cancer and suppresses metastasis by inhibiting EMT [198, 199].
- Knockdown of the *DAXX* gene in gastric cancer cells encourages cell survival, as well as enhances the expression of stem cell markers such as *CD44* and *Oct4,* and promotes tumor development. Overexpression of *DAXX* inhibits the EMT *via* downregulation of *SNAI3* transcription and the probable reason behind the downregulation is the translocation of HDAC-1 from the cytoplasm to the nucleus [199].
- In breast cancer, it acts as a potent inhibitor by repressing pluripotent and EMT genes by potentially binding promoters of pluripotent tumor-initiating cells [TIC] associated genes [199].

CONCLUSION

Abundant studies regarding cancer genes and their function have been done. Cancer genes studied may not necessarily be linked to an individual gene but could also involve various gene mutations. Genetic mutations can be acquired by an individual either due to errors in cell division or due to exposure to certain carcinogenic substances that would damage DNA. Cancer genetic studies are conducted initially by predicting an individual's risk of cancer, then diagnosing and treating cancer. It is important to understand how genetic mutations occur and their influence on cancer development. Having this information increases the potential for early detection, risk reduction, and survival chances and also enhances gene-specific therapies. Many therapy and drugs have been developed to target some of the genes in specific cancers. Also, several techniques for checking the presence of inherited mutations, such as DNA sequencing, are being used.

However, there are a lot of genes on chromosome 6 yet to be studied for their oncogenic potential and genetic mutation.

REFERENCES

[1] Saito S, Matsushima M, Shirahama S, *et al.* Complete genomic structure DNA polymorphisms, and alternative splicing of the human AF-6 gene. DNA Res 1998; 5(2): 115-20.
[http://dx.doi.org/10.1093/dnares/5.2.115] [PMID: 9679199]

[2] Deshpande AJ, Chen L, Fazio M, *et al.* Leukemic transformation by the MLL-AF6 fusion oncogene requires the H3K79 methyltransferase Dot1l. Blood 2013; 121(13): 2533-41.
[http://dx.doi.org/10.1182/blood-2012-11-465120] [PMID: 23361907]

[3] Fournier G, Cabaud O, Josselin E, *et al.* Loss of AF6/afadin, a marker of poor outcome in breast cancer, induces cell migration, invasiveness and tumor growth. Oncogene 2011; 30(36): 3862-74.
[http://dx.doi.org/10.1038/onc.2011.106] [PMID: 21478912]

[4] Elloul S, Kedrin D, Knoblauch NW, *et al.* The Adherens Junction Protein Afadin Is an AKT Substrate that Regulates Breast Cancer Cell Migration 2014.
[http://dx.doi.org/10.1158/1541-7786.MCR-13-0398]

[5] Zhang X, Wang H, Li Q, Li T. CLDN2 inhibits the metastasis of osteosarcoma cells *via* down-regulating the afadin/ERK signaling pathway. Cancer Cell Int 2018; 18(1): 160.
[http://dx.doi.org/10.1186/s12935-018-0662-4] [PMID: 30349422]

[6] Lai Y, Xu P, Liu J, *et al.* Decreased expression of the long non-coding RNA MLLT4 antisense RNA 1 is a potential biomarker and an indicator of a poor prognosis for gastric cancer. Oncol Lett 2017; 14(3): 2629-34.
[http://dx.doi.org/10.3892/ol.2017.6478] [PMID: 28927028]

[7] Marques MS, Melo J, Cavadas B, *et al.* Afadin Downregulation by *Helicobacter pylori* Induces Epithelial to Mesenchymal Transition in Gastric Cells. Front Microbiol 2018; 9: 2712.
[http://dx.doi.org/10.3389/fmicb.2018.02712] [PMID: 30473688]

[8] Sun TT, Wang Y, Cheng H, *et al.* Disrupted interaction between CFTR and AF-6/afadin aggravates malignant phenotypes of colon cancer. Biochim Biophys Acta Mol Cell Res 2014; 1843(3): 618-28.
[http://dx.doi.org/10.1016/j.bbamcr.2013.12.013] [PMID: 24373847]

[9] Xu Y, Chang R, Peng Z, *et al.* Loss of polarity protein AF6 promotes pancreatic cancer metastasis by inducing Snail expression. Nat Commun 2015; 6(1): 7184.
[http://dx.doi.org/10.1038/ncomms8184] [PMID: 26013125]

[10] Yamamoto T, Mori T, Sawada M, *et al.* Loss of AF-6/afadin induces cell invasion, suppresses the formation of glandular structures and might be a predictive marker of resistance to chemotherapy in endometrial cancer. BMC Cancer 2015; 15(1): 275.
[http://dx.doi.org/10.1186/s12885-015-1286-x] [PMID: 25879875]

[11] Paderova J, Orlic-Milacic M, Yoshimoto M, da Cunha Santos G, Gallie B, Squire JA. Novel 6p rearrangements and recurrent translocation breakpoints in retinoblastoma cell lines identified by spectral karyotyping and mBAND analyses. Cancer Genet Cytogenet 2007; 179(2): 102-11.
[http://dx.doi.org/10.1016/j.cancergencyto.2007.08.014] [PMID: 18036396]

[12] Orlic M, Spencer CE, Wang L, Gallie BL. Expression analysis of 6p22 genomic gain in retinoblastoma. Genes Chromosomes Cancer 2006; 45(1): 72-82.
[http://dx.doi.org/10.1002/gcc.20263] [PMID: 16180235]

[13] Evans AJ, Gallie BL, Jewett MAS, *et al.* Defining a 0.5-mb region of genomic gain on chromosome 6p22 in bladder cancer by quantitative-multiplex polymerase chain reaction. Am J Pathol 2004; 164(1): 285-93.
[http://dx.doi.org/10.1016/S0002-9440(10)63118-5] [PMID: 14695341]

[14] Sandahl JD, Coenen EA, Forestier E, *et al.* t(6;9)(p22;q34)/DEK-NUP214-rearranged pediatric myeloid leukemia: an international study of 62 patients. Haematologica 2014; 99(5): 865-72. [http://dx.doi.org/10.3324/haematol.2013.098517] [PMID: 24441146]

[15] Ishida K, Nakashima T, Shibata T, Hara A, Tomita H. Role of the DEK oncogene in the development of squamous cell carcinoma. Int J Clin Oncol 2020; 25(9): 1563-9. [http://dx.doi.org/10.1007/s10147-020-01735-5] [PMID: 32656741]

[16] Privette Vinnedge LM, McClaine R, Wagh PK, Wikenheiser-Brokamp KA, Waltz SE, Wells SI. The human DEK oncogene stimulates β-catenin signaling, invasion and mammosphere formation in breast cancer. Oncogene 2011; 30(24): 2741-52. [http://dx.doi.org/10.1038/onc.2011.2] [PMID: 21317931]

[17] Cifdaloz M, Osterloh L, Graña O, *et al.* Systems analysis identifies melanoma-enriched pro-oncogenic networks controlled by the RNA binding protein CELF1. Nat Commun 2017; 8(1): 2249. [http://dx.doi.org/10.1038/s41467-017-02353-y] [PMID: 29269732]

[18] Ogura H, Nagatake-Kobayashi Y, Adachi J, Tomonaga T, Fujita N, Katayama R. TKI-addicted ROS1-rearranged cells are destined to survival or death by the intensity of ROS1 kinase activity. Sci Rep 2017; 7(1): 5519. [http://dx.doi.org/10.1038/s41598-017-05736-9] [PMID: 28717217]

[19] Stumpfova M, Jänne PA. Zeroing in on ROS1 Rearrangements in Non–Small Cell Lung CancerROS1 in NSCLC. Clin Cancer Res. 2012; 18(16): 4222-4.

[20] Rimkunas VM, Crosby KE, Li D, *et al.* Analysis of Receptor Tyrosine Kinase ROS1-Positive Tumors in Non–Small Cell Lung Cancer: Identification of a FIG-ROS1 Fusion. Clin Cancer Res 2012; 18: 4449 LP – 4457.

[21] Lin JJ, Shaw AT. Recent Advances in Targeting ROS1 in Lung Cancer. J Thorac Oncol 2017; 12(11): 1611-25. [http://dx.doi.org/10.1016/j.jtho.2017.08.002] [PMID: 28818606]

[22] Chiang NJ, Hsu C, Chen JS, *et al.* Expression levels of ROS1/ALK/c-MET and therapeutic efficacy of cetuximab plus chemotherapy in advanced biliary tract cancer. Sci Rep 2016; 6(1): 25369. [http://dx.doi.org/10.1038/srep25369] [PMID: 27136744]

[23] Coccé MC, Mardin BR, Bens S, *et al.* Identification of *ZCCHC8* as fusion partner of *ROS1* in a case of congenital glioblastoma multiforme with a t(6;12)(q21;q24.3). Genes Chromosomes Cancer 2016; 55(9): 677-87. [http://dx.doi.org/10.1002/gcc.22369] [PMID: 27121553]

[24] Lee J, Lee SE, Kang SY, *et al.* Identification of *ROS1* rearrangement in gastric adenocarcinoma. Cancer 2013; 119(9): 1627-35. [http://dx.doi.org/10.1002/cncr.27967] [PMID: 23400546]

[25] Cilloni D, Carturan S, Bracco E, *et al.* Aberrant activation of ROS1 represents a new molecular defect in chronic myelomonocytic leukemia. Leuk Res 2013; 37(5): 520-30. [http://dx.doi.org/10.1016/j.leukres.2013.01.014] [PMID: 23415111]

[26] Morgan GJ, He J, Tytarenko R, *et al.* Kinase domain activation through gene rearrangement in multiple myeloma. Leukemia 2018; 32(11): 2435-44. [http://dx.doi.org/10.1038/s41375-018-0108-y] [PMID: 29654269]

[27] Shih C-H, Chang Y-J, Huang W-C, *et al.* EZH2-mediated upregulation of ROS1 oncogene promotes oral cancer metastasis. Oncogene 2017; 36(47): 6542-54. [http://dx.doi.org/10.1038/onc.2017.262] [PMID: 28759046]

[28] Lopez-Nunez O, John I, Panasiti RN, *et al.* Infantile inflammatory myofibroblastic tumors: clinicopathological and molecular characterization of 12 cases. Mod Pathol 2020; 33(4): 576-90. [http://dx.doi.org/10.1038/s41379-019-0406-6] [PMID: 31690781]

[29]   Martín-Garcia D, Navarro A, Valdés-Mas R, *et al.* *CCND2* and *CCND3* hijack immunoglobulin light-chain enhancers in cyclin D1⁻ mantle cell lymphoma. Blood 2019; 133(9): 940-51.
[http://dx.doi.org/10.1182/blood-2018-07-862151] [PMID: 30538135]

[30]   Curiel-Olmo S, Mondéjar R, Almaraz C, *et al.* Splenic diffuse red pulp small B-cell lymphoma displays increased expression of cyclin D3 and recurrent CCND3 mutations. Blood 2017; 129(8): 1042-5.
[http://dx.doi.org/10.1182/blood-2016-11-751024] [PMID: 28069605]

[31]   Schmitz R, Young RM, Ceribelli M, *et al.* Burkitt lymphoma pathogenesis and therapeutic targets from structural and functional genomics. Nature 2012; 490(7418): 116-20.
[http://dx.doi.org/10.1038/nature11378] [PMID: 22885699]

[32]   Rohde M, Bonn BR, Zimmermann M, *et al.* Relevance of ID3-TCF3-CCND3 pathway mutations in pediatric aggressive B-cell lymphoma treated according to the non-Hodgkin Lymphoma Berlin-Frankfurt-Münster protocols. Haematologica 2017; 102(6): 1091-8.
[http://dx.doi.org/10.3324/haematol.2016.156885] [PMID: 28209658]

[33]   Fabris S, Agnelli L, Mattioli M, *et al.* Characterization of oncogene dysregulation in multiple myeloma by combined FISH and DNA microarray analyses. Genes Chromosomes Cancer 2005; 42(2): 117-27.
[http://dx.doi.org/10.1002/gcc.20123] [PMID: 15543617]

[34]   Tanami H, Tsuda H, Okabe S, *et al.* Involvement of cyclin D3 in liver metastasis of colorectal cancer, revealed by genome-wide copy-number analysis. Lab Invest 2005; 85(9): 1118-29.
[http://dx.doi.org/10.1038/labinvest.3700312] [PMID: 15980885]

[35]   Hua Y, Ma X, Liu X, Yuan X, Qin H, Zhang X. Identification of the potential biomarkers for the metastasis of rectal adenocarcinoma. Acta Pathol Microbiol Scand Suppl 2017; 125(2): 93-100.
[http://dx.doi.org/10.1111/apm.12633] [PMID: 28028826]

[36]   Wang G, Zhang W, Meng W, *et al.* Expression and clinical significance of connective tissue growth factor in thyroid carcinomas. J Int Med Res 2013; 41(4): 1214-20.
[http://dx.doi.org/10.1177/0300060513476595] [PMID: 23847295]

[37]   Li J, Ye L, Owen S, Weeks HP, Zhang Z, Jiang WG. Emerging role of CCN family proteins in tumorigenesis and cancer metastasis (Review). Int J Mol Med 2015; 36(6): 1451-63.
[http://dx.doi.org/10.3892/ijmm.2015.2390] [PMID: 26498181]

[38]   Zirn B, Hartmann O, Samans B, *et al.* Expression profiling of Wilms tumors reveals new candidate genes for different clinical parameters. Int J Cancer 2006; 118(8): 1954-62.
[http://dx.doi.org/10.1002/ijc.21564] [PMID: 16287080]

[39]   Hou CH, Yang R, Tsao YT. Connective tissue growth factor stimulates osteosarcoma cell migration and induces osteosarcoma metastasis by upregulating VCAM-1 expression. Biochem Pharmacol 2018; 155: 71-81.
[http://dx.doi.org/10.1016/j.bcp.2018.06.015] [PMID: 29909077]

[40]   Yu X, Zhen Y, Yang H, *et al.* Loss of connective tissue growth factor as an unfavorable prognosis factor activates miR-18b by PI3K/AKT/C-Jun and C-Myc and promotes cell growth in nasopharyngeal carcinoma. Cell Death Dis 2013; 4(5): e634-4.
[http://dx.doi.org/10.1038/cddis.2013.153] [PMID: 23681229]

[41]   Kang W, Huang T, Zhou Y, *et al.* miR-375 is involved in Hippo pathway by targeting YAP1/TEAD4-CTGF axis in gastric carcinogenesis. Cell Death Dis 2018; 9(2): 92.
[http://dx.doi.org/10.1038/s41419-017-0134-0] [PMID: 29367737]

[42]   Richardson TE, Tang K, Vasudevaraja V, *et al.* GOPC-ROS1 Fusion Due to Microdeletion at 6q22 Is an Oncogenic Driver in a Subset of Pediatric Gliomas and Glioneuronal Tumors. J Neuropathol Exp Neurol 2019; 78(12): 1089-99.
[http://dx.doi.org/10.1093/jnen/nlz093] [PMID: 31626289]

[43]   Kiehna EN, Arnush MR, Tamrazi B, *et al.* Novel GOPC(FIG)-ROS1 fusion in a pediatric high-grade glioma survivor. J Neurosurg Pediatr 2017; 20(1): 51-5.
       [http://dx.doi.org/10.3171/2017.2.PEDS16679] [PMID: 28387643]

[44]   Zeng L, Yang N, Zhang Y. GOPC-ROS1 Rearrangement as an Acquired Resistance Mechanism to Osimertinib and Responding to Crizotinib Combined Treatments in Lung Adenocarcinoma. J Thorac Oncol 2018; 13(7): e114-6.
       [http://dx.doi.org/10.1016/j.jtho.2018.02.005] [PMID: 29935846]

[45]   Ohara N, Haraguchi N, Koseki J, *et al.* Low expression of the GOPC is a poor prognostic marker in colorectal cancer. Oncol Lett 2017; 14(4): 4483-90.
       [http://dx.doi.org/10.3892/ol.2017.6817] [PMID: 29085445]

[46]   Stark MS, Woods SL, Gartside MG, *et al.* Frequent somatic mutations in MAP3K5 and MAP3K9 in metastatic melanoma identified by exome sequencing. Nat Genet 2012; 44(2): 165-9.
       [http://dx.doi.org/10.1038/ng.1041] [PMID: 22197930]

[47]   Prickett TD, Zerlanko B, Gartner JJ, *et al.* Somatic mutations in MAP3K5 attenuate its proapoptotic function in melanoma through increased binding to thioredoxin. J Invest Dermatol 2014; 134(2): 452-60.
       [http://dx.doi.org/10.1038/jid.2013.365] [PMID: 24008424]

[48]   Pressinotti NC, Klocker H, Schäfer G, *et al.* Differential expression of apoptotic genes PDIA3 and MAP3K5 distinguishes between low- and high-risk prostate cancer. Mol Cancer 2009; 8(1): 130.
       [http://dx.doi.org/10.1186/1476-4598-8-130] [PMID: 20035634]

[49]   Sabapathi N, Sabarimurugan S, Madurantakam Royam M, *et al.* Prognostic Significance of FOXC1 in Various Cancers: A Systematic Review and Meta-Analysis. Mol Diagn Ther 2019; 23(6): 695-706.
       [http://dx.doi.org/10.1007/s40291-019-00416-y] [PMID: 31372939]

[50]   Yang Z, Jiang S, Cheng Y, *et al.* FOXC1 in cancer development and therapy: deciphering its emerging and divergent roles. Ther Adv Med Oncol 2017; 9(12): 797-816.
       [http://dx.doi.org/10.1177/1758834017742576] [PMID: 29449899]

[51]   Elian FA, Yan E, Walter MA. FOXC1, the new player in the cancer sandbox. Oncotarget 2018; 9(8): 8165-78.
       [http://dx.doi.org/10.18632/oncotarget.22742] [PMID: 29487724]

[52]   Han B, Bhowmick N, Qu Y, Chung S, Giuliano AE, Cui X. FOXC1: an emerging marker and therapeutic target for cancer. Oncogene 2017; 36(28): 3957-63.
       [http://dx.doi.org/10.1038/onc.2017.48] [PMID: 28288141]

[53]   Zhang Y, Liao Y, Chen C, *et al.* p38-regulated FOXC1 stability is required for colorectal cancer metastasis. J Pathol 2020; 250(2): 217-30.
       [http://dx.doi.org/10.1002/path.5362] [PMID: 31650548]

[54]   Li Q, Wei P, Wu J, *et al.* The FOXC1/FBP1 signaling axis promotes colorectal cancer proliferation by enhancing the Warburg effect. Oncogene 2019; 38(4): 483-96.
       [http://dx.doi.org/10.1038/s41388-018-0469-8] [PMID: 30171256]

[55]   Cao S, Wang Z, Gao X, *et al.* FOXC1 induces cancer stem cell-like properties through upregulation of beta-catenin in NSCLC. J Exp Clin Cancer Res 2018; 37(1): 220.
       [http://dx.doi.org/10.1186/s13046-018-0894-0] [PMID: 30189871]

[56]   Subramani R, Camacho FA, Levin CI, *et al.* FOXC1 plays a crucial role in the growth of pancreatic cancer. Oncogenesis 2018; 7(7): 52.
       [http://dx.doi.org/10.1038/s41389-018-0061-7] [PMID: 29976975]

[57]   Bossi D, Carlomagno F, Pallavicini I, *et al.* Functional characterization of a novel FGFR1OP-RET rearrangement in hematopoietic malignancies. Mol Oncol 2014; 8(2): 221-31.
       [http://dx.doi.org/10.1016/j.molonc.2013.11.004] [PMID: 24315414]

[58]   Vizmanos JL, Hernández R, Vidal MJ, *et al.* Clinical variability of patients with the t(6;8)(q27;p12) and FGFR1OP-FGFR1 fusion: two further cases. Hematol J 2004; 5(6): 534-7.
[http://dx.doi.org/10.1038/sj.thj.6200561] [PMID: 15570299]

[59]   Kang X, Liu H, Onaitis MW, *et al.* Polymorphisms of the centrosomal gene (*FGFR1OP*) and lung cancer risk: a meta-analysis of 14 463 cases and 44 188 controls. Carcinogenesis 2016; 37(3): 280-9.
[http://dx.doi.org/10.1093/carcin/bgw014] [PMID: 26905588]

[60]   Mano Y, Takahashi K, Ishikawa N, *et al.* Fibroblast growth factor receptor 1 oncogene partner as a novel prognostic biomarker and therapeutic target for lung cancer. Cancer Sci 2007; 98(12): 1902-13.
[http://dx.doi.org/10.1111/j.1349-7006.2007.00610.x] [PMID: 17888034]

[61]   Dror S, Sander L, Schwartz H, *et al.* Melanoma miRNA trafficking controls tumour primary niche formation. Nat Cell Biol 2016; 18(9): 1006-17.
[http://dx.doi.org/10.1038/ncb3399] [PMID: 27548915]

[62]   Martin-Kleiner I, Gall Troselj K. Mannose-6-phosphate/insulin-like growth factor 2 receptor (M6P/IGF2R) in carcinogenesis. Cancer Lett 2010; 289(1): 11-22.
[http://dx.doi.org/10.1016/j.canlet.2009.06.036] [PMID: 19646808]

[63]   Ou JM, Lian WS, Qiu MK, *et al.* Knockdown of IGF2R suppresses proliferation and induces apoptosis in hemangioma cells *in vitro* and *in vivo*. Int J Oncol 2014; 45(3): 1241-9.
[http://dx.doi.org/10.3892/ijo.2014.2512] [PMID: 24968760]

[64]   Hoyo C, Schildkraut JM, Murphy SK, *et al. IGF2R* polymorphisms and risk of esophageal and gastric adenocarcinomas. Int J Cancer 2009; 125(11): 2673-8.
[http://dx.doi.org/10.1002/ijc.24623] [PMID: 19626700]

[65]   Lautem A, Simon F, Hoppe-Lotichius M, *et al.* Expression and prognostic significance of insulin-like growth factor-2 receptor in human hepatocellular carcinoma and the influence of transarterial chemoembolization. Oncol Rep 2019; 41(4): 2299-310.
[http://dx.doi.org/10.3892/or.2019.6995] [PMID: 30720132]

[66]   Takeda T, Komatsu M, Chiwaki F, *et al.* Upregulation of IGF2R evades lysosomal dysfunction-induced apoptosis of cervical cancer cells *via* transport of cathepsins. Cell Death Dis 2019; 10(12): 876.
[http://dx.doi.org/10.1038/s41419-019-2117-9] [PMID: 31748500]

[67]   Trent JM, Stanbridge EJ, McBride HL, *et al.* Tumorigenicity in human melanoma cell lines controlled by introduction of human chromosome 6. Science (80-) 1990; 247: 568 LP – 571.

[68]   Hoshimoto S, Kuo CT, Chong KK, *et al.* AIM1 and LINE-1 epigenetic aberrations in tumor and serum relate to melanoma progression and disease outcome. J Invest Dermatol 2012; 132(6): 1689-97.
[http://dx.doi.org/10.1038/jid.2012.36] [PMID: 22402438]

[69]   Rosenbaum E, Begum S, Brait M, *et al.* AIM1 promoter hypermethylation as a predictor of decreased risk of recurrence following radical prostatectomy. Prostate 2012; 72(10): 1133-9.
[http://dx.doi.org/10.1002/pros.22461] [PMID: 22127895]

[70]   Haffner MC, Esopi DM, Chaux A, *et al.* AIM1 is an actin-binding protein that suppresses cell migration and micrometastatic dissemination. Nat Commun 2017; 8(1): 142.
[http://dx.doi.org/10.1038/s41467-017-00084-8] [PMID: 28747635]

[71]   El-Naggar AM, Clarkson PW, Negri GL, *et al.* HACE1 is a potential tumor suppressor in osteosarcoma. Cell Death Dis 2019; 10(1): 21.
[http://dx.doi.org/10.1038/s41419-018-1276-4] [PMID: 30622235]

[72]   Slade I, Stephens P, Douglas J, *et al.* Constitutional translocation breakpoint mapping by genome-wide paired-end sequencing identifies HACE1 as a putative Wilms tumour susceptibility gene. J Med Genet. 2010; 47(5): 342-7.

[73]   El-Hachem N, Habel N, Naiken T, *et al.* Uncovering and deciphering the pro-invasive role of HACE1

in melanoma cells. Cell Death Differ 2018; 25(11): 2010-22.
[http://dx.doi.org/10.1038/s41418-018-0090-y] [PMID: 29515254]

[74]   McCormick KD, Ghosh A, Trivedi S, *et al.* Innate immune signaling through differential RIPK1 expression promote tumor progression in head and neck squamous cell carcinoma. Carcinogenesis 2016; 37(5): 522-9.
[http://dx.doi.org/10.1093/carcin/bgw032] [PMID: 26992898]

[75]   Park S, Hatanpaa KJ, Xie Y, *et al.* The receptor interacting protein 1 inhibits p53 induction through NF-kappaB activation and confers a worse prognosis in glioblastoma. Cancer Res 2009; 69(7): 2809-16.
[http://dx.doi.org/10.1158/0008-5472.CAN-08-4079] [PMID: 19339267]

[76]   Karami-Tehrani F, Malek AR, Shahsavari Z, Atri M. Evaluation of RIP1K and RIP3K expressions in the malignant and benign breast tumors. Tumour Biol 2016; 37(7): 8849-56.
[http://dx.doi.org/10.1007/s13277-015-4762-7] [PMID: 26749282]

[77]   Zeng F, Chen X, Cui W, *et al.* RIPK1 Binds MCU to Mediate Induction of Mitochondrial Ca2+ Uptake and Promotes Colorectal OncogenesisRIPK1 and MCU Promote Colorectal Cancer Progression. Cancer Res. 2018; 78(11): 2876-85.

[78]   Schneider AT, Gautheron J, Feoktistova M, *et al.* RIPK1 Suppresses a TRAF2-Dependent Pathway to Liver Cancer. Cancer Cell 2017; 31(1): 94-109.
[http://dx.doi.org/10.1016/j.ccell.2016.11.009] [PMID: 28017612]

[79]   Zhang J, Hao N, Liu W, *et al.* In-depth proteomic analysis of tissue interstitial fluid for hepatocellular carcinoma serum biomarker discovery. Br J Cancer 2017; 117(11): 1676-84.
[http://dx.doi.org/10.1038/bjc.2017.344] [PMID: 29024941]

[80]   Czckierdowski A, Czekierdowska S, Danilos J, *et al.* Microvessel density and CpG island methylation of the THBS2 gene in malignant ovarian tumors. J Physiol Pharmacol 2008; 59 (Suppl. 4): 53-65.
[PMID: 18955754]

[81]   Nezu Y, Hagiwara K, Yamamoto Y, *et al.* miR-135b, a key regulator of malignancy, is linked to poor prognosis in human myxoid liposarcoma. Oncogene 2016; 35(48): 6177-88.
[http://dx.doi.org/10.1038/onc.2016.157] [PMID: 27157622]

[82]   Zhuo C, Li X, Zhuang H, *et al.* Elevated THBS2, COL1A2, and SPP1 Expression Levels as Predictors of Gastric Cancer Prognosis. Cell Physiol Biochem 2016; 40(6): 1316-24.
[http://dx.doi.org/10.1159/000453184] [PMID: 27997896]

[83]   Ao R, Guan L, Wang Y, Wang JN. *Retracted* : Silencing of COL1A2, COL6A3, and THBS2 inhibits gastric cancer cell proliferation, migration, and invasion while promoting apoptosis through the PI3k-Akt signaling pathway. J Cell Biochem 2018; 119(6): 4420-34.
[http://dx.doi.org/10.1002/jcb.26524] [PMID: 29143985]

[84]   Wei WF, Zhou CF, Wu XG, *et al.* MicroRNA-221-3p, a TWIST2 target, promotes cervical cancer metastasis by directly targeting THBS2. Cell Death Dis 2017; 8(12): 3220.
[http://dx.doi.org/10.1038/s41419-017-0077-5] [PMID: 29242498]

[85]   Wang X, Zhang L, Li H, Sun W, Zhang H, Lai M. THBS2 is a Potential Prognostic Biomarker in Colorectal Cancer. Sci Rep 2016; 6(1): 33366.
[http://dx.doi.org/10.1038/srep33366] [PMID: 27632935]

[86]   Świerczewska M, Sterzyńska K, Wojtowicz K, *et al.* PTPRK Expression Is Downregulated in Drug Resistant Ovarian Cancer Cell Lines, and Especially in ALDH1A1 Positive CSCs-Like Populations. Int J Mol Sci 2019; 20(8): 2053.
[http://dx.doi.org/10.3390/ijms20082053] [PMID: 31027318]

[87]   Sekine S, Yamashita S, Tanabe T, *et al.* Frequent *PTPRK-RSPO3* fusions and *RNF43* mutations in colorectal traditional serrated adenoma. J Pathol 2016; 239(2): 133-8.
[http://dx.doi.org/10.1002/path.4709] [PMID: 26924569]

[88]　Matsushita M, Mori Y, Uchiumi K, *et al.* PTPRK suppresses progression and chemo-resistance of colon cancer cells via direct inhibition of pro-oncogenic CD 133. FEBS Open Bio 2019; 9(5): 935-46.
[http://dx.doi.org/10.1002/2211-5463.12636] [PMID: 30947381]

[89]　Xu L, Xu X, Huang H, *et al.* MiR-1260b promotes the migration and invasion in non-small cell lung cancer *via* targeting PTPRK. Pathol Res Pract 2018; 214(5): 776-83.
[http://dx.doi.org/10.1016/j.prp.2018.02.002] [PMID: 29628123]

[90]　Sun PH, Ye L, Mason MD, Jiang WG. Receptor-like protein tyrosine phosphatase κ negatively regulates the apoptosis of prostate cancer cells *via* the JNK pathway. Int J Oncol 2013; 43(5): 1560-8.
[http://dx.doi.org/10.3892/ijo.2013.2082] [PMID: 24002526]

[91]　Hamamoto R, Toyokawa G, Nakakido M, Ueda K, Nakamura Y. SMYD2-dependent HSP90 methylation promotes cancer cell proliferation by regulating the chaperone complex formation. Cancer Lett 2014; 351(1): 126-33.
[http://dx.doi.org/10.1016/j.canlet.2014.05.014] [PMID: 24880080]

[92]　Wang H, Deng G, Ai M, *et al.* Hsp90ab1 stabilizes LRP5 to promote epithelial–mesenchymal transition *via* activating of AKT and Wnt/β-catenin signaling pathways in gastric cancer progression. Oncogene 2019; 38(9): 1489-507.
[http://dx.doi.org/10.1038/s41388-018-0532-5] [PMID: 30305727]

[93]　Pira G, Uva P, Scanu AM, *et al.* Landscape of transcriptome variations uncovering known and novel driver events in colorectal carcinoma. Sci Rep 2020; 10(1): 432.
[http://dx.doi.org/10.1038/s41598-019-57311-z] [PMID: 31949199]

[94]　Liu K, Kang M, Li J, Qin W, Wang R. Prognostic value of the mRNA expression of members of the HSP90 family in non-small cell lung cancer. Exp Ther Med 2019; 17(4): 2657-65.
[http://dx.doi.org/10.3892/etm.2019.7228] [PMID: 30930968]

[95]　Wang M, Feng L, Li P, Han N, Gao Y, Xiao T. [Hsp90AB1 Protein is Overexpressed in Non-small Cell Lung Cancer Tissues and Associated with Poor Prognosis in Lung Adenocarcinoma Patients]. Zhongguo Fei Ai Za Zhi 2016; 19(2): 64-9. [Hsp90AB1 Protein is Overexpressed in Non-small Cell Lung Cancer Tissues and Associated with Poor Prognosis in Lung Adenocarcinoma Patients].
[PMID: 26903158]

[96]　Kosinsky RL, Helms M, Zerche M, *et al.* USP22-dependent HSP90AB1 expression promotes resistance to HSP90 inhibition in mammary and colorectal cancer. Cell Death Dis 2019; 10(12): 911.
[http://dx.doi.org/10.1038/s41419-019-2141-9] [PMID: 31801945]

[97]　Ohguchi H, Hideshima T, Bhasin MK, *et al.* The KDM3A–KLF2–IRF4 axis maintains myeloma cell survival. Nat Commun 2016; 7(1): 10258.
[http://dx.doi.org/10.1038/ncomms10258] [PMID: 26728187]

[98]　Cho SY, Lim G, Oh SH, *et al.* Primary Plasma Cell Leukemia Associated with t(6;14)(p21;q32) and IGH Rearrangement: A Case Study and Review of the Literature. Ann Clin Lab Sci 2011; 41(3): 277-81.
[PMID: 22075513]

[99]　Qian Y, Du Z, Xing Y, Zhou T, Chen T, Shi M. Interferon regulatory factor 4 (IRF4) is overexpressed in human non-small cell lung cancer (NSCLC) and activates the Notch signaling pathway. Mol Med Rep 2017; 16(5): 6034-40.
[http://dx.doi.org/10.3892/mmr.2017.7319] [PMID: 28849037]

[100]　Yamashita M, Toyota M, Suzuki H, *et al.* DNA methylation of interferon regulatory factors in gastric cancer and noncancerous gastric mucosae. Cancer Sci 2010; 101(7): 1708-16.
[http://dx.doi.org/10.1111/j.1349-7006.2010.01581.x] [PMID: 20507321]

[101]　Asslaber D, Qi Y, Maeding N, *et al.* B-cell–specific IRF4 deletion accelerates chronic lymphocytic leukemia development by enhanced tumor immune evasion. Blood 2019; 134(20): 1717-29.
[http://dx.doi.org/10.1182/blood.2019000973] [PMID: 31537531]

[102] Havelange V, Pekarsky Y, Nakamura T, *et al.* IRF4 mutations in chronic lymphocytic leukemia. Blood 2011; 118(10): 2827-9.
[http://dx.doi.org/10.1182/blood-2011-04-350579] [PMID: 21791429]

[103] Tang B, Yong X, Xie R, Li QW, Yang SM. Vasoactive intestinal peptide receptor-based imaging and treatment of tumors. Int J Oncol 2014; 44(4): 1023-31.
[http://dx.doi.org/10.3892/ijo.2014.2276] [PMID: 24481544]

[104] Moody TW, Nuche-Berenguer B, Jensen RT. Vasoactive intestinal peptide/pituitary adenylate cyclase activating polypeptide, and their receptors and cancer. Curr Opin Endocrinol Diabetes Obes 2016; 23(1): 38-47.
[http://dx.doi.org/10.1097/MED.0000000000000218] [PMID: 26702849]

[105] Tang B, Wu J, Zhu MX, *et al.* VPAC1 couples with TRPV4 channel to promote calcium-dependent gastric cancer progression *via* a novel autocrine mechanism. Oncogene 2019; 38(20): 3946-61.
[http://dx.doi.org/10.1038/s41388-019-0709-6] [PMID: 30692637]

[106] Wang Y, Hu L, Zheng Y, Guo L. HMGA1 in cancer: Cancer classification by location. J Cell Mol Med 2019; 23(4): 2293-302.
[http://dx.doi.org/10.1111/jcmm.14082] [PMID: 30614613]

[107] Drabsch Y, Hugo H, Zhang R, *et al.* Mechanism of and requirement for estrogen-regulated *MYB* expression in estrogen-receptor-positive breast cancer cells. Proc Natl Acad Sci USA 2007; 104(34): 13762-7.
[http://dx.doi.org/10.1073/pnas.0700104104] [PMID: 17690249]

[108] Ramsay RG, Gonda TJ. MYB function in normal and cancer cells. Nat Rev Cancer 2008; 8(7): 523-34.
[http://dx.doi.org/10.1038/nrc2439] [PMID: 18574464]

[109] Stenman G, Andersson MK, Andrén Y. New tricks from an old oncogene. Cell Cycle 2010; 9(15): 3058-67.
[http://dx.doi.org/10.4161/cc.9.15.12515] [PMID: 20647765]

[110] Yang H, Zhang H, Ge S, *et al.* RETRACTED: Exosome-Derived miR-130a Activates Angiogenesis in Gastric Cancer by Targeting C-MYB in Vascular Endothelial Cells. Mol Ther 2018; 26(10): 2466-75.
[http://dx.doi.org/10.1016/j.ymthe.2018.07.023] [PMID: 30120059]

[111] Wang X, Lin Y. Tumor necrosis factor and cancer, buddies or foes? Acta Pharmacol Sin 2008; 29(11): 1275-88.
[http://dx.doi.org/10.1111/j.1745-7254.2008.00889.x] [PMID: 18954521]

[112] Powrózek T, Mlak R, Brzozowska A, Mazurek M, Gołębiowski P, Małecka-Massalska T. Relationship between TNF-α −1031T/C gene polymorphism, plasma level of TNF-α, and risk of cachexia in head and neck cancer patients. J Cancer Res Clin Oncol 2018; 144(8): 1423-34.
[http://dx.doi.org/10.1007/s00432-018-2679-4] [PMID: 29802455]

[113] Wajant H. The Role of TNF in Cancer BT - Death Receptors and Cognate Ligands in Cancer.1-15.

[114] Tse BWC, Scott KF, Russell PJ. Paradoxical roles of tumour necrosis factor-alpha in prostate cancer biology. Prostate Cancer 2012; 2012: 1-8.
[http://dx.doi.org/10.1155/2012/128965] [PMID: 23326670]

[115] Zhao P, Zhang Z. TNF-α promotes colon cancer cell migration and invasion by upregulating TROP-2. Oncol Lett 2018; 15(3): 3820-7.
[http://dx.doi.org/10.3892/ol.2018.7735] [PMID: 29467899]

[116] Gautrey H, Jackson C, Dittrich AL, Browell D, Lennard T, Tyson-Capper A. SRSF3 and hnRNP H1 regulate a splicing hotspot of *HER2* in breast cancer cells. RNA Biol 2015; 12(10): 1139-51.
[http://dx.doi.org/10.1080/15476286.2015.1076610] [PMID: 26367347]

[117] Ke H, Zhao L, Zhang H, *et al.* Loss of TDP43 inhibits progression of triple-negative breast cancer in

coordination with SRSF3. Proc Natl Acad Sci USA 2018; 115(15): E3426-35.
[http://dx.doi.org/10.1073/pnas.1714573115] [PMID: 29581274]

[118] Lin JC, Lee YC, Tan TH, *et al.* RBM4-SRSF3-MAP4K4 splicing cascade modulates the metastatic signature of colorectal cancer cell. Biochim Biophys Acta Mol Cell Res 2018; 1865(2): 259-72.
[http://dx.doi.org/10.1016/j.bbamcr.2017.11.005] [PMID: 29138007]

[119] Peiqi L, Zhaozhong G, Yaotian Y, Jun J, Jihua G, Rong J. Expression of SRSF3 is Correlated with Carcinogenesis and Progression of Oral Squamous Cell Carcinoma. Int J Med Sci 2016; 13(7): 533-9.
[http://dx.doi.org/10.7150/ijms.14871] [PMID: 27429590]

[120] Corbo C, Orrù S, Salvatore F. SRp20: An overview of its role in human diseases. Biochem Biophys Res Commun 2013; 436(1): 1-5.
[http://dx.doi.org/10.1016/j.bbrc.2013.05.027] [PMID: 23685143]

[121] Tarhriz V, Bandehpour M, Dastmalchi S, Ouladsahebmadarek E, Zarredar H, Eyvazi S. Overview of CD24 as a new molecular marker in ovarian cancer. J Cell Physiol 2019; 234(3): 2134-42.
[http://dx.doi.org/10.1002/jcp.27581] [PMID: 30317611]

[122] Eyvazi S, Kazemi B, Dastmalchi S, Bandehpour M. Involvement of CD24 in Multiple Cancer Related Pathways Makes It an Interesting New Target for Cancer Therapy. Curr Cancer Drug Targets 2018; 18(4): 328-36.
[http://dx.doi.org/10.2174/1570163814666170818125036] [PMID: 28820056]

[123] Weng CC, Ding PY, Liu YH, *et al.* Mutant Kras-induced upregulation of CD24 enhances prostate cancer stemness and bone metastasis. Oncogene 2019; 38(12): 2005-19.
[http://dx.doi.org/10.1038/s41388-018-0575-7] [PMID: 30467381]

[124] Zhang P, Zheng P, Liu Y. Amplification of the *CD24* Gene Is an Independent Predictor for Poor Prognosis of Breast Cancer. Front Genet 2019; 10: 560.
[http://dx.doi.org/10.3389/fgene.2019.00560] [PMID: 31244889]

[125] Jang K, Kim M, Gilbert CA, Simpkins F, Ince TA, Slingerland JM. VEGFA activates an epigenetic pathway upregulating ovarian cancer-initiating cells. EMBO Mol Med 2017; 9(3): 304-18.
[http://dx.doi.org/10.15252/emmm.201606840] [PMID: 28179359]

[126] Kim M, Jang K, Miller P, *et al.* VEGFA links self-renewal and metastasis by inducing Sox2 to repress miR-452, driving Slug. Oncogene 2017; 36(36): 5199-211.
[http://dx.doi.org/10.1038/onc.2017.4] [PMID: 28504716]

[127] Ferrara N, Mass RD, Campa C, Kim R. Targeting VEGF-A to treat cancer and age-related macular degeneration. Annu Rev Med 2007; 58(1): 491-504.
[http://dx.doi.org/10.1146/annurev.med.58.061705.145635] [PMID: 17052163]

[128] Takei K, Ikeda S, Arai T, Tanaka N, Muramatsu M, Sawabe M. Lymphotoxin-alpha polymorphisms and presence of cancer in 1,536 consecutive autopsy cases. BMC Cancer 2008; 8(1): 235.
[http://dx.doi.org/10.1186/1471-2407-8-235] [PMID: 18700950]

[129] Mou X, Sheng D, Bao Z, *et al.* Correlation Between Genotypes and Allele Frequency of Lymphotoxin-Alpha and Gastric Cancer *via* Magnetic Separation Dual-Color Fluorescent Genotyping. Nanosci Nanotechnol Lett 2019; 11(10): 1457-63.
[http://dx.doi.org/10.1166/nnl.2019.3031]

[130] Huang Y, Yu X, Wang L, *et al.* Four genetic polymorphisms of lymphotoxin-alpha gene and cancer risk: a systematic review and meta-analysis. PLoS One 2013; 8(12): e82519-9.
[http://dx.doi.org/10.1371/journal.pone.0082519] [PMID: 24349304]

[131] Cerhan JR, Liu-Mares W, Fredericksen ZS, *et al.* Genetic variation in tumor necrosis factor and the nuclear factor-kappaB canonical pathway and risk of non-Hodgkin's lymphoma. Cancer Epidemiol Biomarkers Prev 2008; 17(11): 3161-9.
[http://dx.doi.org/10.1158/1055-9965.EPI-08-0536] [PMID: 18990758]

[132] Skibola CF, Bracci PM, Nieters A, *et al.* Tumor necrosis factor (TNF) and lymphotoxin-α (LTA)

polymorphisms and risk of non-Hodgkin lymphoma in the InterLymph Consortium. Am J Epidemiol 2010; 171(3): 267-76.
[http://dx.doi.org/10.1093/aje/kwp383] [PMID: 20047977]

[133]   King CE, Cuatrecasas M, Castells A, Sepulveda AR, Lee JS, Rustgi AK. LIN28B promotes colon cancer progression and metastasis. Cancer Res 2011; 71(12): 4260-8.
[http://dx.doi.org/10.1158/0008-5472.CAN-10-4637] [PMID: 21512136]

[134]   Zhou J, Ng S-B, Chng W-J. LIN28/LIN28B: an emerging oncogenic driver in cancer stem cells. Int J Biochem & cell Biol 2013; 45: 973–978.

[135]   Lin X, Shen J, Dan Peng , *et al.* RNA-binding protein LIN28B inhibits apoptosis through regulation of the AKT2/FOXO3A/BIM axis in ovarian cancer cells. Signal Transduct Target Ther 2018; 3(1): 23.
[http://dx.doi.org/10.1038/s41392-018-0026-5] [PMID: 30174831]

[136]   Wang C, Gu Y, Zhang E, *et al.* A cancer-testis non-coding RNA LIN28B-AS1 activates driver gene LIN28B by interacting with IGF2BP1 in lung adenocarcinoma. Oncogene 2019; 38(10): 1611-24.
[http://dx.doi.org/10.1038/s41388-018-0548-x] [PMID: 30353165]

[137]   Kugel S, Sebastián C, Fitamant J, *et al.* SIRT6 Suppresses Pancreatic Cancer through Control of Lin28b. Cell 2016; 165(6): 1401-15.
[http://dx.doi.org/10.1016/j.cell.2016.04.033] [PMID: 27180906]

[138]   Li K, Guo Q, Zhang X, *et al.* Oral cancer-associated tertiary lymphoid structures: gene expression profile and prognostic value. Clin Exp Immunol 2020; 199(2): 172-81.
[http://dx.doi.org/10.1111/cei.13389] [PMID: 31652350]

[139]   Martinet L, Filleron T, Le Guellec S, et al. High Endothelial Venule Blood Vessels for Tumor-Infiltrating Lymphocytes Are Associated with Lymphotoxin β–Producing Dendritic Cells in Human Breast Cancer. J Immunol 2013; 191: 2001 LP – 2008.

[140]   Das R, Coupar J, saleh A, et al. Abstract 358: LTB and LTBR mediates alternative Nf-kB activation through NIk and RELB/NF-kB2 to promote cell migration of HNSCC. Cancer Res 2017; 77: 358 LP – 358.

[141]   Yeung B, Ho KC, Yang X. WWP1 E3 ligase targets LATS1 for ubiquitin-mediated degradation in breast cancer cells. PLoS One 2013; 8(4): e61027-7.
[http://dx.doi.org/10.1371/journal.pone.0061027] [PMID: 23573293]

[142]   Takahashi Y, Miyoshi Y, Takahata C, *et al.* Down-regulation of LATS1 and LATS2 mRNA expression by promoter hypermethylation and its association with biologically aggressive phenotype in human breast cancers. Clin Cancer Res. 2005; 11(4): 1380-5.

[143]   Wierzbicki PM, Adrych K, Kartanowicz D, *et al.* Underexpression of *LATS1* TSG in colorectal cancer is associated with promoter hypermethylation. World J Gastroenterol 2013; 19(27): 4363-73.
[http://dx.doi.org/10.3748/wjg.v19.i27.4363] [PMID: 23885148]

[144]   Li Y, Cao ZY, Sun B, *et al.* Effects of IL-17A on the occurrence of lung adenocarcinoma. Cancer Biol Ther 2011; 12(7): 610-6.
[http://dx.doi.org/10.4161/cbt.12.7.16302] [PMID: 21785272]

[145]   Cochaud S, Giustiniani J, Thomas C, *et al.* IL-17A is produced by breast cancer TILs and promotes chemoresistance and proliferation through ERK1/2. Sci Rep 2013; 3(1): 3456.
[http://dx.doi.org/10.1038/srep03456] [PMID: 24316750]

[146]   Arisawa T, Tahara T, Shiroeda H, *et al.* Genetic polymorphisms of IL17A and pri-microRNA-938, targeting IL17A 3′-UTR, influence susceptibility to gastric cancer. Hum Immunol 2012; 73(7): 747-52.
[http://dx.doi.org/10.1016/j.humimm.2012.04.011] [PMID: 22537748]

[147]   Reppert S, Boross I, Koslowski M, *et al.* A role for T-bet-mediated tumour immune surveillance in anti-IL-17A treatment of lung cancer. Nat Commun 2011; 2(1): 600.
[http://dx.doi.org/10.1038/ncomms1609] [PMID: 22186896]

[148] Wu X, Zeng Z, Xu L, *et al.* Increased expression of IL17A in human gastric cancer and its potential roles in gastric carcinogenesis. Tumour Biol 2014; 35(6): 5347-56.
[http://dx.doi.org/10.1007/s13277-014-1697-3] [PMID: 24570184]

[149] Hanieh H, Ahmed EA, Vishnubalaji R, Alajez NM. SOX4: Epigenetic regulation and role in tumorigenesis. Semin Cancer Biol 2020; 67(Pt 1): 91-104.
[http://dx.doi.org/10.1016/j.semcancer.2019.06.022] [PMID: 31271889]

[150] Moreno CS. SOX4: The unappreciated oncogene. Semin Cancer Biol 2020; 67(Pt 1): 57-64.
[http://dx.doi.org/10.1016/j.semcancer.2019.08.027] [PMID: 31445218]

[151] Lei JT, Shao J, Zhang J, *et al.* Functional Annotation of ESR1 Gene Fusions in Estrogen Receptor-Positive Breast Cancer. Cell Rep 2018; 24(6): 1434-1444.e7.
[http://dx.doi.org/10.1016/j.celrep.2018.07.009] [PMID: 30089255]

[152] Doherty JA, Rossing MA, Cushing-Haugen KL, *et al.* ESR1/SYNE1 polymorphism and invasive epithelial ovarian cancer risk: an Ovarian Cancer Association Consortium study. Cancer Epidemiol Biomarkers Prev 2010; 19(1): 245-50.
[http://dx.doi.org/10.1158/1055-9965.EPI-09-0729] [PMID: 20056644]

[153] Sun H, Deng Q, Pan Y, *et al.* Association between estrogen receptor 1 (ESR1) genetic variations and cancer risk: a meta-analysis. J BUON 2015; 20(1): 296-308.
[PMID: 25778331]

[154] Zhai Y, Bommer GT, Feng Y, Wiese AB, Fearon ER, Cho KR. Loss of estrogen receptor 1 enhances cervical cancer invasion. Am J Pathol 2010; 177(2): 884-95.
[http://dx.doi.org/10.2353/ajpath.2010.091166] [PMID: 20581058]

[155] Li LC, Shiina H, Deguchi M, *et al.* Age-dependent methylation of ESR1 gene in prostate cancer. Biochem Biophys Res Commun 2004; 321(2): 455-61.
[http://dx.doi.org/10.1016/j.bbrc.2004.06.164] [PMID: 15358197]

[156] Lei JT, Gou X, Seker S, Ellis MJ. *ESR1* alterations and metastasis in estrogen receptor positive breast cancer. J Cancer Metastasis Treat 2019; 2019: 38.
[http://dx.doi.org/10.20517/2394-4722.2019.12] [PMID: 31106278]

[157] Kreis N-N, Louwen F, Yuan J. The Multifaceted p21 (Cip1/Waf1/*CDKN1A*) in Cell Differentiation, Migration and Cancer Therapy. Cancers (Basel) 2019; 11(9): 1220.
[http://dx.doi.org/10.3390/cancers11091220] [PMID: 31438587]

[158] Kreis N-N, Friemel A, Ritter A, *et al.* Function of p21 (Cip1/Waf1/*CDKN1A*) in Migration and Invasion of Cancer and Trophoblastic Cells. Cancers (Basel) 2019; 11(7): 989.
[http://dx.doi.org/10.3390/cancers11070989] [PMID: 31311187]

[159] Ding J, Li J, Wang H, *et al.* Long noncoding RNA CRNDE promotes colorectal cancer cell proliferation *via* epigenetically silencing DUSP5/CDKN1A expression. Cell Death Dis 2017; 8(8): e2997-7.
[http://dx.doi.org/10.1038/cddis.2017.328] [PMID: 28796262]

[160] Liu J, Ben Q, Lu E, *et al.* Long noncoding RNA PANDAR blocks CDKN1A gene transcription by competitive interaction with p53 protein in gastric cancer. Cell Death Dis 2018; 9(2): 168.
[http://dx.doi.org/10.1038/s41419-017-0246-6] [PMID: 29416011]

[161] Zhang X, Li F, Zhu L. Clinical significance and functions of microRNA-93/CDKN1A axis in human cervical cancer. Life Sci 2018; 209: 242-8.
[http://dx.doi.org/10.1016/j.lfs.2018.08.021] [PMID: 30098344]

[162] Wu Z, Liu K, Wang Y, Xu Z, Meng J, Gu S. Upregulation of microRNA-96 and its oncogenic functions by targeting CDKN1A in bladder cancer. Cancer Cell Int 2015; 15(1): 107.
[http://dx.doi.org/10.1186/s12935-015-0235-8] [PMID: 26582573]

[163] Zhang Y, Feng Y, Ji D, *et al.* TRIM27 functions as an oncogene by activating epithelial-mesenchymal

transition and p-AKT in colorectal cancer. Int J Oncol 2018; 53(2): 620-32.
[http://dx.doi.org/10.3892/ijo.2018.4408] [PMID: 29767249]

[164] Zhang HX, Xu ZS, Lin H, *et al.* TRIM27 mediates STAT3 activation at retromer-positive structures to promote colitis and colitis-associated carcinogenesis. Nat Commun 2018; 9(1): 3441.
[http://dx.doi.org/10.1038/s41467-018-05796-z] [PMID: 30143645]

[165] Ma L, Yao N, Chen P, Zhuang Z. TRIM27 promotes the development of esophagus cancer *via* regulating PTEN/AKT signaling pathway. Cancer Cell Int 2019; 19(1): 283.
[http://dx.doi.org/10.1186/s12935-019-0998-4] [PMID: 31719796]

[166] Ma Y, Wei Z, Bast RC Jr, *et al.* Downregulation of TRIM27 expression inhibits the proliferation of ovarian cancer cells *in vitro* and *in vivo*. Lab Invest 2016; 96(1): 37-48.
[http://dx.doi.org/10.1038/labinvest.2015.132] [PMID: 26568293]

[167] Ji X, Lin L, Shen S, *et al.* Epigenetic–smoking interaction reveals histologically heterogeneous effects of *TRIM27* DNA methylation on overall survival among early-stage NSCLC patients. Mol Oncol 2020; 14(11): 2759-74.
[http://dx.doi.org/10.1002/1878-0261.12785] [PMID: 33448640]

[168] Vega-Benedetti AF, Saucedo C, Zavattari P, Vanni R, Zugaza JL, Parada LA. PLAGL1: an important player in diverse pathological processes. J Appl Genet 2017; 58(1): 71-8.
[http://dx.doi.org/10.1007/s13353-016-0355-4] [PMID: 27311313]

[169] Vega-Benedetti AF, Saucedo CN, Zavattari P, *et al. PLAGL1* gene function during hepatoma cells proliferation. Oncotarget 2018; 9(67): 32775-94.
[http://dx.doi.org/10.18632/oncotarget.25996] [PMID: 30214684]

[170] Kowalczyk A, Krazinski B, Godlewski J, *et al.* Altered expression of the PLAGL1 (ZAC1/LOT1) gene in colorectal cancer: Correlations to the clinicopathological parameters. Int J Oncol 2015; 47(3): 951-62.
[http://dx.doi.org/10.3892/ijo.2015.3067] [PMID: 26134521]

[171] Godlewski J, Krazinski BE, Kowalczyk AE, *et al.* PLAGL1 (ZAC1/LOT1) Expression in Clear Cell Renal Cell Carcinoma: Correlations with Disease Progression and Unfavorable Prognosis. Anticancer Res 2016; 36(2): 617-24.
[PMID: 26851016]

[172] Valleley EMA, Cordery SF, Carr IM, et al. Loss of expression of ZAC/PLAGL1 in diffuse large B-cell lymphoma is independent of promoter hypermethylation. Genes, Chromosom & cancer 2010; 49: 480–486.

[173] Wu G, Chen Z, Li J, *et al.* NOTCH4 Is a Novel Prognostic Marker that Correlates with Colorectal Cancer Progression and Prognosis. J Cancer 2018; 9(13): 2374-9.
[http://dx.doi.org/10.7150/jca.26359] [PMID: 30026833]

[174] Wang JW, Wei XL, Dou XW, Huang WH, Du CW, Zhang GJ. The association between Notch4 expression, and clinicopathological characteristics and clinical outcomes in patients with breast cancer. Oncol Lett 2018; 15(6): 8749-55.
[http://dx.doi.org/10.3892/ol.2018.8442] [PMID: 29805613]

[175] Zhang J, Kuang Y, Wang Y, Xu Q, Ren Q. Notch-4 silencing inhibits prostate cancer growth and EMT *via* the NF-κB pathway. Apoptosis 2017; 22(6): 877-84.
[http://dx.doi.org/10.1007/s10495-017-1368-0] [PMID: 28374086]

[176] Fukusumi T, Guo TW, Sakai A, *et al.* The *NOTCH4 – HEY1* Pathway Induces Epithelial–Mesenchymal Transition in Head and Neck Squamous Cell Carcinoma. Clin Cancer Res 2018; 24(3): 619-33.
[http://dx.doi.org/10.1158/1078-0432.CCR-17-1366] [PMID: 29146722]

[177] Qian C, Liu F, Ye B, Zhang X, Liang Y, Yao J. Notch4 promotes gastric cancer growth through activation of Wnt1/β-catenin signaling. Mol Cell Biochem 2015; 401(1-2): 165-74.

[http://dx.doi.org/10.1007/s11010-014-2304-z] [PMID: 25511451]

[178] Shagisultanova E, Gaponova AV, Gabbasov R, Nicolas E, Golemis EA. Preclinical and clinical studies of the NEDD9 scaffold protein in cancer and other diseases. Gene 2015; 567(1): 1-11.
[http://dx.doi.org/10.1016/j.gene.2015.04.086] [PMID: 25967390]

[179] Sima N, Cheng X, Ye F, Ma D, Xie X, Lü W. The overexpression of scaffolding protein NEDD9 promotes migration and invasion in cervical cancer *via* tyrosine phosphorylated FAK and SRC. PLoS One 2013; 8(9): e74594-4.
[http://dx.doi.org/10.1371/journal.pone.0074594] [PMID: 24058594]

[180] Zhao S, Min P, Liu L, *et al*. NEDD9 Facilitates Hypoxia-Induced Gastric Cancer Cell Migration *via* MICAL1 Related Rac1 Activation. Front Pharmacol 2019; 10: 291.
[http://dx.doi.org/10.3389/fphar.2019.00291] [PMID: 31019460]

[181] Liu J, Yu X, Yu H, *et al*. Knockdown of MAPK14 inhibits the proliferation and migration of clear cell renal cell carcinoma by downregulating the expression of CDC25B. Cancer Med 2020; 9(3): 1183-95.
[http://dx.doi.org/10.1002/cam4.2795] [PMID: 31856414]

[182] Planchard D, Camara-Clayette V, Dorvault N, Soria JC, Fouret P. p38 mitogen-activated protein kinase signaling, ERCC1 expression, and viability of lung cancer cells from never or light smoker patients. Cancer 2012; 118(20): 5015-25.
[http://dx.doi.org/10.1002/cncr.27510] [PMID: 22415779]

[183] Hedrick E, Safe S. Transforming Growth Factor β/NR4A1-Inducible Breast Cancer Cell Migration and Epithelial-to-Mesenchymal Transition Is p38α (Mitogen-Activated Protein Kinase 14) Dependent. Mol Cell Biol 2017; 37(18): e00306-17.
[http://dx.doi.org/10.1128/MCB.00306-17] [PMID: 28674186]

[184] Igea A, Nebreda AR. The Stress Kinase p38α as a Target for Cancer Therapy 2015.
[http://dx.doi.org/10.1158/0008-5472.CAN-15-0173]

[185] Zhang Z, Jiang D, Wang C, *et al*. Polymorphisms in oxidative stress pathway genes and prostate cancer risk. Cancer Causes Control 2019; 30(12): 1365-75.
[http://dx.doi.org/10.1007/s10552-019-01242-7] [PMID: 31667711]

[186] Chatterjee A, Gupta S. The multifaceted role of glutathione S-transferases in cancer. Cancer Lett 2018; 433: 33-42.
[http://dx.doi.org/10.1016/j.canlet.2018.06.028] [PMID: 29959055]

[187] Wang W, Liu F, Wang C, Wang C, Tang Y, Jiang Z. Glutathione S-transferase A1 mediates nicotine-induced lung cancer cell metastasis by promoting epithelial-mesenchymal transition. Exp Ther Med 2017; 14(2): 1783-8.
[http://dx.doi.org/10.3892/etm.2017.4663] [PMID: 28810650]

[188] Liu H, Yang Z, Zang L, *et al*. Downregulation of Glutathione S-transferase A1 suppressed tumor growth and induced cell apoptosis in A549 cell line. Oncol Lett 2018; 16(1): 467-74.
[http://dx.doi.org/10.3892/ol.2018.8608] [PMID: 29928434]

[189] McIlwain CC, Townsend DM, Tew KD. Glutathione S-transferase polymorphisms: cancer incidence and therapy. Oncogene 2006; 25(11): 1639-48.
[http://dx.doi.org/10.1038/sj.onc.1209373] [PMID: 16550164]

[190] Liu X, Sui X, Zhang C, *et al*. Glutathione S-transferase A1 suppresses tumor progression and indicates better prognosis of human primary hepatocellular carcinoma. J Cancer 2020; 11(1): 83-91.
[http://dx.doi.org/10.7150/jca.36495] [PMID: 31892975]

[191] Akhdar H, El Shamieh S, Musso O, *et al*. The rs3957357C>T SNP in GSTA1 Is Associated with a Higher Risk of Occurrence of Hepatocellular Carcinoma in European Individuals. PLoS One 2016; 11(12): e0167543-.
[http://dx.doi.org/10.1371/journal.pone.0167543] [PMID: 27936036]

[192] Chen MK, Tsai HT, Chung TT, *et al*. Glutathione S-transferase P1 and alpha gene variants; role in

susceptibility and tumor size development of oral cancer. Head Neck 2010; 32(8): 1079-87.
[http://dx.doi.org/10.1002/hed.21297] [PMID: 19953622]

[193]   Busby M, Hallett M, Plante I. The Complex Subtype-Dependent Role of Connexin 43 (GJA1) in Breast Cancer. Int J Mol Sci 2018; 19(3): 693.
[http://dx.doi.org/10.3390/ijms19030693] [PMID: 29495625]

[194]   Wang Y, Guo W, Xu H, *et al.* An extensive study of the mechanism of prostate cancer metastasis. Neoplasma 2018; 65(2): 253-61.
[http://dx.doi.org/10.4149/neo_2018_161217N648] [PMID: 29534587]

[195]   Falck E, Klinga-Levan K. Expression patterns of Phf5a/PHF5A and Gja1/GJA1 in rat and human endometrial cancer. Cancer Cell Int 2013; 13(1): 43.
[http://dx.doi.org/10.1186/1475-2867-13-43] [PMID: 23675859]

[196]   Ruch R. Connexin43 Suppresses Lung Cancer Stem Cells. Cancers (Basel) 2019; 11(2): 175.
[http://dx.doi.org/10.3390/cancers11020175] [PMID: 30717421]

[197]   Zhao X, Yu C, Zheng M, Sun J. Prognostic value of the mRNA expression of gap junction α members in patients with gastric cancer. Oncol Lett 2019; 18(2): 1669-78.
[http://dx.doi.org/10.3892/ol.2019.10516] [PMID: 31423234]

[198]   Mahmud I, Liao D. DAXX in cancer: phenomena, processes, mechanisms and regulation. Nucleic Acids Res 2019; 47(15): 7734-52.
[http://dx.doi.org/10.1093/nar/gkz634] [PMID: 31350900]

[199]   Wu C, Ding H, Wang S, *et al.* DAXX inhibits cancer stemness and epithelial–mesenchymal transition in gastric cancer. Br J Cancer 2020; 122(10): 1477-85.
[http://dx.doi.org/10.1038/s41416-020-0800-3] [PMID: 32203224]

Cancer Genes, 2023, *Vol. 1*, 223-242

CHAPTER 7

Chromosome 7

Muthu Vijai Bharath Vairamani[1], **Harini Hariharan**[1] and **Satish Ramalingam**[1,*]

[1] *Department of Genetic Engineering, School of Bioengineering, SRM Institute of Science and Technology, Kattankulathur, India*

Abstract: Chromosome 7 consists of 159 million base pairs, and around 950 genes, representing at least 5 percent of the entire DNA in a cell. Various genes that regulate cell division and cellular growth are present in Chromosome 7. Aberrations in these genes can therefore lead to tumorigenesis. Lymphomas and Leukemia have been frequently correlated with abnormalities on chromosome 7. Aberrations in chromosome 7, such as aneusomy in prostate cancer, gene amplifications in gastric cancer, and chromosomal gain in glioblastoma, are some of the starkly real ramifications of genetic abnormalities on chromosome 7. Numerous essential genes from Chromosome 7, including ABCB5, BRAF, CDK6, EGFR, ETV1, EZH2, IL6, and TWIST1, involved in cancer have been explained in this chapter.

Keywords: Liver cancer, Breast cancer, Colorectal cancer, Esophageal cancer, Gastric cancer, Leukemia, Lymphoma, Melanoma, Ovarian cancer, Pancreatic cancer, Prostate cancer, Renal cancer.

1.1. ABCB5 - ATP BINDING CASSETTE SUBFAMILY B MEMBER 5 LOCATION: CHROMOSOME 7; 7p21.1

This gene encodes for a member of the ATP-binding cassette [ABC] transporter superfamily of integral membrane proteins. These proteins participate in ATP-dependent transmembrane transport of structurally diverse molecules, ranging from small ions, sugars, and peptides to more complex organic molecules [1]. This ABCB5 protein is said to promote the invasiveness and metastasis of cancer cells in both breast and colorectal cancer [2, 3]. This protein has also been proven to regulate a Pro-Inflammatory Cytokine Signalling Circuit and thereby maintain melanoma-initiating cells [4].

---

* **Corresponding author Satish Ramalingam**: Department of Genetic Engineering, School of Bioengineering, SRM Institute of Science and Technology, Kattankulathur, India; E-mail: rsatish76@gmail.com

Satish Ramalingam (Ed.)

1.2. ACTB – ACTIN BETA LOCATION: CHROMOSOME 7; 7p22.1

This gene encodes one of six different actin proteins. Actins are highly conserved proteins involved in cell motility, structure, integrity, and intercellular signaling [5]. The ACTB protein has been used as a reference gene to measure the expression levels of many tumors. Abnormal expression of ACTB has also been reported in liver, melanoma, renal, colorectal, gastric, pancreatic, esophageal, lung, breast, prostate, ovarian cancers, leukemia and lymphoma. These abnormal levels of ACTB are said to improve the invasiveness of tumors and help in cancer metastasis [6 - 8].

1.3. AGR2 - ANTERIOR GRADIENT 2 LOCATION: CHROMOSOME 7; 7p21.1

This gene encodes a member of the disulfide isomerase [PDI] family of endoplasmic reticulum [ER] proteins that catalyze protein folding and thiol-disulfide interchange reactions. This protein plays a role in cell migration, cellular transformation, and metastasis and is a p53 inhibitor [9]. As a p53 inhibitor, ARG2 has been implicated in many cancers, including breast and non-small lung cancer, as a metastasis promoter [10 - 12].

1.4. AKAP9 - A-KINASE ANCHORING PROTEIN 9 LOCATION: CHROMOSOME 7; 7q21.2

The A-kinase anchor proteins [AKAPs] are a group of structurally diverse proteins with the everyday function of binding to the regulatory subunit of protein kinase A [PKA] and confining the holoenzyme to discrete locations within the cell. This gene encodes a member of the AKAP family [13]. AKAP9 proteins have been implicated in thyroid, colorectal, gastric, and breast cancer [14]. The gene resulting from the fusion of AKAP9 and BRAF has been said to activate thyroid cancer by manipulating the MAPK pathway [15].

1.5. AMPH – AMPHIPHYSIN LOCATION: CHROMOSOME 7; 7p14.1

This gene encodes a protein associated with the cytoplasmic surface of synaptic vesicles [16]. APMH is also a critical protein for breast cancer progression [17]. It is also said to manipulate the Ras-Raf-MEK-ERK signal pathway and originally acted as a tumor suppressor for non-small cell lung cancer. Still, mutations in the gene can help activate cancer [18].

1.6. AQP1 - AQUAPORIN 1 LOCATION: CHROMOSOME 7; 7p14.3

This gene encodes a small integral membrane protein with six bilayer-spanning domains that function as a water channel protein. This protein permits passive water transport along an osmotic gradient [19]. AQP1 is said to be overexpressed in both lung cancers and a particular subgroup of basal-like breast cancers [20, 21]. It was also observed that when AQP1 was knocked down in human ovarian cancer cells, it inhibited their growth and invasiveness [22].

1.7. BRAF - B-RAF PROTO-ONCOGENE, SERINE/THREONINE KINASE LOCATION: CHROMOSOME 7; 7q34

This gene encodes a protein belonging to the RAF family of serine/threonine protein kinases. This protein regulates the MAP kinase/ERK signaling pathway, which affects cell division, differentiation, and secretion [23]. The BRAF protein regulates the Ras-Raf-MEK-ERK signal pathway. Therefore, mutations in this gene lead to the progression of multiple cancer types [24]. Multiple cancer progression resulting from the fusion of AKAP9 and BRAF has been said to activate thyroid cancer by manipulating the MAPK pathway [15, 25].

1.8. CARD11 - CASPASE RECRUITMENT DOMAIN FAMILY MEMBER 11 LOCATION: CHROMOSOME 7; 7p22.2

The protein encoded by this gene (Fig. **1**) belongs to the membrane-associated guanylate kinase [MAGUK] family, a class of proteins that functions as molecular scaffolds for the assembly of multiprotein complexes at specialized regions of the plasma membrane [26]. Mutations in the CARD11 gene are responsible for the progression of Cutaneous Squamous Cell Carcinoma [27]. CARD11 has also been associated with Human Diffuse Large B Cell Lymphoma [28].

1.9. CCM2 - CCM2 SCAFFOLD PROTEIN LOCATION: CHROMOSOME 7; 7p13

This gene (Fig. **1**) encodes a scaffold protein that functions in the stress-activated p38 Mitogen-activated protein kinase [MAPK] signaling cascade. The protein interacts with SMAD-specific E3 ubiquitin-protein ligase 1 [also known as SMUR-F1] *via* a phosphotyrosine binding domain to promote RhoA degradation.

The protein is required for endothelial cell's normal cytoskeletal structure, cell-cell interactions, and lumen formation [29]. CCM2 has been implicated in the tumorigenesis of many cancers.

It is also hypothesized that the CCM2 protein can be a biomarker for various cancers [30].

Chromosome 7

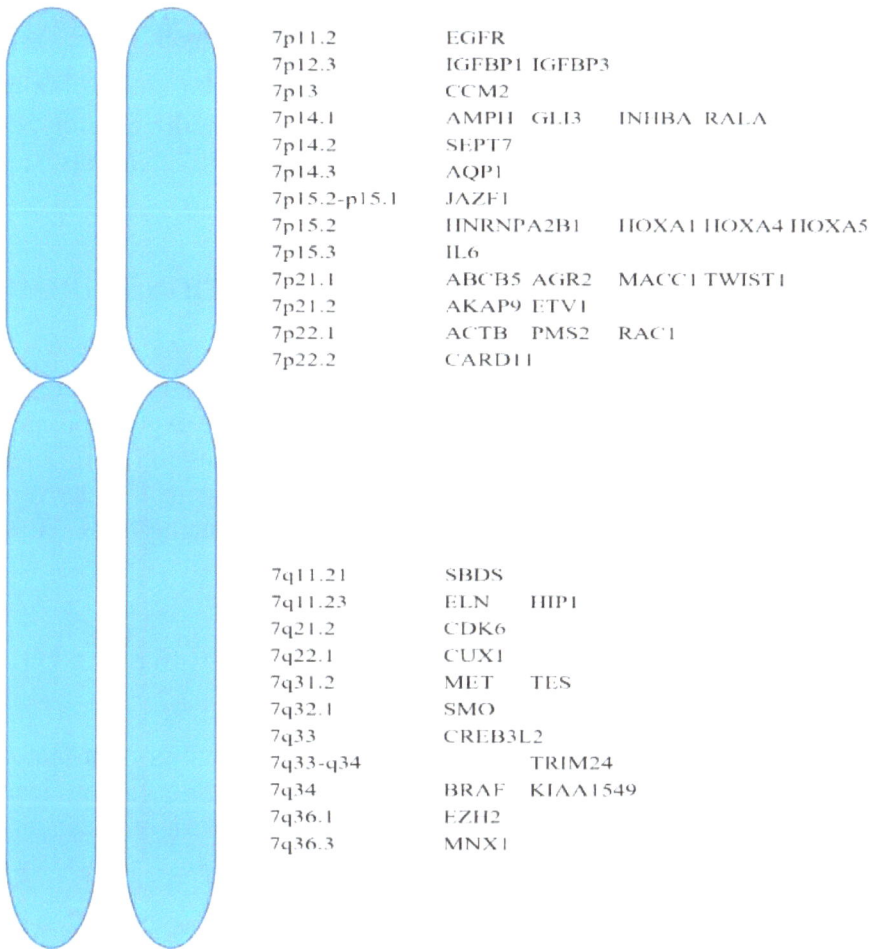

7p11.2	EGFR
7p12.3	IGFBP1 IGFBP3
7p13	CCM2
7p14.1	AMPH GLI3 INHBA RALA
7p14.2	SEPT7
7p14.3	AQP1
7p15.2-p15.1	JAZF1
7p15.2	HNRNPA2B1 HOXA1 HOXA4 HOXA5
7p15.3	IL6
7p21.1	ABCB5 AGR2 MACC1 TWIST1
7p21.2	AKAP9 ETV1
7p22.1	ACTB PMS2 RAC1
7p22.2	CARD11
7q11.21	SBDS
7q11.23	ELN HIP1
7q21.2	CDK6
7q22.1	CUX1
7q31.2	MET TES
7q32.1	SMO
7q33	CREB3L2
7q33-q34	TRIM24
7q34	BRAF KIAA1549
7q36.1	EZH2
7q36.3	MNX1

Fig. (1). This figure displays the loci of the genes from Chromosome 7 whose roles in cancer have been explained in this chapter. Sayooj Madhusoodanan designs this diagram.

1.10. CDK6 - CYCLIN-DEPENDENT KINASE 6 LOCATION: CHROMOSOME 7; 7q21.2

The protein encoded by this gene (Fig. **1**) is a member of the CMGC family of serine/threonine protein kinases. This kinase is a catalytic subunit of the protein kinase complex that is important for cell cycle G1 phase progression and G1/S transition [31]. CDK6 has been implicated in many cancers. It has also been the target for many cancer therapies like using Abemaciclib to inhibit CDK6 to fight against breast cancer, non–small cell lung cancer, and other solid tumors [32, 33].

1.11. CREB3L2 - CAMP RESPONSIVE ELEMENT BINDING PROTEIN THREE LIKE 2 LOCATION: CHROMOSOME 7; 7q33

This gene (Fig. **1**) encodes a member of the oasis bZIP transcription factor family. Members of this family can dimerize but form homodimers only. The encoded protein is a transcriptional activator [34]. The CREB3L2 gene has been implicated in sarcomas and skin cancer [35].

1.12. CUX1 - CUT LIKE HOMEOBOX 1 LOCATION: CHROMOSOME 7; 7q22.1

The protein encoded by this gene (Fig. **1**) is a member of the homeodomain family of DNA-binding proteins. It may regulate gene expression, morphogenesis and differentiation and play a role in cell cycle progression [36]. The CUX1 gene is a haplo-insufficiently expressed tumor suppressor gene that is overexpressed in certain advanced cancers [37]. But targeting and silencing these CUX1 mutations also seem to promote tumorigenesis [38].

1.13. EGFR - EPIDERMAL GROWTH FACTOR RECEPTOR LOCATION: CHROMOSOME 7; 7p11.2

EGFR is a cell surface protein that binds to epidermal growth factor, thus inducing receptor dimerization and tyrosine autophosphorylation leading to cell proliferation. Mutations in this gene are associated with lung cancer [39]. EGFR signaling has been associated with lung, esophageal, colorectal, cervical, and brain tumors [40, 41].

1.14. ELN – ELASTIN LOCATION: CHROMOSOME 7; 7q11.23

This gene (Fig. **1**) encodes a protein that is one of the two components of elastic fibers. Elastic fibers comprise part of the extracellular matrix and confer elasticity to organs and tissues, including the heart, skin, lungs, ligaments, and blood vessels [42]. Elastin is a critical factor in tumor development in colorectal cancer [43].

1.15. ETV1 - ETS VARIANT TRANSCRIPTION FACTOR 1 LOCATION: CHROMOSOME 7; 7p21.2

This gene encodes a member of the ETS [E twenty-six] family of transcription factors. The ETS proteins regulate many target genes that modulate biological processes like cell growth, angiogenesis, migration, proliferation, and diffe-rentiation [44]. ETV1 has been implicated in prostate cancer and melanomas [45, 46]. It is said to improve the metastasis capabilities of pancreatic cancer cells [47].

1.16. EZH2 - ENHANCER OF ZESTE 2 POLYCOMB REPRESSIVE COMPLEX 2 SUBUNIT LOCATION: CHROMOSOME 7; 7q36.1

This gene encodes a member of the Polycomb-group [PcG] family. PcG family members form multimeric protein complexes, which maintain the trans-criptionally repressive state of genes over successive cell generations. This protein is associated with the embryonic ectoderm development protein, the VAV1 oncoprotein, and the X-linked nuclear protein [48]. The EZH2 protein has been implicated in a wide range of cancers for tumorigenesis [49]. It has also been the target for cancer treatment [50, 51].

1.17. GLI3 - GLI FAMILY ZINC FINGER 3 LOCATION: CHROMOSOME 7; 7p14.1

This gene encodes a protein that belongs to the C2H2-type zinc finger proteins subclass of the Gli family. They are DNA-binding transcription factors and mediators of Sonic hedgehog [Shh] signaling [52]. GLI3 has been implicated in pancreatic and cervical cancers [53]. It has also been found that suppressing the GLI3 gene reduces cancer progression [54].

1.18. HIP1 - HUNTINGTIN INTERACTING PROTEIN 1 LOCATION: CHROMOSOME 7; 7q11.23

This gene is a membrane-associated protein that functions in clathrin-mediated endocytosis and protein trafficking within the cell. The encoded protein binds to the huntingtin protein in the brain; this interaction is lost in Huntington's disease [55]. The HIP1 protein has been implemented in prostate and colon cancer [56]. It has also been expressed as a fusion gene with ALK in non-small cell lung cancer [57]. Furthermore, suppressing the HIP1 gene is an effective cancer treatment in prostate cancer [58].

1.19. HNRNPA2B1 - HETEROGENEOUS NUCLEAR RIBONUCLEOPR-OTEIN A2/B1 LOCATION: CHROMOSOME 7; 7p15.2

This gene belongs to the A/B subfamily of ubiquitously expressed heterogeneous nuclear ribonucleoproteins [hnRNPs]. The hnRNPs are RNA-binding proteins, complex with heterogeneous nuclear RNA [hnRNA]. These proteins are associated with pre-mRNAs in the nucleus and appear to influence pre-mRNA processing and other aspects of mRNA metabolism and transport [59]. This gene has been implicated as an EMT promoter in pancreatic cancer by regulating the ERK/snail signaling pathway [60]. It has also been overexpressed in lung and ovarian cancer [61, 62].

1.20. HOXA1 - HOMEOBOX A1 LOCATION: CHROMOSOME 7; 7p15.2

Along with other HOXA genes, this gene encodes the class of transcription factors called homeobox genes, found in clusters A, B, C, and D on four separate chromosomes. The expression of these proteins is spatially and temporally regulated during embryonic development [63]. The over-expression of the HOXA1 gene has been found to promote cell proliferation, invasion, and metastasis in prostate cancer [64]. It has also been implicated in small cell cancer and gastric cancer [65, 66].

1.21. HOXA4 - HOMEOBOX A4 LOCATION: CHROMOSOME 7; 7p15.2

This gene, along with other HOXA genes, encodes transcription factors called homeobox genes, found in clusters A and D on four separate chromosomes. The expression of these proteins is spatially and temporally regulated during embryonic development [67]. It has been found that the downregulation of HOXA4 in Lung cancer inhibits the growth, motility, and invasion of the cancer cells [68]. It has also been found that its overexpression promotes self-renewal and contributes to colon cancer stem cell overpopulation [69].

1.22. HOXA5 - HOMEOBOX A5 LOCATION: CHROMOSOME 7; 7p15.2

Along with other HOXA genes, this gene encodes the class of transcription factors called homeobox genes, found in clusters A, B, C, and D on four separate chromosomes. The expression of these proteins is spatially and temporally regulated during embryonic development [70]. HOXA5 has been found to alter the homeostasis of p53 in breast cancer by binding to the anti-apoptotic protein Twist [71]. It also regulates the plasticity of lung cancer stem-like cells [72].

1.23. IGFBP1 - INSULININSULIN-LIKE FACTOR BINDING PROTEIN 1 LOCATION: CHROMOSOME 7; 7p12.3

This gene is a member of the insulin-like growth factor binding protein [IGFBP] family and encodes a protein with an IGFBP N-terminal domain and a thyroglobulin type-I domain. The encoded protein, mainly expressed in the liver, circulates in the plasma and binds insulin-like growth factors [IGFs] I and II, prolonging their half-lives and altering their interaction with cell surface receptors [73]. This gene is a predictive factor for hematogenous metastasis in gastric cancer [74]. It has also been implicated in prostate and ovarian cancer [75, 76].

1.24. IGFBP3 - INSULIN-LIKE GROWTH FACTOR BINDING PROTEIN 3 LOCATION: CHROMOSOME 7; 7p12.3

This gene is a member of the insulin-like growth factor binding protein [IGFBP] family and encodes a protein with an IGFBP domain and a thyroglobulin type-I domain. The protein forms a ternary complex with an insulin-like growth factor acid-labile subunit [IGFALS] and either insulin-like growth factor [IGF] I or II [77]. It has been found that the tumor suppressor protein p53 interacts with IGFBP3 to induce apoptosis [78]. So, mutations in the p53 gene can cause overexpression of the IGFBP3 protein and lead to cancer. This protein has also been said to have an essential role in cancer initiation in breast cancer [79].

1.25. IL6 - INTERLEUKIN 6 LOCATION: CHROMOSOME 7; 7p15.3

This gene encodes a cytokine that functions in inflammation and the maturation of B cells. In addition, the encoded protein is an endogenous pyrogen capable of inducing fever in people with autoimmune diseases or infections. The protein is primarily produced at sites of acute and chronic inflammation [80]. IL6 has been found overexpressed in almost all cancer types. It promotes tumorigenesis by regulating all hallmarks of cancer and multiple signaling pathways, including apoptosis, survival, proliferation, angiogenesis, less metastasis, and, most importantly, metabolism [81 - 83].

1.26. INHBA - INHIBIN SUBUNIT BETA A LOCATION: CHROMOSOME 7; 7p14.1

This gene encodes a member of the TGF-be proteins TGF-beta [transforming growth factor-beta] superfamily encoded preproprotein and is proteolytically processed to generate a subunit of the dimeric activin and inhibin protein complexes. These complexes activate and inhibit respele stimulating hormone secretion from the pituitary gland [84]. The INBHA protein has been associated with gastric and colorectal cancers [85]. It has also been noted that the silencing of INHBA inhibits gastric cancer cell migration and invasion by impeding activation of the TGF-β signaling pathway [86].

1.27. JAZF1 - JAZF ZINC FINGER 1 LOCATION: CHROMOSOME 7; 7P15.2-p15.1

This gene encodes a nuclear protein with three C2H2-type zinc fingers and functions as a transcriptional repressor. Chromosomal aberrations involving this genes are associated with endometrial stromal tumors [87]. The fusion of JAZF1 and BCORL1 has been observed in endometrial stromal sarcoma [88]. It is also said to promote prostate cancer progression by regulating the JNK/Slug pathway, and I also implicated in gastric cancers [89, 90].

1.28. KIAA1549 - KIAA1549 PROTEIN LOCATION: CHROMOSOME 7; 7q34

The protein encoded by this gene belongs to the UPF0606 family. This gene is fused to the BRAF oncogene in many cases of pilocytic astrocytoma [91, 92]. The fused KIAA149-BRAF gene has also been observed in other brain tumors like Pediatric Low-Grade Astrocytomas and Pediatric Low-Grade Gliomas [93, 94].

1.29. MACC1 - MET TRANSCRIPTIONAL REGULATOR MACC1 LOCATION: CHROMOSOME 7; 7p21.1

MACC1 is a key regulator of the hepatocyte growth factor [HGF] receptor pathway, which is involved in cellular growth, epithelial-mesenchymal transition, angiogenesis, cell motility, invasiveness, and metastasis. MACC1 has been implicated in many cancers because of its role as an HGF receptor pathway regulator [95]. The overexpression of MACC1 has been associated with cancer progression in breast cancers [96]. Furthermore, it has been found that circulating MACC1 can be used as a novel diagnostic and prognostic biomarker for non-small cell lung cancer [97]. MACC1 has also been identified as a novel target for solid tumors [98].

1.30. MET - MET PROTO-ONCOGENE, RECEPTOR TYROSINE KINASE LOCATION: CHROMOSOME 7; 7q31.2

This gene encodes a member of the receptor tyrosine kinase family of proteins and the product of the proto-oncogene MET. The binding of its ligand, the hepatocyte growth factor, induces dimerization and activation of the receptor, which plays a role in cellular survival, embryogenesis, and cellular migration and invasion [99]. Mutations in this gene are associated with papillary renal cell carcinoma, hepatocellular carcinoma, and various head and neck cancers. The MET protein is a novel target for cancer therapy [100, 101].

1.31. MNX1 - MOTOR NEURON AND PANCREAS HOMEOBOX 1 LOCATION: CHROMOSOME 7; 7q36.3

This gene encodes a nuclear protein, which contains a homeobox domain and is a transcription factor. Mutations in this gene result in Currarino syndrome, an autosomal dominant congenital malformation [102]. The MNX1 protein is onto-genically upregulated in prostate cancer [103]. It has also been found that the fusion of the MNX1 and AS1 induces EMT in breast cancer [104]. It was also found that the knockdown of the long noncoding RNA MNX1-AS1 inhibits cell proliferation and migration in ovarian cancer [105].

1.32. PMS2 - PMS1 HOMOLOG 2, MISMATCH REPAIR SYSTEM COMPONENT LOCATION: CHROMOSOME 7; 7p22.1

The protein encoded by this gene is a key component of the mismatch repair system that functions to correct DNA mismatches and small insertions and deletions that can occur during DNA replication and homologous recombination [106]. Mutations in the PMS2 protein have been implicated in colorectal cancers through Immuno-histochemical analysis [107]. PMS2 protein defects have also been implicated in Lynch syndrome-associated cancers [108].

1.33. RAC1 - RAC FAMILY SMALL GTPASE 1 LOCATION: CHROMOSOME 7; 7p22.1

The protein encoded by this gene is a GTPase which belongs to the RAS superfamily of small GTP-binding proteins. Members of this superfamily appear to regulate a diverse array of cellular events, including the control of cell growth, cytoskeletal reorganization, and the activation of protein kinases [109]. The overexpression of RAC1 has been found in breast cancers [110]. This protein is said to promote cancer metastasis by regulating the Twist1 [111]. Therefore, RAC1 has been a potential target for cancer therapy for targeting cancer angio-genesis and metastasis [112].

1.34. RALA - RAS LIKE PROTO-ONCOGENE A LOCATION: CHROMOSOME 7; 7p14.1

The product of this gene belongs to the small GTPase superfamily, the Ras family of proteins. GTP-binding proteins mediate the transmembrane signaling initiated by the occupancy of certain cell surface receptors [113]. RALA has been implicated in several cancers, such as colorectal cancer, ovarian cancer and non-small cell lung cancer [114]. Furthermore, the inhibition of the RALA pathway has been crucial in non-small cell lung cancer treatment [115]. It has also been determined that the activation of RALA is a necessary part of cancer tumorigenesis in humans [116].

1.35. SBDS - SBDS RIBOSOME MATURATION FACTOR LOCATION: CHROMOSOME 7; 7q11.21

This gene encodes a highly conserved protein that plays an essential role in ribosome biogenesis. Mutations within this gene are associated with the auto-somal recessive disorder Shwachman-Bodian-Diamond syndrome [117]. SBDS has been implicated in the bad prognosis of a broad spectrum of cancers as it is said to regulate the P53 tumor suppression protein [118].

1.36. SEPT7 - SEPTIN 7 LOCATION: CHROMOSOME 7; 7p14.2

This gene encodes a protein that is highly similar to the CDC10 protein of Saccharomyces cerevisiae. This human protein functions in gliomagenesis and the suppression of glioma cell growth, and it is required for the association of centromere-associated protein E with the kinetochore [119]. It has been found that human breast cancer cells require MEK/ERK activation, which is regulated by the SEPT7 protein [120]. It has also been found that the downregulation of SEPT7 leads to suppressed cell growth in hepatocellular carcinomas [121].

1.37. SMO - SMOOTHENED, FRIZZLED CLASS RECEPTOR LOCATION: CHROMOSOME 7; 7q32.1

The protein encoded by this gene is a G protein-coupled receptor that interacts with the patched protein, a receptor for hedgehog proteins. The encoded protein transduces signals to other proteins after activation by a hedgehog protein/patched protein complex [122]. The inhibition of SMO has been found to modulate Cellular Plasticity and Invasiveness in Colorectal Cancer [123]. It has also been found that SMO can be used to inhibit breast cancer cells by targeting the Hedgehog/PLI pathway [124].

1.38. TES - TESTIN LIM DOMAIN PROTEIN LOCATION: CHROMOSOME 7; 7q31.2

This protein is a negative regulator of cell growth and may act as a tumor suppressor. This scaffold protein may also play a role in cell adhesion, cell spreading, and the reorganization of the actin cytoskeleton [125]. The expression of the TES protein is high in epithelial ovarian cancer [126]. It is also worth noting that the regulation of TES protein by CFP suppresses the growth of breast cancer cells [127].

1.39. TRIM24 - TRIPARTITE MOTIF-CONTAINING 24 LOCATION: CHROMOSOME 7; 7Q33-q34

The protein encoded by this gene mediates transcriptional control by interaction with the activation function 2 [AF2] region of several nuclear receptors, including the estrogen, retinoic acid, and vitamin D3 receptors. The protein localizes to nuclear bodies and is thought to associate with chromatin and heterochromatin-associated factors. The protein is a member of the tripartite motif [TRIM] family [128]. TRIM24 has been implicated in a wide variety of cancers [129]. It is said to link a non-canonical histone signature to breast cancer and is said to be an Oncogenic Transcriptional Activator in Prostate Cancer [130, 131].

1.40. TWIST1 - TWIST FAMILY BHLH TRANSCRIPTION FACTOR 1 LOCATION: CHROMOSOME 7; 7p21.1

This gene encodes a basic helix-loop-helix [bHLH] transcription factor that plays an important role in embryonic development. The encoded protein forms both homodimers and heterodimers that bind to DNA E box sequences and regulate the transcription of genes involved in cranial suture closure during skull development [132]. This TWIST1 protein has been implicated in a lot of cancers since it is used to regulate the TWIST1 pathway. TWIST1 is the key regulator of cancer-associated fibroblasts [133]. It has also been implicated in the tumor progression of breast cancer [134].

CONCLUSION

So far, research has elucidated many genes on chromosome 7 associated with cancer initiation, progression, and metastasis. The underlying mechanisms of cancer can be further explicated by focusing on the abrupt intra-cellular changes caused by the mutations in these genes in a cancerous cell.

More research is yet to be conducted to discover new genes on Chromosome 7, which may play more critical roles in fostering carcinogenesis.

REFERENCES

[1]   ABCB5 ATP binding cassette subfamily B member 5 [Homo sapiens (human)] - Gene - NCBI, https://www.ncbi.nlm.nih.gov/gene/340273 (accessed 17 January 2021).

[2]   Yao J, Yao X, Tian T, *et al.* ABCB5-ZEB1 axis promotes invasion and metastasis in breast cancer cells. Oncol Res 2017; 25(3): 305-16.
[http://dx.doi.org/10.3727/096504016X14734149559061] [PMID: 28281973]

[3]   Guo Q, Grimmig T, Gonzalez G, *et al.* ATP-binding cassette member B5 (ABCB5) promotes tumor cell invasiveness in human colorectal cancer. J Biol Chem 2018; 293(28): 11166-78.
[http://dx.doi.org/10.1074/jbc.RA118.003187] [PMID: 29789423]

[4]   Wilson BJ, Saab KR, Ma J, *et al.* ABCB5 maintains melanoma-initiating cells through a proinflammatory cytokine signaling circuit. Cancer Res 2014; 74(15): 4196-207.
[http://dx.doi.org/10.1158/0008-5472.CAN-14-0582] [PMID: 24934811]

[5]   ACTB actin beta [Homo sapiens (human)] - Gene - NCBI https://www.ncbi.nlm.nih.gov/gene/60 (accessed 17 January 2021).

[6]   Guo C, Liu S, Wang J, Sun MZ, Greenaway FT. ACTB in cancer. Clin Chim Acta 2013; 417: 39-44.
[http://dx.doi.org/10.1016/j.cca.2012.12.012] [PMID: 23266771]

[7]   Majidzadeh-A K, Esmaeili R, Abdoli N. TFRC and ACTB as the best reference genes to quantify Urokinase Plasminogen Activator in breast cancer. BMC Res Notes 2011; 4(1): 215.
[http://dx.doi.org/10.1186/1756-0500-4-215] [PMID: 21702980]

[8]   Walter RFH, Werner R, Vollbrecht C, *et al.* ACTB, CDKN1B, GAPDH, GRB2, RHOA and SDCBP Were Identified as Reference Genes in Neuroendocrine Lung Cancer *via* the nCounter Technology. PLoS One 2016; 11(11): e0165181.
[http://dx.doi.org/10.1371/journal.pone.0165181] [PMID: 27802291]

[9]   AGR2 anterior gradient 2, protein disulphide isomerase family member [Homo sapiens (human)] - Gene - NCBI, https://www.ncbi.nlm.nih.gov/gene/10551 (accessed 17 January 2021).

[10]   Digitum: Repositorio Institucional de la Universidad de Murcia: Expression of AGR2 in non small cell lung cancer, https://digitum.um.es/digitum/handle/10201/27610 (accessed 17 January 2021).

[11]   Fritzsche FR, Dahl E, Pahl S, *et al.* Prognostic relevance of AGR2 expression in breast cancer. Clin Cancer Res 2006; 12(6): 1728-34.
[http://dx.doi.org/10.1158/1078-0432.CCR-05-2057] [PMID: 16551856]

[12]   Innes HE, Liu D, Barraclough R, *et al.* Significance of the metastasis-inducing protein AGR2 for outcome in hormonally treated breast cancer patients. Br J Cancer 2006; 94(7): 1057-65.
[http://dx.doi.org/10.1038/sj.bjc.6603065] [PMID: 16598187]

[13]   AKAP9 A-kinase anchoring protein 9 [Homo sapiens (human)] - Gene - NCBI, https://www.ncbi.nlm.nih.gov/gene/10142 (accessed 17 January 2021).

[14]   Hu ZY, Liu YP, Xie LY, *et al.* AKAP-9 promotes colorectal cancer development by regulating Cdc42 interacting protein 4. Biochim Biophys Acta Mol Basis Dis 2016; 1862(6): 1172-81.
[http://dx.doi.org/10.1016/j.bbadis.2016.03.012] [PMID: 27039663]

[15]   Ciampi R, Knauf JA, Kerler R, *et al.* Oncogenic AKAP9-BRAF fusion is a novel mechanism of MAPK pathway activation in thyroid cancer. J Clin Invest 2005; 115(1): 94-101.
[http://dx.doi.org/10.1172/JCI23237] [PMID: 15630448]

[16]   AMPH amphiphysin [Homo sapiens (human)] - Gene - NCBI, https://www.ncbi.nlm.nih.gov/gene/273 (accessed 17 January 2021).

[17]   Chen Y, Liu J, Li L, Xia H, Lin Z, Zhong T. AMPH-1 is critical for breast cancer progression. J Cancer 2018; 9(12): 2175-82.
[http://dx.doi.org/10.7150/jca.25428] [PMID: 29937937]

[18]   Yang H, Wan Z, Huang C, Yin H, Song D. AMPH-1 is a tumor suppressor of lung cancer by inhibiting Ras-Raf-MEK-ERK signal pathway. Lasers Med Sci 2019; 34(3): 473-8.
[http://dx.doi.org/10.1007/s10103-018-2616-4] [PMID: 30143925]

[19]   AQP1 aquaporin 1 (Colton blood group) [Homo sapiens (human)] - Gene - NCBI, https://www.ncbi.nlm.nih.gov/gene/358 (accessed 17 January 2021).

[20]   Otterbach F, Callies R, Adamzik M, *et al.* Aquaporin 1 (AQP1) expression is a novel characteristic feature of a particularly aggressive subgroup of basal-like breast carcinomas. Breast Cancer Res Treat 2010; 120(1): 67-76.
[http://dx.doi.org/10.1007/s10549-009-0370-9] [PMID: 19306058]

[21]   Hoque MO, Soria JC, Woo J, *et al.* Aquaporin 1 is overexpressed in lung cancer and stimulates NIH-3T3 cell proliferation and anchorage-independent growth. Am J Pathol 2006; 168(4): 1345-53.
[http://dx.doi.org/10.2353/ajpath.2006.050596] [PMID: 16565507]

[22]   Wang Y, Fan Y, Zheng C, Zhang X. Knockdown of AQP1 inhibits growth and invasion of human ovarian cancer cells. Mol Med Rep 2017; 16(4): 5499-504.
[http://dx.doi.org/10.3892/mmr.2017.7282] [PMID: 28849036]

[23]   BRAF B-Raf proto-oncogene, serine/threonine kinase [Homo sapiens (human)] - Gene - NCBI, https://www.ncbi.nlm.nih.gov/gene/673 (accessed 17 January 2021).

[24]   Davies H, Bignell GR, Cox C, *et al.* Mutations of the BRAF gene in human cancer. Nature 2002; 417(6892): 949-54.
[http://dx.doi.org/10.1038/nature00766] [PMID: 12068308]

[25]   Xing M. BRAF mutation in thyroid cancer. Endocr Relat Cancer 2005; 12(2): 245-62.
[http://dx.doi.org/10.1677/erc.1.0978] [PMID: 15947100]

[26]   CARD11 caspase recruitment domain family member 11 [Homo sapiens (human)] - Gene - NCBI, https://www.ncbi.nlm.nih.gov/gene/84433 (accessed 17 January 2021).

[27]   Watt SA, Purdie KJ, den Breems NY, *et al.* Novel CARD11 Mutations in Human Cutaneous Squamous Cell Carcinoma Lead to Aberrant NF-κB Regulation. Am J Pathol 2015; 185(9): 2354-63.
[http://dx.doi.org/10.1016/j.ajpath.2015.05.018] [PMID: 26212909]

[28]   Lenz G, Davis RE, Ngo VN, et al. Oncogenic CARD11 mutations in human diffuse large B cell lymphoma. Science (80-) 2008; 319: 1676–1679.

[29]   CCM2 CCM2 scaffold protein [Homo sapiens (human)] - Gene - NCBI, https: //www. ncbi.nlm.nih.gov/gene/ 83605 (accessed 17 January 2021).

[30]   Abou-Fadel J, Qu Y, Gonzalez E, Smith M, Zhang J. Emerging roles of CCM genes during tumorigenesis with potential application as novel biomarkers across major types of cancers. Oncol Rep 2020; 43(6): 1945-63.
[http://dx.doi.org/10.3892/or.2020.7550] [PMID: 32186778]

[31]   CDK6 cyclin dependent kinase 6 [Homo sapiens (human)]-Gene-NCBI, https://www.ncbi.nlm.nih.gov/gene/1021 (accessed 17 January 2021).

[32]   Tadesse S, Yu M, Kumarasiri M, Le BT, Wang S. Targeting CDK6 in cancer: State of the art and new insights. Cell Cycle 2015; 14(20): 3220-30.
[http://dx.doi.org/10.1080/15384101.2015.1084445] [PMID: 26315616]

[33]   Patnaik A, Rosen LS, Tolaney SM, *et al.* Efficacy and safety of Abemaciclib, an inhibitor of CDK4 and CDK6, for patients with breast cancer, non–small cell lung cancer, and other solid tumors. Cancer Discov 2016; 6(7): 740-53.
[http://dx.doi.org/10.1158/2159-8290.CD-16-0095] [PMID: 27217383]

[34]   CREB3L2 cAMP responsive element binding protein 3 like 2 [Homo sapiens (human)] - Gene - NCBI, https://www.ncbi.nlm.nih.gov/gene/64764 (accessed 17 January 2021).

[35]   Möller E, Hornick JL, Magnusson L, Veerla S, Domanski HA, Mertens F. FUS-CREB3L2/L1-positive
       sarcomas show a specific gene expression profile with upregulation of CD24 and FOXL1. Clin Cancer
       Res 2011; 17(9): 2646-56.
       [http://dx.doi.org/10.1158/1078-0432.CCR-11-0145] [PMID: 21536545]

[36]   CUX1 cut like homeobox 1 [Homo sapiens (human)]-Gene-NCBI, https://www.ncbi.nlm.
       nih.gov/gene/1523 (accessed 17 January 2021).

[37]   Ramdzan ZM, Nepveu A. CUX1, a haploinsufficient tumour suppressor gene overexpressed in
       advanced cancers. Nat Rev Cancer 2014; 14(10): 673-82.
       [http://dx.doi.org/10.1038/nrc3805] [PMID: 25190083]

[38]   Wong CC, Martincorena I, Rust AG, *et al.* Inactivating CUX1 mutations promote tumorigenesis. Nat
       Genet 2014; 46(1): 33-8.
       [http://dx.doi.org/10.1038/ng.2846] [PMID: 24316979]

[39]   EGFR epidermal growth factor receptor [Homo sapiens (human)]-Gene-NCBI, https://www.ncbi.
       nlm.nih.gov/gene/1956 (accessed 17 January 2021).

[40]   Seshacharyulu P, Ponnusamy MP, Haridas D, Jain M, Ganti AK, Batra SK. Targeting the EGFR
       signaling pathway in cancer therapy. Expert Opin Ther Targets 2012; 16(1): 15-31.
       [http://dx.doi.org/10.1517/14728222.2011.648617] [PMID: 22239438]

[41]   Yarden Y. The EGFR family and its ligands in human cancer. Eur J Cancer 2001; 37 (Suppl. 4): 3-8.
       [http://dx.doi.org/10.1016/S0959-8049(01)00230-1] [PMID: 11597398]

[42]   Tassabehji M, Metcalfe K, Donnai D, *et al.* Elastin: genomic structure and point mutations in patients
       with supravalvular aortic stenosis. Hum Mol Genet 1997; 6(7): 1029-36.
       [http://dx.doi.org/10.1093/hmg/6.7.1029] [PMID: 9215671]

[43]   Li J, Xu X, Jiang Y, *et al.* Elastin is a key factor of tumor development in colorectal cancer. BMC
       Cancer 2020; 20(1): 217.
       [http://dx.doi.org/10.1186/s12885-020-6686-x] [PMID: 32171282]

[44]   ETV1 ETS variant transcription factor 1 [Homo sapiens (human)]-Gene -NCBI, https://www.ncbi.
       nlm.nih.gov/gene/2115 (accessed 26 January 2021).

[45]   Jané-Valbuena J, Widlund HR, Perner S, *et al.* An oncogenic role for ETV1 in melanoma. Cancer Res
       2010; 70(5): 2075-84.
       [http://dx.doi.org/10.1158/0008-5472.CAN-09-3092] [PMID: 20160028]

[46]   Baena E, Shao Z, Linn DE, *et al.* ETV1 directs androgen metabolism and confers aggressive prostate
       cancer in targeted mice and patients. Genes Dev 2013; 27(6): 683-98.
       [http://dx.doi.org/10.1101/gad.211011.112] [PMID: 23512661]

[47]   Heeg S, Das KK, Reichert M, *et al.* ETS-Transcription Factor ETV1 Regulates Stromal Expansion and
       Metastasis in Pancreatic Cancer. Gastroenterology 2016; 151(3): 540-553.e14.
       [http://dx.doi.org/10.1053/j.gastro.2016.06.005] [PMID: 27318148]

[48]   EZH2 enhancer of zeste 2 polycomb repressive complex 2 subunit [Homo sapiens (human)] - Gene -
       NCBI, https://www.ncbi.nlm.nih.gov/gene/2146 (accessed 26 January 2021).

[49]   Chang C-J, Hung M-C. The role of EZH2 in tumour progression. Br J Cancer 2012; 106(2): 243-7.
       [http://dx.doi.org/10.1038/bjc.2011.551] [PMID: 22187039]

[50]   Duan R, Du W, Guo W. EZH2: a novel target for cancer treatment. J Hematol Oncol. 2020; 13(1):
       104.
       [http://dx.doi.org/10.1186/s13045-020-00937-8]

[51]   Yamagishi M, Uchimaru K. Targeting EZH2 in cancer therapy. Curr Opin Oncol 2017; 29(5): 375-81.
       [http://dx.doi.org/10.1097/CCO.0000000000000390] [PMID: 28665819]

[52]   GLI3 GLI family zinc finger 3 [Homo sapiens (human)]-Gene-NCBI https://www.ncbi.nlm.nih.

gov/gene/2737 (accessed 26 January 2021).

[53]   Steg A, Amm HM, Novak Z, Frost AR, Johnson MR. Gli3 mediates cell survival and sensitivity to cyclopamine in pancreatic cancer. Cancer Biol Ther 2010; 10(9): 893-902.
[http://dx.doi.org/10.4161/cbt.10.9.13252] [PMID: 20814245]

[54]   Wen S-Y, Lin Y, Yu Y-Q, *et al.* miR-506 acts as a tumor suppressor by directly targeting the hedgehog pathway transcription factor Gli3 in human cervical cancer. Oncogene 2015; 34(6): 717-25.
[http://dx.doi.org/10.1038/onc.2014.9] [PMID: 24608427]

[55]   HIP1 huntingtin interacting protein 1 [Homo sapiens (human)]-Gene-NCBI, https://www.ncbi.nlm.nih.gov/gene/3092 (accessed 27 January 2021).

[56]   Rao DS, Hyun TS, Kumar PD, *et al.* Huntingtin-interacting protein 1 is overexpressed in prostate and colon cancer and is critical for cellular survival. J Clin Invest 2002; 110(3): 351-60.
[http://dx.doi.org/10.1172/JCI0215529] [PMID: 12163454]

[57]   Ou SHI, Klempner SJ, Greenbowe JR, *et al.* Identification of a novel HIP1-ALK fusion variant in Non-Small-Cell Lung Cancer (NSCLC) and discovery of ALK I1171 (I1171N/S) mutations in two ALK-rearranged NSCLC patients with resistance to Alectinib. J Thorac Oncol 2014; 9(12): 1821-5.
[http://dx.doi.org/10.1097/JTO.0000000000000368] [PMID: 25393796]

[58]   Rotundo F, Cominetti D, El Bezawy R, *et al.* *miR-1272* Exerts Tumor-Suppressive Functions in Prostate Cancer *via HIP1* Suppression. Cells 2020; 9(2): 435.
[http://dx.doi.org/10.3390/cells9020435] [PMID: 32069895]

[59]   HNRNPA2B1 heterogeneous nuclear ribonucleoprotein A2/B1 [Homo sapiens (human)] - Gene - NCBI, https://www.ncbi.nlm.nih.gov/gene/3181 (accessed 27 January 2021).

[60]   Dai S, Zhang J, Huang S, *et al.* HNRNPA2B1 regulates the epithelial–mesenchymal transition in pancreatic cancer cells through the ERK/snail signalling pathway. Cancer Cell Int 2017; 17(1): 12.
[http://dx.doi.org/10.1186/s12935-016-0368-4] [PMID: 28077929]

[61]   Yang Y, Wei Q, Tang Y, *et al.* Loss of hnRNPA2B1 inhibits malignant capability and promotes apoptosis *via* down-regulating Lin28B expression in ovarian cancer. Cancer Lett 2020; 475: 43-52.
[http://dx.doi.org/10.1016/j.canlet.2020.01.029] [PMID: 32006618]

[62]   Dowling P, Pollard D, Larkin A, *et al.* Abnormal levels of heterogeneous nuclear ribonucleoprotein A2B1 (hnRNPA2B1) in tumour tissue and blood samples from patients diagnosed with lung cancer. Mol Biosyst 2015; 11(3): 743-52.
[http://dx.doi.org/10.1039/C4MB00384E] [PMID: 25483567]

[63]   HOXA1 homeobox A1 [Homo sapiens (human)]-Gene-NCBI, https://www.ncbi.nlm.nih.gov/gene/3198 (accessed 27 January 2021).

[64]   Wang H, Liu G, Shen D, *et al.* HOXA1 enhances the cell proliferation, invasion and metastasis of prostate cancer cells. Oncol Rep 2015; 34(3): 1203-10.
[http://dx.doi.org/10.3892/or.2015.4085] [PMID: 26135141]

[65]   Yuan C, Zhu X, Han Y, *et al.* Elevated HOXA1 expression correlates with accelerated tumor cell proliferation and poor prognosis in gastric cancer partly *via* cyclin D1. J Exp Clin Cancer Res 2016; 35(1): 15.
[http://dx.doi.org/10.1186/s13046-016-0294-2] [PMID: 26791264]

[66]   Xiao F, Bai Y, Chen Z, *et al.* Downregulation of HOXA1 gene affects small cell lung cancer cell survival and chemoresistance under the regulation of miR-100. Eur J Cancer 2014; 50(8): 1541-54.
[http://dx.doi.org/10.1016/j.ejca.2014.01.024] [PMID: 24559685]

[67]   HOXA4 homeobox A4 [Homo sapiens (human)]-Gene-NCBI, https://www.ncbi.nlm.nih.gov/gene/3201 (accessed 27 January 2021).

[68]   Cheng S, Qian F, Huang Q, Wei L, Fu Y, Du Y. HOXA4, down-regulated in lung cancer, inhibits the growth, motility and invasion of lung cancer cells. Cell Death Dis 2018; 9(5): 465.

[http://dx.doi.org/10.1038/s41419-018-0497-x] [PMID: 29700285]

[69]   Bhatlekar S, Viswanathan V, Fields JZ, Boman BM. Overexpression of HOXA4 and HOXA9 genes promotes self-renewal and contributes to colon cancer stem cell overpopulation. J Cell Physiol 2018; 233(2): 727-35.
[http://dx.doi.org/10.1002/jcp.25981] [PMID: 28464221]

[70]   HOXA5 homeobox A5 [Homo sapiens (human)]-Gene-NCBI, https://www.ncbi.nlm.nih.gov/gene /3202 (accessed 27 January 2021).

[71]   Stasinopoulos IA, Mironchik Y, Raman A, Wildes F, Winnard P Jr, Raman V. HOXA5-twist interaction alters p53 homeostasis in breast cancer cells. J Biol Chem 2005; 280(3): 2294-9.
[http://dx.doi.org/10.1074/jbc.M411018200] [PMID: 15545268]

[72]   Saijo H, Hirohashi Y, Torigoe T, *et al.* Plasticity of lung cancer stem-like cells is regulated by the transcription factor *HOXA5* that is induced by oxidative stress. Oncotarget 2016; 7(31): 50043-56.
[http://dx.doi.org/10.18632/oncotarget.10571] [PMID: 27418136]

[73]   IGFBP1 insulin like growth factor binding protein 1 [Homo sapiens (human)] - Gene - NCBI, https://www.ncbi.nlm.nih.gov/gene/3484 (accessed 27 January 2021).

[74]   Sato Y, Inokuchi M, Takagi Y, Kojima K. IGFBP1 is a predictive factor for haematogenous metastasis in patients with gastric cancer. Anticancer Res 2019; 39(6): 2829-37.
[http://dx.doi.org/10.21873/anticanres.13411] [PMID: 31177120]

[75]   Terry KL, Tworoger SS, Gates MA, Cramer DW, Hankinson SE. Common genetic variation in IGF1, IGFBP1 and IGFBP3 and ovarian cancer risk. Carcinogenesis 2009; 30(12): 2042-6.
[http://dx.doi.org/10.1093/carcin/bgp257] [PMID: 19858071]

[76]   Cao Y, Nimptsch K, Shui IM, *et al.* Prediagnostic plasma IGFBP-1, IGF-1 and risk of prostate cancer. Int J Cancer 2015; 136(10): 2418-26.
[http://dx.doi.org/10.1002/ijc.29295] [PMID: 25348852]

[77]   IGFBP3 insulin like growth factor binding protein 3 [Homo sapiens (human)] - Gene - NCBI, https://www.ncbi.nlm.nih.gov/gene/3486 (accessed 27 January 2021).

[78]   Grimberg A. P53 and IGFBP-3: apoptosis and cancer protection. Mol Genet Metab 2000; 70(2): 85-98.
[http://dx.doi.org/10.1006/mgme.2000.3008] [PMID: 10873390]

[79]   Burger AM, Leyland-Jones B, Banerjee K, Spyropoulos DD, Seth AK. Essential roles of IGFBP-3 and IGFBP-rP1 in breast cancer. Eur J Cancer 2005; 41(11): 1515-27.
[http://dx.doi.org/10.1016/j.ejca.2005.04.023] [PMID: 15979304]

[80]   IL6 interleukin 6 [Homo sapiens (human)] - Gene - NCBI, https://www.ncbi.nlm.nih.gov/gene/3569 (accessed 27 January 2021).

[81]   Knüpfer H, Preiß R. Significance of interleukin-6 (IL-6) in breast cancer (review). Breast Cancer Res Treat 2007; 102(2): 129-35.
[http://dx.doi.org/10.1007/s10549-006-9328-3] [PMID: 16927176]

[82]   Kumari N, Dwarakanath BS, Das A, Bhatt AN. Role of interleukin-6 in cancer progression and therapeutic resistance. Tumour Biol 2016; 37(9): 11553-72.
[http://dx.doi.org/10.1007/s13277-016-5098-7] [PMID: 27260630]

[83]   Guo Y, Xu F, Lu T, Duan Z, Zhang Z. Interleukin-6 signaling pathway in targeted therapy for cancer. Cancer Treat Rev 2012; 38(7): 904-10.
[http://dx.doi.org/10.1016/j.ctrv.2012.04.007] [PMID: 22651903]

[84]   INHBA inhibin subunit beta A [Homo sapiens (human)]-Gene-NCBI, https://www.ncbi.nlm.nih. gov/gene/3624 (accessed 10 February 2021).

[85]   Okano M, Yamamoto H, Ohkuma H, *et al.* Significance of INHBA expression in human colorectal cancer. Oncol Rep 2013; 30(6): 2903-8.

[http://dx.doi.org/10.3892/or.2013.2761] [PMID: 24085226]

[86] Chen ZL, Qin L, Peng XB, Hu Y, Liu B. INHBA gene silencing inhibits gastric cancer cell migration and invasion by impeding activation of the TGF-β signaling pathway. J Cell Physiol 2019; 234(10): 18065-74.
[http://dx.doi.org/10.1002/jcp.28439] [PMID: 30963572]

[87] JAZF1 JAZF zinc finger 1 [Homo sapiens (human)]-Gene-NCBI, https://www.ncbi.nlm.nih.gov/gene/221895 (accessed 10 February 2021).

[88] Allen AJ, Ali SM, Gowen K, Elvin JA, Pejovic T. A recurrent endometrial stromal sarcoma harbors the novel fusion *JAZF1-BCORL1*. Gynecol Oncol Rep 2017; 20: 51-3.
[http://dx.doi.org/10.1016/j.gore.2017.03.002] [PMID: 28331900]

[89] Mei JW, Yang ZY, Xiang HG, *et al.* MicroRNA-1275 inhibits cell migration and invasion in gastric cancer by regulating vimentin and E-cadherin *via* JAZF1. BMC Cancer 2019; 19(1): 740.
[http://dx.doi.org/10.1186/s12885-019-5929-1] [PMID: 31357957]

[90] Sung Y, Park S, Park SJ, *et al.* Jazf1 promotes prostate cancer progression by activating JNK/Slug. Oncotarget 2018; 9(1): 755-65.
[http://dx.doi.org/10.18632/oncotarget.23146] [PMID: 29416651]

[91] KIAA1549 KIAA1549 [Homo sapiens (human)]-Gene-NCBI, https://www.ncbi.nlm.nih.gov/gene/57670 (accessed 16 February 2021).

[92] Antonelli M, Badiali M, Moi L, *et al. KIAA1549:BRAF* fusion gene in pediatric brain tumors of various histogenesis. Pediatr Blood Cancer 2015; 62(4): 724-7.
[http://dx.doi.org/10.1002/pbc.25272] [PMID: 25382612]

[93] Tian Y, Rich BE, Vena N, *et al.* Detection of KIAA1549-BRAF fusion transcripts in formalin-fixed paraffin-embedded pediatric low-grade gliomas. J Mol Diagn 2011; 13(6): 669-77.
[http://dx.doi.org/10.1016/j.jmoldx.2011.07.002] [PMID: 21884820]

[94] Hawkins C, Walker E, Mohamed N, *et al.* BRAF-KIAA1549 fusion predicts better clinical outcome in pediatric low-grade astrocytoma. Clin Cancer Res 2011; 17(14): 4790-8.
[http://dx.doi.org/10.1158/1078-0432.CCR-11-0034] [PMID: 21610142]

[95] MACC1 MET transcriptional regulator MACC1 [Homo sapiens (human)] - Gene - NCBI, https://www.ncbi.nlm.nih.gov/gene/346389 (accessed 16 February 2021).

[96] Huang Y, Zhang H, Cai J, *et al.* Overexpression of MACC1 and Its significance in human Breast Cancer Progression. Cell Biosci 2013; 3(1): 16.
[http://dx.doi.org/10.1186/2045-3701-3-16] [PMID: 23497677]

[97] Wang Z, Cai M, Weng Y, *et al.* Circulating MACC1 as a novel diagnostic and prognostic biomarker for nonsmall cell lung cancer. J Cancer Res Clin Oncol 2015; 141(8): 1353-61.
[http://dx.doi.org/10.1007/s00432-014-1903-0] [PMID: 25544672]

[98] Stein U. MACC1 – a novel target for solid cancers. Expert Opin Ther Targets 2013; 17(9): 1039-52.
[http://dx.doi.org/10.1517/14728222.2013.815727] [PMID: 23815185]

[99] MET MET proto-oncogene, receptor tyrosine kinase [Homo sapiens (human)] - Gene - NCBI, https://www.ncbi.nlm.nih.gov/gene/4233 (accessed 16 February 2021).

[100] Drilon A, Cappuzzo F, Ou SHI, Camidge DR. Targeting MET in Lung Cancer: Will Expectations Finally Be MET? J Thorac Oncol 2017; 12(1): 15-26.
[http://dx.doi.org/10.1016/j.jtho.2016.10.014] [PMID: 27794501]

[101] Cecchi F, Rabe DC, Bottaro DP. Targeting the HGF/Met signalling pathway in cancer. Eur J Cancer 2010; 46(7): 1260-70.
[http://dx.doi.org/10.1016/j.ejca.2010.02.028] [PMID: 20303741]

[102] MNX1 motor neuron and pancreas homeobox 1 [Homo sapiens (human)] - Gene - NCBI, https://www.ncbi.nlm.nih.gov/gene/3110 (accessed 18 February 2021).

[103] Zhang L, Wang J, Wang Y, *et al.* MNX1 is oncogenically upregulated in African-American prostate cancer. Cancer Res 2016; 76(21): 6290-8.
[http://dx.doi.org/10.1158/0008-5472.CAN-16-0087] [PMID: 27578002]

[104] Cheng Y, Pan Y, Pan Y, Wang O. MNX1-AS1 is a functional oncogene that induces EMT and activates the AKT/mTOR pathway and MNX1 in breast cancer. Cancer Manag Res 2019; 11: 803-12.
[http://dx.doi.org/10.2147/CMAR.S188007] [PMID: 30697072]

[105] Lv Y, Li H, Li F, Liu P, Zhao X. Long Noncoding RNA MNX1-AS1 Knockdown Inhibits Cell Proliferation and Migration in Ovarian Cancer. Cancer Biother Radiopharm 2017; 32(3): 91-9.
[http://dx.doi.org/10.1089/cbr.2017.2178] [PMID: 28414551]

[106] PMS2 PMS1 homolog 2, mismatch repair system component [Homo sapiens (human)] - Gene - NCBI, https://www.ncbi.nlm.nih.gov/gene/5395 (accessed 18 February 2021).

[107] Truninger K, Menigatti M, Luz J, *et al.* Immunohistochemical analysis reveals high frequency of PMS2 defects in colorectal cancer. Gastroenterology 2005; 128(5): 1160-71.
[http://dx.doi.org/10.1053/j.gastro.2005.01.056] [PMID: 15887099]

[108] Broeke SWT, Klift HMV, Tops CMJ, *et al.* Cancer Risks for PMS2-associated lynch syndrom.Journal of Clinical Oncology. 2961-8.

[109] RAC1 Rac family small GTPase 1 [Homo sapiens (human)]-Gene-NCBI, https://www.ncbi.nlm.nih.gov/gene/5879 (accessed 18 February 2021).

[110] Schnelzer A, Prechtel D, Knaus U, *et al.* Rac1 in human breast cancer: overexpression, mutation analysis, and characterization of a new isoform, Rac1b. Oncogene 2000; 19(26): 3013-20.
[http://dx.doi.org/10.1038/sj.onc.1203621] [PMID: 10871853]

[111] Yang WH, Lan HY, Huang CH, *et al.* RAC1 activation mediates Twist1-induced cancer cell migration. Nat Cell Biol 2012; 14(4): 366-74.
[http://dx.doi.org/10.1038/ncb2455] [PMID: 22407364]

[112] Bid HK, Roberts RD, Manchanda PK, Houghton PJ. RAC1: an emerging therapeutic option for targeting cancer angiogenesis and metastasis. Mol Cancer Ther 2013; 12(10): 1925-34.
[http://dx.doi.org/10.1158/1535-7163.MCT-13-0164] [PMID: 24072884]

[113] RALA RAS like proto-oncogene A [Homo sapiens (human)]-Gene-NCBI, https://www.ncbi.nlm.nih.gov/gene/5898 (accessed 18 February 2021).

[114] Martin TD, Der CJ. Differential involvement of RalA and RalB in colorectal cancer. Small GTPases 2012; 3(2): 126-30.
[http://dx.doi.org/10.4161/sgtp.19571] [PMID: 22790202]

[115] Male H, Patel V, Jacob MA, *et al.* Inhibition of RalA signaling pathway in treatment of non-small cell lung cancer. Lung Cancer 2012; 77(2): 252-9.
[http://dx.doi.org/10.1016/j.lungcan.2012.03.007] [PMID: 22498113]

[116] Lim KH, Baines AT, Fiordalisi JJ, *et al.* Activation of RalA is critical for Ras-induced tumorigenesis of human cells. Cancer Cell 2005; 7(6): 533-45.
[http://dx.doi.org/10.1016/j.ccr.2005.04.030] [PMID: 15950903]

[117] SBDS SBDS ribosome maturation factor [Homo sapiens (human)]-Gene-NCBI, https://www.ncbi.nlm.nih.gov/gene/51119 (accessed 18 February 2021).

[118] Hao Q, Wang J, Chen Y, *et al.* Dual regulation of p53 by the ribosome maturation factor SBDS. Cell Death Dis 2020; 11(3): 197.
[http://dx.doi.org/10.1038/s41419-020-2393-4] [PMID: 32198344]

[119] SEPTIN7 septin 7 [Homo sapiens (human)] - Gene - NCBI, https://www.ncbi.nlm.nih.gov/gene/989 (accessed 18 February 2021).

[120] Zhang N, Liu L, Fan N, *et al.* The requirement of SEPT2 and SEPT7 for migration and invasion in

human breast cancer *via* MEK/ERK activation. Oncotarget 2016; 7(38): 61587-600.
[http://dx.doi.org/10.18632/oncotarget.11402] [PMID: 27557506]

[121] Zhou J, Lu S, Yang S, *et al.* MicroRNA-127 post-transcriptionally downregulates Sept7 and suppresses cell growth in hepatocellular carcinoma cells. Cell Physiol Biochem 2014; 33(5): 1537-46.
[http://dx.doi.org/10.1159/000358717] [PMID: 24854842]

[122] SMO smoothened, frizzled class receptor [Homo sapiens (human)]-Gene-NCBI, https://www.ncbi.nlm.nih.gov/gene/6608 (accessed 18 February 2021).

[123] Magistri P, Battistelli C, Strippoli R, *et al.* SMO Inhibition Modulates Cellular Plasticity and Invasiveness in Colorectal Cancer. Front Pharmacol 2018; 8: 956.
[http://dx.doi.org/10.3389/fphar.2017.00956] [PMID: 29456503]

[124] Benvenuto M, Masuelli L, De Smaele E, *et al. In vitro* and *in vivo* inhibition of breast cancer cell growth by targeting the Hedgehog/GLI pathway with SMO (GDC-0449) or GLI (GANT-61) inhibitors. Oncotarget 2016; 7(8): 9250-70.
[http://dx.doi.org/10.18632/oncotarget.7062] [PMID: 26843616]

[125] TES testin LIM domain protein [Homo sapiens (human)]-Gene-NCBI, https://www.ncbi.nlm.nih.gov/gene/26136 (accessed 18 February 2021).

[126] Tammela J, Uenaka A, Ono T, *et al.* OY-TES-1 expression and serum immunoreactivity in epithelial ovarian cancer. Int J Oncol 2006; 29(4): 903-10.
[http://dx.doi.org/10.3892/ijo.29.4.903] [PMID: 16964386]

[127] Block I, Müller C, Sdogati D, *et al.* CFP suppresses breast cancer cell growth by TES-mediated upregulation of the transcription factor DDIT3. Oncogene 2019; 38(23): 4560-73.
[http://dx.doi.org/10.1038/s41388-019-0739-0] [PMID: 30755730]

[128] TRIM24 tripartite motif containing 24 [Homo sapiens (human)]-Genc-NCBI, https://www.ncbi.nlm.nih.gov/gene/8805 (accessed 18 February 2021).

[129] Appikonda S, Thakkar KN, Barton MC. Regulation of gene expression in human cancers by TRIM24. Drug Discov Today Technol 2016; 19: 57-63.
[http://dx.doi.org/10.1016/j.ddtec.2016.05.001] [PMID: 27769359]

[130] Groner AC, Cato L, de Tribolet-Hardy J, *et al.* TRIM24 Is an Oncogenic Transcriptional Activator in Prostate Cancer. Cancer Cell 2016; 29(6): 846-58.
[http://dx.doi.org/10.1016/j.ccell.2016.04.012] [PMID: 27238081]

[131] Tsai WW, Wang Z, Yiu TT, *et al.* TRIM24 links a non-canonical histone signature to breast cancer. Nature 2010; 468(7326): 927-32.
[http://dx.doi.org/10.1038/nature09542] [PMID: 21164480]

[132] TWIST1 twist family bHLH transcription factor 1 [Homo sapiens (human)] - Gene - NCBI, https://www.ncbi.nlm.nih.gov/gene/7291 (accessed 18 February 2021).

[133] Lee KW, Yeo SY, Sung CO, Kim SH. Twist1 is a key regulator of cancer-associated fibroblasts. Cancer Res 2015; 75(1): 73-85.
[http://dx.doi.org/10.1158/0008-5472.CAN-14-0350] [PMID: 25368021]

[134] Gort EH, Suijkerbuijk KPM, Roothaan SM, *et al.* Methylation of the TWIST1 promoter, TWIST1 mRNA levels, and immunohistochemical expression of TWIST1 in breast cancer. Cancer Epidemiol Biomarkers Prev 2008; 17(12): 3325-30.
[http://dx.doi.org/10.1158/1055-9965.EPI-08-0472] [PMID: 19064546]

Cancer Genes, 2023, *Vol. 1*, 243-286

CHAPTER 8

Chromosome 8

Muthu Vijai Bharat Vairamani[1]**, Harini Hariharan**[1] **and Satish Ramalingam**[1],*

[1] *Department of Genetic Engineering, School of Bioengineering, SRM Institute of Science and Technology, Kattankulathur, India*

Abstract: Chromosome 8 spans more than 146 million DNA base pairs, and represents between 4.5 and 5 percent of the total DNA in cells. Sixteen percent of these genes and their mutations have been identified to play a role in cancer development. Cancer is a genetic disease at the somatic cell level. Multiple gene mutations usually precede them throughout one's life. Oncogenes such as Myc, Lyn, Atad2, *etc.*, from chromosome 8 promoted cancer cell proliferation, invasion, and migration. The increased expression of these proteins can transform a normal cell into a cancer cell. Chromosome 8 also houses multiple tumor suppressor genes, such as Dlc1, E2f5, Gata4, Ido1, *etc.* These proteins, when expressed, reduce the chances of tumor initiation within cells. Thus, mutations leading to the reduced expression of these genes are associated with multiple cancers. Mutation of other functional genes like Ank1, Ctsb, Ext1, Il7, *etc.*, has also been implicated in various cancers for their role in increasing the invasive nature of cancers by regulating angiogenesis and facilitating cancer metastasis. Cancers can also stem from the translocational mutations of genes in chromosome 8. This chapter explains essential cancer genes, genetic mutations, and gene variations that can cause an increased risk of cancer and its progression.

Keywords: A Cancer stem cell, Chromosome 6, Deletion, Gene Mutations, Oncogenes, Tumor suppressor genes.

1.1. ADAM28: ADAM METALLOPEPTIDASE DOMAIN 28 CHROMOSOME 8; 8p21.2

This gene encodes a member of the ADAM (a disintegrin and metalloprotease domain) family. Members of this family are membrane-anchored proteins structurally related to snake venom disintegrins and have been implicated in various biological processes involving cell-cell and cell-matrix interactions, including fertilization, muscle development, and neurogenesis [1]. ADAM28 is

* **Corresponding author Satish Ramalingam**: Department of Genetic Engineering, School of Bioengineering, SRM Institute of Science and Technology, Kattankulathur, India; E-mail: rsatish76@gmail.com

overexpressed in non-small cell lung carcinomas and has also been proven to correlate with cancer cell proliferation and lymph node metastasis [2].

ADAM28 has also been associated with the proliferation of human breast carcinoma cells through the cleavage of insulin-like growth factor binding protein-3 [3].

1.2. ADAM32: ADAM METALLOPEPTIDASE DOMAIN 32 CHROMOS-OME 8; 8p11.22

This gene encodes a member of the disintegrin family of membrane-anchored proteins that play a role in diverse biological processes, such as brain development, fertilization, tumor development, and inflammation. This gene is predominantly expressed in the testis. The encoded protein undergoes proteolytic processing to generate a mature polypeptide comprised of a metalloprotease, disintegrin, and epidermal growth factor-like domains [4]. ADAM32 has been suspected of having a role in multiple carcinomas for its ectodomain-shedding activity of several proteins like Tumour necrosis factor (TNF)-α [5]. GNMTF predictions have also shown that ADAM32 can act as a driver gene for cancer cell proliferation [6].

1.3. ADAM7: ADAM METALLOPEPTIDASE DOMAIN 7 CHROMOS-OME 8; 8p21.2

This gene encodes a member of the ADAMs family of zinc proteases. These transmembrane proteins play roles in multiple processes, including cell signaling, adhesion, and migration. The encoded protein lacks protease activity and may play roles in protein-protein interactions and cell adhesion processes, including sperm-egg fusion [7]. Mutations in the ADAM7 gene have been associated with the development of melanomas [8]. It has also been identified as one of 7 biomarker genes in high-risk prostate cancer [9].

1.4. ADAM9: ADAM METALLOPEPTIDASE DOMAIN 9 CHROMOS-OME 8; 8p11.22

This gene encodes a member of the ADAM [a disintegrin and metalloprotease domain] family. Members of this family are membrane-anchored proteins structurally related to snake venom disintegrins and have been implicated in various biological processes involving cell-cell and cell-matrix interactions, including fertilization, muscle development, and neurogenesis [10]. Elevated

ADAM9 expression has been detected during the transition of human LNCaP prostate cancer cells from an androgen-dependent to an androgen-independent and metastatic state [11] and *In vivo* targeting of ADAM9 gene expression using lentivirus-delivered shRNA has been shown to suppress prostate cancer growth [12]. ADAM9 has also been shown to be highly expressed in pancreatic cancer [13], human breast cancer [14], and renal cell cancer [15].

1.5. ADGRB1: ADHESION G PROTEIN-COUPLED RECEPTOR B1 CHROMOSOME 8; 8q24.3

ADGRB1, also known as BAI1 (Brain-specific Angiogenesis Inhibitor), contains at least one 'functional' p53-binding site within an intron, and its expression is induced by wildtype p53. There are two other brain-specific angiogenesis inhibitor genes, designated BAI2 and BAI3, which, along with BAI1, have similar tissue specificities and structures; however, only BAI1 is transcriptionally regulated by p53. BAI1 is postulated to be a member of the secretin receptor family, an inhibitor of angiogenesis, and a growth suppressor of glioblastomas [16]. ADGRB1 prevents the formation of Medulloblastomas by protecting p53 from mdm2-mediated degradation [17]. It has also been implicated to have in hepatocellular carcinoma [18]

1.6. ADHFE1: ALCOHOL DEHYDROGENASE IRON CONTAINING 1 CHROMOSOME 8; 8q13.1

The ADHFE1 gene encodes hydroxy acid-oxoacid transhydrogenase [EC 1.1.99.24], which is responsible for the oxidation of 4-hydroxybutyrate in mammalian tissues [19]. ADHFE1 is a breast cancer oncogene and promotes orthotopic tumor growth [20]. It has also been found that the hyper-methylation of the ADHFE1 gene can cause colorectal cancer [21 - 23].

1.7. AGO2: ARGONAUTE RISC CATALYTIC COMPONENT 2 CHROMOSOME 8; 8q24.3

This gene encodes a member of the Argonaute family of proteins which play a role in RNA interference. The encoded protein is fundamental and contains aAZ and PIWI domains. It may interact with dicer1 and play a role in short-interfering-RNA-mediated gene silencing. Multiple transcript variants encoding different isoforms have been found for this gene [24]. The AGO2 gene has a high incidence of gene alterations across cancer types, including invasive breast carcinoma [23.30%], colon and rectum adenocarcinoma [12.3%], bladder urothelial carcinoma [20.8%], and prostate adenocarcinoma [20.7%] and hence can serve as a cancer biomarker [25 - 28].

1.8. ANGPT1: ANGIOPOIETIN 1 CHROMOSOME 8; 8q23.1

This gene encodes a secreted glycoprotein that belongs to the angiopoietin family. Members of this family play important roles in vascular development and angiogenesis. It is critical in mediating reciprocal interactions between the endothelium and surrounding matrix and mesenchyme and inhibits endothelial permeability [29]. ANGPT1 has been identified as a VEG-F-independent angiogenic gene in Breast cancer [30] and colorectal cancer [31]. This is further supported by the fact that dual targeting of ANGPT1 and TGFBR2 genes by miR-204 miRNA controls angiogenesis in Breast cancer [32].

1.9. ANGPT2: ANGIOPOIETIN 2 CHROMOSOME 8; 8p23.1

The protein encoded by this gene is an antagonist of angiopoietin 1 [Ang-1], and both [Ang-1 and Ang-2] are ligands for the endothelial tyrosine kinase receptor [Tie2]. These two ligands affect angiogenesis during embryogenesis and tumorigenesis. The encoded protein disrupts the vascular remodeling ability of Ang-1 and may induce endothelial cell apoptosis [33]. The methylation of this ANGPT2 gene has been strongly associated with gene expression and prognosis in chronic lymphocytic leukemia [34]. ANGPT2, when regulated by DARPP-32 protein, has been found to promote angiogenesis in gastric tumors [35]. This gene has also been found to be remodeled by the ADAM9 protein in lung cancers [36].

1.10. ANK1: ANKYRIN 1 CHROMOSOME 8; 8p11.21

Ankyrin 1, the prototype of the Ankyrins family of proteins, was first discovered in the erythrocytes but has since been found in the brain and muscles. Mutations in erythrocytic ankyrin 1 have been associated with approximately half of all patients with hereditary spherocytosis. Complex patterns of alternative splicing in the regulatory domain have been described, giving rise to different isoforms of ankyrin 1 [37]. Overexpression of ankyrin 1 has been found to promote pancreatic cancer cell growth [38]. Aberrant methylation of the ANK1 promoter was found to be highly prevalent in oral squamous cell carcinoma and contributes to oral carcinogenesis [39], and has also been found to promote lung cancer growth [40].

1.11. ANKRD46: ANKYRIN REPEAT DOMAIN 46 CHROMOSOME 8; 8q22.3

This gene (Fig. **1**) encodes a protein containing multiple ankyrin repeats. Ankyrin domains function in protein-protein interactions in a variety of cellular processes. Alternative splicing results in multiple transcript variants. It is expressed ubiquitously in the brain and adrenal gland, among other tissues [41]. The ANKRD46 gene is upregulated in gastric cancer [42]. But the same gene is targeted by miR-21 in human breast cancer, and its expression is reduced [43].

1.12. ANXA13: ANNEXIN A13 CHROMOSOME 8; 8q24.13

This gene (Fig. **1**) encodes a member of the annexin family. Members of this calcium-dependent phospholipid-binding protein family play a role in regulating cellular growth and signal transduction pathways. The specific function of this gene has not yet been determined; however, it is associated with the plasma membrane of undifferentiated, proliferating endothelial cells and differentiated villus enterocytes [44]. The overexpression of ANXA13 has been found to promote tumor growth, cell invasion, and metastasis in human colorectal cancer [45]. It has also been found tressed in oesophageal cancer [46]. Furthermore, the targeted knockdown of the ANXA13 has been found to impair the growth and proliferation of cancer cells in colon cancer [47].

1.13. ARC: ACTIVITY REGULATED CYTOSKELETON ASSOCIATED PROTEIN CHROMOSOME 8; 8q24.3

ARC protein is released from neurons in extracellular vesicles that mediate the transfer of ARC mRNA into new target cells, where ARC mRNA can undergo activity-dependent translation. ARC capsids are endocytosed and can transfer ARC mRNA into the cytoplasm of neurons. It acts as a critical key regulator of synaptic plasticity [48]. The ARC gene is overexpressed in glioma patients. The apoptosis inhibitor ARC is induced by hypoxia-inducible factor 1, which leads to the inhibition of apoptosis in several cancer types like colon and Renal cancer [49 - 51].

1.14. ARFGEF1: ADP RIBOSYLATION FACTOR GUANINE NUCLEO-TIDE EXCHANGE FACTOR 1 CHROMOSOME 8; 8q13.2

ADP-ribosylation factors [ARFs] play an important role in intracellular vesicular trafficking. The protein encoded by this gene activates ARFs by accelerating the replacement of bound GDP with GTP. It has also been proposed to be involved in establishing resistance of cell polarity during directed cell movement in wound healing [52]. The overexpression of this has been shown in both breast cancer and thyroid cancer [53, 54]. Furthermore, targeting this ARFGEF1 gene with the miR-215 mRNA showed suppressed proliferation, migration, and invasion [55].

1.15. ARHGEF10: RHO GUANINE NUCLEOTIDE EXCHANGE FACTOR 10 CHROMOSOME 8; 8p23.3

This gene (Fig. **1**) encodes a Rho guanine nucleotide exchange factor [GEF]. Rho GEFs regulate the activity of small Rho GTPases by stimulating the exchange of guanine diphosphate [GDP] for guanine triphosphate [GTP] and may play a role in neural morphogenesis. This gene mutation is associated with slowed nerve conduction velocity [SNCV] [56]. The SRHGEF10 genes have been implicated in multiple carcinogeneses [57]. Mutations and Homozygous deletions in this gene have been shown in Bladder cancer, making it a potential tumor suppressor gene [58].

1.16. ASAH1: N-ACYLSPHINGOSINE AMIDOHYDROLASE 1 CHROM-OSOME 8; 8p22

This gene (Fig. **1**) encodes a member of the acid ceramidase family of proteins. Alternative splicing results in multiple transcript variants, at least one of which encodes a preproprotein that is proteolytically processed. Processing this preproprotein generates alpha and beta subunits that heterodimerize to form the mature lysosomal enzyme, which catalyzes the degradation of ceramide into sphingosine and free fatty acid. This enzyme is overexpressed in multiple human cancers and may play a role in cancer progression [59]. Some cancers that have an overexpression of this gene are Breast cancer, thyroid cancer, renal cancer, and melanoma [60 - 62].

1.17. ASAP1: ARFGAP WITH SH3 DOMAIN, ANKYRIN REPEAT, AND PH DOMAIN 1 CHROMOSOME 8; 8q24.21-q24.22

This gene (Fig. **1**) encodes an ADP-ribosylation factor [ARF] GTPase-activating protein. The GTPase-activating activity is stimulated by phosphatidylinositol 4,5-biphosphate [PIP2], and is greater towards ARF1 and ARF5, and lesser for ARF6. This gene may regulate membrane trafficking and cytoskeleton remodeling [63]. The ASAP1 gene is found to be overexpressed in epithelial ovarian cancer [64, 65]. It is also said to increase tumor cell motility and invasiveness and stimulates metastasis in colorectal cancer [66].

1.18. ASH2L: ASH2-LIKE, HISTONE LYSINE METHYLTRANSFERASE COMPLEX SUBUNIT CHROMOSOME 8; 8p11.23

The ASH2L gene (Fig. **1**) encodes for the histone lysine methyltransferase complex subunit. It is a component of the Set1/Ash2 histone methyltransferase [HMT] complex, which methylates explicitly 'Lys-4' of histone H3, but not if the neighboring 'Lys-9' residue is already methylated. As part of the MLL1/MLL complex, it is involved in methylation and dimethylation at 'Lys-4' of histone H3. It may function as a transcriptional regulator and play a role in hematopoiesis [66]. The ASH2L gene is said to be involved in tumor progression in pancreatic ductal adenocarcinoma [67]. Reducing the expression of the ASH2L gene has also been found to reduce acute myeloid leukemia [68].

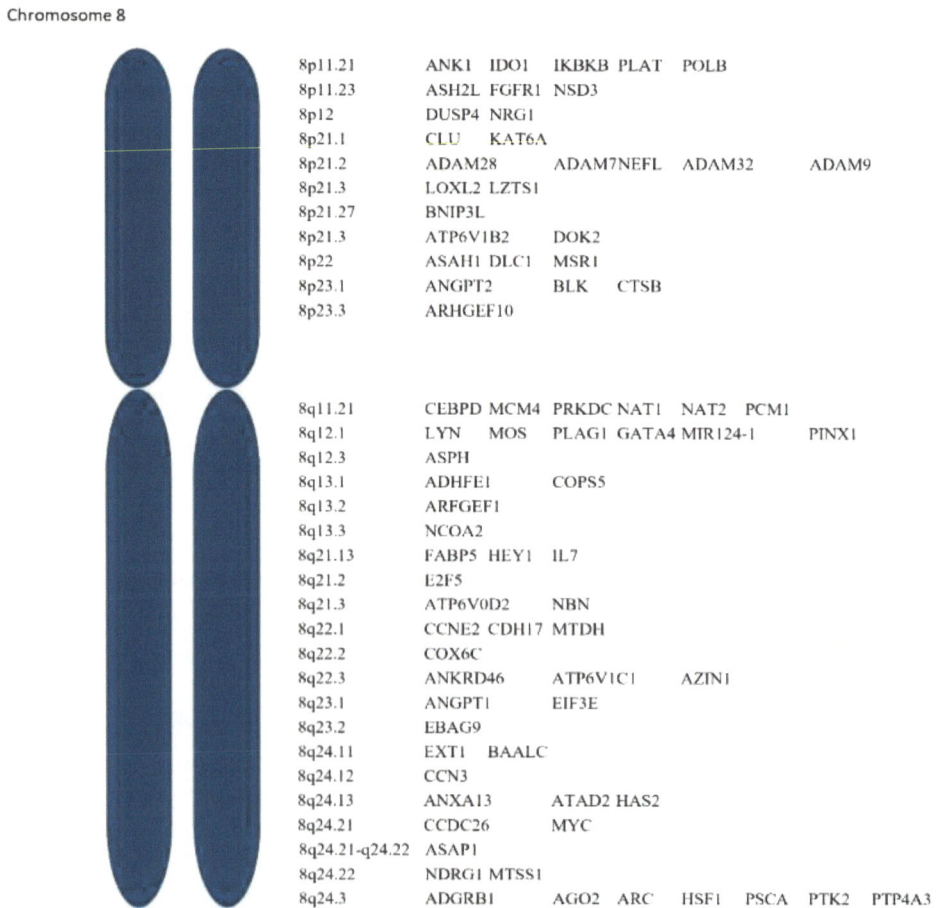

Chromosome 8

8p11.21	ANK1	IDO1	IKBKB	PLAT	POLB	
8p11.23	ASH2L	FGFR1	NSD3			
8p12	DUSP4	NRG1				
8p21.1	CLU	KAT6A				
8p21.2	ADAM28		ADAM7	NEFL	ADAM32	ADAM9
8p21.3	LOXL2	LZTS1				
8p21.27	BNIP3L					
8p21.3	ATP6V1B2	DOK2				
8p22	ASAH1	DLC1	MSR1			
8p23.1	ANGPT2		BLK	CTSB		
8p23.3	ARHGEF10					
8q11.21	CEBPD	MCM4	PRKDC	NAT1	NAT2	PCM1
8q12.1	LYN	MOS	PLAG1	GATA4	MIR124-1	PINX1
8q12.3	ASPH					
8q13.1	ADHFE1		COPS5			
8q13.2	ARFGEF1					
8q13.3	NCOA2					
8q21.13	FABP5	HEY1	IL7			
8q21.2	E2F5					
8q21.3	ATP6V0D2	NBN				
8q22.1	CCNE2	CDH17	MTDH			
8q22.2	COX6C					
8q22.3	ANKRD46		ATP6V1C1	AZIN1		
8q23.1	ANGPT1		EIF3E			
8q23.2	EBAG9					
8q24.11	EXT1	BAALC				
8q24.12	CCN3					
8q24.13	ANXA13		ATAD2	HAS2		
8q24.21	CCDC26		MYC			
8q24.21-q24.22	ASAP1					
8q24.22	NDRG1	MTSS1				
8q24.3	ADGRB1		AGO2	ARC	HSF1	PSCA PTK2 PTP4A3

Fig. (1). This figure represents all those genes from Chromosome 8 whose involvement in cancer has been explained in this chapter. Sayooj Madhusoodanan designed this diagram.

1.19. ASPH: ASPARTATE BETA-HYDROXYLASE CHROMOSOME 8; 8q12.3

This gene (Fig. **1**) is thought to play an important role in calcium homeostasis. The gene is expressed from two promoters and undergoes extensive alternative splicing. The encoded set of proteins share varying amounts of overlap near their N-termini but have substantial variations in their C-terminal domains resulting in distinct functional properties [69]. ASPH gene has been implicated in pancreatic cancer [70]. It has also been implicated as a therapeutic target in human malignant gliomas [71].

1.20. ATAD2: ATPASE FAMILY AAA DOMAIN CONTAINING 2 CHROMOSOME 8; 8q24.13

A large family of ATPases has been described, whose key feature is that they share a conserved region of about 220 amino acids that contains an ATP-binding site. The proteins in this family either have one or two AAA [ATPases Associated with diverse cellular Activities] domains. AAA family proteins often perform chaperone-like functions that assist in the assembly, operation, or disassembly of protein complexes [72]. ATAD2 is an oncogene that promotes cell proliferation, invasion, and migration in Cervical cancer [73]. It has also been associated with malignancy in pancreatic tumors and is also a novel cofactor of Myc [74, 75].

1.21. ATP6V0D2: ATPASE H+ TRANSPORTING V0 SUBUNIT D2 CHROMOSOME 8; 8q21.3

It is a subunit of the integral membrane V0 complex of vacuolar ATPase. Vacuolar ATPase is responsible for acidifying a variety of intracellular compartments in eukaryotic cells, thus providing most of the energy required for transport processes in the vacuolar system. It may also play a role in the coupling of proton transport and ATP hydrolysis [76]. The expression of ATP6V0D2 in tumor-associated macrophages is inhibited by lactate and increases tumor progression [77].

1.22. ATP6V1B2: ATPASE H+ TRANSPORTING V1 SUBUNIT B2 CHROMOSOME 8; 8p21.3

This gene encodes a component of vacuolar ATPase [V-ATPase], a multisubunit enzyme that mediates the acidification of eukaryotic intracellular organelles. V-ATPase-dependent organelle acidification is necessary for such intracellular processes as protein sorting, zymogen activation, receptor-mediated endocytosis, and synaptic vesicle proton gradient generation [78]. Somatic mutations in the ATP6V1B2 have been said to cause follicular lymphoma tumors in 22% of the cases [79, 80].

1.23. ATP6V1C1: ATPASE H+ TRANSPORTING V1 SUBUNIT C1 CHROMOSOME 8; 8q22.3

This gene encodes a component of vacuolar ATPase [V-ATPase], a multisubunit enzyme that mediates the acidification of intracellular compartments of eukaryotic cells. V-ATPase-dependent acidification is necessary for such intracellular processes such as protein sorting, zymogen activation, receptor-mediated endocytosis, and synaptic vesicle proton gradient generation. V-ATPase comprises cytosolic V1 and transmembrane V0 domains [81]. The ATP6V1C1 gene is overexpressed in breast cancer [82, 83]. Furthermore, the silencing of this gene results in decreased growth of breast cancer cells and prevents bone metastasis [84].

1.24. AZIN1: ANTIZYME INHIBITOR 1 CHROMOSOME 8; 8q22.3

The protein encoded by this gene belongs to the antizyme inhibitor family, which plays a role in cell growth and proliferation by maintaining polyamine homeostasis within the cell. Antizyme inhibitors are homologs of ornithine decarboxylase [ODC, the key enzyme in polyamine biosynthesis] that have lost the ability to decarboxylase ornithine; however, they retain the ability to bind to antizymes [85]. The AZIN1 gene has been found to increase the oncogenic potential of colorectal cancer by editing the stemness of cancer cells [86]. It also, along with ADAR1, is said to be an important prognostic marker in gastric cancer [87]. This evidence makes it a potential carcinogenic molecule in multiple cancer types [88].

1.25. BAALC: BAALC BINDER OF MAP3K1 AND KLF4 CHROMOSOME 8; 8q22.3

This gene was identified by gene expression studies in patients with acute myeloid leukemia [AML]. The gene is conserved among mammals and is not found in lower organisms. Tissues that express this gene develop from the neuroectoderm. Multiple alternatively spliced transcript variants that encode different proteins have been described for this gene; however, some of the transcript variants are found only in AML cell lines [89]. BAALC is overexpressed in both Acute lymphoblastic leukemia [90, 91] and Acute myeloid leukemia [92], hence considered a prognostic marker for both.

1.26. BLK: BLK PROTO-ONCOGENE, SRC FAMILY TYROSINE KINASE CHROMOSOME 8; 8p23.1

This gene encodes a non-receptor tyrosine-kinase of the src family of proto-oncogenes typically involved in cell proliferation and differentiation.

The protein has a role in B-cell receptor signaling and B-cell development. The protein also stimulates insulin synthesis and secretion in response to glucose and enhances the expression of several pancreatic beta-cell transcription factors [93]. The BLK gene has been regarded as an oncogene for cutaneous T-cell lymphoma [CTCL] [94, 95]. But it is also said to have tumor suppressor properties in chronic myeloid leukemia stem cells [96].

1.27. BNIP3L: BCL2 INTERACTING PROTEIN 3 LIKE CHROMOSOME 8; 8p21.27

Also known as NIX and BNIP3a, this gene encodes a protein that belongs to the pro-apoptotic subfamily within the Bcl-2 family of proteins. The encoded protein binds to Bcl-2 and possesses the BH3 domain. The protein directly targets mitochondria and causes apoptotic changes, including loss of membrane potential and the release of cytochrome-c [97]. The BNIP3L gene is involved in multiple cancers. It is a tumor suppressor in breast and ovarian cancer [98]. It has also been implicated in hepatocellular carcinomas, renal cell carcinomas, and pancreatic cancer [99 - 101].

1.28. CCDC26: CCDC26 LONG NON-CODING RNA CHROMOSOME 8; 8q24.21

CCDC26, also known as RAM, is a type of long non-coding RNA that plays an important role in brain development [102]. It is also a retinoic acid modulator of differentiation and death. A single nucleotide polymorphism is said to cause multiple gliomas and brain cancers in children, including brainstem glioma, astrocytoma, and other brain tumors [103 - 105].

1.29. CCNE2: CYCLIN NE2 CHROMOSOME 8; 8q22.1

The protein encoded by this gene belongs to the highly conserved cyclin family, whose members are characterized by a dramatic periodicity in protein abundance through the cell cycle. Cyclins function as regulators of CDK kinases. Different cyclins exhibit distinct expression and degradation patterns that contribute to each mitotic event's temporal coordination. This cyclin forms a complex with and functions as a regulatory subunit of CDK2 [106]. CCNE2 is implicated in breast cancer and was found to play an important role in resistance to trastuzumab therapy [107]. It was also found that suppressing the expression of the CCNE2 gene in non-small cell lung cancer and castration-resistant prostate cancer suggests that it was over-expressed in these cancers [108, 109].

1.30. CDH17: CADHERIN 17 CHROMOSOME 8; 8q22.1

This gene is a member of the cadherin superfamily, genes encoding calcium-dependent, membrane-associated glycoproteins. The encoded protein is cadherin-like, consisting of an extracellular region, containing 7 cadherin domains, and a transmembrane region but lacking the conserved cytoplasmic domain [110]. CDH17 is a prognostic marker for early-stage gastric cancer [111]. It is also implicated in hepatocellular carcinoma [112]. The silencing of CDH17 has been found to enhance apoptosis and inhibits autophagy in colorectal cancer [113].

1.31. CEBPD: CCAAT ENHANCER BINDING PROTEIN DELTA CHROMOSOME 8; 8q11.21

The protein encoded by this intronless gene is a bZIP transcription factor that can bind to specific DNA regulatory regions as a homodimer. It can also form heterodimers with the related protein CEBP-alpha. The encoded protein is important in regulating genes involved in immune and inflammatory responses. It may be involved in regulating genes associated with the activation and differentiation of macrophages [114]. The CEBPD gene has been implicated in human breast cancer cell lines and other primary breast tumors [115]. They have also been implicated in acute myeloid leukemia and prostate cancer [116, 117]

1.32. CLU: CLUSTERIN CHROMOSOME 8; 8p21.1

The protein encoded by this gene is a secreted chaperone that can also be found in the cell cytosol under some stress conditions. It has been suggested to be involved in several basic biological events such as cell death, tumor progression, and neurodegenerative disorders. Alternate splicing results in both coding and non-coding variants [118]. Differential regulation of the CLU gene has been Implicated in Prostate cancer [119]. It has also been involved in breast and human ovarian cancer [120, 121].

1.33. COPS5: COP9 SIGNALOSOME SUBUNIT 5 CHROMOSOME 8; 8q13.1

The protein encoded by this gene is one of the eight subunits of COP9 signalosome, a highly conserved protein complex that functions as an essential regulator in multiple signaling pathways. The structure and function of COP9 signalosome are similar to that of the 19S regulatory particle of 26S proteasome. COP9 signalosome has been shown to interact with SCF-type E3 ubiquitin ligases and act as a positive regulator of E3 ubiquitin ligases [122]. Targeting the COPS5 gene and silencing it has reduced metastasis and angiogenesis in breast and nasopharyngeal cancer [123, 124]. It has also been implicated in lung cancer [125].

1.34. COX6C: CYTOCHROME C OXIDASE SUBUNIT 6C CHROMOSOME 8; 8q22.2

Cytochrome c oxidase, the terminal enzyme of the mitochondrial respiratory chain, catalyzes the electron transfer from reduced cytochrome c to oxygen. It is a heteromeric complex consisting of 3 catalytic subunits encoded by mitochondrial genes and multiple structural subunits encoded by nuclear genes. The mitochondrially-encoded subunits function in electron transfer, and the nuclear-encoded subunits may regulate and assemble the complex [126]. Gene fusion of COX6C and HMGIC has led to uterine leiomyoma [127]. It has also been implicated in breast cancer [128].

1.35. CTSB: CATHEPSIN B CHROMOSOME 8; 8p23.1

This gene encodes a member of the C1 family of peptidases. Alternative splicing of this gene results in multiple transcript variants. At least one of these variants encodes a proteolytically processed preproprotein to generate multiple protein products. These products include the cathepsin B light and heavy chains, which can dimerize to form the double chain form of the enzyme. This enzyme is a lysosomal cysteine protease with both endopeptidase and exopeptidase activity that may play a role in protein turnover [129]. Mutations in the CTSB gene has been implicated in Human gastric adenocarcinoma [130]. Overexpression of CTSB has been found to lead to oesophageal adenocarcinoma and breast cancer [131, 132].

1.36. DLC1: DLC1 RHO GTPASE ACTIVATING PROTEIN CHROMOSOME 8; 8p22

This gene encodes a GTPase-activating protein [GAP] that is a member of the rhoGAP family of proteins that play a role in regulating small GTP-binding proteins. GAP family proteins participate in signaling pathways that regulate cell processes involved in cytoskeletal changes [133]. The DCL1 gene acts as a tumor suppressor and inhibits the growth of hepatocellular carcinoma and lung cancer [134, 135]. It also acts as an estrogen-induced tumor suppressor in Breast cancer [136].

1.37. DOK2: DOCKING PROTEIN 2 CHROMOSOME 8; 8p21.3

The protein encoded by this gene is constitutively tyrosine phosphorylated in hematopoietic progenitors isolated from chronic myelogenous leukemia [CML] patients in the chronic phase. It may be a critical substrate for p210[bcr/abl], a chimeric protein whose presence is associated with CML. This encoded protein binds p120 [RasGAP] from CML cells [137]. DOK2 gene has been implicated in lung adenocarcinoma and acute myeloid leukemia [138, 139]. It has also been found to be a tumor suppressor in gastric and colorectal cancers [140].

1.38. DUSP4: DUAL SPECIFICITY PHOSPHATASE 4 CHROMOSOME 8; 8p12

The protein encoded by this gene is a member of the dual specificity protein phosphatase subfamily. These phosphatases inactivate their target kinases by dephosphorylating phosphoserine/threonine and phosphotyrosine residues. They negatively regulate members of the mitogen-activated protein [MAP] kinase superfamily [MAPK/ERK, SAPK/JNK, p38], which are associated with cellular proliferation and differentiation [141]. The expression of DUSP4 has been associated with increased cell proliferation in colorectal cancer [142]. It has also been found that the decreased expression of DUSP4 leads to metastasis of Colorectal cancer cells to the liver and lungs [143]. DUSP4 has also been associated with breast cancer [144].

1.39. E2F5: E2F TRANSCRIPTION FACTOR 5 CHROMOSOME 8; 8q21.2

The protein encoded by this gene is a member of the E2F family of transcription factors. The E2F family plays a crucial role in the control of the cell cycle and the action of tumor suppressor proteins and is also a target of the transforming proteins of small DNA tumor viruses. The E2F pro-teins contain several evolutionarily conserved domains present in most family members [145]. The competitive binding of E2F5 with MiR-98 has been found to contribute to the migration of breast cancer cells [146]. It has also been found that the silencing of the E2F5 gene can lead to the suppression of colorectal and prostate cancers [147, 148].

1.40. EBAG9: ESTROGEN RECEPTOR BINDING SITE ASSOCIATED ANTIGEN 9 CHROMOSOME 8; 8q23.2

This gene was identified as an estrogen-responsive gene. Regulation of transcription by estrogen is mediated by the estrogen receptor, which binds to the estrogen-responsive element found in the 5'-flanking region of this gene. The encoded protein is a tumor-associated antigen expressed at high frequency in various cancers [149]. The expression of EBAG9 has been associated with the advanced form of human epithelial ovarian cancer [150]. The over-expression of the gene in the uterine cells can also indicate the early stages of uterine leiomyoma [151]. It has also been implicated in the early stages of breast cancer [152].

1.41. EIF3E: EUKARYOTIC TRANSLATION INITIATION FACTOR 3 SUBUNIT E CHROMOSOME 8; 8q23.1

Component of the eukaryotic translation initiation factor 3 [eIF-3] complex, which is required for several steps in the initiation of protein synthesis. The eIF-3 complex associates with the 40S ribosome and facilitates the recruitment of eIF-1, eIF-1A, eIF-2:GTP:methionyl-tRNAi and eIF-5 to form the 43S pre-initiation complex [43S PIC]. The eIF-3 complex stimulates mRNA recruitment to the 43S PIC and scanning of the mRNA for AUG recognition [153]. It has been found that decreased expression of EIF3E in breast cancer cells mediates the Epithelial Mesenchymal transition, thereby metastasizing cancer [154]. It has also been implicated in Lung and Prostate cancer [155, 156].

1.42. EXT1: EXOSTOSIN GLYCOSYLTRANSFERASE 1 CHROMOSO-ME 8; 8q24.11

This gene encodes an endoplasmic reticulum-resident type II transmembrane glycosyltransferase involved in the chain elongation step of heparan sulfate biosynthesis. Mutations in this gene cause the type I form of multiple exostoses [157]. The mutations in the EXT1 gene are the cause of multiple hereditary exostoses [HME] [158]. It has also been implicated in osteosarcoma and osteochondroma [159, 160].

1.43. FABP5: FATTY ACID BINDING PROTEIN 5 CHROMOSOME 8; 8q21.13

This gene encodes the fatty acid binding protein found in epidermal cells and was first identified as upregulated in psoriasis tissue. Fatty acid-binding proteins are a family of small, highly conserved, cytoplasmic proteins that bind long-chain fatty acids and other hydrophobic ligands. FABPs may play roles in fatty acid uptake, transport, and metabolism. Polymorphisms in this gene are associated with type 2 diabetes. The human genome contains many pseudogenes similar to this locus [161]. The FABP5 gene has been found to promote tumor angiogenesis in hepatocellular carcinoma [162]. It has been related to poor survivability in human breast cancer [163]. It has also been regulated epigenetically in human prostate cancer [164].

1.44. FGFR1: FIBROBLAST GROWTH FACTOR RECEPTOR 1 CHROMOSOME 8; 8p11.23

The protein encoded by this gene is a member of the fibroblast growth factor receptor [FGFR] family, where the amino acid sequence is highly conserved between members and throughout evolution. FGFR family members differ in their ligand affinities and tissue distribution [165]. FGFR1 expression has been found to induce epithelial to mesenchymal transition in non-small cell lung carcinoma [166]. The FGFR1 expression has also been implicated in breast cancer and pediatric low-grade gliomas [167, 168].

1.45. GATA4: GATA BINDING PROTEIN 4 CHROMOSOME 8; 8p23.1

This gene encodes a member of the GATA family of zinc-finger transcription factors. Members of this family recognize the GATA motif which is present in the promoters of many genes. This protein is thought to regulate genes involved in embryogenesis and myocardial differentiation and function and is necessary for normal testicular development. Mutations in this gene have been associated with cardiac septal defects [169]. Restoring the expression of GATA4 in breast cancer has been found to impede cancer progression [170]. A tumor suppressor gene in lung and ovarian cancer [171, 172].

1.46. HAS2: HYALURONAN SYNTHASE 2 CHROMOSOME 8; 8q24.13

Hyaluronan or hyaluronic acid [HA] is a high molecular weight unbranched polysaccharide synthesized by various organisms, from bacteria to mammals, and is a constituent of the extracellular matrix. It consists of alternating glucuronic acid and N-acetylglucosamine residues that are linked by beta-1-3 and beta-1-4 glycosidic bonds. HA is synthesized by membrane-bound synthase at the inner surface of the plasma membrane, and the chains are extruded through pore-like structures into the extracellular space [173]. The expression of the HAS2 gene in breast cancer cells is said to induce epithelial-to-mesenchymal transition [174]. It has also been implicated in bladder cancers and other urinary system cancers [175, 176].

1.47. HEY1: HE'S A RELATED FAMILY BHLH TRANSCRIPTION FACTOR WITH YRPW MOTIF 1 CHROMOSOME 8; 8q21.13

This gene encodes a nuclear protein belonging to the hairy and enhancer of split-related [HESR] family of basic helix-loop-helix [bHLH]-type transcriptional repressors. Expression of this gene is induced by the Notch and c-Jun signal transduction pathways. Two similar and redundant genes in mice are required for embryonic cardiovascular development and are also implicated in neurogenesis and somitogenesis [177]. The upregulated expression of the HEY1 gene has been implicated in the epithelial-to-mesenchymal transition in breast cancer [178]. It has also been implicated in multiple bone cancers like mesenchymal chondro-sarcoma [179, 180].

1.48. HSF1: HEAT SHOCK TRANSCRIPTION FACTOR 1 CHROMOSOME 8; 8q24.3

The product of this gene is a transcription factor that is rapidly induced after temperature stress and binds heat shock promoter elements [HSE]. This protein plays a role in the regulation of lifespan. Expression of this gene is repressed by phosphorylation, which promotes binding by heat shock protein 90 [181]. The overexpression of the HSF1 gene has been implicated in breast cancer [182]. Downregulating the HSF1 gene has been found to impede cancer progression in hepatocellular carcinoma [183]. It has also been found that the expression of HSF1 in melanomas increases cancer resistance to drugs like doxorubicin and paclitaxel [184].

1.49. IDO1: INDOLEAMINE 2,3-DIOXYGENASE 1 CHROMOSOME 8; 8p11.21

This gene encodes indoleamine 2,3-dioxygenase [IDO] - a heme enzyme that catalyzes the first and rate-limiting step in tryptophan catabolism to N-formyl-kynurenine. This enzyme acts on multiple tryptophan substrates, including D-tryptophan, L-tryptophan, 5-hydroxy-tryptophan, tryptamine, and serotonin. This enzyme is thought to play a role in a variety of pathophysiological processes, such as antimicrobial and antitumor defense, neuropathology, immunoregulation, and antioxidant activity [185]. The IDO1 gene has been found to promote cancer cell proliferation and inhibit apoptosis in colorectal cancer by activating the PI3K-Akt signaling [186]. It has also been found to have tumor suppression roles in prostate cancer and Hodgkin's lymphoma [187, 188].

1.50. IKBKB: INHIBITOR OF NUCLEAR FACTOR KAPPA B KINASE SUBUNIT BETA CHROMOSOME 8; 8p11.21

The protein encoded by this gene phosphorylates the inhibitor in the inhibitor/NF-kappa-B complex, causing dissociation of the inhibitor and activation of NF-kappa-B. The encoded protein itself is found in a complex of proteins. Several transcript variants, some protein-coding and some not, have been found for this gene [189]. This gene has been found to activate the Akt and NF-kB pathways in castration-resistant prostate cancer [190]. It has also been implicated as a driving agent in Kaposi sarcoma and skin cancers [191, 192].

1.51. IL7: INTERLEUKIN 7 CHROMOSOME 8; 8q21.13

The protein encoded by this gene is a cytokine important for B and T cell development. This cytokine and the hepatocyte growth factor [HGF] form a heterodimer that functions as a pre-pro-B cell growth-stimulating factor. This cytokine is found to be a cofactor for V[D]J rearrangement of the T cell receptor beta [TCRB] during early T cell development [193]. Mutations in the IL7 gene have been implicated to gain oncogenic functions and promote T-cell acute lymphoblastic leukemia in children [194]. The overexpression of IL7 has also been found in the formation of osteoclasts or early-stage prostate cancer [195, 196].

1.52. KAT6A: LYSINE ACETYLTRANSFERASE 6A CHROMOSOME 8; 8p11.21

This gene encodes a member of the MOZ, YBFR2, SAS2, and TIP60 family of histone acetyltransferases. The protein is composed of a nuclear localization domain, a double C2H2 zinc finger domain that binds to acetylated histone tails, a histone acetyl-transferase domain, a glutamate/aspartate-rich region, and a serine- and methionine-rich transactivation domain [197]. Translocation of the KAT6A gene with the CREBBP gene in chromosome 16 has been found to cause acute myeloid leukemia [198]. It has also been implicated in several hematological malignancies [199].

1.53. LOXL2: LYSYL OXIDASE-LIKE 2 CHROMOSOME 8; 8p21.3

This gene encodes a member of the lysyl oxidase gene family. The prototypic member of the family is essential to the biogenesis of connective tissue, encoding an extracellular copper-dependent amine oxidase that catalyzes the first step in the formation of crosslinks in collagens and elastin. A highly conserved amino acid sequence at the C-terminus end appears to be sufficient for amine oxidase activity, suggesting that each family member may retain this function [200]. It has been found that the up-regulation of LOXL2 in a hypoxic tumor environment promotes vasculogenic mimicry formation in hepatocellular carcinoma [201]. It has also been found to promote lung metastasis of breast cancer [202].

1.54. LYN: LYN PROTO-ONCOGENE, SRC FAMILY TYROSINE KINASE CHROMOSOME 8; 8q12.1

This gene encodes a tyrosine-protein kinase, which may be involved in the regulation of mast cell degranulation, and erythroid differentiation. Alternatively, spliced transcript variants encoding different isoforms have been found for this gene [203]. The LYN gene has been found to promote Epithelial to mesenchymal transition in Breast cancer and is said to be a target of dasatinib [204]. It has also been implicated in chronic lymphocytic leukemia and chronic myelogenous leukemia [205, 206].

1.55. LZTS1: LEUCINE ZIPPER TUMOR SUPPRESSOR 1 CHROMOSOME 8; 8p21.3

This gene encodes a tumor suppressor protein that is ubiquitously expressed in normal tissues. In uveal melanomas, expression of this protein is silenced in rapidly metastasizing and metastatic tumor cells but has normal expression in slowly metastasizing or non-metastasizing tumor cells [207]. The downregulation of the LZTS1 gene has been found to increase cancer cell resistance to paclitaxel and is associated with poor prognosis of breast cancer [208]. It has also been found that LZTS1 functions as a tumor suppressor in prostate cancer [209].

1.56. MCM4: MINICHROMOSOME MAINTENANCE COMPLEX COMPONENT 4 CHROMOSOME 8; 8q11.21

The protein encoded by this gene is one of the highly conserved minichromosome maintenance proteins [MCM] that are essential for the initiation of eukaryotic genome replication. The hexameric protein complex formed by MCM proteins is a key component of the pre-replication complex [pre_RC] and may be involved in the formation of replication forks and the recruitment of other DNA replication-related proteins [210]. The expression of MCM4 has been found in lung adenocarcinomas and gastric cancer [42, 211]. It has also been found that mutated MCM4 expression was observed in human melanoma cells [212].

1.57. MIR124-1: MICRORNA 124-1 CHROMOSOME 8; 8p23.1

microRNAs [miRNAs] are short [20-24 nt] non-coding RNAs that are involved in the post-transcriptional regulation of gene expression in multicellular organisms by affecting both the stability and translation of mRNAs. The mature miRNA is incorporated into an RNA-induced silencing complex [RISC], which recognizes target mRNAs through imperfect base pairing with the miRNA and most commonly results in translational inhibition or destabilization of the target mRNA [213]. It has been found that the miR124-1 acts as a tumor suppressor for gliomas, and the silencing of the miRNA cause gliomas in children [214, 215]. It has also been implicated in gastric cancers [216].

1.58. MOS: MOS PROTO-ONCOGENE, SERINE/THREONINE KINASE CHROMOSOME 8; 8q12.1

MOS is a serine/threonine kinase that activates the MAP kinase cascade through direct phosphorylation of the MAP kinase activator MEK [217]. The MOS gene is an oncogene for human breast cancer [218]. It has also been found that MOS has elevated expression levels in gastric cancers [219].

1.59. MSR1: MACROPHAGE SCAVENGER RECEPTOR 1 CHROMOS-OME 8; 8p22

This gene encodes the class-A macrophage scavenger receptors, which include three different types [1 - 3] generated by alternative splicing of this gene. These receptors or isoforms are macrophage-specific trimeric integral membrane glyco-proteins and have been implicated in many macrophage-associated physiological and pathological processes, including atherosclerosis, Alzheimer's disease, and host defense [220]. Elevated levels of MSR1 have been found in prostate cancers and breast cancers [221, 222].

1.60. MTDH: METADHERIN CHROMOSOME 8; 8q22.1

The MTDH gene downregulates SLC1A2/EAAT2 promoter activity when expressed ectopically. It also activates the nuclear factor kappa-B [NF-kappa-B] transcription factor. It promotes anchorage-independent growth of immortalized melanocytes and astrocytes, which is a key component in tumor cell expansion. It also promotes lung metastasis and also affects bone and brain metastasis, possibly by enhancing the seeding of tumor cells to the target organ endothelium. It induces chemoresistance [223]. When targeted by miRNAs, the silencing of the MTDH gene reduces the proliferation of lung squamous cell carcinoma and decreases the chemoresistance of breast cancer [224, 225]. And it has been found that the overexpression of MTDH has been found to increase liver cancer cell proliferation [226].

1.61. MTSS1: MTSS I-BAR DOMAIN CONTAINING 1 CHROMOSOME 8; 8q24.13

MTSS1 [MTSS I-BAR Domain Containing 1] is a Protein Coding gene. Diseases associated with MTSS1 include Mitochondrial Complex I Deficiency, Nuclear Type 24 and Lung Giant Cell Carcinoma. Among its related pathways are Hedgehog signaling events mediated by Gli proteins and Cytoskeletal Signalling [227]. The MTSS1 gene expression has been related to metastasis in hepatitis B-related hepatocellular carcinoma and lung adenocarcinoma [228, 229]. It has also been implicated in colorectal cancers [230].

1.62. MYC: MYC PROTO-ONCOGENE, BHLH TRANSCRIPTION FACTOR CHROMOSOME 8; 8q24.21

This gene is a proto-oncogene and encodes a nuclear phosphoprotein that plays a role in cell cycle progression, apoptosis, and cellular transformation. The encoded protein forms a heterodimer with the related transcription factor MAX. This complex binds to the E-box DNA consensus sequence and regulates the transcription of specific target genes. Amplification of this gene is frequently observed in numerous human cancers [231]. The MYC gene has been implicated in multiple cancers such as breast, liver, colorectal, lung, *etc* [232, 233].

1.63. NAT1: N-ACETYLTRANSFERASE 1 CHROMOSOME 8; 8p22

This gene is one of two arylamines N-acetyltransferase [NAT] genes in the human genome and is orthologous to the mouse and rat Nat2 genes. The enzyme encoded by this gene catalyzes the transfer of an acetyl group from acetyl-CoA to various arylamine and hydrazine substrates. This enzyme helps metabolize drugs and other xenobiotics, and functions in folate catabolism [234]. Overexpression of NAT1 has been implicated in bladder cancers and breast cancers [235, 236]. Mutations in the NAT1 gene have been found to cause colorectal cancers [237].

1.64. NAT2: N-ACETYLTRANSFERASE 2 CHROMOSOME 8; 8p22

This gene encodes an enzyme that functions to both activate and deactivate arylamine and hydrazine drugs and carcinogens. Polymorphisms in this gene are responsible for the N-acetylation polymorphism in which human populations segregate into rapid, intermediate, and slow acetylator phenotypes. Polymorphisms in this gene are also associated with higher incidences of cancer and drug toxicity [238]. Overexpression of NAT1 has been implicated in bladder cancers and breast cancers [236, 239]. Mutations in the NAT1 gene have been found to cause colorectal cancers [237].

1.65. NBN: NIBRIN CHROMOSOME 8; 8q21.3

Mutations in this gene are associated with Nijmegen breakage syndrome, an autosomal recessive chromosomal instability syndrome characterized by microcephaly, growth retardation, immunodeficiency, and cancer predisposition. The encoded protein is a member of the MRE11/RAD50 double-strand break repair complex, consisting of 5 proteins [240]. The mutated NBN gene is responsible for inherited prostate and ovarian cancer [241, 242]. It has also been implicated in breast cancer [243].

1.66. NCOA2: NUCLEAR RECEPTOR COACTIVATOR 2 CHROMOSOME 8; 8q13.3

The protein encoded by this gene functions as a transcriptional coactivator for nuclear hormone receptors, including steroid, thyroid, retinoid, and vitamin D receptors. The encoded protein acts as an intermediary factor for the ligand-dependent activity of these nuclear receptors, which regulate their target genes upon binding of cognate response elements [244]. Fusion of NCOA2 and other genes has been observed to cause congenital spindle cell rhabdomyosarcoma in infants [245]. The fusion of NCOA2 and HEY1 is expressed in mesenchymal chindrosarcoma [179]. The NCOA2 gene has also been implicated as a therapeutic target in clinically aggressive prostate cancer [246].

1.67. NDRG1: N-MYC DOWNSTREAM REGULATED 1 CHROMOSOME 8; 8q24.22

This gene is a member of the N-myc downregulated gene family, which belongs to the alpha/beta hydrolase superfamily. The protein encoded by this gene is a cytoplasmic protein involved in stress responses, hormone responses, cell growth, and differentiation. The encoded protein is necessary for p53-mediated caspase activation and apoptosis [247]. Aberrant NDRG1 gene expression has been implicated in breast cancer and hepatocellular carcinoma [248, 249]. It has also been observed as a metastasis suppressor for prostate cancer [250].

1.68. NEFL: NEUROFILAMENT LIGHT CHROMOSOME 8; 8p21.2

Neurofilaments are type IV intermediate filament heteropolymers composed of light, medium, and heavy chains. Neurofilaments comprise the exoskeleton and they functionally maintain the neuronal caliber. They may also play a role in intracellular transport to axons and dendrites. This gene encodes the light chain neurofilament protein [251]. The NEFL gene has been found to inhibit cancer cell proliferation and invasion in childhood gliomas [252]. It has also been implicated in prostate and breast cancer [253, 254].

1.69. CCN3: CELLULAR COMMUNICATION NETWORK FACTOR 3 CHROMOSOME 8; 8q24.12

Also named NOV, the protein encoded by this gene are a small secreted cysteine-rich protein and a member of the CCN family of regulatory proteins. CNN family proteins associate with the extracellular matrix and play an essential role in cardiovascular and skeletal development, fibrosis, and cancer development [255]. The CCN3 gene has been implicated in prostate cancer bone metastasis [256]. It has also been implicated in Wilm's tumors and breast cancer [257, 258].

1.70. NRG1: NEUREGULIN 1 CHROMOSOME 8; 8p12

The protein encoded by this gene is a membrane glycoprotein that mediates cell-cell signaling and plays a critical role in the growth and development of multiple organ systems. An extraordinary variety of different isoforms are produced from this gene through alternative promoter usage and splicing [259]. NRG1 expression in breast cancer cells is said to be associated with chemo resistance [260]. The fusion of NRG1 and CD74 has been implicated in lung adenocarcinomas [261].

1.71. NSD3: NUCLEAR RECEPTOR BINDING SET DOMAIN PROTEIN 3 CHROMOSOME 8; 8p11.23

This gene is related to the Wolf-Hirschhorn syndrome candidate-1 gene and encodes a protein with PWWP [proline-tryptophan-tryptophan-proline] domains. This protein methylates histone H3 at lysine residues 4 and 27, which represses gene transcription. Two alternatively spliced variants have been described [262].

The NSD3 gene is a common driver for breast cancer, lung cancer, and pancreatic adenocarcinomas [263]. It has also been implicated in non-small cell lung adenocarcinomas [264].

1.72. PCM1: PERICENTRIOLAR MATERIAL 1 CHROMOSOME 8; 8p22

The protein encoded by this gene is a component of centriolar satellites, which are electron-dense granules scattered around centrosomes. Inhibition studies show that this protein is essential for the correct localization of several centrosomal proteins and for anchoring microtubules to the centrosome. Chromosomal aberrations involving this gene are associated with papillary thyroid carcinomas and a variety of hematological malignancies, including atypical chronic myeloid leukemia and T-cell lymphoma [265]. The fusion of PCM1 and JAK2 has been implicated in acute myeloid leukemia, acute erythroid leukemia, and myeloid neoplasms [266 - 268].

1.73. PINX1: PIN2 [TERF1] INTERACTING TELOMERASE INHIBITOR 1 CHROMOSOME 8; 8p23.1

PINX1 [PIN2 [TERF1] Interacting Telomerase Inhibitor 1] is a Protein Coding gene. Diseases associated with PINX1 include Inflammatory Bowel Disease 22 and Thrombophlebitis Migrans. Among its related pathways is the Regulation of Telomerase. Gene Ontology [GO] annotations related to this gene include nucleic acid binding and telomerase RNA binding [269]. The PINX1 gene inhibits and reduces the telomerase activity in human breast cancer and gastric cancer and impedes cancer progression and metastasis [270, 271]. It has also been implicated in hepatocellular carcinoma [272].

1.74. PLAG1: PLEOMORPHIC ADENOMA G1 ZINC FINGER CHROMOSOME 8; 8q12.1

Pleomorphic adenoma gene 1 encodes a zinc finger protein with 2 putative nuclear localization signals. PLAG1, which is developmentally regulated, is consistently rearranged in pleomorphic adenomas of the salivary glands. PLAG1 is activated by the reciprocal chromosomal translocations involving 8q12 in a subset of salivary gland pleomorphic adenomas [273 - 275].

1.75. PLAT: PLASMINOGEN ACTIVATOR, TISSUE TYPE CHROMOS-OME 8; 8p11.21

This gene encodes tissue-type plasminogen activator, a secreted serine protease that converts the proenzyme plasminogen to plasmin, a fibrinolytic enzyme. The encoded preproprotein is proteolytically processed by plasmin or trypsin to generate heavy and light chains. These chains associate *via* disulfide linkages to form the heterodimeric enzyme [276]. The amplification of the PLAT gene has been observed in Breast and Ovarian cancer [277]. It has also been implicated in pancreatic and prostate cancer [278, 279].

1.76. POLB: DNA POLYMERASE BETA CHROMOSOME 8; 8p11.21

The protein encoded by this gene is a DNA polymerase involved in base excision and repair, also called gap-filling DNA synthesis. The encoded protein, acting as a monomer, is normally found in the cytoplasm, but it translocates to the nucleus upon DNA damage. Several transcript variants of this gene exist, but the full-length nature of only one has been described to date [280]. Mutations in the POLB gene is expressed in colorectal and bladder cancer [281, 282]. It has also been implicated as a predictive marker in lung adenocarcinoma [283].

1.77. PRKDC: PROTEIN KINASE, DNA-ACTIVATED, CATALYTIC SUBUNIT CHROMOSOME 8; 8q11.21

This gene encodes the catalytic subunit of the DNA-dependent protein kinase [DNA-PK]. It functions with the Ku70/Ku80 heterodimer protein in DNA double-strand break repair and recombination. The protein encoded is a member of the PI3/PI4-kinase family [284]. Mutations in the PRKDC gene have been implicated in brain stem gliomas in children [285]. It has also been found to regulate chemosensitivity and is a predictive marker in breast cancer [286]. This gene has also been expressed in non-small cell lung adenocarcinomas [287].

1.78. PSCA: PROSTATE STEM CELL ANTIGEN CHROMOSOME 8; 8q24.3

This gene encodes a glycosylphosphatidylinositol-anchored cell membrane glycoprotein. In addition to being highly expressed in the prostate, it is also expressed in the bladder, placenta, colon, kidney, and stomach [288]. The PSCA gene has been proven to be highly expressed in prostate cancers, gall bladder cancers, and stomach cancers, although the exact role it plays concerning the initiation and progression of the cancer is unknown [289, 290]. It has also been implicated in metastatic prostate cancer [291].

1.79. PTK2: PROTEIN TYROSINE KINASE 2 CHROMOSOME 8; 8q24.3

The PTK2 gene, also known as the FAK gene [Focal Adhesion Kinase], encodes a cytoplasmic protein tyrosine kinase, concentrated in the focal adhesions that form between cells growing in the presence of extracellular matrix constituents. The encoded protein is a member of the FAK subfamily of protein tyrosine kinases but lacks significant sequence similarity to kinases from other subfamilies [292]. The FAK protein is said to get phosphorylated by the G-protein coupled estrogen receptors in the breast and is said to lead to the progression of triple-negative breast cancer and lung cancer [293, 138]. It has also been said that the PTK2 protein regulates the Wnt/β-catenin signaling pathway and promotes the proliferation of hepatocellular carcinoma [294].

1.80. PTP4A3: PROTEIN TYROSINE PHOSPHATASE 4A3 CHROMOSOME 8; 8q24.3

This gene encodes a member of the protein-tyrosine phosphatase family. Protein tyrosine phosphatases are cell signaling molecules that play regulatory roles in a variety of cellular processes. Studies of this class of protein tyrosine phosphatase in mice demonstrate that they are prenylated *in vivo*, suggesting their association with the cell plasma membrane [295]. The PTP4A3 gene is said to cause the progression of gastric cancers by regulating the Wnt/β-catenin pathway [296]. The upregulation of the PTP4A3 gene has also been associated with increased tumor differentiation in hepatocellular carcinoma [297]. The targeted deletion of the PTP4A3 gene has also been found to suppress colon cancer in rat models [298].

CONCLUSION

Numerous studies on chromosome 8 show that these genes play a vital role in cancer. Mutations, genetic alterations, and chromosomal translocation of these genes can be directly or indirectly linked to the initiation, cancer's initiation, progression, and invasion of cancer. The oncogenes and non-expression/low expression of tumor suppressor genes should be noted in particular. Any effort to cure or control the spread of cancer would benefit by targeting these genes, either by suppressing or boosting the expression of these genes. Furthermore, understanding how these different genes that contribute to the same type of cancer, interact with each other could provide us with more information about cancer pathways. It should also be noted that this list does not comprise all cancer-causing genes in chromosome 8. More research trying to find more genes that contribute to cancer progression should be encouraged.

REFERENCES

[1]   ADAM28 ADAM metallopeptidase domain 28 [Homo sapiens (human)]-Gene-NCBI,

https://www.ncbi.nlm.nih.gov/gene?Db=gene&Cmd=ShowDetailView&TermToSearch=10863

[2]   Ohtsuka T, Shiomi T, Shimoda M, *et al.* ADAM28 is overexpressed in human non-small cell lung carcinomas and correlates with cell proliferation and lymph node metastasis. Int J Cancer 2006; 118(2): 263-73.
[http://dx.doi.org/10.1002/ijc.21324] [PMID: 16052521]

[3]   Mitsui Y, Mochizuki S, Kodama T, *et al.* ADAM28 is overexpressed in human breast carcinomas: implications for carcinoma cell proliferation through cleavage of insulin-like growth factor binding protein-3. Cancer Res 2006; 66(20): 9913-20.
[http://dx.doi.org/10.1158/0008-5472.CAN-06-0377] [PMID: 17047053]

[4]   ADAM32 ADAM metallopeptidase domain 32 [Homo sapiens (human)]-Gene-NCBI, https://www.ncbi.nlm.nih.gov/gene/203102 (accessed 1 March 2020).

[5]   Marczok S, Bortz B, Wang C, Pospisil H. Comprehensive analysis of genome rearrangements in eight human malignant tumor tissues. PLoS One 2016; 11(7): e0158995.
[http://dx.doi.org/10.1371/journal.pone.0158995] [PMID: 27391163]

[6]   Gligorijević V, Malod-Dognin N, Pržulj N. Patient-specific data fusion for cancer stratification and personalised treatment. Pacific Symposium on Biocomputing. 321-32.
[http://dx.doi.org/10.1142/9789814749411_0030]

[7]   ADAM7 ADAM metallopeptidase domain 7 [Homo sapiens (human)]-Gene-NCBI, https://www.ncbi.nlm.nih.gov/gene/8756 (accessed 1 March 2020).

[8]   Wei X, Moncada-Pazos A, Cal S, *et al.* Analysis of the disintegrin-metalloproteinases family reveals ADAM29 and ADAM7 are often mutated in melanoma. Hum Mutat 2011; 32(6): E2148-75.
[http://dx.doi.org/10.1002/humu.21477] [PMID: 21618342]

[9]   Rajan P, Stockley J, Sudbery IM, *et al.* Identification of a candidate prognostic gene signature by transcriptome analysis of matched pre-and post-treatment prostatic biopsies from patients with advanced prostate cancer. BMC Cancer 2014; 14(1): 977.
[http://dx.doi.org/10.1186/1471-2407-14-977] [PMID: 25519703]

[10]   ADAM9 ADAM metallopeptidase domain 9 [Homo sapiens (human)]-Gene-NCBI, https://www.ncbi.nlm.nih.gov/gene/8754 (accessed 31 March 2020).

[11]   Sung SY, Kubo H, Shigemura K, *et al.* Oxidative stress induces ADAM9 protein expression in human prostate cancer cells. Cancer Res 2006; 66(19): 9519-26.
[http://dx.doi.org/10.1158/0008-5472.CAN-05-4375] [PMID: 17018608]

[12]   Liu CM, Hsieh CL, He YC, *et al.* *In vivo* targeting of ADAM9 gene expression using lentivirus-delivered shRNA suppresses prostate cancer growth by regulating REG4 dependent cell cycle progression. PLoS One 2013; 8(1): e53795.
[http://dx.doi.org/10.1371/journal.pone.0053795] [PMID: 23342005]

[13]   Grützmann R, Lüttges J, Sipos B, *et al.* ADAM9 expression in pancreatic cancer is associated with tumour type and is a prognostic factor in ductal adenocarcinoma. Br J Cancer 2004; 90(5): 1053-8.
[http://dx.doi.org/10.1038/sj.bjc.6601645] [PMID: 14997207]

[14]   O'Shea C, McKie N, Buggy Y, *et al.* Expression of ADAM-9 mRNA and protein in human breast cancer. Int J Cancer 2003; 105(6): 754-61.
[http://dx.doi.org/10.1002/ijc.11161] [PMID: 12767059]

[15]   Fritzsche FR, Wassermann K, Jung M, *et al.* ADAM9 is highly expressed in renal cell cancer and is associated with tumour progression. BMC Cancer 2008; 8(1): 179.
[http://dx.doi.org/10.1186/1471-2407-8-179] [PMID: 18582378]

[16]   ADGRB1 adhesion G protein-coupled receptor B1 [Homo sapiens (human)]-Gene-NCBI, https://www.ncbi.nlm.nih.gov/gene/575 (accessed 31 March 2020).

[17]   Zhu D, Osuka S, Zhang Z, *et al.* BAI1 Suppresses Medulloblastoma Formation by Protecting p53 from

Mdm2-Mediated Degradation. Cancer Cell 2018; 33(6): 1004-1016.e5.
[http://dx.doi.org/10.1016/j.ccell.2018.05.006] [PMID: 29894688]

[18] Zhang W, He H, Zang M, *et al.* Genetic Features of Aflatoxin-Associated Hepatocellular Carcinoma. Gastroenterology 2017; 153(1): 249-262.e2.
[http://dx.doi.org/10.1053/j.gastro.2017.03.024] [PMID: 28363643]

[19] ADHFE1 alcohol dehydrogenase iron containing 1 [Homo sapiens (human)]-Gene-NCBI, https://www.ncbi.nlm.nih.gov/gene/137872 (accessed 5 April 2020).

[20] Mishra P, Tang W, Putluri V, *et al.* ADHFE1 is a breast cancer oncogene and induces metabolic reprogramming. J Clin Invest 2017; 128(1): 323-40.
[http://dx.doi.org/10.1172/JCI93815] [PMID: 29202474]

[21] Moon JW, Lee SK, Lee YW, *et al.* Alcohol induces cell proliferation *via* hypermethylation of ADHFE1 in colorectal cancer cells. BMC Cancer 2014; 14(1): 377.
[http://dx.doi.org/10.1186/1471-2407-14-377] [PMID: 24886599]

[22] Tae CH, Ryu KJ, Kim SH, *et al.* Alcohol dehydrogenase, iron containing, 1promoter hypermethylation associated with colorectal cancer differentiation. BMC Cancer 2013; 13(1): 142.
[http://dx.doi.org/10.1186/1471-2407-13-142] [PMID: 23517143]

[23] Hu YH, Ma S, Zhang XN, *et al.* Hypermethylation of ADHFE1 promotes the proliferation of colorectal cancer cell *via* modulating cell cycle progression. OncoTargets Ther 2019; 12: 8105-15.
[http://dx.doi.org/10.2147/OTT.S223423] [PMID: 31632063]

[24] AGO2 argonaute RISC catalytic component 2 [Homo sapiens (human)]-Gene-NCBI, https://www.ncbi.nlm.nih.gov/gene/27161 (accessed 5 April 2020).

[25] Huang JT, Wang J, Srivastava V, Sen S, Liu SM. MicroRNA machinery genes as novel biomarkers for cancer. Front Oncol 2014; 4: 113.
[http://dx.doi.org/10.3389/fonc.2014.00113] [PMID: 24904827]

[26] Ye Z, Jin H, Qian Q. Argonaute 2: A novel rising star in cancer research. J Cancer 2015; 6(9): 877-82.
[http://dx.doi.org/10.7150/jca.11735] [PMID: 26284139]

[27] Kim MS, Oh JE, Kim YR, *et al.* Somatic mutations and losses of expression of microRNA regulation-related genes *AGO2* and *TNRC6A* in gastric and colorectal cancers. J Pathol 2010; 221(2): 139-46.
[http://dx.doi.org/10.1002/path.2683] [PMID: 20198652]

[28] Aporntewan C, Phokaew C, Piriyapongsa J, *et al.* Hypomethylation of intragenic LINE-1 represses transcription in cancer cells through AGO2. PLoS One 2011; 6(3): e17934.
[http://dx.doi.org/10.1371/journal.pone.0017934] [PMID: 21423624]

[29] ANGPT1 angiopoietin 1 [Homo sapiens (human)]-Gene-NCBI, https://www.ncbi.nlm.nih.gov /gene/284 (accessed 5 April 2020).

[30] Makhoul I, Todorova VK, Siegel ER, *et al.* Germline genetic variants in TEK, ANGPT1, ANGPT2, MMP9, FGF2 and VEGFA are associated with pathologic complete response to bevacizumab in breast cancer patients. PLoS One 2017; 12(1): e0168550.
[http://dx.doi.org/10.1371/journal.pone.0168550] [PMID: 28045923]

[31] Dai J, Wan S, Zhou F, *et al.* Genetic polymorphism in a VEGF-independent angiogenesis gene ANGPT1 and overall survival of colorectal cancer patients after surgical resection. PLoS One 2012; 7(4): e34758.
[http://dx.doi.org/10.1371/journal.pone.0034758] [PMID: 22496856]

[32] Flores-Pérez A, Marchat LA, Rodríguez-Cuevas S, *et al.* Dual targeting of ANGPT1 and TGFBR2 genes by miR-204 controls angiogenesis in breast cancer. Sci Rep 2016; 6(1): 34504.
[http://dx.doi.org/10.1038/srep34504] [PMID: 27703260]

[33] ANGPT2 angiopoietin 2 [Homo sapiens (human)]-Gene-NCBI, https://www.ncbi.nlm.nih.gov/gene /285 (accessed 6 April 2020).

[34] Martinelli S, Kanduri M, Maffei R, *et al.* *ANGPT2* promoter methylation is strongly associated with gene expression and prognosis in chronic lymphocytic leukemia. Epigenetics 2013; 8(7): 720-9. [http://dx.doi.org/10.4161/epi.24947] [PMID: 23803577]

[35] Chen Z, Zhu S, Hong J, *et al.* Gastric tumour-derived ANGPT2 regulation by DARPP-32 promotes angiogenesis. Gut 2016; 65(6): 925-34. [http://dx.doi.org/10.1136/gutjnl-2014-308416] [PMID: 25779598]

[36] Lin CY, Cho CF, Bai ST, *et al.* ADAM9 promotes lung cancer progression through vascular remodeling by VEGFA, ANGPT2, and PLAT. Sci Rep 2017; 7(1): 15108. [http://dx.doi.org/10.1038/s41598-017-15159-1] [PMID: 29118335]

[37] ANK1 ankyrin 1 [Homo sapiens (human)]-Gene-NCBI, https://www.ncbi.nlm.nih.gov/gene/286 (accessed 6 April 2020).

[38] Omura N, Mizuma M, MacGregor A, *et al.* Overexpression of *ankyrin1* promotes pancreatic cancer cell growth. Oncotarget 2016; 7(23): 34977-87. [http://dx.doi.org/10.18632/oncotarget.9009] [PMID: 27144336]

[39] Chou ST, Peng HY, Mo KC, *et al.* MicroRNA-486-3p functions as a tumor suppressor in oral cancer by targeting DDR1. J Exp Clin Cancer Res 2019; 38(1): 281. [http://dx.doi.org/10.1186/s13046-019-1283-z] [PMID: 31253192]

[40] Tessema M, Yingling CM, Picchi MA, *et al.* ANK1 Methylation regulates expression of MicroRNA-486-5p and discriminates lung tumors by histology and smoking status. Cancer Lett 2017; 410: 191-200. [http://dx.doi.org/10.1016/j.canlet.2017.09.038] [PMID: 28965852]

[41] ANKRD46 ankyrin repeat domain 46 [Homo sapiens (human)]-Gene-NCBI, https://www.ncbi.nlm.nih.gov/gene/157567#gene-expression (accessed 7 April 2020).

[42] Cheng L, Wang P, Yang S, *et al.* Identification of genes with a correlation between copy number and expression in gastric cancer. BMC Med Genomics 2012; 5(1): 14. [http://dx.doi.org/10.1186/1755-8794-5-14] [PMID: 22559327]

[43] Yan LX, Wu QN, Zhang Y, *et al.* Knockdown of miR-21 in human breast cancer cell lines inhibits proliferation, *in vitro* migration and in vivotumor growth. Breast Cancer Res 2011; 13(1): R2. [http://dx.doi.org/10.1186/bcr2803] [PMID: 21219636]

[44] ANXA13 annexin A13 [Homo sapiens (human)]-Gene-NCBI, https://www.ncbi.nlm.nih.gov/gene/?term=Homo+sapiens+annexin+A13 (accessed 13 May 2020).

[45] Jiang G, Wang P, Wang W, Li W, Dai L, Chen K. Annexin A13 promotes tumor cell invasion *in vitro* and is associated with metastasis in human colorectal cancer. Oncotarget 2017; 8(13): 21663-73. [http://dx.doi.org/10.18632/oncotarget.15523] [PMID: 28423508]

[46] Bo H, Ghazizadeh M, Shimizu H, *et al.* Effect of ionizing irradiation on human esophageal cancer cell lines by cDNA microarray gene expression analysis. J Nippon Med Sch 2004; 71(3): 172-80. [http://dx.doi.org/10.1272/jnms.71.172] [PMID: 15226608]

[47] Moss AC, Lawlor G, Murray D, *et al.* ETV4 and Myeov knockdown impairs colon cancer cell line proliferation and invasion. Biochem Biophys Res Commun 2006; 345(1): 216-21. [http://dx.doi.org/10.1016/j.bbrc.2006.04.094] [PMID: 16678123]

[48] ARC protein expression summary - The Human Protein Atlas, https://www.proteinatlas.org/ENSG00000198576-ARC (accessed 13 May 2020).

[49] Ao J, Kuang L, Zhou Y, Zhao R, Yang C. Hypoxia-inducible Factor 1 regulated ARC expression mediated hypoxia induced inactivation of the intrinsic death pathway in p53 deficient human colon cancer cells. Biochem Biophys Res Commun 2012; 420(4): 913-7. [http://dx.doi.org/10.1016/j.bbrc.2012.03.101] [PMID: 22475487]

[50] Razorenova OV, Castellini L, Colavitti R, *et al.* The apoptosis repressor with a CARD domain (ARC)

gene is a direct hypoxia-inducible factor 1 target gene and promotes survival and proliferation of VHL-deficient renal cancer cells. Mol Cell Biol 2014; 34(4): 739-51.
[http://dx.doi.org/10.1128/MCB.00644-12] [PMID: 24344197]

[51]   Zhang YQ, Herman B. Expression and modification of ARC (apoptosis repressor with a CARD domain) is distinctly regulated by oxidative stress in cancer cells. J Cell Biochem 2008; 104(3): 818-25.
[http://dx.doi.org/10.1002/jcb.21666] [PMID: 18172857]

[52]   ARFGEF1 ADP ribosylation factor guanine nucleotide exchange factor 1 [Homo sapiens (human)]-Gene - NCBI, https://www.ncbi.nlm.nih.gov/gene/10565 (accessed 13 May 2020).

[53]   Callari M, Cappelletti V, De Cecco L, *et al.* Gene expression analysis reveals a different transcriptomic landscape in female and male breast cancer. Breast Cancer Res Treat 2011; 127(3): 601-10.
[http://dx.doi.org/10.1007/s10549-010-1015-8] [PMID: 20625818]

[54]   Kim JH, Kim TW, Kim SJ. Downregulation of ARFGEF1 and CAMK2B by promoter hypermethylation in breast cancer cells. BMB Rep 2011; 44(8): 523-8.
[http://dx.doi.org/10.5483/BMBRep.2011.44.8.523] [PMID: 21871176]

[55]   Han J, Zhang M, Nie C, *et al.* miR-215 suppresses papillary thyroid cancer proliferation, migration, and invasion through the AKT/GSK-3β/Snail signaling by targeting ARFGEF1. Cell Death Dis 2019; 10(3): 195.
[http://dx.doi.org/10.1038/s41419-019-1444-1]

[56]   ARHGEF10 Rho guanine nucleotide exchange factor 10 [Homo sapiens (human)]-Gene-NCBI, https://www.ncbi.nlm.nih.gov/gene/9639 (accessed 13 May 2020).

[57]   Cooke SL, Pole JCM, Chin SF, Ellis IO, Caldas C, Edwards PAW. High-resolution array CGH clarifies events occurring on 8p in carcinogenesis. BMC Cancer 2008; 8(1): 288.
[http://dx.doi.org/10.1186/1471-2407-8-288] [PMID: 18840272]

[58]   Williams SV, Taylor C, Platt F, Hurst CD, Aveyard J, Knowles MA. Mutation and homozygous deletion of ARHGEF10 in bladder cancer; a candidate tumour suppressor gene at 8p23.3. Cancer Genet Cytogenet 2010; 203(1): 68.
[http://dx.doi.org/10.1016/j.cancergencyto.2010.07.053]

[59]   ASAH1 N-acylsphingosine amidohydrolase 1 [Homo sapiens (human)]-Gene-NCBI, https://www.ncbi.nlm.nih.gov/gene/427 (accessed 13 May 2020).

[60]   Sänger N, Ruckhäberle E, Györffy B, *et al.* Acid ceramidase is associated with an improved prognosis in both DCIS and invasive breast cancer. Mol Oncol 2015; 9(1): 58-67.
[http://dx.doi.org/10.1016/j.molonc.2014.07.016] [PMID: 25131496]

[61]   Lucki NC, Sewer MB. Genistein stimulates MCF-7 breast cancer cell growth by inducing acid ceramidase (ASAH1) gene expression. J Biol Chem 2011; 286(22): 19399-409.
[http://dx.doi.org/10.1074/jbc.M110.195826] [PMID: 21493710]

[62]   Zhang H, Li D, Su Y, *et al.* Identification of the *N*-acylsphingosine amidohydrolase 1 gene *(ASAH1)* for susceptibility to schizophrenia in a Han Chinese population. World J Biol Psychiatry 2012; 13(2): 106-13.
[http://dx.doi.org/10.3109/15622975.2011.559273] [PMID: 21375364]

[63]   ASAP1 ArfGAP with SH3 domain, ankyrin repeat and PH domain 1 [Homo sapiens (human)]-Gen-NCBI, https://www.ncbi.nlm.nih.gov/gene/50807 (accessed 13 May 2020).

[64]   Fu Y, Biglia N, Wang Z, *et al.* Long non-coding RNAs, ASAP1-IT1, FAM215A, and LINC00472, in epithelial ovarian cancer. Gynecol Oncol 2016; 143(3): 642-9.
[http://dx.doi.org/10.1016/j.ygyno.2016.09.021] [PMID: 27667152]

[65]   Hou T, Yang C, Tong C, Zhang H, Xiao J, Li J. Overexpression of ASAP1 is associated with poor prognosis in epithelial ovarian cancer. Int J Clin Exp Pathol 2013; 7(1): 280-7.

[PMID: 24427349]

[66]   Müller T, Stein U, Poletti A, *et al.* ASAP1 promotes tumor cell motility and invasiveness, stimulates metastasis formation *in vivo*, and correlates with poor survival in colorectal cancer patients. Oncogene 2010; 29(16): 2393-403.
[http://dx.doi.org/10.1038/onc.2010.6] [PMID: 20154719]

[67]   Chen Y, Li Z, Zhang M, *et al.* Circ-ASH2L promotes tumor progression by sponging miR-34a to regulate Notch1 in pancreatic ductal adenocarcinoma. J Exp Clin Cancer Res 2019; 38(1): 466.
[http://dx.doi.org/10.1186/s13046-019-1436-0] [PMID: 31718694]

[68]   Butler JS, Qiu YH, Zhang N, *et al.* Low expression of ASH2L protein correlates with a favorable outcome in acute myeloid leukemia. Leuk Lymphoma 2017; 58(5): 1207-18.
[http://dx.doi.org/10.1080/10428194.2016.1235272] [PMID: 28185526]

[69]   ASPH aspartate beta-hydroxylase [Homo sapiens (human)]-Gene-NCBI, https://www.ncbi.nlm.nih.gov/gene/444 (accessed 13 May 2020).

[70]   Hou G, Xu B, Bi Y, *et al.* Recent advances in research on aspartate β-hydroxylase (ASPH) in pancreatic cancer: A brief update. Bosn J Basic Med Sci 2018; 18(4): 297-304.
[http://dx.doi.org/10.17305/bjbms.2018.3539] [PMID: 30179586]

[71]   Sturla LM, Tong M, Hebda N, *et al.* Aspartate-β-hydroxylase (ASPH): A potential therapeutic target in human malignant gliomas. Heliyon 2016; 2(12): e00203.
[http://dx.doi.org/10.1016/j.heliyon.2016.e00203] [PMID: 27981247]

[72]   ATAD2 ATPase family AAA domain containing 2 [Homo sapiens (human)]-Gene-NCBI, https://www.ncbi.nlm.nih.gov/gene/29028 (accessed 13 May 2020).

[73]   Zheng L, Li T, Zhang Y, *et al.* Oncogene ATAD2 promotes cell proliferation, invasion and migration in cervical cancer. Oncol Rep 2015; 33(5): 2337-44.
[http://dx.doi.org/10.3892/or.2015.3867] [PMID: 25813398]

[74]   Liu N, Funasaka K, Obayashi T, *et al.* ATAD2 is associated with malignant characteristics of pancreatic cancer cells. Oncol Lett 2019; 17(3): 3489-94.
[http://dx.doi.org/10.3892/ol.2019.9960] [PMID: 30867788]

[75]   Ciró M, Prosperini E, Quarto M, *et al.* ATAD2 is a novel cofactor for MYC, overexpressed and amplified in aggressive tumors. Cancer Res 2009; 69(21): 8491-8.
[http://dx.doi.org/10.1158/0008-5472.CAN-09-2131] [PMID: 19843847]

[76]   ATP6V0D2 ATPase H+ transporting V0 subunit d2 [Homo sapiens (human)]-Gene-NCBI, https://www.ncbi.nlm.nih.gov/gene/245972 (accessed 13 May 2020).

[77]   Liu N, Luo J, Kuang D, *et al.* Lactate inhibits ATP6V0d2 expression in tumor-associated macrophages to promote HIF-2α–mediated tumor progression. J Clin Invest 2019; 129(2): 631-46.
[http://dx.doi.org/10.1172/JCI123027] [PMID: 30431439]

[78]   ATP6V1B2 ATPase H+ transporting V1 subunit B2 [Homo sapiens (human)]-Gene-NCBI, https://www.ncbi.nlm.nih.gov/gene/526 (accessed 14 May 2020).

[79]   Wang F, Gatica D, Ying ZX, *et al.* Follicular lymphoma–associated mutations in vacuolar ATPase ATP6V1B2 activate autophagic flux and mTOR. J Clin Invest 2019; 129(4): 1626-40.
[http://dx.doi.org/10.1172/JCI98288] [PMID: 30720463]

[80]   ATP6V1B2 Gene - Somatic Mutations in Cancer, https://cancer.sanger.ac.uk/cosmic/gene/analysis?ln=ATP6V1B2 (accessed 14 May 2020).

[81]   ATP6V1C1 ATPase H+ transporting V1 subunit C1 [Homo sapiens (human)]-Gene-NCBI, https://www.ncbi.nlm.nih.gov/gene/528 (accessed 14 May 2020).

[82]   ATP6V1C1 is highly expressed in human breast cancer cells, and ATP6V1C1... | Download Scientific Diagram, https://www.researchgate.net/figure/ATP6V1C1-is-highly-expressed-in-human- (accessed 14 May 2020).

[83]   McConnell M, Feng S, Chen W, *et al.* Osteoclast proton pump regulator Atp6v1c1 enhances breast cancer growth by activating the mTORC1 pathway and bone metastasis by increasing V-ATPase activity. Oncotarget 2017; 8(29): 47675-90.
[http://dx.doi.org/10.18632/oncotarget.17544] [PMID: 28504970]

[84]   Feng S, Zhu G, McConnell M, *et al.* Silencing of atp6v1c1 prevents breast cancer growth and bone metastasis. Int J Biol Sci 2013; 9(8): 853-62.
[http://dx.doi.org/10.7150/ijbs.6030] [PMID: 24155661]

[85]   AZIN1 antizyme inhibitor 1 [Homo sapiens (human)]-Gene-NCBI, https://www.ncbi.nlm.nih .gov/gene/51582 (accessed 14 May 2020).

[86]   Shigeyasu K, Okugawa Y, Toden S, *et al.* AZIN1 RNA editing confers cancer stemness and enhances oncogenic potential in colorectal cancer. JCI Insight 2018; 3(12): e99976.
[http://dx.doi.org/10.1172/jci.insight.99976] [PMID: 29925690]

[87]   Okugawa Y, Toiyama Y, Shigeyasu K, *et al.* Enhanced AZIN1 RNA editing and overexpression of its regulatory enzyme ADAR1 are important prognostic biomarkers in gastric cancer. J Transl Med 2018; 16(1): 366.
[http://dx.doi.org/10.1186/s12967-018-1740-z] [PMID: 30563560]

[88]   Qiu S, Liu J, Xing F. Antizyme inhibitor 1: a potential carcinogenic molecule. Cancer Sci 2017; 108(2): 163-9.
[http://dx.doi.org/10.1111/cas.13122] [PMID: 27870265]

[89]   BAALC BAALC binder of MAP3K1 and KLF4 [Homo sapiens (human)]-Gene-NCBI, https://www.ncbi.nlm.nih.gov/gene/79870 (accessed 14 May 2020).

[90]   Tanner SM, Austin JL, Leone G, *et al.* BAALC, the human member of a novel mammalian neuroectoderm gene lineage, is implicated in hematopoiesis and acute leukemia. Proc Natl Acad Sci USA 2001; 98(24): 13901-6.
[http://dx.doi.org/10.1073/pnas.241525498] [PMID: 11707601]

[91]   Heesch S, Schlee C, Neumann M, *et al.* BAALC-associated gene expression profiles define IGFBP7 as a novel molecular marker in acute leukemia. Leukemia 2010; 24(8): 1429-36.
[http://dx.doi.org/10.1038/leu.2010.130] [PMID: 20535151]

[92]   Weber S, Alpermann T, Dicker F, *et al.* BAALC expression: a suitable marker for prognostic risk stratification and detection of residual disease in cytogenetically normal acute myeloid leukemia. Blood Cancer J 2014; 4(1): e173.
[http://dx.doi.org/10.1038/bcj.2013.71] [PMID: 24413067]

[93]   BLK BLK proto-oncogene, Src family tyrosine kinase [Homo sapiens (human)]-Gene-NCBI, https://www.ncbi.nlm.nih.gov/gene/640 (accessed 18 May 2020).

[94]   Petersen DL, Krejsgaard T, Berthelsen J, *et al.* B-lymphoid tyrosine kinase (Blk) is an oncogene and a potential target for therapy with dasatinib in cutaneous T-cell lymphoma (CTCL). Leukemia 2014; 28(10): 2109-12.
[http://dx.doi.org/10.1038/leu.2014.192] [PMID: 24919804]

[95]   Petersen DL, Berthelsen J, Willerslev-Olsen A, *et al.* A novel BLK-induced tumor model. Tumour Biol 2017; 39(7).
[http://dx.doi.org/10.1177/1010428317714196] [PMID: 28670978]

[96]   Zhang H, Peng C, Hu Y, *et al.* The Blk pathway functions as a tumor suppressor in chronic myeloid leukemia stem cells. Nat Genet 2012; 44(8): 861-71.
[http://dx.doi.org/10.1038/ng.2350] [PMID: 22797726]

[97]   BNIP3L BCL2 interacting protein 3 like [Homo sapiens (human)]-Gene-NCBI, https://www.ncbi. nlm.nih.gov/gene?Db=gene&Cmd=DetailsSearch&Term=665 (accessed 17 Jun .(2020).

[98] Lai J, Flanagan J, Phillips WA, Chenevix-Trench G, Arnold J. Analysis of the candidate 8p21 tumour suppressor, BNIP3L, in breast and ovarian cancer. Br J Cancer 2003; 88(2): 270-6.
[http://dx.doi.org/10.1038/sj.bjc.6600674] [PMID: 12610513]

[99] Calvisi DF, Ladu S, Gorden A, *et al.* Mechanistic and prognostic significance of aberrant methylation in the molecular pathogenesis of human hepatocellular carcinoma. J Clin Invest 2007; 117(9): 2713-22.
[http://dx.doi.org/10.1172/JCI31457] [PMID: 17717605]

[100] Jin X, Wu XX, Jin C, Inui M, Sugimoto M, Kakehi Y. Delineation of apoptotic genes for synergistic apoptosis of lexatumumab and anthracyclines in human renal cell carcinoma cells by polymerase chain reaction array. Anticancer Drugs 2012; 23(4): 445-54.
[http://dx.doi.org/10.1097/CAD.0b013e32834fd796] [PMID: 22205156]

[101] Niedergethmann M, Alves F, Neff JK, *et al.* Gene expression profiling of liver metastases and tumour invasion in pancreatic cancer using an orthotopic SCID mouse model. Br J Cancer 2007; 97(10): 1432-40.
[http://dx.doi.org/10.1038/sj.bjc.6604031] [PMID: 17940512]

[102] CCDC26 CCDC26 long non-coding RNA [Homo sapiens (human)]-Gene-NCBI, https://www.ncbi.nlm.nih.gov/gene/137196 (accessed 17 June 2020).

[103] Wei XB, Jin TB, Li G, *et al.* CCDC26 gene polymorphism and glioblastoma risk in the Han Chinese population. Asian Pac J Cancer Prev 2014; 15(8): 3629-33.
[http://dx.doi.org/10.7314/APJCP.2014.15.8.3629] [PMID: 24870769]

[104] Adel Fahmideh M, Lavebratt C, Schüz J, *et al.* *CCDC26, CDKN2BAS, RTEL1* and *TERT* Polymorphisms in pediatric brain tumor susceptibility. Carcinogenesis 2015; 36(8): 876-82.
[http://dx.doi.org/10.1093/carcin/bgv074] [PMID: 26014354]

[105] González-Castro TB, Juárez-Rojop IE, López-Narváez ML, *et al.* Genetic Polymorphisms of CCDC26 rs891835, rs6470745, and rs55705857 in Glioma Risk: A Systematic Review and Meta-analysis. Biochem Genet 2019; 57(4): 583-605.
[http://dx.doi.org/10.1007/s10528-019-09911-7] [PMID: 30778791]

[106] CCNE2 cyclin E2 [Homo sapiens (human)]-Gene-NCBI https://www.ncbi.nlm.nih.gov/gene/9134 (accessed 17 June 2020).

[107] Tormo E, Adam-Artigues A, Ballester S, *et al.* The role of miR-26a and miR-30b in HER2+ breast cancer trastuzumab resistance and regulation of the CCNE2 gene. Sci Rep 2017; 7(1): 41309.
[http://dx.doi.org/10.1038/srep41309] [PMID: 28120942]

[108] Gao P, Wang H, Yu J, *et al.* miR-3607-3p suppresses non-small cell lung cancer (NSCLC) by targeting TGFBR1 and CCNE2. PLoS Genet 2018; 14(12): e1007790.
[http://dx.doi.org/10.1371/journal.pgen.1007790] [PMID: 30557355]

[109] Zhang L, Zhang XW, Liu CH, *et al.* miRNA-30a functions as a tumor suppressor by downregulating cyclin E2 expression in castration-resistant prostate cancer. Mol Med Rep 2016; 14(3): 2077-84.
[http://dx.doi.org/10.3892/mmr.2016.5469] [PMID: 27431942]

[110] CDH17 cadherin 17 [Homo sapiens (human)]-Gene-NCBI, https://www.ncbi.nlm.nih.gov/gene /1015 (accessed 17 June 2020).

[111] Lee HJ, Nam KT, Park HS, *et al.* Gene expression profiling of metaplastic lineages identifies CDH17 as a prognostic marker in early stage gastric cancer. Gastroenterology 2010; 139(1): 213-225.e3.
[http://dx.doi.org/10.1053/j.gastro.2010.04.008] [PMID: 20398667]

[112] Shek FH, Luo R, Lam BYH, *et al.* Serine peptidase inhibitor Kazal type 1 (SPINK1) as novel downstream effector of the cadherin-17/β-catenin axis in hepatocellular carcinoma. Cell Oncol (Dordr) 2017; 40(5): 443-56.
[http://dx.doi.org/10.1007/s13402-017-0332-x] [PMID: 28631187]

[113] Tian X, Han Z, Zhu Q, *et al.* Silencing of cadherin-17 enhances apoptosis and inhibits autophagy in colorectal cancer cells. Biomed Pharmacother 2018; 108: 331-7.
[http://dx.doi.org/10.1016/j.biopha.2018.09.020] [PMID: 30227326]

[114] CEBPD CCAAT enhancer binding protein delta [Homo sapiens (human)]-Gene-NCBI, https://www.ncbi.nlm.nih.gov/gene/1052 (accessed 17 June 2020).

[115] Tang D, Sivko GS, DeWille JW. Promoter methylation reduces C/EBPδ (CEBPD) gene expression in the SUM-52PE human breast cancer cell line and in primary breast tumors. Breast Cancer Res Treat 2006; 95(2): 161-70.
[http://dx.doi.org/10.1007/s10549-005-9061-3] [PMID: 16322893]

[116] Chuang C-H, Wang W-J, Li C-F, *et al.* The combination of the prodrugs perforin-CEBPD and perforin-granzyme B efficiently enhances the activation of caspase signaling and kills prostate cancer. Cell Death Dis 2014; 5(5): e1220.
[http://dx.doi.org/10.1038/cddis.2014.106] [PMID: 24810056]

[117] Marchwicka A, Marcinkowska E. Regulation of Expression of CEBP Genes by Variably Expressed Vitamin D Receptor and Retinoic Acid Receptor α in Human Acute Myeloid Leukemia Cell Lines. Int J Mol Sci 2018; 19(7): 1918.
[http://dx.doi.org/10.3390/ijms19071918] [PMID: 29966306]

[118] CLU clusterin [Homo sapiens (human)]-Gene-NCBI, https://www.ncbi.nlm.nih.gov/gene/1191 (accessed 17 June 2020).

[119] Bouaouiche S, Magadoux L, Dondaine L, *et al.* Glyceryl trinitrate-induced cytotoxicity of docetaxel-resistant prostatic cancer cells is associated with differential regulation of clusterin Int J Oncol 2019; 54(4): 1446-56.
[http://dx.doi.org/10.3892/ijo.2019.4708] [PMID: 30720069]

[120] Karaca B, Atmaca H, Bozkurt E, *et al.* Combination of AT-101/cisplatin overcomes chemoresistance by inducing apoptosis and modulating epigenetics in human ovarian cancer cells. Mol Biol Rep 2013; 40(6): 3925-33.
[http://dx.doi.org/10.1007/s11033-012-2469-z] [PMID: 23269627]

[121] Zografos E, Anagnostopoulos AK, Papadopoulou A, *et al.* Serum Proteomic Signatures of Male Breast Cancer. Cancer Genomics Proteomics 2019; 16(2): 129-37.
[http://dx.doi.org/10.21873/cgp.20118] [PMID: 30850364]

[122] COPS5 COP9 signalosome subunit 5 [Homo sapiens (human)]-Gene-NCBI, https://www.ncbi.nlm.nih.gov/gene/10987 (accessed 17 June 2020).

[123] Pan Y, Claret FX. Targeting Jab1/CSN5 in nasopharyngeal carcinoma. Cancer Lett 2012; 326(2): 155-60.
[http://dx.doi.org/10.1016/j.canlet.2012.07.033] [PMID: 22867945]

[124] Wei Y, Liu G, Wu B, Yuan Y, Pan Y. Let-7d inhibits growth and metastasis in breast cancer by targeting Jab1/Cops5. Cell Physiol Biochem 2018; 47(5): 2126-35.
[http://dx.doi.org/10.1159/000491523] [PMID: 29975923]

[125] El-aarag SA, Mahmoud A, Hashem MH, Abd Elkader H, Hemeida AE, ElHefnawi M. In silico identification of potential key regulatory factors in smoking-induced lung cancer. BMC Med Genomics 2017; 10(1): 40.
[http://dx.doi.org/10.1186/s12920-017-0284-z] [PMID: 28592245]

[126] COX6C cytochrome c oxidase subunit 6C [Homo sapiens (human)]-Gene-NCBI, https://www.ncbi.nlm.nih.gov/gene/1345 (accessed 17 June 2020).

[127] Kurose K, Mine N, Doi D, *et al.* Novel gene fusion ofCOX6C at 8q22-23 toHMGIC at 12q15 in a uterine leiomyoma. Genes Chromosomes Cancer 2000; 27(3): 303-7.
[http://dx.doi.org/10.1002/(SICI)1098-2264(200003)27:3<303::AID-GCC11>3.0.CO;2-3] [PMID: 10679920]

[128] Chang FW, Fan HC, Liu JM, *et al.* Estrogen enhances the expression of the multidrug transporter gene ABCG2—increasing drug resistance of breast cancer cells through estrogen receptors. Int J Mol Sci 2017; 18(1): 163.
[http://dx.doi.org/10.3390/ijms18010163] [PMID: 28098816]

[129] CTSB cathepsin B [Homo sapiens (human)]-Gene-NCBI, https://www.ncbi.nlm.nih.gov/gene/1508 (accessed 17 June 2020).

[130] Cao L, Taggart RT, Berquin IM, Moin K, Fong D, Sloane BF. Human gastric adenocarcinoma cathepsin B: isolation and sequencing of full-length cDNAs and polymorphisms of the gene. Gene 1994; 139(2): 163-9.
[http://dx.doi.org/10.1016/0378-1119(94)90750-1] [PMID: 8112600]

[131] Zacharakis N, Chinnasamy H, Black M, *et al.* Immune recognition of somatic mutations leading to complete durable regression in metastatic breast cancer. Nat Med 2018; 24(6): 724-30.
[http://dx.doi.org/10.1038/s41591-018-0040-8] [PMID: 29867227]

[132] Hughes SJ, Glover TW, Zhu XX, *et al.* A novel amplicon at 8p22–23 results in overexpression of cathepsin B in esophageal adenocarcinoma. Proc Natl Acad Sci USA 1998; 95(21): 12410-5.
[http://dx.doi.org/10.1073/pnas.95.21.12410] [PMID: 9770500]

[133] DLC1 DLC1 Rho GTPase activating protein [Homo sapiens (human)]-Gene-NCBI, https://www.ncbi.nlm.nih.gov/gene/10395 (accessed 17 June 2020).

[134] Du X, Qian X, Papageorge A, *et al.* Functional interaction of tumor suppressor DLC1 and caveolin-1 in cancer cells. Cancer Res 2012; 72(17): 4405-16.
[http://dx.doi.org/10.1158/0008-5472.CAN-12-0777] [PMID: 22693251]

[135] Wu HT, Xie CR, Lv J, *et al.* The tumor suppressor DLC1 inhibits cancer progression and oncogenic autophagy in hepatocellular carcinoma. Lab Invest 2018; 98(8): 1014-24.
[http://dx.doi.org/10.1038/s41374-018-0062-3] [PMID: 29785050]

[136] Chi D, Singhal H, Li L, *et al.* Estrogen receptor signaling is reprogrammed during breast tumorigenesis. Proc Natl Acad Sci USA 2019; 116(23): 11437-43.
[http://dx.doi.org/10.1073/pnas.1819155116] [PMID: 31110002]

[137] DOK2 docking protein 2 [Homo sapiens (human)]-Gene-NCBI, https://www.ncbi.nlm.nih.gov/gene/9046 (accessed 17 June 2020).

[138] Bidkhori G, Narimani Z, Hosseini Ashtiani S, Moeini A, Nowzari-Dalini A, Masoudi-Nejad A. Reconstruction of an integrated genome-scale co-expression network reveals key modules involved in lung adenocarcinoma. PLoS One 2013; 8(7): e67552.
[http://dx.doi.org/10.1371/journal.pone.0067552] [PMID: 23874428]

[139] He PF, Xu ZJ, Zhou JD, *et al.* Methylation-associated DOK1 and DOK2 down-regulation: Potential biomarkers for predicting adverse prognosis in acute myeloid leukemia J Cell Physiol 2018; 233(9): 6604-14.
[http://dx.doi.org/10.1002/jcp.26271] [PMID: 29150948]

[140] an CH, Kim MS, Yoo NJ, Lee SH. Mutational and expressional analysis of a haploinsufficient tumor suppressor gene DOK2 in gastric and colorectal cancers. Acta Pathol Microbiol Scand Suppl 2011; 119(8): 562-4.
[http://dx.doi.org/10.1111/j.1600-0463.2011.02749.x] [PMID: 21749457]

[141] DUSP4 dual specificity phosphatase 4 [Homo sapiens (human)]-Gene-NCBI, https://www.ncbi.nlm.nih.gov/gene/1846 (accessed 17 June 2020).

[142] Gröschl B, Bettstetter M, Giedl C, *et al.* Expression of the MAP kinase phosphatase DUSP4 is associated with microsatellite instability in colorectal cancer (CRC) and causes increased cell proliferation. Int J Cancer 2013; 132(7): 1537-46.
[http://dx.doi.org/10.1002/ijc.27834] [PMID: 22965873]

[143] Saigusa S, Inoue Y, Tanaka K, *et al.* Decreased expression of DUSP4 is associated with liver and lung metastases in colorectal cancer. Med Oncol 2013; 30(3): 620.
[http://dx.doi.org/10.1007/s12032-013-0620-x] [PMID: 23749251]

[144] Xue Z, Vis DJ, Bruna A, *et al.* MAP3K1 and MAP2K4 mutations are associated with sensitivity to MEK inhibitors in multiple cancer models. Cell Res 2018; 28(7): 719-29.
[http://dx.doi.org/10.1038/s41422-018-0044-4] [PMID: 29795445]

[145] E2F5 E2F transcription factor 5 [Homo sapiens (human)]-Gene-NCBI, https://www.ncbi.nlm.nih.gov/gene/1875 (accessed 17 June 2020).

[146] Cai C, Huo Q, Wang X, Chen B, Yang Q. SNHG16 contributes to breast cancer cell migration by competitively binding miR-98 with E2F5. Biochem Biophys Res Commun 2017; 485(2): 272-8.
[http://dx.doi.org/10.1016/j.bbrc.2017.02.094] [PMID: 28232182]

[147] Li SM, Wu HL, Yu X, *et al.* The putative tumour suppressor miR-1-3p modulates prostate cancer cell aggressiveness by repressing E2F5 and PFTK1. J Exp Clin Cancer Res 2018; 37(1): 219.
[http://dx.doi.org/10.1186/s13046-018-0895-z] [PMID: 30185212]

[148] Lu G, Sun Y, An S, *et al.* MicroRNA-34a targets FMNL2 and E2F5 and suppresses the progression of colorectal cancer. Exp Mol Pathol 2015; 99(1): 173-9.
[http://dx.doi.org/10.1016/j.yexmp.2015.06.014] [PMID: 26103003]

[149] EBAG9 estrogen receptor binding site associated antigen 9 [Homo sapiens (human)]-Gene-NCBI, https://www.ncbi.nlm.nih.gov/gene/9166 (accessed 17 June 2020).

[150] Akahira J, Aoki M, Suzuki T, *et al.* Expression of EBAG9/RCAS1 is associated with advanced disease in human epithelial ovarian cancer. Br J Cancer 2004; 90(11): 2197-202.
[http://dx.doi.org/10.1038/sj.bjc.6601832] [PMID: 15164121]

[151] Wicherek L. Alterations in RCAS1 serum concentration levels during menstrual cycle in patients with uterine leiomyoma and lack of analogical changes in adenomyosis. Gynecol Obstet Invest 2009; 67(3): 195-201.
[http://dx.doi.org/10.1159/000188045] [PMID: 19122463]

[152] Tsuneizumi M, Emi M, Nagai H, *et al.* Overrepresentation of the EBAG9 gene at 8q23 associated with early-stage breast cancers. Clin Cancer Res 2001; 7(11): 3526-32.
[PMID: 11705872]

[153] EIF3E eukaryotic translation initiation factor 3 subunit E [Homo sapiens (human)]-Gene-NCBI, https://www.ncbi.nlm.nih.gov/gene/3646 (accessed 17 June 2020).

[154] Desnoyers G, Frost LD, Courteau L, Wall ML, Lewis SM. Decreased eIF3e expression can mediate epithelial-to-mesenchymal transition through activation of the TGFβ signaling pathway. Mol Cancer Res 2015; 13(10): 1421-30.
[http://dx.doi.org/10.1158/1541-7786.MCR-14-0645] [PMID: 26056130]

[155] Lin S, Choe J, Du P, Triboulet R, Gregory RI. The m6A Methyltransferase METTL3 Promotes Translation in Human Cancer Cells. Mol Cell 2016; 62(3): 335-45.
[http://dx.doi.org/10.1016/j.molcel.2016.03.021] [PMID: 27117702]

[156] Hu J, Luo H, Xu Y, *et al.* The Prognostic Significance of *EIF3C* Gene during the Tumorigenesis of Prostate Cancer. Cancer Invest 2019; 37(4-5): 199-208.
[http://dx.doi.org/10.1080/07357907.2019.1618322] [PMID: 31181967]

[157] EXT1 exostosin glycosyltransferase 1 [Homo sapiens (human)]-Gene-NCBI, https://www.ncbi.nlm.nih.gov/gene/2131 (accessed 18 June 2020).

[158] Pacifici M. Hereditary Multiple Exostoses: New Insights into Pathogenesis, Clinical Complications, and Potential Treatments. Curr Osteoporos Rep 2017; 15(3): 142-52.
[http://dx.doi.org/10.1007/s11914-017-0355-2] [PMID: 28466453]

[159] Tsuda Y, Gregory JJ, Fujiwara T, Abudu S. Secondary chondrosarcoma arising from osteochondroma.

Bone Joint J 2019; 101-B(10): 1313-20.
[http://dx.doi.org/10.1302/0301-620X.101B9.BJJ-2019-0190.R1] [PMID: 31564158]

[160] Bovée JVMG, Sakkers RJB, Geirnaerdt MJA, Taminiau AHM, Hogendoorn PCW. Intermediate grade osteosarcoma and chondrosarcoma arising in an osteochondroma. A case report of a patient with hereditary multiple exostoses. J Clin Pathol 2002; 55(3): 226-9.
[http://dx.doi.org/10.1136/jcp.55.3.226] [PMID: 11896078]

[161] FABP5 fatty acid binding protein 5 [Homo sapiens (human)]-Gene-NCBI, https://www.ncbi.nlm.nih.gov/gene/2171 (accessed 18 June 2020).

[162] Pan L, Xiao H, Liao R, *et al.* Fatty acid binding protein 5 promotes tumor angiogenesis and activates the IL6/STAT3/VEGFA pathway in hepatocellular carcinoma. Biomed Pharmacother 2018; 106: 68-76.
[http://dx.doi.org/10.1016/j.biopha.2018.06.040] [PMID: 29957468]

[163] Liu RZ, Graham K, Glubrecht DD, Germain DR, Mackey JR, Godbout R. Association of FABP5 expression with poor survival in triple-negative breast cancer: implication for retinoic acid therapy. Am J Pathol 2011; 178(3): 997-1008.
[http://dx.doi.org/10.1016/j.ajpath.2010.11.075] [PMID: 21356353]

[164] Kawaguchi K, Kinameri A, Suzuki S, Senga S, Ke Y, Fujii H. The cancer-promoting gene fatty acid-binding protein 5 (*FABP5*) is epigenetically regulated during human prostate carcinogenesis. Biochem J 2016; 473(4): 449-61.
[http://dx.doi.org/10.1042/BJ20150926] [PMID: 26614767]

[165] FGFR1 fibroblast growth factor receptor 1 [Homo sapiens (human)]-Gene-NCBI, https://www.ncbi.nlm.nih.gov/gene/2260 (accessed 18 June 2020).

[166] Vad-Nielsen J, Gammelgaard KR, Daugaard TF, Nielsen AL. Cause-and-Effect relationship between FGFR1 expression and epithelial-mesenchymal transition in EGFR-mutated non-small cell lung cancer cells. Lung Cancer 2019; 132: 132-40.
[http://dx.doi.org/10.1016/j.lungcan.2019.04.023] [PMID: 31097086]

[167] Chioni AM, Grose R. FGFR1 cleavage and nuclear translocation regulates breast cancer cell behavior. J Cell Biol 2012; 197(6): 801-17.
[http://dx.doi.org/10.1083/jcb.201108077] [PMID: 22665522]

[168] Zhang J, Wu G, Miller CP, *et al.* Whole-genome sequencing identifies genetic alterations in pediatric low-grade gliomas. Nat Genet 2013; 45(6): 602-12.
[http://dx.doi.org/10.1038/ng.2611] [PMID: 23583981]

[169] GATA4 GATA binding protein 4 [Homo sapiens (human)]-Gene-NCBI, https://www.ncbi.nlm.nih.gov/gene/2626 (accessed 18 June 2020).

[170] Han X, Tang J, Chen T, Ren G. Restoration of GATA4 expression impedes breast cancer progression by transcriptional repression of ReLA and inhibition of NF-κB signaling J Cell Biochem 2019; 120(1): 917-27.
[http://dx.doi.org/10.1002/jcb.27455] [PMID: 30187949]

[171] Gao L, Hu Y, Tian Y, *et al.* Lung cancer deficient in the tumor suppressor GATA4 is sensitive to TGFBR1 inhibition. Nat Commun 2019; 10(1): 1665.
[http://dx.doi.org/10.1038/s41467-019-09295-7] [PMID: 30971692]

[172] Anttonen M, Pihlajoki M, Andersson N, *et al.* FOXL2, GATA4, and SMAD3 co-operatively modulate gene expression, cell viability and apoptosis in ovarian granulosa cell tumor cells. PLoS One 2014; 9(1): e85545.
[http://dx.doi.org/10.1371/journal.pone.0085545] [PMID: 24416423]

[173] HAS2 hyaluronan synthase 2 [Homo sapiens (human)] - Gene - NCBI, https://www.ncbi.nlm.nih.gov/gene/3037 (accessed 18 June 2020).

[174] Kolliopoulos C, Lin CY, Heldin CH, Moustakas A, Heldin P. Has2 natural antisense RNA and Hmga2

promote Has2 expression during TGFβ-induced EMT in breast cancer. Matrix Biol 2019; 80: 29-45.
[http://dx.doi.org/10.1016/j.matbio.2018.09.002] [PMID: 30194979]

[175]   Guin S, Ru Y, Agarwal N, *et al.* Loss of Glycogen Debranching Enzyme AGL Drives Bladder Tumor
         Growth *via* Induction of Hyaluronic Acid Synthesis. Clin Cancer Res 2016; 22(5): 1274-83.
         [http://dx.doi.org/10.1158/1078-0432.CCR-15-1706] [PMID: 26490312]

[176]   Golshani R, Hautmann SH, Estrella V, *et al.* HAS1 expression in bladder cancer and its relation to
         urinary HA test. Int J Cancer 2007; 120(8): 1712-20.
         [http://dx.doi.org/10.1002/ijc.22222] [PMID: 17230515]

[177]   HEY1 hes related family bHLH transcription factor with YRPW motif 1 [Homo sapiens (human)]-
         Gene-NCBI, https://www.ncbi.nlm.nih.gov/gene/23462 (accessed 18 June 2020).

[178]   Ibrahim SA, Gadalla R, El-Ghonaimy EA, *et al.* Syndecan-1 is a novel molecular marker for triple
         negative inflammatory breast cancer and modulates the cancer stem cell phenotype *via* the IL-
         6/STAT3, Notch and EGFR signaling pathways. Mol Cancer 2017; 16(1): 57.
         [http://dx.doi.org/10.1186/s12943-017-0621-z] [PMID: 28270211]

[179]   Panagopoulos I, Gorunova L, Bjerkehagen B, Boye K, Heim S. Chromosome aberrations and HEY1-
         NCOA2 fusion gene in a mesenchymal chondrosarcoma. Oncol Rep 2014; 32(1): 40-4.
         [http://dx.doi.org/10.3892/or.2014.3180] [PMID: 24839999]

[180]   Toki S, Motoi T, Miyake M, Kobayashi E, Kawai A, Yoshida A. Minute mesenchymal
         chondrosarcoma within osteochondroma: an unexpected diagnosis confirmed by HEY1-NCOA2
         fusion. Hum Pathol 2018; 81: 255-60.
         [http://dx.doi.org/10.1016/j.humpath.2018.03.014] [PMID: 29596896]

[181]   HSF1 heat shock transcription factor 1 [Homo sapiens (human)]-Gene-NCBI, https://www.ncbi.nlm
         .nih.gov/gene/3297 (accessed 18 June 2020).

[182]   Yang X, Wang J, Liu S, Yan Q. HSF1 and Sp1 regulate FUT4 gene expression and cell proliferation in
         breast cancer cells. J Cell Biochem 2014; 115(1): 168-78.
         [http://dx.doi.org/10.1002/jcb.24645] [PMID: 23959823]

[183]   Liang W, Liao Y, Li Z, *et al.* MicroRNA-644a promotes apoptosis of hepatocellular carcinoma cells
         by downregulating the expression of heat shock factor 1. Cell Commun Signal 2018; 16(1): 30.
         [http://dx.doi.org/10.1186/s12964-018-0244-z] [PMID: 29898735]

[184]   Vydra N, Toma A, Glowala-Kosinska M, Gogler-Piglowska A, Widlak W. Overexpression of heat
         shock transcription factor 1 enhances the resistance of melanoma cells to doxorubicin and paclitaxel.
         BMC Cancer 2013; 13(1): 504.
         [http://dx.doi.org/10.1186/1471-2407-13-504] [PMID: 24165036]

[185]   IDO1 indoleamine 2,3-dioxygenase 1 [Homo sapiens (human)]-Gene-NCBI, https://www.ncbi.nlm.
         nih.gov/gene/3620 (accessed 18 June 2020).

[186]   Bishnupuri KS, Alvarado DM, Khouri AN, *et al.* IDO1 and kynurenine pathway metabolites activate
         PI3K-Akt signaling in the neoplastic colon epithelium to promote cancer cell proliferation and inhibit
         apoptosis. Cancer Res 2019; 79(6): 1138-50.
         [http://dx.doi.org/10.1158/0008-5472.CAN-18-0668] [PMID: 30679179]

[187]   Noonepalle SK, Gu F, Lee EJ, *et al.* Promoter Methylation Modulates Indoleamine 2,3-Dioxygenase 1
         Induction by Activated T Cells in Human Breast Cancers. Cancer Immunol Res 2017; 5(4): 330-44.
         [http://dx.doi.org/10.1158/2326-6066.CIR-16-0182] [PMID: 28264810]

[188]   Xu P, Sun C, Cao X, *et al.* Immune Characteristics of Chinese Diffuse Large B-Cell Lymphoma
         Patients: Implications for Cancer Immunotherapies. EBioMedicine 2018; 33: 94-104.
         [http://dx.doi.org/10.1016/j.ebiom.2018.06.010] [PMID: 29936139]

[189]   IKBKB inhibitor of nuclear factor kappa B kinase subunit beta [Homo sapiens (human)]-Gene-NCBI,
         https://www.ncbi.nlm.nih.gov/gene/3551 (accessed 18 June 2020).

[190] Shang Z, Yu J, Sun L, *et al.* LncRNA PCAT1 activates AKT and NF-κB signaling in castration-resistant prostate cancer by regulating the PHLPP/FKBP51/IKKα complex. Nucleic Acids Res 2019; 47(8): 4211-25.
[http://dx.doi.org/10.1093/nar/gkz108] [PMID: 30773595]

[191] Quan XX, Hawk NV, Chen W, *et al.* Targeting Notch1 and IKKα Enhanced NF-κB Activation in CD133⁺ Skin Cancer Stem Cells. Mol Cancer Ther 2018; 17(9): 2034-48.
[http://dx.doi.org/10.1158/1535-7163.MCT-17-0421] [PMID: 29959199]

[192] Matta H, Gopalakrishnan R, Graham C, *et al.* Kaposi's sarcoma associated herpesvirus encoded viral FLICE inhibitory protein K13 activates NF-κB pathway independent of TRAF6, TAK1 and LUBAC. PLoS One 2012; 7(5): e36601.
[http://dx.doi.org/10.1371/journal.pone.0036601] [PMID: 22590573]

[193] IL7 interleukin 7 [Homo sapiens (human)]-Gene-NCBI, https://www.ncbi.nlm.nih.gov/gene/3574 (accessed 18 June 2020).

[194] Zenatti PP, Ribeiro D, Li W, *et al.* Oncogenic IL7R gain-of-function mutations in childhood T-cell acute lymphoblastic leukemia. Nat Genet 2011; 43(10): 932-9.
[http://dx.doi.org/10.1038/ng.924] [PMID: 21892159]

[195] Mengus C, Le Magnen C, Trella E, *et al.* Elevated levels of circulating IL-7 and IL-15 in patients with early stage prostate cancer. J Transl Med 2011; 9(1): 162.
[http://dx.doi.org/10.1186/1479-5876-9-162] [PMID: 21943235]

[196] Roato I, Brunetti G, Gorassini E, *et al.* IL-7 up-regulates TNF-alpha-dependent osteoclastogenesis in patients affected by solid tumor. PLoS One 2006; 1(1): e124.
[http://dx.doi.org/10.1371/journal.pone.0000124] [PMID: 17205128]

[197] KAT6A lysine acetyltransferase 6A [Homo sapiens (human)] - Gene - NCBI, https://www.ncbi.nlm.nih.gov/gene/7994 (accessed 18 June 2020).

[198] Xie W, Hu S, Xu J, Chen Z, Medeiros LJ, Tang G. Acute myeloid leukemia with t(8;16)(p11.2;p13.3)/KAT6A-CREBBP in adults. Ann Hematol 2019; 98(5): 1149-57.
[http://dx.doi.org/10. 1007/s00277-019-03637-7] [PMID: 30759270]

[199] Baldazzi C, Luatti S, Paolini S, *et al.* FGFR1 and KAT6A rearrangements in patients with hematological malignancies and chromosome 8p11 abnormalities: biological and clinical features. Am J Hematol 2016; 91(3): E14-6.
[http://dx.doi.org/10.1002/ajh.24276] [PMID: 26667788]

[200] LOXL2 lysyl oxidase like 2 [Homo sapiens (human)]-Gene-NCBI, https://www.ncbi.nlm.nih.gov/gene/4017 (accessed 18 June 2020).

[201] Wang M, Zhao X, Zhu D, *et al.* HIF-1α promoted vasculogenic mimicry formation in hepatocellular carcinoma through LOXL2 up-regulation in hypoxic tumor microenvironment. J Exp Clin Cancer Res 2017; 36(1): 60.
[http://dx.doi.org/10.1186/s13046-017-0533-1] [PMID: 28449718]

[202] Salvador F, Martin A, López-Menéndez C, *et al.* Lysyl oxidase-like protein LOXL2 promotes lung metastasis of breast cancer. Cancer Res 2017; 77(21): 5846-59.
[http://dx.doi.org/10.1158/0008-5472.CAN-16-3152] [PMID: 28720577]

[203] LYN LYN proto-oncogene, Src family tyrosine kinase [Homo sapiens (human)]-Gene-NCBI, https://www.ncbi.nlm.nih.gov/gene/4067 (accessed 18 June 2020).

[204] Tornillo G, Knowlson C, Kendrick H, *et al.* Dual Mechanisms of LYN Kinase Dysregulation Drive Aggressive Behavior in Breast Cancer Cells. Cell Rep 2018; 25(13): 3674-3692.e10.
[http://dx.doi.org/10.1016/j.celrep.2018.11.103] [PMID: 30590041]

[205] Ferri C, Bianchini M, Bengió R, Larripa I. Expression of LYN and PTEN genes in chronic myeloid leukemia and their importance in therapeutic strategy. Blood Cells Mol Dis 2014; 52(2-3): 121-5.

[http://dx.doi.org/10.1016/j.bcmd.2013.09.002] [PMID: 24091144]

[206] Seda V, Mraz M. B-cell receptor signalling and its crosstalk with other pathways in normal and malignant cells. Eur J Haematol 2015; 94(3): 193-205.
[http://dx.doi.org/10.1111/ejh.12427] [PMID: 25080849]

[207] LZTS1 leucine zipper tumor suppressor 1 [Homo sapiens (human)]-Gene-NCBI, https://www.ncbi.nlm.nih.gov/gene/11178 (accessed 18 June 2020).

[208] Lovat F, Ishii H, Schiappacassi M, *et al.* LZTS1 downregulation confers paclitaxel resistance and is associated with worse prognosis in breast cancer. Oncotarget 2014; 5(4): 970-7.
[http://dx.doi.org/10.18632/oncotarget.1630] [PMID: 24448468]

[209] Cabeza-Arvelaiz Y, Sepulveda JL, Lebovitz RM, Thompson TC, Chinault AC. Functional identification of LZTS1 as a candidate prostate tumor suppressor gene on human chromosome 8p22. Oncogene 2001; 20(31): 4169-79.
[http://dx.doi.org/10.1038/sj.onc.1204539] [PMID: 11464283]

[210] MCM4 minichromosome maintenance complex component 4 [Homo sapiens (human)]-Gene-NCBI, https://www.ncbi.nlm.nih.gov/gene/4173 (accessed 18 June 2020).

[211] Cao Y, Zhu W, Chen W, Wu J, Hou G, Li Y. Prognostic Value of BIRC5 in Lung Adenocarcinoma Lacking EGFR, KRAS, and ALK Mutations by Integrated Bioinformatics Analysis. Dis Markers 2019; 2019: 1-12.
[http://dx.doi.org/10.1155/2019/5451290] [PMID: 31093306]

[212] Ishimi Y, Irie D. G364R mutation of MCM4 detected in human skin cancer cells affects DNA helicase activity of MCM4/6/7 complex. J Biochem 2015; 157(6): 561-9.
[http://dx.doi.org/10.1093/jb/mvv015] [PMID: 25661590]

[213] MIR124-1 microRNA 124-1 [Homo sapiens (human)]-Gene-NCBI, https://www.ncbi.nlm.nih.gov/gene/406907 (accessed 18 June 2020).

[214] Lu J, Ji H, Tang H, Xu Z. microRNA-124a suppresses PHF19 over-expression, EZH2 hyper-activation, and aberrant cell proliferation in human glioma. Biochem Biophys Res Commun 2018; 503(3): 1610-7.
[http://dx.doi.org/10.1016/j.bbrc.2018.07.089] [PMID: 30131250]

[215] Tivnan A, Zhao J, Johns TG, *et al.* The tumor suppressor microRNA, miR-124a, is regulated by epigenetic silencing and by the transcriptional factor, REST in glioblastoma. Tumour Biol 2014; 35(2): 1459-65.
[http://dx.doi.org/10.1007/s13277-013-1200-6] [PMID: 24068568]

[216] Tahara T, Tahara S, Horiguchi N, *et al.* Gastric Mucosal Microarchitectures Associated with Irreversibility with *Helicobacter pylori* Eradication and Downregulation of Micro RNA (miR)-124a. Cancer Invest 2019; 37(9): 417-26.
[http://dx.doi.org/10.1080/07357907.2019.1663207] [PMID: 31483161]

[217] MOS MOS proto-oncogene, serine/threonine kinase [Homo sapiens (human)]-Gene-NCBI, https://www.ncbi.nlm.nih.gov/gene/?term=Homo+sapiens+MOS+proto-oncogene%2C+serine%2Fthreonine+kinase (accessed 18 June 2020).

[218] Hall JM, Zuppan PJ, Anderson LA, Huey B, Carter C, King MC. Oncogenes and human breast cancer. Am J Hum Genet 1989; 44(4): 577-84.
[PMID: 2564734]

[219] Yoon H, Kim N, Shin CM, *et al.* Risk Factors for Metachronous Gastric Neoplasms in Patients Who Underwent Endoscopic Resection of a Gastric Neoplasm. Gut Liver 2016; 10(2): 228-36.
[http://dx.doi.org/10.5009/gnl14472] [PMID: 26087797]

[220] MSR1 macrophage scavenger receptor 1 [Homo sapiens (human)]-Gene-NCBI, https://www.ncbi.nlm.nih.gov/gene/4481 (accessed 18 June 2020).

[221] Hsing AW, Sakoda LC, Chen J, *et al.* MSR1 variants and the risks of prostate cancer and benign prostatic hyperplasia: a population-based study in China. Carcinogenesis 2007; 28(12): 2530-6. [http://dx.doi.org/10.1093/carcin/bgm196] [PMID: 17768178]

[222] Rose AM, Krishan A, Chakarova CF, *et al.* MSR1 repeats modulate gene expression and affect risk of breast and prostate cancer. Ann Oncol 2018; 29(5): 1292-303. [http://dx.doi.org/10.1093/annonc/mdy082] [PMID: 29509840]

[223] MTDH metadherin [Homo sapiens (human)]-Gene-NCBI, https://www.ncbi.nlm .nih.gov/gene/92140 (accessed 18 June 2020).

[224] Mataki H, Seki N, Mizuno K, *et al.* Dual-strand tumor-suppressor *microRNA-145* (*miR-145-5p* and *miR-145-3p*) coordinately targeted *MTDH* in lung squamous cell carcinoma. Oncotarget 2016; 7(44): 72084-98. [http://dx.doi.org/10.18632/oncotarget.12290] [PMID: 27765924]

[225] Yang L, Tian Y, Leong WS, *et al.* Efficient and tumor-specific knockdown of MTDH gene attenuates paclitaxel resistance of breast cancer cells both *in vivo* and *in vitro*. Breast Cancer Res 2018; 20(1): 113. [http://dx.doi.org/10.1186/s13058-018-1042-7] [PMID: 30227879]

[226] Li W, Dai H, Ou Q, Zuo G, Liu C. Overexpression of microRNA-30a-5p inhibits liver cancer cell proliferation and induces apoptosis by targeting MTDH/PTEN/AKT pathway. Tumour Biol 2016; 37(5): 5885-95. [http://dx.doi.org/10.1007/s13277-015-4456-1] [PMID: 26589417]

[227] MTSS1 MTSS I-BAR domain containing 1 [Homo sapiens (human)]-Gene-NCBI, https://www. ncbi.nlm.nih.gov/gene/9788 (accessed 18 June 2020).

[228] Huang XY, Huang ZL, Xu B, *et al.* Elevated MTSS1 expression associated with metastasis and poor prognosis of residual hepatitis B-related hepatocellular carcinoma. J Exp Clin Cancer Res 2016; 35(1): 85. [http://dx.doi.org/10.1186/s13046-016-0361-8] [PMID: 27230279]

[229] Taylor MD, Bollt O, Iyer SC, Robertson GP. Metastasis suppressor 1 (MTSS1) expression is associated with reduced *in-vivo* metastasis and enhanced patient survival in lung adenocarcinoma. Clin Exp Metastasis 2018; 35(1-2): 15-23. [http://dx.doi.org/10.1007/s10585-017-9869-3] [PMID: 29218652]

[230] Tang X, Yang M, Wang Z, Wu X, Wang D. MicroRNA-23a promotes colorectal cancer cell migration and proliferation by targeting at MARK1. Acta Biochim Biophys Sin (Shanghai) 2019; 51(7): 661-8. [http://dx.doi.org/10.1093/abbs/gmz047] [PMID: 31281935]

[231] MYC MYC proto-oncogene, bHLH transcription factor [Homo sapiens (human)]-Gene-NCBI, https://www.ncbi.nlm.nih.gov/gene/4609 (accessed 18 June 2020).

[232] Stine ZE, Walton ZE, Altman BJ, et al. MYC, Metabolism, and Cancer. AACR. Epub ahead of print 2015. DOI: 10.1158/2159-8290.CD-15-0507. [http://dx.doi.org/10.1158/2159-8290.CD-15-0507]

[233] Cell CD-, 2012 undefined. MYC on the path to cancer. Elsevier, https://www.sciencedirect.com/ science/article/pii/S0092867412002966 (accessed 18 June 2020).

[234] NAT1 N-acetyltransferase 1 [Homo sapiens (human)]-Gene-NCBI, https://www.ncbi.nlm .nih.gov/gene/9 (accessed 18 June 2020).

[235] Dhaini HR, El Hafi B, Khamis AM. NAT1 genotypic and phenotypic contribution to urinary bladder cancer risk: a systematic review and meta-analysis. Drug Metab Rev 2018; 50(2): 208-19. [http://dx.doi.org/10.1080/03602532.2017.1415928] [PMID: 29258340]

[236] Lee KM, Park SK, Kim SU, *et al.* N-acetyltransferase (NAT1, NAT2) and glutathione S-transferase (GSTM1, GSTT1) polymorphisms in breast cancer. Cancer Lett 2003; 196(2): 179-86.

[http://dx.doi.org/10.1016/S0304-3835(03)00311-2] [PMID: 12860276]

[237] Lilla C, Verla-Tebit E, Risch A, *et al.* Effect of NAT1 and NAT2 genetic polymorphisms on colorectal cancer risk associated with exposure to tobacco smoke and meat consumption. Cancer Epidemiol Biomarkers Prev 2006; 15(1): 99-107.
[http://dx.doi.org/10.1158/1055-9965.EPI-05-0618] [PMID: 16434594]

[238] NAT2 N-acetyltransferase 2 [Homo sapiens (human)]-Gene-NCBI, https://www.ncbi.nlm.nih.gov/gene/10 (accessed 18 June 2020).

[239] Blaszkewicz M. Highlight report: N-acetyltransferase 2 and urinary bladder cancer risk. Arch Toxicol 2017; 91(9): 3205-6.
[http://dx.doi.org/10.1007/s00204-017-2001-2] [PMID: 28577040]

[240] NBN nibrin [Homo sapiens (human)]-Gene-NCBI, https://www.ncbi.nlm.nih.gov/gene/4683 (accessed 18 June 2020).

[241] Rusak B, Kluźniak W, Wokołorczykv D, *et al.* Inherited NBN Mutations and Prostate Cancer Risk and Survival. Cancer Res Treat 2019; 51(3): 1180-7.
[http://dx.doi.org/10.4143/crt.2018.532] [PMID: 30590007]

[242] Ramus SJ, Song H, Dicks E, *et al.* Germline mutations in the BRIP1, BARD1, PALB2, and NBN genes in women with ovarian cancer. J Natl Cancer Inst 2015; 107(11): djv214.
[http://dx.doi.org/10.1093/jnci/djv214] [PMID: 26315354]

[243] Kurian AW, Ward KC, Howlader N, *et al.* Genetic testing and results in a population-based cohort of breast cancer patients and ovarian cancer patients. J Clin Oncol 2019; 37(15): 1305-15.
[http://dx.doi.org/10.1200/JCO.18.01854] [PMID: 30964716]

[244] NCOA2 nuclear receptor coactivator 2 [Homo sapiens (human)]-Gene-NCBI, https://www.ncbi.nlm.nih.gov/gene/10499 (accessed 18 June 2020).

[245] Whittle SB, Hicks MJ, Roy A, Vasudevan SA, Reddy K, Venkatramani R. Congenital spindle cell rhabdomyosarcoma. Pediatr Blood Cancer 2019; 66(11): e27935.
[http://dx.doi.org/10.1002/pbc.27935] [PMID: 31339226]

[246] Silva MP, Barros-Silva JD, Vieira J, *et al. NCOA2* is a candidate target gene of 8q gain associated with clinically aggressive prostate cancer. Genes Chromosomes Cancer 2016; 55(4): 365-74.
[http://dx.doi.org/10.1002/gcc.22340] [PMID: 26799514]

[247] NDRG1 N-myc downstream regulated 1 [Homo sapiens (human)]-Gene-NCBI, https://www.ncbi.nlm.nih.gov/gene/10397 (accessed 19 June 2020).

[248] Liu Y, Wang D, Li Y, *et al.* Long noncoding RNA CCAT2 promotes hepatocellular carcinoma proliferation and metastasis through up-regulation of NDRG1. Exp Cell Res 2019; 379(1): 19-29.
[http://dx.doi.org/10.1016/j.yexcr.2019.03.029] [PMID: 30922920]

[249] Yeh CC, Luo JL, Nhut Phan N, *et al.* Different effects of long noncoding RNA *NDRG1-OT1* fragments on *NDRG1* transcription in breast cancer cells under hypoxia. RNA Biol 2018; 15(12): 1487-98.
[http://dx.doi.org/10.1080/15476286.2018.1553480] [PMID: 30497328]

[250] Park KC, Menezes SV, Kalinowski DS, *et al.* Identification of differential phosphorylation and sub-cellular localization of the metastasis suppressor, NDRG1. Biochim Biophys Acta Mol Basis Dis 2018; 1864(8): 2644-63.
[http://dx.doi.org/10.1016/j.bbadis.2018.04.011] [PMID: 29679718]

[251] NEFL neurofilament light [Homo sapiens (human)]-Gene-NCBI, https://www.ncbi.nlm.nih.gov/gene/4747 (accessed 19 June 2020).

[252] Wang Z, Xiong J, Zhang S, Wang J, Gong Z, Dai M. Up-Regulation of microRNA-183 Promotes Cell Proliferation and Invasion in Glioma By Directly Targeting NEFL. Cell Mol Neurobiol 2016; 36(8): 1303-10.

[http://dx.doi.org/10.1007/s10571-016-0328-5] [PMID: 26879754]

[253] Kang S, Kim B, Park SB, *et al.* Stage-specific methylome screen identifies that NEFL is downregulated by promoter hypermethylation in breast cancer. Int J Oncol 2013; 43(5): 1659-65.
[http://dx.doi.org/10.3892/ijo.2013.2094] [PMID: 24026393]

[254] Häggman MJ, Wojno KJ, Pearsall CP, Macoska JA. Allelic loss of 8p sequences in prostatic intraepithelial neoplasia and carcinoma. Urology 1997; 50(4): 643-7.
[http://dx.doi.org/10.1016/S0090-4295(97)00304-X] [PMID: 9338751]

[255] CCN3 cellular communication network factor 3 [Homo sapiens (human)]-Gene-NCBI, https://www.ncbi.nlm.nih.gov/gene/4856 (accessed 19 June 2020).

[256] Dankner M, Ouellet V, Communal L, *et al.* CCN3/Nephroblastoma Overexpressed Is a Functional Mediator of Prostate Cancer Bone Metastasis That Is Associated with Poor Patient Prognosis. Am J Pathol 2019; 189(7): 1451-61.
[http://dx.doi.org/10.1016/j.ajpath.2019.04.006] [PMID: 31202437]

[257] Jiang WG, Watkins G, Fodstad O, Douglas-Jones A, Mokbel K, Mansel RE. Differential expression of the CCN family members Cyr61, CTGF and Nov in human breast cancer. Endocr Relat Cancer 2004; 11(4): 781-91.
[http://dx.doi.org/10.1677/erc.1.00825] [PMID: 15613452]

[258] Liu C, Liu XJ, Crowe PD, *et al.* Nephroblastoma overexpressed gene (NOV) codes for a growth factor that induces protein tyrosine phosphorylation. Gene 1999; 238(2): 471-8.
[http://dx.doi.org/10.1016/S0378-1119(99)00364-9] [PMID: 10570975]

[259] NRG1 neuregulin 1 [Homo sapiens (human)]-Gene-NCBI, https://www.ncbi.nlm.nih.gov/gene/3084 (accessed 19 June 2020).

[260] Yang L, Li Y, Shen E, *et al.* NRG1-dependent activation of HER3 induces primary resistance to trastuzumab in HER2-overexpressing breast cancer cells. Int J Oncol 2017; 51(5): 1553-62.
[http://dx.doi.org/10.3892/ijo.2017.4130] [PMID: 29048656]

[261] Fernandez-Cuesta L, Plenker D, Osada H, *et al.* CD74-NRG1 fusions in lung adenocarcinoma. Cancer Discov 2014; 4(4): 415-22.
[http://dx.doi.org/10.1158/2159-8290.CD-13-0633] [PMID: 24469108]

[262] NSD3 nuclear receptor binding SET domain protein 3 [Homo sapiens (human)]-Gene-NCBI, https://www.ncbi.nlm.nih.gov/gene/54904 (accessed 19 June 2020).

[263] Mahmood SF, Gruel N, Nicolle R, *et al.* PPAPDC1B and WHSC1L1 are common drivers of the 8p11-12 amplicon, not only in breast tumors but also in pancreatic adenocarcinomas and lung tumors. Am J Pathol 2013; 183(5): 1634-44.
[http://dx.doi.org/10.1016/j.ajpath.2013.07.028] [PMID: 24051013]

[264] Dutt A, Ramos AH, Hammerman PS, *et al.* Inhibitor-sensitive FGFR1 amplification in human non-small cell lung cancer. PLoS One 2011; 6(6): e20351.
[http://dx.doi.org/10.1371/journal.pone.0020351] [PMID: 21666749]

[265] PCM1 pericentriolar material 1 [Homo sapiens (human)]-Gene-NCBI, https://www.ncbi.nlm.nih.gov/gene/5108 (accessed 19 June 2020).

[266] Lee JM, Lee J, Han E, *et al.* PCM1-JAK2 fusion in a patient with acute myeloid leukemia. Ann Lab Med 2018; 38(5): 492-4.
[http://dx.doi.org/10.3343/alm.2018.38.5.492] [PMID: 29797824]

[267] Murati A, Gelsi-Boyer V, Adélaïde J, *et al.* PCM1-JAK2 fusion in myeloproliferative disorders and acute erythroid leukemia with t(8;9) translocation. Leukemia 2005; 19(9): 1692-6.
[http://dx.doi.org/10.1038/sj.leu.2403879] [PMID: 16034466]

[268] Rumi E, Milosevic JD, Selleslag D, *et al.* Efficacy of ruxolitinib in myeloid neoplasms with PCM1-JAK2 fusion gene. Ann Hematol 2015; 94(11): 1927-8.

[http://dx.doi.org/10.1007/s00277-015-2451-7] [PMID: 26202607]

[269] PINX1 PIN2 (TERF1) interacting telomerase inhibitor 1 [Homo sapiens (human)]-Gene-NCBI, https://www.ncbi.nlm.nih.gov/gene/54984 (accessed 19 June 2020).

[270] Wang H, Wang X, Zhou G, *et al.* PinX1 inhibits telomerase activity in gastric cancer cells through Mad1/c-Myc pathway. J Gastrointest Surg 2010; 14(8): 1227-34.
[http://dx.doi.org/10.1007/s11605-010-1253-4] [PMID: 20544396]

[271] Shi M, Cao M, Song J, *et al.* PinX1 inhibits the invasion and metastasis of human breast cancer *via* suppressing NF-κB/MMP-9 signaling pathway. Mol Cancer 2015; 14(1): 66.
[http://dx.doi.org/10.1186/s12943-015-0332-2] [PMID: 25888829]

[272] Sriprapun M, Chuaypen N, Khlaiphuengsin A, Pinjaroen N, Payungporn S, Tangkijvanich P. Association of PINX1 but not TEP1 polymorphisms with progression to hepatocellular carcinoma in thai patients with chronic hepatitis B virus infection. Asian Pac J Cancer Prev 2016; 17(4): 2019-25.
[http://dx.doi.org/10.7314/APJCP.2016.17.4.2019] [PMID: 27221889]

[273] PLAG1 PLAG1 zinc finger [Homo sapiens (human)]-Gene-NCBI, https://www.ncbi.nlm.nih.gov/gene/5324 (accessed 19 June 2020).

[274] Wasserman JK, Dickson BC, Smith A, Swanson D, Purgina BM, Weinreb I. Metastasizing Pleomorphic Adenoma. Am J Surg Pathol 2019; 43(8): 1145-51.
[http://dx.doi.org/10.1097/PAS.0000000000001280] [PMID: 31094927]

[275] Katabi N, Xu B, Jungbluth AA, *et al.* PLAG1 immunohistochemistry is a sensitive marker for pleomorphic adenoma: a comparative study with *PLAG1* genetic abnormalities. Histopathology 2018; 72(2): 285-93.
[http://dx.doi.org/10.1111/his.13341] [PMID: 28796899]

[276] PLAT plasminogen activator, tissue type [Homo sapiens (human)]-Gene-NCBI, https://www.ncbi.nlm.nih.gov/gene/5327 (accessed 19 June 2020).

[277] Theillet C, Adelaide J, Louason G, *et al.* FGFRI andPLAT genes and DNA amplification at 8p 12 in breast and ovarian cancers. Genes Chromosomes Cancer 1993; 7(4): 219-26.
[http://dx.doi.org/10.1002/gcc.2870070407] [PMID: 7692948]

[278] König JJ, Teubel W, van Steenbrugge GJ, Romijn JC, Hagemeijer A. Characterization of chromosome 8 aberrations in the prostate cancer cell line LNCaP-FGC and sublines. Urol Res 1999; 27(1): 3-8.
[http://dx.doi.org/10.1007/s002400050082] [PMID: 10092147]

[279] Lu Y, Li C, Chen H, Zhong W. Identification of hub genes and analysis of prognostic values in pancreatic ductal adenocarcinoma by integrated bioinformatics methods. Mol Biol Rep 2018; 45(6): 1799-807.
[http://dx.doi.org/10.1007/s11033-018-4325-2] [PMID: 30173393]

[280] POLB DNA polymerase beta [Homo sapiens (human)]-Gene-NCBI, https://www.ncbi.nlm.nih.gov/gene/5423 (accessed 19 June 2020).

[281] Eydmann ME, Knowles MA. Mutation analysis of 8p genes POLB and PPP2CB in bladder cancer. Cancer Genet Cytogenet 1997; 93(2): 167-71.
[http://dx.doi.org/10.1016/S0165-4608(96)00200-2] [PMID: 9078303]

[282] Iwatsuki M, Mimori K, Yokobori T, *et al.* A platinum agent resistance gene, *POLB*, is a prognostic indicator in colorectal cancer. J Surg Oncol 2009; 100(3): 261-6.
[http://dx.doi.org/10.1002/jso.21275] [PMID: 19330779]

[283] Chang JG, Chen CC, Wu YY, *et al.* Uncovering synthetic lethal interactions for therapeutic targets and predictive markers in lung adenocarcinoma. Oncotarget 2016; 7(45): 73664-80.
[http://dx.doi.org/10.18632/oncotarget.12046] [PMID: 27655641]

[284] PRKDC protein kinase, DNA-activated, catalytic subunit [Homo sapiens (human)]-Gene-NCBI, https://www.ncbi.nlm.nih.gov/gene/5591 (accessed 19 June 2020).

[285] Hu M, Du J, Cui L, *et al. IL-10* and *PRKDC* polymorphisms are associated with glioma patient survival. Oncotarget 2016; 7(49): 80680-7.
[http://dx.doi.org/10.18632/oncotarget.13028] [PMID: 27811370]

[286] Sun G, Yang L, Dong C, Ma B, Shan M, Ma B. PRKDC regulates chemosensitivity and is a potential prognostic and predictive marker of response to adjuvant chemotherapy in breast cancer patients. Oncol Rep 2017; 37(6): 3536-42.
[http://dx.doi.org/10.3892/or.2017.5634] [PMID: 28498431]

[287] Kita K, Fukuda K, Takahashi H, *et al.* Patient-derived xenograft models of non-small cell lung cancer for evaluating targeted drug sensitivity and resistance Cancer Sci 2019; 110(10): 3215-24.
[http://dx.doi.org/10.1111/cas.14171] [PMID: 31432603]

[288] PSCA prostate stem cell antigen [Homo sapiens (human)]-Gene-NCBI, https://www.ncbi.nlm.nih.gov/gene/8000 (accessed 28 August 2020).

[289] Heinrichs SKM, Hess T, Becker J, *et al.* Evidence for *PTGER4, PSCA,* and *MBOAT7* as risk genes for gastric cancer on the genome and transcriptome level. Cancer Med 2018; 7(10): 5057-65.
[http://dx.doi.org/10.1002/cam4.1719] [PMID: 30191681]

[290] Heinrich MC, Göbel C, Kluth M, *et al.* PSCA expression is associated with favorable tumor features and reduced PSA recurrence in operated prostate cancer. BMC Cancer 2018; 18(1): 612.
[http://dx.doi.org/10.1186/s12885-018-4547-7] [PMID: 29855276]

[291] Saeki N, Gu J, Yoshida T, Wu X. Prostate stem cell antigen: a Jekyll and Hyde molecule? Clin Cancer Res 2010; 16(14): 3533-8.
[http://dx.doi.org/10.1158/1078-0432.CCR-09-3169] [PMID: 20501618]

[292] PTK2 | Cancer Genetics Web, http://www.cancerindex.org/geneweb/PTK2.htm (accessed 28 August 2020).

[293] Rigiracciolo DC, Santolla MF, Lappano R, *et al.* Focal adhesion kinase (FAK) activation by estrogens involves GPER in triple-negative breast cancer cells. J Exp Clin Cancer Res 2019; 38(1): 58.
[http://dx.doi.org/10.1186/s13046-019-1056-8] [PMID: 30728047]

[294] Fan Z, Duan J, Wang L, *et al.* PTK2 promotes cancer stem cell traits in hepatocellular carcinoma by activating Wnt/β-catenin signaling. Cancer Lett 2019; 450: 132-43.
[http://dx.doi.org/10.1016/j.canlet.2019.02.040] [PMID: 30849480]

[295] PTP4A3 | Cancer Genetics Web, http://www.cancerindex.org/geneweb//PTP4A3.htm (accessed 28 August 2020).

[296] Wang L, Yu T, Li W, *et al.* The miR-29c-KIAA1199 axis regulates gastric cancer migration by binding with WBP11 and PTP4A3. Oncogene 2019; 38(17): 3134-50.
[http://dx.doi.org/10.1038/s41388-018-0642-0] [PMID: 30626935]

[297] Mayinuer A, Yasen M, Mogushi K, *et al.* Upregulation of protein tyrosine phosphatase type IVA member 3 (PTP4A3/PRL-3) is associated with tumor differentiation and a poor prognosis in human hepatocellular carcinoma. Ann Surg Oncol 2013; 20(1): 305-17.
[http://dx.doi.org/10.1245/s10434-012-2395-2] [PMID: 23064776]

[298] Zimmerman MW, Homanics GE, Lazo JS. Targeted deletion of the metastasis-associated phosphatase Ptp4a3 (PRL-3) suppresses murine colon cancer. PLoS One 2013; 8(3): e58300.
[http://dx.doi.org/10.1371/journal.pone.0058300] [PMID: 23555575]

CHAPTER 9

Chromosome 9

Thilaga Thirugnanam[1], **Yamini Chandrapraksh**[1,#], **Sivasankari Ramadurai**[1,#], **Abhishek Mitra**[1,#], **Ravi Gor**[1], **Saurav Panicker**[1] and **Satish Ramalingam**[1,*]

[1] *Department of Genetic Engineering, School of Bioengineering, SRM Institute of Science and Technology, Kattankulathur, India*

Abstract: Chromosome 9 represents approximately 4.5 percent of the total DNA in cells, and it's a submetacentric type of chromosome. Chromosomal abnormalities in chromosome 9 have been reported in different kinds of cancer, for example, deletion of the long-q arm, a fusion of ABL1 with BCR results in the ABL1-BCR fusion gene, *etc*. Bladder cancer, chronic myeloid leukemia, *etc*., are several cancer types resulting from genetic changes in the genes present in chromosome 9. Dysregulation of the tumor suppressor genes or activation of the oncogene from chromosome 9 has supported the normal cell's transformation. Here, we have listed a few top genes reappearing themselves as causative agent for cancer development in cancer and types of cancer.

Keywords: ABL1-BCR, Bladder Cancer, Chromosomal Abnormalities, Chronic Myeloid Leukemia, Fusion Gene, Genetic Change, Oncogene, q-arm, Submetacentric, Tumor Suppressor.

1.1. ABCA1 - ATP-BINDING CASSETTE, SUBFAMILY A, MEMBER 1 CHROMOSOME 9; 9q31.1

ABCA1 belongs to the ATP-binding cassette transporter (ABC) superfamily [1]. It is involved in the reverse transport of the cholesterol pathway, which helps translocate the phospholipids and cholesterol from the cytoplasm to the cell surface embedded with apolipoproteins and monitors the pathway [1]. Several mutations in this gene lead to a high-density lipoprotein deficiency disorder called Tangier disease, which further causes atherosclerosis [1]. Disruptions in *ABCA1* expression cause cancer and tumor progression [2]. A study observed the correlation between ABCA1 and cholesterol in colorectal cancer where the upregulation of ABCA1 resulted in cell invasion, cell proliferation, and Epithe-

---

[*] **Corresponding author Satish Ramalingam**: Department of Genetic Engineering, School of Bioengineering, SRM Institute of Science and Technology, Kattankulathur, India; E-mail: rsatish76@gmail.com
[#] Equal authorship and equal contribution status.

lial-Mesenchymal transition away from the primary location [2]. In addition, ABCA1 might induce metastasis and growth of tumors [2]. *ABCA1* gene expression might be a potential biomarker for the prognosis of colorectal cancer [2].

1.2. ANXA1 - ANNEXIN A1 CHROMOSOME 9; 9q21.13

ANXA1 belongs to the superfamily of annexin proteins which binds to phospholipids on cell membranes involving physiological functions such as cellular differentiation, membrane trafficking, proliferation, and signal trans-duction [3]. In addition, expression of ANXA1 is reported in various cancers, including bladder, liver, lung, skin, prostate, pancreatic, colorectal, endometrial, esophageal, melanoma, cervical cancer, and oral cancer [4]. In prostate cancer, ANXA1 was downregulated under hypoxic conditions resulting in cell invasion and metastasis of the prostate cancer cell line, indicating that ANXA1 might be a useful therapeutic marker for prostate cancer undergoing metastasis [5]. In colorectal cancer, the expression of ANXA1 was increased, leading to early metastasis of lymph nodes and invasion, suggesting that ANXA1 could serve as a biomarker for colorectal cancer prognosis [4].

1.3. AQP3 - AQUAPORIN 3 CHROMOSOME 9; 9p13.3

AQP3 is a water channel protein belonging to the aquaporin protein family that regulates the influx and efflux of water in cells [6]. This protein is expressed in the membrane of chorions in the amniotic fluid and placenta in humans to maintain amniotic fluid homeostasis [6]. Apart from water homeostasis, AQP3 also regulates the flow of solutes of neutral charges, such as urea and glycerol [6]. AQP3 is expressed in normal tissues like the brain, lungs, pancreas, prostate, epithelial cells, breast, liver, ovary, and bladder [7]. Moreover, the expression of AQP3 is increased in pancreatic, colon, hepatocellular carcinoma, and lung cancer [7]. This protein induces proliferation, migration, and invasion of cancer cells, and promotes epithelial-mesenchymal transition [7].

1.4. BAG1 - BCL2- ASSOCIATED ANTHANOGENE 1 CHROMOSOME 9; 9p13.3

BCL2- associated anthanogene 1 (*BAG1*) is widely involved in the development, progression, and metastasis of cancer; overexpression of BCL2- associated anthanogene 1 (BAG1) is reported in breast cancer, it consists of the development of lesions, tumor development, cancer progression, and metastasis [8].

1.5. BRINP1 - BONE MORPHOGENETIC PROTEIN/RETINOIC ACID-INDUCIBLE NEURAL-SPECIFIC PROTEIN 1 CHROMOSOME 9; 9q33.1

This gene is commonly known as Deleted in Bladder Cancer Chromosome 1 (*DBCC1*), which is widely seen in patients with Bladder and Lung cancer, and the effect of this gene is seen lesser in the early stages of lung cancer; this gene is further silenced so that proliferation, migration, invasion of the cancer cells can be controlled, and Lung cancer can be reduced and prevented. Downregulation of Deleted in Bladder Cancer Chromosome 1 (*DBCC1*) is done by DNA methylation [9].

1.6. CA9 - CARBONIC ANHYDRASE 9 CHROMOSOME 9; 9p13.3

Acid transport is significant in cancer cell progression, transport metabolons, cancer invasion, and cell migration; an acid vehicle is seen between bicarbonate and Carbonic anhydrase (*CA9*), which alters the pH, acid, and bases level, which leads to the progression of cancer [10].

1.7. CCL19 - C-C MOTIF CHEMOKINE LIGAND 19 CHROMOSOME 9; 9p13.3

CCL19 is associated with cervical cancer and is also involved in epithelial to mesenchymal transition cervical cancer. The overexpression of the C-C motif ligand 19 (CCL19) leads to the progression of cervical cancer and is also abnormally expressed, which involves tumor development [11].

1.8. CCL21 - C-C MOTIF CHEMOKINE LIGAND 21 CHROMOSOME 9; 9p13.3

CCL21 is expressed during the formation of lymphoid organs and vessels, interacting with glycosaminoglycans and embedding the proteins on endothelial cell surfaces [12]. The CCL21 induces breast cancer proliferation, and this ligand is responsible for the metastasis and progression of tumors in the breast cells and tissues [12].

1.9. CD274 - MOLECULE PROGRAMMED CELL DEATH 1 LIGAND 1 CHROMOSOME 9; 9p24.1

CD274 is also known as PD-1 or Programmed death 1, which regulates the suppression of the immune response to Th1 cytotoxicity *via* negative feedback [12]. This protein is also involved in various cancer, such as Hodgkin's lymphoma, renal cell carcinoma, melanoma, bladder cancer, and non-small cell lung carcinoma, where it is expressed on the cell membrane of immune cells and tumors [12]. In colorectal cancer, CD274 is expressed in the cell membrane and cytoplasm of colorectal cancer cells regulating the densities of T-cells [13].

1.10. CDK9 - CYCLIN-DEPENDENT KINASE 9 CHROMOSOME 9; 9q34.11

Cyclin-dependent kinase 9 (CDK9) is responsible for the formation and inducing of different cancers, the progression of cancer occurs due to the transcription of Myc, which is a proto-oncogene accountable for the development of malignancy, the commonly caused cancer from the Cyclin-dependent kinase 9, (CDK9) pathway are seen in the Hematopoietic and Lymphoid tissue developing regions, which later forms different forms of Leukaemia, Lymphomas, Hodgkin's disease [14].

1.11. CDKN2B - CYCLIN-DEPENDENT KINASE INHIBITOR 2B CHROMOSOME 9; 9p21.3

This gene encoding cyclin-dependent kinase inhibitor protein inhibits the expression of cyclin-dependent kinases to regulate the cell cycle G1 progression [15]. CDKN2B is downregulated in T-acute lymphoblastic leukemia due to deletion or hypermethylation [15]. Further, the loss of *CDKN2A-CDKN2B* was associated with shorter survival in cutaneous T-cell lymphoma CTCL patients [16]. Hence, these deletions can be used to access individuals with an aggressive form of epidermotropic CTCLs [16]. Similarly, this gene was also altered more frequently in upper tract urothelial carcinoma [17].

1.12. CDKN2B-AS1- CDKN2B ANTISENSE RNA 1 CHROMOSOME 9; 9p21.3

ANRIL, also known as *p15AS, PCAT12, CDKN2BAS, CDKN2B-AS,* and *NCRNA-00089*, regulates epigenetic gene silencing [18]. *ANRIL* is involved in cardiovascular disease, Alzheimer's disease, type-2 diabetes, intracranial aneurysm, glaucoma, periodontitis, and endometriosis [18]. In cervical cancer, *CDKN2B-AS1* inhibited apoptosis and senescence inhibition and promoted tumor growth by activating the CDKN2B-AS1/miR-181a-5p/TGFβI axis [18]. Hence, this knockdown can help overcome the development of cervical cancer [18]. Similarly, *CDKN2B-AS1* also induced CDKN2B-AS1/miR-141/Cyclin D axis in renal cell carcinoma and regulated the EMT-driven metastasis. Hence, this axis might be a promising therapeutic target in renal cell carcinoma [19].

1.13. CKS2 - CDC28 PROTEIN KINASE REGULATORY SUBUNIT 2 CHROMOSOME 9; 9q22.2

CKS2 is upregulated in malignant phenotypes of hepatocellular carcinoma (HCC) where downregulation of CKS2 suppressed cell proliferation, colony formation, chemoresistance, cell migration, and cell invasion of HCC tumor cells, indicating that CSK2 is a novel prognostic biomarker and therapeutic target of HCC [20]. In colorectal cancer, *CSK2* was reported as a Wnt/β-catenin target gene that induced metastasis, cell migration, and epithelial-mesenchymal transition [21]. This gene was crosstalk with other downstream signaling systems to activate metastasis-promoting genes [21]. Similarly, the CSK2 was upregulated in the bladder and muscle-invasive cancer cells, suggesting a role as a potential therapeutic target for bladder and muscle-invasive cancer [22]. Androgen-independent metastatic tumors in prostate cancer were found to have increased *CKS2* expression indicating an aggressive form of prostate cancer [23].

1.14. DAB2IP - DAB2 INTERACTING PROTEIN CHROMOSOME 9; 9q33.2

This name is also known as AIP1, AIP-1, AF9Q34, and DIP1/2. This gene is a GTPase-activating protein that acts as a tumor suppressor [24]. Due to methylation, *DAB2IP* is silenced in several cancers, including prostate and breast cancer [24]. The expression of DAB2IP resulted in chemoresistance in castration-resistant prostate cancer [24]. Further, this gene is a potential tumor suppressor that, on inhibition, activates the mutant p53 due to high insulin levels in type 2 diabetes patients leading to the development of cancer [25]. In urothelial carcinoma, the downregulation of DAB2IP resulted in the activation of ERK and Akt pathways leading to the expression of epithelial to mesenchymal transition biomarkers resulting in cell proliferation, migration, and invasion of bladder cancer [26].

1.15. DAPK1-DEATH-ASSOCIATED PROTEIN KINASE 1 CHROMOSOME 9; 9q21.33

As *DAPK* or *ROCO3* is a tumor suppressor, it is associated with apoptosis [27]. The promoter of the gene *DAPK1* was methylated in cervical cancer (CC) based on the histological tumor type [27]. These methylation markers may be useful in the early identification of CC precursor lesions and human papillomavirus in infected women [27]. Likewise, promoter methylation of the *DAPK1* gene is linked to the progression of breast cancer cells and decreased breast cancer survival rate in Indian women [28]. Cytochrome P450 1B1 (*CYP1B1*) promotes the development of renal cell carcinoma by inducing the CDC20 and by inhibiting the downregulation of *DAPK1* [29]. Hence, CYP1B1 is a potential therapeutic biomarker for renal cell carcinoma [29].

1.16. DEC1- DELETED IN ESOPHAGEAL CANCER 1 CHROMOSOME 9; 9q33.1

DEC1 is situated in a locus usually deleted in esophageal squamous cell carcinoma leading to no or reduced expression. It also functions as a tumor suppressor for esophageal squamous cell carcinomas [30]. Decreased expression of *DEC1* induces metastasis in head and neck squamous cell carcinoma [30]. In addition, the trimethylation of H3 K27 regulates the expression of DEC1 [30]. In breast cancer cells, increased expression of DEC1 affected the cell cycle by disrupting the levels of cyclin E protein [31]. In addition, DEC1 stabilized cyclin E by interacting with it in breast cancer [31]. Further, DEC1 induced epithelial to mesenchymal under transition hypoxic conditions by downregulating E-cadherin in hepatocellular carcinoma [32].

1.17. FOXE1- FORKHEAD BOX E1 CHROMOSOME 9; 9q22.33

FOXE1 is a transcription factor belonging to the forkhead family, which functions as a thyroid transcription factor aiding in thyroid morphogenesis [33]. Mutations in *FOXE1* cause various diseases, including Bamforth-Lazarus syndrome and non-medullary thyroid cancer-4. In papillary thyroid cancer, miR-524-5p interacted with ITGA3 and FOXE1 proteins, which suppressed cell invasion, migration, cell viability, and apoptosis [33]. In contrast, *FOXE1* and *ITGA3* expression was downregulated, disrupting cell cycling and autophagy pathways [33]. A study observed that the FOXE1 promoter was hypermethylated in cutaneous squamous cell carcinoma resulting in decreased or no expression of the *FOXE1* gene [34].

1.18. GALT - GALACTOSE-1-PHOSPHATE URIDYLYLTRANSFERASE CHROMOSOME 9; 9p13.3

GALT is involved in the Leloir pathway of galactose metabolism. It catalyzes the conversion of uridine diphosphate glucose to galactose and the lack of GALT causes galactosemia in humans and is detrimental in newborns. D1 and D2 genotypes of this gene were not associated between galactose intake, ovarian dysfunction, and the risk of epithelial ovarian cancer [35]. Further in breast cancer, GalT I regulated cell adhesion to laminin [36].

1.19. GAS1 - GROWTH ARREST-SPECIFIC 1 CHROMOSOME 9; 9q21.33

Growth arrest-specific 1 protein is a tumor suppressor involved in inhibiting cell growth, which also blocks the cells from entering the S phase [37]. In glioma, upregulation of *GAS1* promoted apoptosis and cell cycle arrest of glioma cells, indicating a potential to treat glioblastoma [37]. In contrast, Gas1 downregulated the AMPK/mTOR/p70S6K signaling axis by targeting FOXM1 resulting in abnormal cancer progression, metastasis, and cancer cell proliferation in colorectal cancer [38]. In addition, this might be used to predict the first two stages of colorectal cancer reoccurrence and metastasis [39].

1.20. JAK2 - JANUS KINASE 2 CHROMOSOME 9; 9p24.1

This gene (Fig. **1**) belongs to the cytokine receptor signaling proteins family, which is essential for responses to gamma interferon [40]. Several mutations in *JAK2* causing a loss of CDKN2A and JAK2 alleles lead to immunotherapy resistance marking the importance of screening *JAK2* deficiency and immune checkpoint blocking therapy [40]. Alterations of *JAK2* were found to activate JAK/STAT signaling in these patients [41].

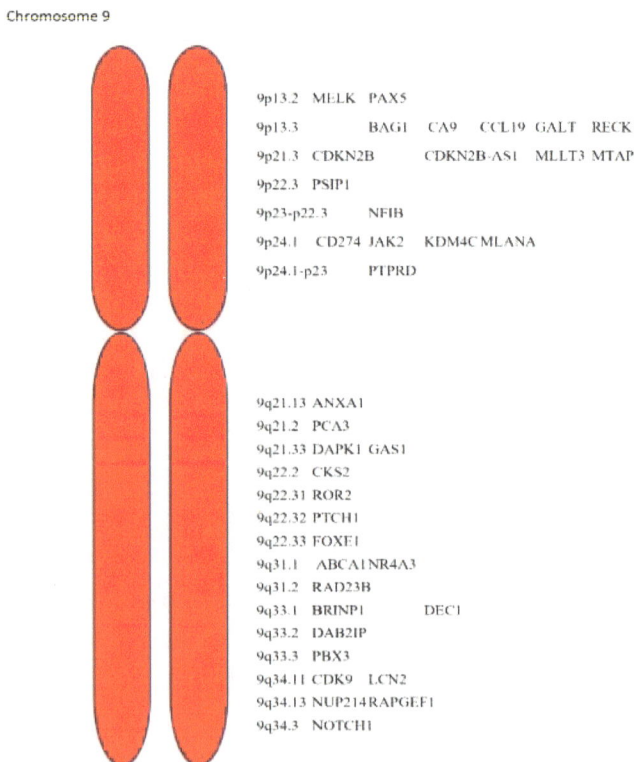

Chromosome 9

Locus	Genes
9p13.2	MELK PAX5
9p13.3	BAG1 CA9 CCL19 GALT RECK
9p21.3	CDKN2B CDKN2B-AS1 MLLT3 MTAP
9p22.3	PSIP1
9p23-p22.3	NFIB
9p24.1	CD274 JAK2 KDM4C MLANA
9p24.1-p23	PTPRD
9q21.13	ANXA1
9q21.2	PCA3
9q21.33	DAPK1 GAS1
9q22.2	CKS2
9q22.31	ROR2
9q22.32	PTCH1
9q22.33	FOXE1
9q31.1	ABCA1 NR4A3
9q31.2	RAD23B
9q33.1	BRINP1 DEC1
9q33.2	DAB2IP
9q33.3	PBX3
9q34.11	CDK9 LCN2
9q34.13	NUP214 RAPGEF1
9q34.3	NOTCH1

Fig. (1). This figure displays the loci of the genes from Chromosome 9 whose roles in cancer have been explained in this chapter. Sayooj Madhusoodanan designed these diagrams.

1.21. KDM4C - KYSINE DEMETHYLASE 4C CHROMOSOME 9; 9p24.1

KDM4C (Fig. **1**) is a nuclear protein belonging to the Jumonji domain 2 proteins involved in catalyzing the demethylation of trimethylated histones [42]. In oesophageal squamous cell carcinoma, chromosomal aberrations are correlated with increased transcriptional expression [42]. Downregulation of KDM4C decreased the tumor progression in pancreatic cancer cells indicating that *KDM4C* is an oncoprotein in pancreatic cancer [43]. A study observed that KDM4C induced cell proliferation by activating AKT and c-Myc in pancreatic cancer [44].

1.22. LCN2 - LIPOCALIN 2 CHROMOSOME 9; 9q34.11

LCN2 belongs to the family of lipocalin proteins and is involved in cell regulation, proliferation, and differentiation by interacting with cell membrane receptors and carrying lipophilic ligands [45]. In addition, LCN2 is involved in pancreatic, thyroid, colon, and ovarian cancers [46]. In breast cancer, upregulation of LCN2 resulted in metastasis, epithelial-mesenchymal transition, and angio-genesis, suggesting that LCN2 might serve as a biomarker for metastasis in breast cancer [46].

1.23. MELK - MATERNAL EMBRYONIC LEUCINE ZIPPER KINASE CHROMOSOME 9; 9p13.2

MELK gene encodes for maternal embryonic leucine zipper kinase in humans that belongs to the AMPK/Snf1 protein kinase family [47]. The expression of MELK is increased in various cancers, indicating a target for pharmacological inhibition [48]. Earlier studies have shown that MELK is essential for cancer cell pro-liferation [48]. However, a recent study has shown that MELK is not essential for cancer cell growth, casting doubt on targeting this protein in patients [48]. Since the results depend on the experimental design, there is a need for further research [48]. Further, upregulation of MELK correlated to tumor progression, cancer aggression, poor prognosis, and radioresistance [49 - 53].

1.24. MLANA - MELAN-A CHROMOSOME 9; 9p24.1

MLANA is an antigen secreted by various cancer cells such as adrenocortical carcinoma, sarcoma, and melanoma and non-melanoma cells, including retinal pigmental cells and skin cells [54]. MLANA is used as a biomarker for cancers like sinonasal melanomas that develop in the neck and head [54]. In head and neck squamous cell carcinoma, upregulation of MLANA resulted in disease progression, which might serve as a biomarker [54].

1.25. MLLT3 - SUPER ELONGATION COMPLEX SUBUNIT CHROMO SOME 9; 9p 21.3

MLLT3 is a proto-oncogene (Fig. 1) and was initially identified in leukemia involving cell differentiation [55], cell fate decision [56], and nervous system development and disease condition [57]. Disruption in MLLT3 was correlated with ataxia, mental retardation, and epilepsy in humans [58]. A study showed that MLLT3 is involved in lymphocytoma [59]. A study by the Calvanese group showed that expression of MLLT3 is essential for regulating hematopoietic stem cells, especially in human fetal, neonatal, and adult hematopoietic stem cells, while downregulated in cultures [60]. A study by Dickinson *et al.* (2016) found that the knockout of the mouse homolog of human MLLT3 is homozygous-lethal among 1,751 knockout alleles [61].

1.26. MTAP - METHYL THIO ADENOSINE PHOSPHORYLASE CHROMO SOME 9; 9p 21.3

MTAP gene encodes for S-methyl-5'- this adenosine phosphorylase involved in the polyamine metabolism [62] where MTAP helps in metabolizing MTA to adenine and methionine and recycling back to MTA [63]. In several cancers, the MTAP enzyme is deleted along with *p16*, a tumor suppressor gene [62]. Though the full length of the MTAP gene is unknown, alternatively spliced transcripts have been identified [62]. *MTAP* is in chromosome 9p21 near *CDKN2A*, a tumor suppressor gene which results in co-deletion of the MTAP gene frequently in human tumors [63].

1.27. NFIB - NUCLEAR FACTOR I B CHROMOSOME 9; 9p23-p22.3

The NFIB gene and three other genes form the NFI gene complex [64, 65]. The NFIB gene is a transcription factor involved in embryonic development for tissue differentiation in the fetus [65]. NFIB is present abundantly in the lungs, skeletal muscle, heart, and also in the developing liver, kidneys, and brain [64]. In melanoma, NFIB induces the expression of EZH2. A study showed that BRN2 regulates NFIB expression to upregulate cell migration and invasion, which might occur due to the up-and-downregulation of EZH2 and MITF, respectively [66].

1.28. NOTCH1 - NOTCH RECEPTOR 1 CHROMOSOME 9; 9q34.3

NOTCH1 is a transmembrane protein involved in Notch signaling to regulate tissue and cell development [67]. This gene mutation leads to aortic valve disease, head and neck squamous cell carcinoma, and chronic and acute lymphoblastic leukemia [68]. Several cancers exhibited oncogenic including the brain, bone, and lymph node [69], and tumor-suppressive effects of Notch signaling were in prostate cancer, disruption in Notch signaling led to the progression of prostate cancer cells [70].

1.29. NR4A3 - NUCLEAR RECEPTOR SUBFAMILY 4 GROUP A MEMBER 3 CHROMOSOME 9; 9q31.1

NR4A3 is a transcription factor that interacts with NGFI-B Response Element (NBRE) and is involved in stress, apoptosis, and cell growth [71]. NR4A3 is present in various tissues, including T-cells, heart, skeletal muscle, brain, adipose, kidney, and liver [71]. In addition, this gene is expressed in diseases such as extraskeletal myxoid chondrosarcomas which are caused due to reciprocal trans-locations in the *NR4A3* gene [71]. In diffuse large B-cell lymphoma, NR4A3 is upregulated, leading to apoptosis during chemotherapy [71].

1.30. NUP214 - NUCLEOPORIN 214 CHROMOSOME 9; 9q34.13

In eukaryotic cells, nucleoporins are part of the nuclear pore complex, and the NUP214 gene, belonging to the FG- repeat-containing nucleoporins family, is essential in the nuclear transport of macromolecules [72], and cell cycle progression [73]. Chromosomal translocations frequently occur in *NUP214* that translocate with the DEK gene on chromosome 6, resulting in myelodysplastic syndrome and acute leukemia [74].

1.31. PAX5 - PAIRED BOX 5 CHROMOSOME 9; 9p13.2

Pax5 is a transcription factor expressed in the development of the brain and other organs in the embryo, cell differentiation, and hematopoiesis [75]. *Pax5* gene variants are described in various cells, such as lymphoid lineage cells and testicles [75]. In addition, Pax5 is expressed different cancers Hodgkin's lymphoma and lymphoblastic leukemia [75]. Mutation in *Pax5* causes disruption in the differentiation of B cells leading to acute lymphoblastic leukemia. In T-cell lymphoblastic leukemia, *Pax5* is hypermethylated, leading to its silencing of it [75].

1.32. PBX3 - PBX HOMEOBOX 3 CHROMOSOME 9; 9q33.3

PBX3 belongs to the family of pre-B cell leukemia transcription factors, involved in early development and certain adult functions [76]. A recent study in gastric cancer showed that PBX3 promotes cell invasion, and metastasis through epithelial-mesenchymal transition [77]. PBX3 is involved in aggressive prostate cancer [78], and colorectal cancer, where it triggers the mitogen-activated protein kinase/extracellular signal-regulated kinase pathway [79].

1.33. PCA3 - PROSTATE CANCER-ASSOCIATED 3 CHROMOSOME 9; 9q21.2

Several studies on *PCA3* have been published due to its potential as a marker for prostate cancer [80]. *PCA3* transcribes to a long non-coding RNA which is expressed in microsomes and the nucleus [80]. The function of PCA3 is unknown, however, in androgen receptor signaling, inhibition of PCA3 promoted apoptosis and inhibition of cell growth [80]. Polymorphic repeats in PCA3 might promote metastasis of prostate cancer. As *PCA3* is upregulated in prostate cancer, it is widely studied to utilize it as a biomarker [81].

1.34. PSIP1 - PC4 AND SFRS1 INTERACTING PROTEIN 1 CHROMOSOME 9; 9p22.3

PSIP1 produces different proteins such as PSIP1/p52 and PSIP1/p75 [82]. They are responsible for DNA repair, transcription, splicing, and inhibition of apoptosis [82]. *PSIP1* is abnormally expressed in leukemia and especially the development of ovarian cancer involving lymphangiogenesis and subcutaneous angiogenesis and is upregulated in breast cancer, liver cancer, colon cancer, prostate cancer, uterus cancer, and thyroid cancer [82]. In addition, PSIP1 is expressed in the proliferation and progression of cancer [82]. In breast cancer, downregulation of PSIP1 resulted in metastasis, cell cycle, cell proliferation, and apoptosis [82].

1.35. PTCH1 - PATCHED 1 CHROMOSOME 9; 9q22.32

PTCH1 belongs to the family of patched proteins that is responsible for the hedgehog signaling pathway during the development of tumors and embryos [83]. Mutations in the *PTCH1* gene cause basal cell nevus syndrome, holopro-sencephaly, trichoepitheliomas, basal cell, and esophageal squamous cell carcinomas of the bladder [83]. Many studies reported the expression of PTCH1 protein in human disorders and tumorigenesis [84 - 86].

1.36. PTPRD - PROTEIN TYROSINE PHOSPHATASE RECEPTOR TYPE D CHROMOSOME 9; 9p24.1-P23

PTP belonging to the tyrosine phosphatase family plays a role in cell differentiation, cancer cell progression, and epithelial-to-mesenchymal transition [87]. In organisms such as chickens and flies, PTP is involved in neuron development, such as neurite growth and regulation of axon guidance [88]. PTPRT is mutated in colorectal cancer, gastric cancer and lung cancer [89]. In head and neck squamous cell carcinoma, mutated PTPRT disrupted the dephosphorylation of the Signal transducer and activator of transcription 3 protein [90].

1.37. RAD23B - RAD23 HOMOLOG B CHROMOSOME 9; 9q31.2

RAD23B is involved in nucleotide excision repair and binds with proteasome through the ubiquitin-like domain in proteasome mechanisms such as ubiquitin-mediated proteolytic pathway and DNA repair pathway [91]. In addition, RAD23B upregulates nucleotide excision of DNA-3-methyladenine glycosylase enzyme, indicating involvement in recognizing the DNA damage during the base excision repair pathway [91].

1.38. RAPGEF1 - RAP GUANINE NUCLEOTIDE EXCHANGE FACTOR 1 CHROMOSOME 9; 9q34.13

RAPGEF1 binds to CRK, activating GTPases in the Ras family, which might play a role in apoptosis, cell transformation, and signal transduction [92]. In fibroblasts, RAPGEF1 upregulation suppressed the anchorage-independent growth that was activated by oncogenes [92]. In addition, RAPGEF1 is also upregulated in small-cell lung carcinomas [93]. RAPGEF1 is silenced by hypermethylation of the promoter squamous cervical cancer and is hypomethylated in gastric and colorectal cancer [94].

1.39. RECK - REVERSION-INDUCING CYSTEINE-RICH PROTEIN WITH KAZAL MOTIFS CHROMOSOME 9; 9p13.3

RECK is a tumor suppressor gene that is expressed in several normal tissues and tumors, positively correlating with overall survival [95]. In glioma, RECK might be involved in blood vessel formation and maturation by VEGF [96, 97]. In addition, the expression of RECK is also associated with VEGF and CD105 in esophageal carcinoma [98]. Under hypoxic conditions, normal RECK expression suppressed cancer cell invasion and migration by binding with HIF-1α and activating RECK promoter [99, 100].

1.40. ROR2 - RECEPTOR TYROSINE KINASE-LIKE ORPHAN RECEPTOR 2 CHROMOSOME 9; 9q22.31

ROR2 gene encodes for tyrosine-protein kinase transmembrane [101]. In colorectal cancer, ROR2 is epigenetically inactivated, where downregulation of ROR2 leads to metastasis, tumor growth, and Wnt signaling activation [102, 103]. In contrast, under hypoxic conditions in melanoma, expression of ROR2 along with Wnt5a increased drug resistance and cell migration [104].

CONCLUSION

Chromosome 9, with many flows in the gene sequence, deletion, fusion of the gene, *etc.*, has shown its involvement in the progression of the disease. Interaction of the gene CDKN2B-AS1 with several microRNAs and cell cycle proteins helps in the development of various cancer, including renal cell carcinoma, cervical cancer, *etc.* Many genes residing on chromosome 9 have features as tumor suppressors. Loss of these genes from the chromosome makes the cell more prone to transform into tumor-progressing cells. The mutations and deletions further support this in the protooncogene, which promotes the various types of cancer. This chromosome also has important genes responsible for cell signaling, and stem cell maintenance like the NOTCH1, JAK2, PTCH1, *etc.* Dysregulation of this has been reported for different types of cancer, including nevoid basal cell carcinoma, colon cancer, *etc.* PCA3 gene expressed in the prostate tissues has shown its overexpression in the development of prostate cancer. Similarly, the other genes from this chromosome are listed with their carcinogenesis in the variety of cancer in this chapter.

REFERENCES

[1]   Oram JF, Lawn RM. ABCA1: the gatekeeper for eliminating excess tissue cholesterol. J Lipid Res 2001; 42(8): 1173-9.
        [http://dx.doi.org/10.1016/S0022-2275(20)31566-2] [PMID: 11483617]

[2]   Aguirre-Portolés C, Feliu J, Reglero G, Ramírez de Molina A. ABCA1 overexpression worsens colorectal cancer prognosis by facilitating tumour growth and caveolin-1-dependent invasiveness, and these effects can be ameliorated using the BET inhibitor apabetalone. Mol Oncol 2018; 12(10): 1735-52.
        [http://dx.doi.org/10.1002/1878-0261.12367] [PMID: 30098223]

[3]   Caron D, Maaroufi H, Michaud S, Tanguay RM, Faure RL. Annexin A1 is regulated by domains cross-talk through post-translational phosphorylation and SUMOYlation. Cell Signal 2013; 25(10): 1962-9.
        [http://dx.doi.org/10.1016/j.cellsig.2013.05.028] [PMID: 23727357]

[4]   Guo C, Liu S, Sun MZ. Potential role of Anxa1 in cancer. Future Oncol 2013; 9(11): 1773-93.
        [http://dx.doi.org/10.2217/fon.13.114] [PMID: 24156336]

[5]   Bizzarro V, Belvedere R, Migliaro V, Romano E, Parente L, Petrella A. Hypoxia regulates ANXA1 expression to support prostate cancer cell invasion and aggressiveness. Cell Adhes Migr 2017; 11(3): 247-60.

[http://dx.doi.org/10.1080/19336918.2016.1259056] [PMID: 27834582]

[6]   Zhu X. Expression of AQP3 protein in hAECs is regulated by Camp-PKA-CREB signalling pathway. Front Biosci 2015; 20(7): 1047-55.
[http://dx.doi.org/10.2741/4357]

[7]   Marlar S, Jensen HH, Login FH, Nejsum LN. Aquaporin-3 in Cancer. Int J Mol Sci 2017; 18(10): 2106.
[http://dx.doi.org/10.3390/ijms18102106] [PMID: 28991174]

[8]   Cutress RI, Townsend PA, Brimmell M, Bateman AC, Hague A, Packham G. BAG-1 expression and function in human cancer. Br J Cancer 2002; 87(8): 834-9.
[http://dx.doi.org/10.1038/sj.bjc.6600538] [PMID: 12373595]

[9]   Zhou G, Ye J, Fang Y, *et al.* Identification of DBCCR1 as a suppressor in the development of lung cancer that is associated with increased DNA methyltransferase 1. Oncotarget 2017; 8(20): 32821-32.
[http://dx.doi.org/10.18632/oncotarget.15826] [PMID: 28427182]

[10] Becker HM. Carbonic anhydrase IX and acid transport in cancer. Br J Cancer 2020; 122(2): 157-67.
[http://dx.doi.org/10.1038/s41416-019-0642-z] [PMID: 31819195]

[11] Zhang X, Wang Y, Cao Y, Zhang X, Zhao H. Increased CCL19 expression is associated with progression in cervical cancer. Oncotarget 2017; 8(43): 73817-25.
[http://dx.doi.org/10.18632/oncotarget.17982] [PMID: 29088748]

[12] Le DT, Uram JN, Wang H, *et al.* PD-1 Blockade in Tumors with Mismatch-Repair Deficiency. N Engl J Med 2015; 372(26): 2509-20.
[http://dx.doi.org/10.1056/NEJMoa1500596] [PMID: 26028255]

[13] Masugi Y, Nishihara R, Yang J, *et al.* Tumour CD274 (PD-L1) expression and T cells in colorectal cancer. Gut 2017; 66(8): 1463-73.
[http://dx.doi.org/10.1136/gutjnl-2016-311421] [PMID: 27196573]

[14] Franco LC, Morales F, Boffo S, Giordano A. CDK9: A key player in cancer and other diseases. J Cell Biochem 2018; 119(2): 1273-84.
[http://dx.doi.org/10.1002/jcb.26293] [PMID: 28722178]

[15] Jang W, Park J, Kwon A, *et al.* CDKN2B downregulation and other genetic characteristics in T-acute lymphoblastic leukemia. Exp Mol Med 2019; 51(1): 1-15.
[http://dx.doi.org/10.1038/s12276-018-0195-x] [PMID: 30635552]

[16] Laharanne E, Chevret E, Idrissi Y, *et al.* CDKN2A–CDKN2B deletion defines an aggressive subset of cutaneous T-cell lymphoma. Mod Pathol 2010; 23(4): 547-58.
[http://dx.doi.org/10.1038/modpathol.2009.196] [PMID: 20118908]

[17] Sfakianos JP, Cha EK, Iyer G, *et al.* Genomic Characterization of Upper Tract Urothelial Carcinoma. Eur Urol 2015; 68(6): 970-7.
[http://dx.doi.org/10.1016/j.eururo.2015.07.039] [PMID: 26278805]

[18] Zhu L, Zhang Q, Li S, Jiang S, Cui J, Dang G. Interference of the long noncoding RNA CDKN2B-AS1 upregulates miR-181a-5p/TGFβI axis to restrain the metastasis and promote apoptosis and senescence of cervical cancer cells. Cancer Med 2019; 8(4): 1721-30.
[http://dx.doi.org/10.1002/cam4.2040] [PMID: 30884187]

[19] Dasgupta P, Kulkarni P, Majid S, *et al.* LncRNA CDKN2B-AS1/miR-141/cyclin D network regulates tumor progression and metastasis of renal cell carcinoma. Cell Death Dis 2020; 11(8): 660.
[http://dx.doi.org/10.1038/s41419-020-02877-0] [PMID: 32814766]

[20] Zhang J, Song Q, Liu J, Lu L, Xu Y, Zheng W. Cyclin-Dependent Kinase Regulatory Subunit 2 Indicated Poor Prognosis and Facilitated Aggressive Phenotype of Hepatocellular Carcinoma. Dis Markers 2019; 2019: 1-13.
[http://dx.doi.org/10.1155/2019/8964015] [PMID: 31781310]

[21]   Qi J, Yu Y, Akilli Öztürk Ö, *et al*. New Wnt/β-catenin target genes promote experimental metastasis and migration of colorectal cancer cells through different signals. Gut 2016; 65(10): 1690-701.
[http://dx.doi.org/10.1136/gutjnl-2014-307900] [PMID: 26156959]

[22]   Chen R, Feng C, Xu Y. Cyclin-dependent kinase-associated protein Cks2 is associated with bladder cancer progression. J Int Med Res 2011; 39(2): 533-40.
[http://dx.doi.org/10.1177/147323001103900222] [PMID: 21672358]

[23]   Stanbrough M, Bubley GJ, Ross K, *et al*. Increased expression of genes converting adrenal androgens to testosterone in androgen-independent prostate cancer. Cancer Res 2006; 66(5): 2815-25.
[http://dx.doi.org/10.1158/0008-5472.CAN-05-4000] [PMID: 16510604]

[24]   Wu K, Xie D, Zou Y, *et al*. The mechanism of DAB2IP in chemoresistance of prostate cancer cells. Clin Cancer Res 2013; 19(17): 4740-9.
[http://dx.doi.org/10.1158/1078-0432.CCR-13-0954] [PMID: 23838317]

[25]   Valentino E, Bellazzo A, Di Minin G, *et al*. Mutant p53 potentiates the oncogenic effects of insulin by inhibiting the tumor suppressor DAB2IP. Proc Natl Acad Sci USA 2017; 114(29): 7623-8.
[http://dx.doi.org/10.1073/pnas.1700996114] [PMID: 28667123]

[26]   Shen YJ, Kong ZL, Wan FN, *et al*. Downregulation of DAB 2 IP results in cell proliferation and invasion and contributes to unfavorable outcomes in bladder cancer. Cancer Sci 2014; 105(6): 704-12.
[http://dx.doi.org/10.1111/cas.12407] [PMID: 24684735]

[27]   Agodi A, Barchitta M, Quattrocchi A, Maugeri A, Vinciguerra M. DAPK1 Promoter Methylation and Cervical Cancer Risk: A Systematic Review and a Meta-Analysis. PLoS One 2015; 10(8): e0135078.
[http://dx.doi.org/10.1371/journal.pone.0135078] [PMID: 26267895]

[28]   Yadav P, Masroor M, Nandi K, *et al*. Promoter Methylation of BRCA1, DAPK1 and RASSF1A is Associated with Increased Mortality among Indian Women with Breast Cancer. Asian Pac J Cancer Prev 2018; 19(2): 443-8.
[PMID: 29480000]

[29]   Mitsui Y, Chang I, Fukuhara S, *et al*. CYP1B1 promotes tumorigenesis *via* altered expression of CDC20 and DAPK1 genes in renal cell carcinoma. BMC Cancer 2015; 15(1): 942.
[http://dx.doi.org/10.1186/s12885-015-1951-0] [PMID: 26626260]

[30]   Kunimoto Y, Nakano S, Kataoka H, Shimada Y, Oshimura M, Kitano H. Deleted in Esophageal Cancer 1(DEC1) is down-regulated and contributes to migration in head and neck squamous cell carcinoma cell lines. ORL J Otorhinolaryngol Relat Spec 2011; 73(1): 17-23.
[http://dx.doi.org/10.1159/000320997] [PMID: 20975315]

[31]   Bi H, Li S, Qu X, *et al*. DEC1 regulates breast cancer cell proliferation by stabilizing cyclin E protein and delays the progression of cell cycle S phase. Cell Death Dis 2015; 6(9): e1891-1.
[http://dx.doi.org/10.1038/cddis.2015.247] [PMID: 26402517]

[32]   Murakami K, Wu Y, Imaizumi T, *et al*. DEC1 promotes hypoxia-induced epithelial-mesenchymal transition (EMT) in human hepatocellular carcinoma cells. Biomed Res 2017; 38(4): 221-7.
[http://dx.doi.org/10.2220/biomedres.38.221] [PMID: 28794399]

[33]   Liu H, Chen X, Lin T, Chen X, Yan J, Jiang S. MicroRNA-524-5p suppresses the progression of papillary thyroid carcinoma cells *via* targeting on FOXE1 and ITGA3 in cell autophagy and cycling pathways. J Cell Physiol 2019; 234(10): 18382-91.
[http://dx.doi.org/10.1002/jcp.28472] [PMID: 30941771]

[34]   Venza I, Visalli M, Tripodo B, *et al*. FOXE1 is a target for aberrant methylation in cutaneous squamous cell carcinoma. Br J Dermatol 2010; 162(5): 1093-7.
[http://dx.doi.org/10.1111/j.1365-2133.2009.09560.x] [PMID: 19845668]

[35]   Merritt MA, Kotsopoulos J, Cramer DW, Hankinson SE, Terry KL, Tworoger SS. Duarte galactose--phosphate uridyl transferase genotypes are not associated with ovarian cancer risk. Fertil Steril 2012; 98(3): 687-91.

[http://dx.doi.org/10.1016/j.fertnstert.2012.05.045] [PMID: 22749219]

[36]   Villegas-Comonfort S, Serna-Marquez N, Galindo-Hernandez O, Navarro-Tito N, Salazar EP. Arachidonic acid induces an increase of β-1,4-galactosyltransferase I expression in MDA-MB-231 breast cancer cells. J Cell Biochem 2012; 113(11): 3330-41.
[http://dx.doi.org/10.1002/jcb.24209] [PMID: 22644815]

[37]   Sánchez-Hernández L, Hernández-Soto J, Vergara P, González RO, Segovia J. Additive effects of the combined expression of soluble forms of GAS1 and PTEN inhibiting glioblastoma growth. Gene Ther 2018; 25(6): 439-49.
[http://dx.doi.org/10.1038/s41434-018-0020-0] [PMID: 29941984]

[38]   Li Q, Qin Y, Wei P, *et al. Gas1* Inhibits Metastatic and Metabolic Phenotypes in Colorectal Carcinoma. Mol Cancer Res 2016; 14(9): 830-40.
[http://dx.doi.org/10.1158/1541-7786.MCR-16-0032] [PMID: 27401611]

[39]   Jiang Z, Xu Y, Cai S. Down-regulated GAS1 expression correlates with recurrence in stage II and III colorectal cancer. Hum Pathol 2011; 42(3): 361-8.
[http://dx.doi.org/10.1016/j.humpath.2010.03.009] [PMID: 21111449]

[40]   Horn S, Leonardelli S, Sucker A, Schadendorf D, Griewank KG, Paschen A. Tumor CDKN2A-Associated JAK2 Loss and Susceptibility to Immunotherapy Resistance. J Natl Cancer Inst 2018; 110(6): 677-81.
[http://dx.doi.org/10.1093/jnci/djx271] [PMID: 29917141]

[41]   Tasian SK, Loh ML, Hunger SP. Philadelphia chromosome–like acute lymphoblastic leukemia. Blood 2017; 130(19): 2064-72.
[http://dx.doi.org/10.1182/blood-2017-06-743252] [PMID: 28972016]

[42]   Boeckel JN, Derlet A, Glaser SF, *et al.* JMJD8 Regulates Angiogenic Sprouting and Cellular Metabolism by Interacting With Pyruvate Kinase M2 in Endothelial Cells. Arterioscler Thromb Vasc Biol 2016; 36(7): 1425-33.
[http://dx.doi.org/10.1161/ATVBAHA.116.307695] [PMID: 27199445]

[43]   Wissmann M, Yin N, Müller JM, *et al.* Cooperative demethylation by JMJD2C and LSD1 promotes androgen receptor-dependent gene expression. Nat Cell Biol 2007; 9(3): 347-53.
[http://dx.doi.org/10.1038/ncb1546] [PMID: 17277772]

[44]   Cantley LC, Neel BG. New insights into tumor suppression: PTEN suppresses tumor formation by restraining the phosphoinositide 3-kinase/AKT pathway. Proc Natl Acad Sci USA 1999; 96(8): 4240-5.
[http://dx.doi.org/10.1073/pnas.96.8.4240] [PMID: 10200246]

[45]   Åkerstrom B, Flower DR, Salier JP. Lipocalins: unity in diversity. Biochim Biophys Acta Protein Struct Mol Enzymol 2000; 1482(1-2): 1-8.
[http://dx.doi.org/10.1016/S0167-4838(00)00137-0] [PMID: 11058742]

[46]   Hu C, Yang K, Li M, Huang W, Zhang F, Wang H. Lipocalin 2: a potential therapeutic target for breast cancer metastasis. OncoTargets Ther 2018; 11: 8099-106.
[http://dx.doi.org/10.2147/OTT.S181223] [PMID: 30519052]

[47]   Heyer BS, Kochanowski H, Solter D. Expression ofMelk, a new protein kinase, during early mouse development. Dev Dyn 1999; 215(4): 344-51.
[http://dx.doi.org/10.1002/(SICI)1097-0177(199908)215:4<344::AID-AJA6>3.0.CO;2-H]   [PMID: 10417823]

[48]   Gray D, Jubb AM, Hogue D, *et al.* Maternal embryonic leucine zipper kinase/murine protein serine-threonine kinase 38 is a promising therapeutic target for multiple cancers. Cancer Res 2005; 65(21): 9751-61.
[http://dx.doi.org/10.1158/0008-5472.CAN-04-4531] [PMID: 16266996]

[49]   Guan S, Lu J, Zhao Y, *et al.* MELK is a novel therapeutic target in high-risk neuroblastoma.

Oncotarget 2018; 9(2): 2591-602.
[http://dx.doi.org/10.18632/oncotarget.23515] [PMID: 29416794]

[50]   Marie SKN, Okamoto OK, Uno M, *et al.* Maternal embryonic leucine zipper kinase transcript abundance correlates with malignancy grade in human astrocytomas. Int J Cancer 2008; 122(4): 807-15.
[http://dx.doi.org/10.1002/ijc.23189] [PMID: 17960622]

[51]   Yamamoto F, Yamamoto M, Soto JL, *et al.* NotI-MseI methylation-sensitive amplified fragment length polymorphism for DNA methylation analysis of human cancers. Electrophoresis 2001; 22(10): 1946-56.
[http://dx.doi.org/10.1002/1522-2683(200106)22:10<1946::AID-ELPS1946>3.0.CO;2-Y]   [PMID: 11465493]

[52]   Suzuki K, Suzuki I, Leodolter A, *et al.* Global DNA demethylation in gastrointestinal cancer is age dependent and precedes genomic damage. Cancer Cell 2006; 9(3): 199-207.
[http://dx.doi.org/10.1016/j.ccr.2006.02.016] [PMID: 16530704]

[53]   Han L, Yue X, Zhou X, *et al.* MicroRNA-21 expression is regulated by β-catenin/STAT3 pathway and promotes glioma cell invasion by direct targeting RECK. CNS Neurosci Ther 2012; 18(7): 573-83.
[http://dx.doi.org/10.1111/j.1755-5949.2012.00344.x] [PMID: 22630347]

[54]   Rodrigues-Junior DM, Tan SS, Lim SK, *et al.* High expression of MLANA in the plasma of patients with head and neck squamous cell carcinoma as a predictor of tumor progression. Head Neck 2019; 41(5): 1199-205.
[http://dx.doi.org/10.1002/hed.25510] [PMID: 30803092]

[55]   Pina C, May G, Soneji S, Hong D, Enver T. MLLT3 regulates early human erythroid and mega-karyocytic cell fate. Cell Stem Cell 2008; 2(3): 264-73.
[http://dx.doi.org/10.1016/j.stem.2008.01.013] [PMID: 18371451]

[56]   Vogel T, Gruss P. Expression of Leukaemia associated transcription factor Af9/Mllt3 in the cerebral cortex of the mouse. Gene Expr Patterns 2009; 9(2): 83-93.
[http://dx.doi.org/10.1016/j.gep.2008.10.004] [PMID: 19000783]

[57]   Büttner N, Johnsen SA, Kügler S, Vogel T. *Af9/Mllt3* interferes with *Tbr1* expression through epigenetic modification of histone H3K79 during development of the cerebral cortex. Proc Natl Acad Sci USA 2010; 107(15): 7042-7.
[http://dx.doi.org/10.1073/pnas.0912041107] [PMID: 20348416]

[58]   Pramparo T, Grosso S, Messa J, *et al.* Loss-of-function mutation of the AF9/MLLT3 gene in a girl with neuromotor development delay, cerebellar ataxia, and epilepsy. Hum Genet 2005; 118(1): 76-81.
[http://dx.doi.org/10.1007/s00439-005-0004-1] [PMID: 16001262]

[59]   Zhang T, Luo Y, Wang T, Yang JY. MicroRNA-297b-5p/3p target Mllt3/Af9 to suppress lymphoma cell proliferation, migration and invasion *in vitro* and tumor growth in nude mice. Leuk Lymphoma 2012; 53(10): 2033-40.
[http://dx.doi.org/10.3109/10428194.2012.678005] [PMID: 22448917]

[60]   Calvanese V, Nguyen AT, Bolan TJ, *et al.* MLLT3 governs human haematopoietic stem-cell self-renewal and engraftment. Nature 2019; 576(7786): 281-6.
[http://dx.doi.org/10.1038/s41586-019-1790-2] [PMID: 31776511]

[61]   Dickinson ME, Flenniken AM, Ji X, *et al.* High-throughput discovery of novel developmental phenotypes. Nature 2016; 537(7621): 508-14.
[http://dx.doi.org/10.1038/nature19356] [PMID: 27626380]

[62]   Schmid M, Sen M, Rosenbach MD, Carrera CJ, Friedman H, Carson DA. A methylthioadenosine phosphorylase (MTAP) fusion transcript identifies a new gene on chromosome 9p21 that is frequently deleted in cancer. Oncogene 2000; 19(50): 5747-54.
[http://dx.doi.org/10.1038/sj.onc.1203942] [PMID: 11126361]

[63]   Mavrakis KJ, McDonald ER, Schlabach MR, *et al.* Disordered methionine metabolism in MTAP/CDKN2A-deleted cancers leads to dependence on PRMT5. Science 2016; 351: 1208–1213. [http://dx.doi.org/10.1126/science.aad5944] [PMID: 26912361]

[64]   Chaudhry AZ, Lyons GE, Gronostajski RM. Expression patterns of the four nuclear factor I genes during mouse embryogenesis indicate a potential role in development. Dev Dyn 1997; 208(3): 313-25. [http://dx.doi.org/10.1002/(SICI)1097-0177(199703)208:3<313::AID-AJA3>3.0.CO;2-L] [PMID: 9056636]

[65]   Gründer A, Ebel TT, Mallo M, *et al.* Nuclear factor I-B (Nfib) deficient mice have severe lung hypoplasia. Mech Dev 2002; 112(1-2): 69-77. [http://dx.doi.org/10.1016/S0925-4773(01)00640-2] [PMID: 11850179]

[66]   Goodall J, Carreira S, Denat L, *et al.* Brn-2 represses microphthalmia-associated transcription factor expression and marks a distinct subpopulation of microphthalmia-associated transcription factor-negative melanoma cells. Cancer Res 2008; 68(19): 7788-94. [http://dx.doi.org/10.1158/0008-5472.CAN-08-1053] [PMID: 18829533]

[67]   Tanigaki K, Nogaki F, Takahashi J, Tashiro K, Kurooka H, Honjo T. Notch1 and Notch3 instructively restrict bFGF-responsive multipotent neural progenitor cells to an astroglial fate. Neuron 2001; 29(1): 45-55. [http://dx.doi.org/10.1016/S0896-6273(01)00179-9] [PMID: 11182080]

[68]   Keilani S, Sugaya K. Reelin induces a radial glial phenotype in human neural progenitor cells by activation of Notch-1. BMC Dev Biol 2008; 8(1): 69. [http://dx.doi.org/10.1186/1471-213X-8-69] [PMID: 18593473]

[69]   Leong KG, Gao WQ. The Notch pathway in prostate development and cancer. Differentiation 2008; 76(6): 699-716. [http://dx.doi.org/10.1111/j.1432-0436.2008.00288.x] [PMID: 18565101]

[70]   Leong KG, Karsan A. Recent insights into the role of Notch signaling in tumorigenesis. Blood 2006; 107(6): 2223-33. [http://dx.doi.org/10.1182/blood-2005-08-3329] [PMID: 16291593]

[71]   Deutsch AJ, Angerer H, Fuchs TE, Neumeister P. The nuclear orphan receptors NR4A as therapeutic target in cancer therapy. Anticancer Agents Med Chem 2012; 12(9): 1001-14. [http://dx.doi.org/10.2174/187152012803529619] [PMID: 22583411]

[72]   Napetschnig J, Blobel G, Hoelz A. Crystal structure of the N-terminal domain of the human protooncogene Nup214/CAN. Proc Natl Acad Sci USA 2007; 104(6): 1783-8. [http://dx.doi.org/10.1073/pnas.0610828104] [PMID: 17264208]

[73]   Napetschnig J, Kassube SA, Debler EW, Wong RW, Blobel G, Hoelz A. Structural and functional analysis of the interaction between the nucleoporin Nup214 and the DEAD-box helicase Ddx19. Proc Natl Acad Sci USA 2009; 106(9): 3089-94. [http://dx.doi.org/10.1073/pnas.0813267106] [PMID: 19208808]

[74]   Liu F, Gao L, Jing Y, *et al.* RETRACTED ARTICLE: Detection and clinical significance of gene rearrangements in Chinese patients with adult acute lymphoblastic leukemia. Leuk Lymphoma 2013; 54(7): 1521-6. [http://dx.doi.org/10.3109/10428194.2012.754888] [PMID: 23210573]

[75]   Hütter G, Kaiser M, Neumann M, *et al.* Epigenetic regulation of PAX5 expression in acute T-cell lymphoblastic leukemia. Leuk Res 2011; 35(5): 614-9. [http://dx.doi.org/10.1016/j.leukres.2010.11.015] [PMID: 21156323]

[76]   Longobardi E, Penkov D, Mateos D, Florian G, Torres M, Blasi F. Biochemistry of the tale transcription factors PREP, MEIS, and PBX in vertebrates. Dev Dyn 2014; 243(1): 59-75. [http://dx.doi.org/10.1002/dvdy.24016] [PMID: 23873833]

[77]   Stoesz SP, Friedl A, Haag JD, Lindstrom MJ, Clark GM, Gould MN. Heterogeneous expression of the

lipocalin NGAL in primary breast cancers. Int J Cancer 1998; 79(6): 565-72.
[http://dx.doi.org/10.1002/(SICI)1097-0215(19981218)79:6<565::AID-IJC3>3.0.CO;2-F]   [PMID: 9842963]

[78]   Wenners AS, Mehta K, Loibl S, *et al.* Neutrophil gelatinase-associated lipocalin (NGAL) predicts response to neoadjuvant chemotherapy and clinical outcome in primary human breast cancer. PLoS One 2012; 7(10): e45826.
[http://dx.doi.org/10.1371/journal.pone.0045826] [PMID: 23056218]

[79]   Nobori T, Takabayashi K, Tran P, *et al.* Genomic cloning of methylthioadenosine phosphorylase: a purine metabolic enzyme deficient in multiple different cancers. Proc Natl Acad Sci USA 1996; 93(12): 6203-8.
[http://dx.doi.org/10.1073/pnas.93.12.6203] [PMID: 8650244]

[80]   Wang Y, Liu X-J, Yao X-D. Function of PCA3 in prostate tissue and clinical research progress on developing a PCA3 score. Chin J Cancer Res 2014; 26(4): 493-500.
[PMID: 25232225]

[81]   Filella X, Foj L, Milà M, Augé JM, Molina R, Jiménez W. PCA3 in the detection and management of early prostate cancer. Tumour Biol 2013; 34(3): 1337-47.
[http://dx.doi.org/10.1007/s13277-013-0739-6] [PMID: 23504524]

[82]   Singh DK, Gholamalamdari O, Jadaliha M, *et al.* PSIP1/p75 promotes tumorigenicity in breast cancer cells by promoting the transcription of cell cycle genes. Carcinogenesis 2017; 38(10): 966-75.
[http://dx.doi.org/10.1093/carcin/bgx062] [PMID: 28633434]

[83]   Ming JE, Kaupas ME, Roessler E, *et al.* Mutations in PATCHED-1, the receptor for SONIC HEDGEHOG, are associated with holoprosencephaly. Hum Genet 2002; 110(4): 297-301.
[http://dx.doi.org/10.1007/s00439-002-0695-5] [PMID: 11941477]

[84]   Kimonis VE, Mehta SG, Digiovanna JJ, Bale SJ, Pastakia B. Radiological features in 82 patients with nevoid basal cell carcinoma (NBCC or Gorlin) syndrome. Genet Med 2004; 6(6): 495-502.
[http://dx.doi.org/10.1097/01.GIM.0000145045.17711.1C] [PMID: 15545745]

[85]   Pan S, Dong Q, Sun LS, Li TJ. Mechanisms of inactivation of PTCH1 gene in nevoid basal cell carcinoma syndrome: modification of the two-hit hypothesis. Clin Cancer Res 2010; 16(2): 442-50.
[http://dx.doi.org/10.1158/1078-0432.CCR-09-2574] [PMID: 20068110]

[86]   Mancuso M, Pazzaglia S, Tanori M, *et al.* Basal cell carcinoma and its development: insights from radiation-induced tumors in Ptch1-deficient mice. Cancer Res 2004; 64(3): 934-41.
[http://dx.doi.org/10.1158/0008-5472.CAN-03-2460] [PMID: 14871823]

[87]   Pulido R, Krueger NX, Serra-Pagès C, Saito H, Streuli M. Molecular characterization of the human transmembrane protein-tyrosine phosphatase δ. Evidence for tissue-specific expression of alternative human transmembrane protein-tyrosine phosphatase δ isoforms. J Biol Chem 1995; 270(12): 6722-8.
[http://dx.doi.org/10.1074/jbc.270.12.6722] [PMID: 7896816]

[88]   Mizuno K, Hasegawa K, Katagiri T, Ogimoto M, Ichikawa T, Yakura H. MPTP delta, a putative murine homolog of HPTP delta, is expressed in specialized regions of the brain and in the B-cell lineage. Mol Cell Biol 1993; 13(9): 5513-23.
[PMID: 8355697]

[89]   Wang Z, Shen D, Parsons DW, et al. Mutational Analysis of the Tyrosine Phosphatome in Colorectal Cancers. Science 2004; 304: 1164-6.
[http://dx.doi.org/10.1126/science.1096096] [PMID: 15155950]

[90]   Lui VWY, Peyser ND, Ng PKS, *et al.* Frequent mutation of receptor protein tyrosine phosphatases provides a mechanism for STAT3 hyperactivation in head and neck cancer. Proc Natl Acad Sci USA 2014; 111(3): 1114-9.
[http://dx.doi.org/10.1073/pnas.1319551111] [PMID: 24395800]

[91]   Schauber C, Chen L, Tongaonkar P, *et al.* Rad23 links DNA repair to the ubiquitin/proteasome

pathway. Nature 1998; 391(6668): 715-8.
[http://dx.doi.org/10.1038/35661] [PMID: 9490418]

[92]   Guerrero C, Martín-Encabo S, Fernández-Medarde A, Santos E. C3G-mediated suppression of oncogene-induced focus formation in fibroblasts involves inhibition of ERK activation, cyclin A expression and alterations of anchorage-independent growth. Oncogene 2004; 23(28): 4885-93.
[http://dx.doi.org/10.1038/sj.onc.1207622] [PMID: 15077165]

[93]   Hirata T, Nagai H, Koizumi K, *et al.* Amplification, up-regulation and over-expression of C3G (CRK SH3 domain-binding guanine nucleotide-releasing factor) in non-small cell lung cancers. J Hum Genet 2004; 49(6): 290-5.
[http://dx.doi.org/10.1007/s10038-004-0148-1] [PMID: 15138850]

[94]   Han HB, Gu J, Ji DB, *et al.* PBX3 promotes migration and invasion of colorectal cancer cells *via* activation of MAPK/ERK signaling pathway. World J Gastroenterol 2014; 20(48): 18260-70.
[http://dx.doi.org/10.3748/wjg.v20.i48.18260] [PMID: 25561793]

[95]   Clark JCM, Thomas DM, Choong PFM, Dass CR. RECK—a newly discovered inhibitor of metastasis with prognostic significance in multiple forms of cancer. Cancer Metastasis Rev 2007; 26(3-4): 675-83.
[http://dx.doi.org/10.1007/s10555-007-9093-8] [PMID: 17828469]

[96]   Rahmah NN, Sakai K, Sano K, Hongo K. Expression of RECK in endothelial cells of glioma: comparison with CD34 and VEGF expressions. J Neurooncol 2012; 107(3): 559-64.
[http://dx.doi.org/10.1007/s11060-011-0778-z] [PMID: 22183444]

[97]   Alexius-Lindgren M, Andersson E, Lindstedt I, Engström W. The RECK gene and biological malignancy--its significance in angiogenesis and inhibition of matrix metalloproteinases. Anticancer Res 2014; 34(8): 3867-73.
[PMID: 25075007]

[98]   Li SL, Gao DL, Zhao ZH, *et al.* Correlation of matrix metalloproteinase suppressor genes RECK, VEGF, and CD105 with angiogenesis and biological behavior in esophageal squamous cell carcinoma. World J Gastroenterol 2007; 13(45): 6076-81.
[http://dx.doi.org/10.3748/wjg.v13.45.6076] [PMID: 18023103]

[99]   Jeon HW, Lee YM. Inhibition of histone deacetylase attenuates hypoxia-induced migration and invasion of cancer cells *via* the restoration of RECK expression. Mol Cancer Ther 2010; 9(5): 1361-70.
[http://dx.doi.org/10.1158/1535-7163.MCT-09-0717] [PMID: 20442303]

[100] Jeon HW, Lee KJ, Lee SH, Kim WH, Lee YM. Attenuated expression and function of the RECK tumor suppressor under hypoxic conditions is mediated by the MAPK signaling pathways. Arch Pharm Res 2011; 34(1): 137-45.
[http://dx.doi.org/10.1007/s12272-011-0116-1] [PMID: 21468925]

[101] Oldridge M, M Fortuna A, Maringa M, *et al.* Dominant mutations in ROR2, encoding an orphan receptor tyrosine kinase, cause brachydactyly type B. Nat Genet 2000; 24(3): 275-8.
[http://dx.doi.org/10.1038/73495] [PMID: 10700182]

[102] Lara E, Calvanese V, Huidobro C, *et al.* Epigenetic repression of ROR2 has a Wnt-mediated, pro-tumourigenic role in colon cancer. Mol Cancer 2010; 9(1): 170.
[http://dx.doi.org/10.1186/1476-4598-9-170] [PMID: 20591152]

[103] Ma SSQ, Srivastava S, Llamosas E, *et al.* ROR2 is epigenetically inactivated in the early stages of colorectal neoplasia and is associated with proliferation and migration. BMC Cancer 2016; 16(1): 508.
[http://dx.doi.org/10.1186/s12885-016-2576-7] [PMID: 27440078]

[104] O'Connell MP, Marchbank K, Webster MR, *et al.* Hypoxia induces phenotypic plasticity and therapy resistance in melanoma *via* the tyrosine kinase receptors ROR1 and ROR2. Cancer Discov 2013; 3(12): 1378-93.
[http://dx.doi.org/10.1158/2159-8290.CD-13-0005] [PMID: 24104062]

CHAPTER 10

Chromosome 10

Saurav Panicker[1] and **Satish Ramalingam**[1,*]

[1] *Department of Genetic Engineering, School of Bioengineering, SRM Institute of Science and Technology, Kattankulathur, India*

Abstract: Chromosome 10 contains various genes that are significantly involved in tumorigenesis. These genes described herein that play roles in cancer comprise receptor tyrosine kinases (FGFR2), proto-oncogenes (FRAT1, RET), tumor suppressor genes (PTEN, KLF6), and also genes involved in signal transduction (MAPK8), gene fusions (CCDC6, KIF5B, VTI1A), developmental processes (GATA3, NODAL), Epithelial-Mesenchymal transition (ZEB1, VIM) and epigenetic regulation (MLLT10). This chapter provides a compilation of many such genes from Chromosome 10 that are associated with cancer, with vivid delineations of the underlying molecular mechanisms of each gene in its contribution to cancer initiation, progression and metastasis. Genes that are insufficiently investigated but implicated in tumorigenesis have also been described in this chapter.

Keywords: Apoptosis, Cell Cycle, Cytogenetic Location, Deletion, Downregulation, Gene, Gene Amplification, Invasion, Malignant, Migration, Mutation, Signal Transduction, Translocation, Tumor Progression, Upregulation.

1.1. ALL1 – ACUTE LYMPHOCYTIC LEUKEMIA LOCATION: CHROMOSOME 10; 10q21

ALL1 protein has been reported in Leukemia. ALL1 gene undergoes translocation with chromosomal band 11q23 [1]. Mutations in this gene have been reported in 5- 10% of Acute Leukemia [1]. ALL gene fusion with chromosome 11 has been reported in 11% of adult *de novo* AML [Acute myeloid leukemia] [2]. ALL1 gene mutation and Trisomy 11 have been frequently correlated in multiple adult AML patients. ALL1 gene undergoes partial tandem duplication of an internal position of itself, thereby triggering leukemogenesis [2]. Various types of self-fusions and tandem duplications among exons of ALL genes have been observed in AML [3]. Such self-fusions and tandem duplication among the exons of the ALL1 gene contribute to genetic instability leading to leukemia [2, 3].

---

[*] **Corresponding author Satish Ramalingam**: Department of Genetic Engineering, School of Bioengineering, SRM Institute of Science and Technology, Kattankulathur, India; E-mail: rsatish76@gmail.com

Satish Ramalingam (Ed.)

1.2. ALOX5 - ARACHIDONATE 5-LIPOXYGENASE LOCATION: CHROMOSOME 10; 10q11.21

ALOX5 gene (Fig. **1**) is off 71.9-kilo base pairs. The gene consists of 14 exons and 13 introns. The ALOX5 protein is of 673 amino acids and has a molecular weight of 78 kilo-dalton. Cells involved in inflammatory responses and allergy express ALOX5 [4]. Such cells include neutrophils, basophils, mast cells, and eosinophils [4]. ALOX5 gene dysregulation has been reported in Chronic Myeloid Leukemia [CML] [5]. ALOX5 is a critical regulator of Cancer Stem Cells [CSC] in CML [5]. ALOX5 promotes the activity of Leukemia Stem Cells in CML [5]. ALOX5 deficiency failed BCR-ABL to induce leukemogenesis in CML [5]. Neutrophils support lung metastasis of breast cancer *via* ALOX5-dependent leukotriene release [4]. Inhibition of ALOX5 using Zileuton inhibited breast cancer's lung metastasis and the activity of Leukemia Stem Cells in CML [4, 5]. Contrary to the theory that ALOX5 is a novel target against CSC, it was further reported that deletion of ALOX5 in the tumor microenvironment could aggravate lung cancer progression [6] since ALOX5 gene products had antitumor roles in the tumor microenvironment *via* T-cell recruitment [6]. Hence, recent research suggests that caution must be taken while targeting ALOX5 though it provides a novel target against CSC [5, 6].

1.3. CAMK1D- CALCIUM/CALMODULIN-DEPENDENT PROTEIN KINASE ID ` LOCATION: CHROMOSOME 10; 10p13

CAMK1D belongs to the CaMK family of Ca2þ/calmodulin-regulated serine/threonine protein kinases [7]. CAMK1D gene is amplified and overexpressed in most breast cancers [7]. CAMK1D overexpression in non-tumorigenic breast epithelial cells indicated EMT [Epithelial Mesenchymal Transition]. CAMK1D is reported to be the driver oncogene in multiple basal-like tumors. CAMK1D is identified to be a novel oncogene that promotes EMT in breast cancer and could be used as a potential therapeutic target for basal-like tumors [7]. CAMK1D is essential for cellular proliferation [7 - 9]. CAMK1D has been shown to promote fibroblast proliferation by activating the cyclin D- 1/CDK4 complex [7, 8]. It's yet to be found if CAMK1D enhances proliferation through the exact mechanism in other cell types. Nevertheless, CAMK1D is associated with CREB pathway activation in basal breast cancers [7]. It's yet to be speculated if CREB protein is a direct target of CAMK1D or if CAMK1D associates with genes containing CREB sequence [7, 8, 10]. Such an example is the CCND1 gene that codes for Cyclin D-1 and contains a CREB sequence in its promoter region [7, 10]. CAMK1D is a new potential target for molecular-targeted therapy since CAMK1D promotes

EMT, which is vital to invasion and metastasis, adding to the fact that kinases have always been used as previous drug targets [7].

Chromosome 10

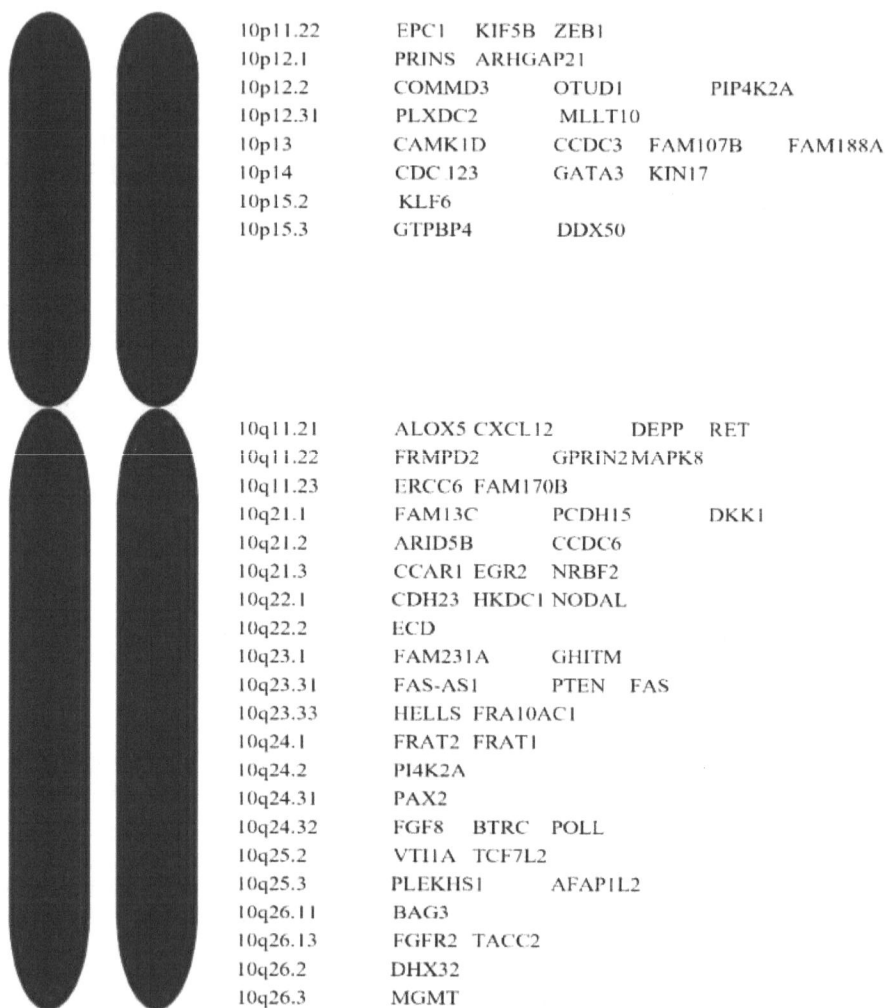

10p11.22	EPC1　KIF5B　ZEB1
10p12.1	PRINS　ARHGAP21
10p12.2	COMMD3　　　OTUD1　　　　　PIP4K2A
10p12.31	PLXDC2　　　MLLT10
10p13	CAMK1D　　　CCDC3　FAM107B　　FAM188A
10p14	CDC 123　　　GATA3　KIN17
10p15.2	KLF6
10p15.3	GTPBP4　　　　DDX50
10q11.21	ALOX5 CXCL12　　　　DEPP　RET
10q11.22	FRMPD2　　　　GPRIN2 MAPK8
10q11.23	ERCC6 FAM170B
10q21.1	FAM13C　　　PCDH15　　　DKK1
10q21.2	ARID5B　　　CCDC6
10q21.3	CCAR1 EGR2　NRBF2
10q22.1	CDH23 HKDC1 NODAL
10q22.2	ECD
10q23.1	FAM231A　　　GHITM
10q23.31	FAS-AS1　　　PTEN　FAS
10q23.33	HELLS FRA10AC1
10q24.1	FRAT2 FRAT1
10q24.2	PI4K2A
10q24.31	PAX2
10q24.32	FGF8　BTRC　POLL
10q25.2	VTI1A TCF7L2
10q25.3	PLEKHS1　　　AFAP1L2
10q26.11	BAG3
10q26.13	FGFR2 TACC2
10q26.2	DHX32
10q26.3	MGMT

Fig. (1). This figure displays the loci of the genes from Chromosome 10 whose roles in cancer have been explained in this chapter. Sayooj Madhusoodanan designed this diagram.

1.4. ARID5B: AT-RICH INTERACTION DOMAIN 5B LOCATION: CHROMOSOME 10; 10q21.2

ARID5B gene mutations have been reported in childhood acute lymphoblastic leukemia [ALL] [11]. ALL is the most common malignancy reported in childhood [12]. Genome-Wide Association Studies [GWAS] have exposed the genetic risk factors [allelic variations] within the ARID5b gene [11 - 13]. ARID5B gene is actively involved in lymphoid differentiation, therefore frequent polymorphisms in this gene effectively increase the risk of obtaining ALL [14]. The 3rd intron of the ARID5b gene has been confirmed to be the mutational hotspot for developing ALL [12, 13]. ALL risk alleles within the ARID5b gene have been identified for multiple ethnic groups [12]. ARID5B actively contributes to T-cell leuke-mogenesis by positively regulating the expression of the oncogenic transcription factor TAL1 [15]. TAL1 induces an anomalous oncogenic transcriptional cascade in T-cell Acute Lymphoblastic Leukemia [T-ALL] to support the growth and survival of T-ALL cells [15]. ARID5B and TAL1 coordinately regulate the expression of the same target genes [15]. Notably, the TAL1 complex and ARID5b positively coordinate with each other in all T-ALL cells [15]. ARID5B gene's enhancer sequence located upstream is activated in T-ALL [T-cell acute lymphoblastic leukemia] since TAL1, and its regulatory partners bind at this enhancer frequently in T-ALL [15]. ARID5B is a prominent oncogenic partner in TAL1's cascade in inducing T-ALL [15]. This is because ARID5B is essentially required for the survival and growth of T- ALL cells [15]. ARID5B overexpression succors the growth and existence of TAL1-positive T-ALL cells [15]. ARID5B knockdown downregulates TAL1 [T-cell acute lymphocytic leukemia protein 1] in cancer cells. ARID5B activates the expression of the oncogene *MYC* in T-ALL cells [15].ARID5B's positive regulation of TAL1-induced transcriptional cascade augments the oncogenic pathways that contribute to T-cell leukemogenesis [15].

1.5.   ARHGAP21 - RHO GTPASE ACTIVATING PROTEIN 21 LOCA-TION: CHROMOSOME 10; 10p12.1 – 10p12.3

ARHGAP21 is Rho-GTPase activating protein [16] (Fig. 1). It is overexpressed in head and neck squamous cell carcinoma [16]. This protein is a major supervisor of actin cytoskeleton dynamics, cell adhesion, cell migration, and other intra-cellular dynamics [16, 17]. ARHGAP21 is a chief regulator of cell-cell junction formation and cell-cell adhesion by governing the recruitment of its partner: alpha-catenin [16 - 18]. Increased cell migration through RhoC overexpression caused by ARHGAP21's underexpression has been implicated in prostate cancer cell lines [16]. ARHGAP21 silencing in glioblastoma cell lines led to an increase in cell migration properties [16]. Silencing of ARHGAP21 reduces proliferation in prostate cancer cells [16]. ARHGAP21 functions as the Rho-GAP for both RhoA and Cdc42, where Cdc42 is important for cadherin-mediated cell-cell adhesion [16, 18]. ARHGAP21 knockdown weakens cell-cell adhesion and increases cell migration [16, 18]. ARHGAP21 controls alpha-tubulin acetylation and promotes epithelial scattering [18]. ARHGAP21's interaction in alpha-tubulin acetylation is important for EMT [18]. RhoC upregulation is seen in EMT, and RhoC upregulation can be caused by ARHGAP21 depletion [16]. Hence, it can be concluded that ARHGAP21 may play a vital role in metastatic progression through EMT [18].

1.6. AFAP1L2 - ACTIN FILAMENT ASSOCIATED PROTEIN 1 LIKE 2 LOCATION: CHROMOSOME 10; 10q25.3

This gene (Fig. **1**) encodes a protein of 818 amino acids which weighs 130 kDa. AFAP1L2 mRNA is highly expressed in the human thyroid and spleen. Its mRNA is moderately expressed in the esophagus, stomach, and lymph nodes. It functions as an adaptor protein for signal transduction. It regulates cell proliferation and survival. AFAP1L2 affects cellular changes by activating kinases which further activate other downstream proteins involved in several signaling pathways [19, 20]. It binds to SH2 domain-containing proteins. It interacts with multiple kinases through its SH2 and SH3 domains, thereby regulating cell homeostasis. It binds to the PI3K and regulates PI3K downstream signaling [21]. Knockdown of this protein reduced cell proliferation. It regulates cell proliferation and cell survival by mediating the PI3K/Akt pathway [19]. Human esophageal squamous carcinoma showed elevated levels of AFAP1L2. Lck is an Src family member that is expressed aberrantly in colorectal cancer cells [21, 22]. AFAP1L2 is found to interact with Lck in colorectal cancer cells. A missense mutation in AFAP1L2 was found in the majority of cancers like the prostate, ovary, skin, lung, and intestine [20, 21]. Elevated expression levels of AFAP1L2 were found in gastric cancer tissues [20].

1.7. CCDC3 - COILED COIL DOMAIN-CONTAINING 3 CHROMOSOME 10; 10p13

Knockdown of CCDC3 attenuated the migration and invasive potential of cervical cancer cells [23]. This proves that CCDC3 expression is required for EMT progression [23]. CCDC3 knockdown using shRNA also inhibited the expression of genes required for EMT [23]. It has been reported that cervical cancer cells cannot attain their maximum migratory and invasive potential to undergo EMT unless CCDC3 is expressed normally [23]. CCDC3 expression is thus required for the metastasis of cervical cancer cells [23]. CCDC3 is hypothesized to have a strong connection with regulating the stemness of cancer stem cells, but it is yet to be proved [23]. CCDC3 is expressed in endothelial cells [23, 24]. CCDC3 inhibits TNF-α-induced NF-κB activation in endothelial cells [25]. CCDC3 over-expression decreased the TNF-alpha-induced expression of VCAM- 1 [25]. CCDC3 knockdown increased the expression of VCAM-1 [25]. We can conclude from these findings that CCDC3 plays a critical role in endothelial inflammation [25]. Moreover, CCDC3 could be a critical interacting component required for EndMT [Endothelial-to-Mesenchymal Transition] [23, 25]. CCDC3 was negatively correlated with tumor suppressor genes APC, PROC, and ATOH1 [23]. CCDC3 is normally highly expressed in the aorta and adipose tissues [23, 25]. CCDC3 is a recently discovered target of TP63 [24]. As a downstream player of the p63 circuit, CCDC3 is a crucial player in liver lipid metabolism [24].

1.8. CCNY - CELL CYCLE PROTEIN CYCLIN Y CHROMOSOME 10; 10p11.21

CCNY is overexpressed in NSCLC human specimens [26]. CCNY mRNA expression strongly correlated with the malignant histologic types of NSCLC [26]. CCNY was found critical in actively promoting the tumorigenic growth of lung cancer cells in NSCLC [26]. CCNY knockdown inhibited cell proliferation and anchorage-independent growth in lung cancer cells [26]. These results prove that CCNY is critical for oncogenesis in NSCLC [26]. CCNY binds to PFTKI kinase, which results in enhanced PFTK1 activity CCNY is required for cancer cell proliferation in NSCLC [26]. Overexpression of CCNY induced rapid proliferation of cancer cells, which resulted in a remarkably increased tumor size [26]. CCNY overexpression caused increased tumorigenicity in NSCLC [26]. CCNY also has a cancer-specific expression in the tumor tissue [26]. Hence, we can conclude that CCNY play a critical role in NSCLC formation and progression [26, 27]. CCNY has been shown to have an effect on Breast Cancer development [27]. PFTK1 is a Cdc-2-related kinase that modulates cell cycle progression [27]. This is how a PFTK1 interacting protein like CCNY directly influences cell growth and proliferation [26, 27].

CCNY is highly overexpressed in human breast cancer samples [27]. CCNY overexpression correlated with lymph node metastasis of breast cancer [27]. CCNY knockdown repressed proliferation in breast cancer cell lines [27]. CCNY underexpression promoted the phosphorylation of Bad and p53 and caspase-3 cleavage, thereby proving CCNY's vital role in regulating apoptosis [27]. It is to be noted that with CCNY's influence on cell growth in cancer cells *via* controlling cell proliferation and apoptosis, CCNY could provide to be an excellent biomarker in the future for NSCLC and breast cancer [26, 27].

1.9. CDC 123 – CELL DIVISION CYCLE PROTEIN 123 CHROMOSOME 10; 10p14-p13

Basal and luminal breast cancers follow different oncogenic pathways. Breast cancer has always been heterogeneous due to multiple genomic alterations contributing to the cancer progression in different tissues [28]. CDC123 was identified to be the potential marker for basal breast cancer [28]. Checking CDC123's expression profile will aid in categorizing the subtype of breast cancer [28].CDC123 was reported to be expressed only in basal breast cancer and CDC123 was never expressed in luminal breast cancer tissue samples [28]. CDC123 was reported to be a newly characterized oncogene that regulates the cell cycle, to be a reliable marker in basal-type breast cancers. Gene amplification at the CDC123 region would be an indicator of carcinogenesis initiation in basal breast cancer types [28].

1.10. CDH23 – CADHERIN RELATED 23 CHROMOSOME 10; 10q22.1

CDH23 is a member of the cadherin superfamily. CDH23 is mainly concerned with defining cell-cell boundaries in tissues [29]. Cell migration was faster when CDH23 was knocked down in cancer cells [29]. CDH23 overexpression resulted in the suppression of cell migration [29]. CDH23 is expressed normally at the cell-cell boundaries and is a major player in cell-cell adhesion [29]. CDH23 silencing blocks cell-cell aggregation [29]. CDH23 depletion results in cancer metastasis [29]. DNA promoter methylation of CDH23 was the main reason behind CDH23 downregulation in metastasis [29]. CDH23 downregulation supports EMT in metastasis [29]. CDH 23 only controls cell-cell adhesion and defines cell-cell boundaries, but CDH23 has no role in cell proliferation [29]. CDH23 also has no role in cell survival and cell viability [29]. CDH23 upregulation is a clear indication of the initial stages of breast cancer metastasis [30]. Since CDH23 has a remarkable influence on cancer cell migration, this gene could serve as potent drug target to prevent metastasis [29]. Intracranial tumors like pituitary adenomas are caused by missense mutations in CDH23 [30]. Missense mutations in CDH23 result in amino acid substitutions in the calcium-binding motif of the CDH23 protein [30]. Mutations in CDH23 have been correlated to cranial tumors, especially pituitary adenomas [PA] [30]. CDH23 has been confirmed as the genetic risk factor in hereditary pituitary tumors [30].CDH23 mutations have been tracked down in all the generations of those families afflicted with pituitary tumors [30].CDH23 mutations promote tumor growth and invasion in PA since CDH23 mutations result in the dysregulation of cell-cell adhesion [30].

1.11. CCAR1- CELL DIVISION CYCLE AND APOPTOSIS REGULATOR 1 CHROMOSOME 10; 10q21.3

It is a perinuclear phosphor protein that plays an active role in modulating cell growth and apoptosis through its interaction with p53, Beta-catenin and activates steroid receptor signaling [31]. CCAR1 is a negative regulator of EGFR signaling [32]. CCAR1 binds to p53 and is an important co-activator of p53 [33]. CCAR1 expression is vital for the chemotherapy-mediated apoptosis of cancer cells [31]. Small molecule inhibitors [SMIs] have been widely used in cancer therapy, and recently SMIs that mimic CCAR1 have been developed [31]. These mimics are called CFMs [CCAR1 Functional Mimetics]. CFMs induce apoptosis in a p53-independent manner and have been found effective against drug-resistant breast cancer cells [31]. CCAR1 regulates NOTCH signaling through its interaction with Par-4 [34]. CFMs have found success in treating Neuroblastoma [35]. CFMs can inhibit Neuroblastoma tumors and demote the metastatic invasiveness and migration of Neuroblastoma cells [35]. Nano-lipid formulation of CFMs provides a bright future in cancer therapy.

1.12. COMMD3: COMM DOMAIN CONTAINING 3 CHROMOSOME 10; 10p12.2

COMMD3 protein is recruited to the promoter region of c-MYC and regulates c-MYC expression [36]. COMMD3 undergoes gene fusion with the BMI1 gene [36]. COMMD3:BMI overexpression is reported in prostate cancer [36]. COMMD3: BMI fusion's overexpression is correlated to the different stages and grades of prostate tumors [36]. Later stages of prostate cancer will have higher expression levels of COMMD3:BMI and its expression levels will be relatively the highest in metastatic prostate tumors [36]. Hence COMMD3 is a reliable prognostic marker in analyzing prostate cancer progression [36]. COMMD3 overexpression increased the migration rate and invasiveness of tumor cells [36]. COMMD3 overexpression results in aberrant c-Myc expression in prostate cancers [36].

1.13. CXCL12: C-X-C CHEMOKINE LIGAND 12 CHROMOSOME 10; 10q11.21

CXCL12 activates multiple signaling pathways, including ERK, RAS, p38, and MAPK [37]. Hence, CXCL12 mutation can cause aberration in all the above signaling pathways. CXCL12 also modulates the expression of Cancer Stem Cells [38]. CXCL12 overexpression causes tumor cells to metastasize [37]. Blocking the CXCL12-CXCR4 axis helps in inhibiting the cell migration rate and metastasis [37]. The expression of CSC markers like CD133 and CD44 requires the support of CXCL12 expression [37]. This suggests that the CXCL12-CXCR4 axis is vital to maintaining the stemness of CSC in many tumors [39]. CXCL12 plays an important role in the communication between tumor cells in the tumor microenvironment [38]. CXCL12/CXCR4 axis has immense potential for tumor therapy [37].

1.14. DDX50: CHROMOSOME 10; 10P15.3

DDX50 is also known as LARP4B (Fig. **1**). LARP4B is an RNA Binding Protein and is a component of the mRNA translation regulatory complex [40, 41]. It functions as a tumor suppressor [40]. LARP4B expression is downregulated in glioma stem cells relative to its expression in neural stem cells [40]. LARP4B was deleted in the majority of glioblastomas [40]. LARP4B overexpression resulted in arresting the proliferation in glioma cells [40]. LARP4B knockdown enhanced the proliferation of glioma cells [40]. LARP4B deregulation is an important early event of tumorigenesis in glioblastomas [41]. Deletions within the LARP4B locus led to tumor initiation [41]. Bcl2 member BAX gets upregulated when LARP4B is overexpressed [41]. LARP4B promotes cell death through apoptosis [41]. LARP4B mediated tumor inhibition contains huge potential in treating glioblastoma [40].

1.15. DEPP: DECIDUAL PROTEIN INDUCED BY PROGESTERONE [DEPP] CHROMOSOME 10; 10q11.21

DEPP is expressed normally in human endometrial stromal cells [42]. DEPP (Fig. **1**) regulates the effects of progesterone expression during endometrial decidualization [42]. DEPP overexpression increased the MAPK phosphorylation manifold levels in colon cancer cells [43]. Baicalein is found to have substantial anti-tumor effects in colon cancer [43]. DEPP plays a major role in Baicalein-induced apoptosis [43]. DEPP expression is required for Baicalein-induced apoptosis [43]. DEPP knockdown inhibited the activation of caspase-3 and caspase-8 in Baicalein-treated tumors [43]. Baicalein upregulates DEPP, which induces MAPK's enhanced phosphorylation rate to trigger elevated levels of apoptosis in human colon cancer cells [43].

1.16. DHX32; DEAH BOX HELICASE 32 CHROMOSOME 10; 10q26.2

DHX32 is a human RNA helicase. DHX32 is overexpressed in colorectal cancer at both mRNA and protein levels [44]. DHX32 overexpression enhances the metastatic invasiveness and migratory potential of colon cancer cells [44]. DHX32 knockdown depleted VEGF levels [44]. DHX32 overexpression down-regulates the ant-apoptotic gene BCL-2 [44]. DHX32 contributes to the rapid proliferation of cancer cells [44]. DHX32 overexpression results in T-cells being unable to respond to apoptotic stimuli. DHX32 deregulates the Wnt pathway to trigger colorectal carcinogenesis [44]. DHX32 provides chemotherapeutic resistance to CRC cells [44]. DHX32 overexpression desensitized the colon cancer cells from 5-FU treatment [44].

1.17. EGR2 – EARLY GROWTH RESPONSE 2 CHROMOSOME 10; 10q21.3

EGR2 (Fig. **1**) is a zinc finger transcription factor and has essential roles in hindbrain development [45]. EGR2 has an immune role in our body and is influenced by the SFRP1 tumor suppressor protein [45]. EGR2 upregulation transactivates BAK and BNIP3L [46]. EGR2 upregulation alters the permeability of the mitochondrial membranes and releases higher levels of caspase-3,7,8 for enhanced apoptotic signal transduction [46]. All these strongly contribute to the PTEN-induced apoptotic pathway by EGR2 [46]. PTEN calls for EGR2, which directly increases BAK and BNIP3L levels [46]. ErbB2 [HER2] mutation-induced breast tumors showed significant upregulation of EGR2 [47]. EGR2 upregulation causes hyper-activation of ErbB2 since EGR2 binds excessively to its binding site in the HER2 promoter to cause HER2 overexpression [45, 47]. EGR2 could be a useful molecule for drug targeting based on its close association with HER2 overexpression and apoptotic induction *via* PTEN [46, 47].

1.18. ECD: HUMAN ECDYSONELESS CHROMOSOME 10; 10q22.2

ECD is a novel cell cycle regulator that plays a role in pancreatic tumorigenesis [48]. ECD specifically regulates cell cycle progression, especially during embryonic development, and its aberration can cause cancer [49]. ECD works through the Rb-E2F pathway [49]. ECD directly interacts with the Rb protein [49]. ECD deficiency causes anomalous cell cycle progression by bringing a block in the G1-S phase transition [49]. ECD overexpression contributes to pancreatic cancer by deregulating the glycolysis pathway in cancer [48]. ECD was highly overexpressed in primary and metastatic pancreatic cancers [48]. ECD modulates the expression of GLUT4 to alter the rates of glucose uptake, lactate metabolism, and ATP production in pancreatic cancer cells [48]. pAkt regulates aerobic glycolysis in tumor cells and ECD depletion *via* knockdown decreased pAkt levels [48]. Aberrant expression of ECD promotes pancreatic tumorigenesis by affecting glucose metabolism [48].

1.19. EPC1 GENE: ENHANCER OF POLYCOMB HOMOLOG 1 CHROMOSOME 10; 10p11.22

EPC1 is a recently discovered protein with a function in DNA damage protection [50]. EPC1 interacts with the E2F1 transcription factor, which is a prominent regulator of the cell cycle and apoptosis [50]. E2F1 binds to the promoter region of EPC1. E2F1-mediated apoptosis can be triggered by EPC1 depletion [50]. Nuclear EPC1 stimulates E2F1, which upregulates BCL-2 to silence death mecha-nisms activated by drugs [50]. EPC1 expression has increased in metastatic cells. EPC1 and E2F1 were vividly upregulated in drug-resistant cancer cells [50]. EPC1 upregulation is favored by cancer cells in attaining drug resistance and silencing drug-induced cell death mechanisms [50]. EPC fusion genes have been reported in uterine mesenchymal cancers [51]. EPC1- PHF has been identified long back in endometrial stromal sarcoma [51].

1.20. ERCC6:COCKAYNE SYNDROME B PROTEIN CHROMOSOME 10; 10q11.23

ERCC6 is an important protein belonging to the helicase-like protein family involved in the DNA repair mechanism [52]. Polymorphisms in the ERCC6 gene that causes the dysregulation of the ERCC6 protein can cause cancer, primarily lung cancer [52]. Myriad types of DNA damage, including irradiation-based dimers, chemical carcinogen-induced adducts, and ROS mutations, are repaired by ERCC6 [52]. ERCC6 is hypersensitive to DNA damage-inducing agents. Hence, ERCC6 is very vital to genome stability and genomic integrity [52]. Mutations in the ERCC6 gene make the patients more vulnerable to being afflicted with cancer in the future [52]. ERCC6 polymorphisms increase the risk of getting lung cancer [52].

1.21. FAM107B CHROMOSOME 10; 10p13

FAM107B deregulation is observed in gliomas and is a major component of glioma tumor progression [53]. FAM107B is a cytoskeleton cross-linker supporting metastatic invasion [53]. More research is yet to be done on FAM107B's role in carcinogenesis [53].

1.22. FAM13C: FAMILY WITH SEQUENCE SIMILARITY 13C CHRO-MOSOME 10; 10q21.1

FAM13C has been reported recently to be a prognostic marker in prostate cancer [54]. FAM13C overexpression is a relevant expression signature for prostate cancer progression [54]. FAM13C is involved in signal transduction pathways important to cancer progression [54]. Elevated levels of FAM13C positively correlated to increased tumor cell proliferation. Cancers without PTEN deletions had a robust expression of FAM13C in the cancer samples [54]. Prognostic predictions based on FAM13C expressions were reliable and remained independent of already established clinical and non-clinical parameters [54]. Shreds of evidence from the gene expression profile of other cancer validate that FAM13C overexpression supported cancer progression [54]. Tumors arising from *TMPRSS2:ERG* fusion gene harbor FAM13C upregulation [54].

1.23.   FAM170B: FAMILY WITH SEQUENCE SIMILARITY 170 MEMBER B CHROMOSOME 10; 10q11.23

Hepatocellular carcinoma [HCC] can be caused by Hepatitis B Virus [HBV] and Hepatitis C virus [HCV] [55]. HCC caused by HBV or HCV is associated with the *FAM170B-AS1* fusion gene [55]. *FAM170B-AS1* is a potent gene that could be responsible for homeostasis imbalance in HCC by allowing cancer cells to be affected by oxidative stress or even dysregulating cancer cell division rates [55].

1.24.   FAM188A: FAMILY WITH SEQUENCE SIMILARITY 188, MEMBER A CHROMOSOME 10; 10p13

FAM188a is also known as MINDY3 (Fig. **1**). This gene functions as a tumor suppressor in lung and gastric cancers [56]. This gene has a caspase-associated recruitment domain [56]. So, this protein may function in apoptosis [56]. Polymorphisms in this gene are associated with an increase in the risk of gastric cancers [56]. More research is yet to be done on this gene and its role in cancer.

1.25. FAM231A: FAMILY MEMBER CHROMOSOME 10; 10q23.1

FAM213 was first identified to function in fetal liver development [57]. FAM213A silencing in oral squamous cell carcinoma reduced oncogenesis [57]. TCF12 transcriptionally suppresses FAM213A [57]. FAM213A is a peroxiredoxin-like anti-oxidative protein [57]. OSCC with elevated TCF12 expression gave patients a riskier chance for survival [57]. FAM213A expression has been associated with carcinogenic progression in head-neck cancers [57]. 4-Nitroquinoline oxide-1 [4NQO], an environmental carcinogen, its administration enhanced the expression of FAM213A by upregulating miR-211 [57]. miR-211 expression is critical to OSCC progression [57]. miR-211 mediated FAM213A upregulation supports OSCC progression by protecting cancer cells from oxidative stress-induced damage [57]. TCF12 downregulates FAM213A and both proteins are inversely proportional to their expression levels [57]. FAM213A was the downstream target of the miR-211-TCF12 axis. TCF12 downregulates FAM213A by binding at the promoter region and inhibits FAM213A transcription [57]. Metastatic invasion and migration promoted by mir-211 in OSCC can be inhibited by FAM213A knockdown [57]. FAM213A depletes ROS-related signals to save cancer cells from oxidative stress [57]. FAM213A has a strong say in OSCC based on its direct interaction with the miR211 axis [57].

1.26. FAS-AS1: FAS ANTISENSE RNA 1 [FAS-AS1] CHROMOSOME 10; 10q23.31

FAS-AS1 has been reported in breast cancer and many other cancers [58, 59]. It is an antisense long non-coding RNA [lnc RNA] [58]. Over the years, multiple reports have stated that FAS-AS1 expression is a prognostic marker for breast cancer and AML [58, 59]. But latest reports have suggested that FAS-AS1 lncRNA expression is not able to distinguish between AML patients and healthy patients, and hence FAS-AS1 is not a reliable biomarker for diagnosis/prognosis [58]. FAS-AS1 normally functions in regulating human erythropoiesis [58]. FAS-AS1 regulates Fas expression in lung cancer cells [59]. There have been contrasting evidence regarding the reliability of FAS-AS1 as a reliable biomarker [58]. More research has to be done to confirm the reliability of FAS-AS1 lncRNA's potential in being called a biomarker [58].

1.27. FGFR2: FIBROBLAST GROWTH FACTOR RECEPTOR 2 CHROMOSOME 10; 10q26

FGFR2 is a transmembrane receptor tyrosine kinase that triggers cell proliferation [60]. Mutations in FGFR2 that activate oncogenesis in several cancers are a frequently observed phenomenon [60]. FGFR2 activates the RAS/MAPK axis. ERK1/2 has a putative phosphorylation site in FGFR2's serine located at the 777th position [called S780]. Mutations that cause FGFR2 to lack S780 have been observed in many cancers [60]. In bladder cancer, S780 has been converted to leucine [missense mutation], hence FGFR2 signaling was aberrantly increased in bladder cancer. Cells with mutations at S780 had faster cell migration rates. ERK1/2's direct phosphorylation of FGFR2 at S780 is a vital feedback loop, and mutations at S780 deactivate this feedback loop, resulting in aberrantly increased FGFR2 signaling activation. This leads to enhanced metastatic migration rates [60]. FGFR2 overexpression has been observed in multiple cancers [61]. FGFR2 overexpression is associated with poor survival in Gastric cancer [61]. FGFR2's reliability as a prognostic marker in solid tumors remains debatable [61]. FGFR2 mutations support gastric cancer progression *via* the PI3K-Akt-mTOR pathway post-downregulation of TSP4 [62].

1.28. FRA10AC1: FRA10A ASSOCIATED CGG REPEAT 1 CHROMO-SOME 10; 10q23.33

Esrrb expression and Esrrb targets have been studied in prostate cancer cells [63]. Esrrb is a nuclear receptor estrogen-related receptor beta [63]. The Esrrb gene has gained widespread attention in recent years owing to its role in iPSC development [63]. Esrrb is downregulated in prostate cancer cells and promotes prostate cancer tumorigenesis [63]. FRA10AC1 is one of the many mRNAs directly regulated by

Esrrb, even in prostate cancer [63]. FRA10AC1 is a nuclear phosphoprotein and its function is yet to be established [63].

1.29. FRAT1: CHROMOSOME 10; 10q24.1

FRAT1 is a proto-oncogene that acts through the Wnt pathway [64]. FRAT1 upregulation at mRNA levels and protein levels has been observed in gastric cancer, esophageal cancer, and colorectal and pancreatic cancer [64, 65]. FRAT1 codes for GSK-3beta binding proteins [64]. FRAT1 mRNA was highly expressed in cervical cancer and CML cell lines [64]. FRAT1 upregulation induces Wnt pathway deregulation, ultimately leading to gastric cancer [64]. Beta-catenin expression and secretion are controlled by FRAT1 [65]. FRAT1 overexpression corresponds to increased malignancy of the cancers [65]. FRAT1 is highly overexpressed in Stage III and Stage IV cancer patients [65]. FRAT1 could be helpful for TNM grading of cancer stages [65]. FRAT2 competes with Axin for binding to GSK-3 beta and thereby controls Wnt pathway transduction [66].

1.30. FRAT2 CHROMOSOME 10; 10q24.1

FRAT2 is encoded by an intronless gene belonging to the GSK-3 beta-binding protein family. It is a positive modulator of the Wnt signaling pathway. Similar to FRAT1, FRAT2 was upregulated in gastric cancer [64]. FRAT2 upregulation coupled with FRAT1 upregulation can deregulate the Wnt pathway to cause gastric cancer [64]. c-Jun phosphorylation and JNK activity are regulated by FRAT2 expression [66]. Defunct FRAT2 functioning can lead to aberrant Wnt signaling [66]. FRAT2 is important for the balance between canonical and non-canonical Wnt signaling pathways since FRAT2 operates at the junction between canonical and non-canonical Wnt pathways [66]. FRAT2 competes with Axin for binding to GSK-3 beta and thereby controls Wnt pathway transduction [66].

1.31. FRMPD2: FERM AND PDZ DOMAIN CONTAINING 2 CHROMOSOME 10; 10q11.22

FRMPD2 is differentially underexpressed in the later stages of Renal cell carcinoma [67] FRMPD2 has a role of binding to 1- phosphatidylinositol [67, 68]. FRMPD2 plays a role in tight junction developments and has been reported to be downregulated in many epithelial cancer cell lines [67, 68]. More research on FRMPD2 in carcinogenesis is still to be exposed.

1.32. GATA3: CHROMOSOME 10; 10p14

GATA3 is expressed in luminal epithelial cells of mammary glands lining the breast ductal structures and is vital to mammary gland development [69]. The luminal transcription program is controlled by GATA3 in determining the luminal cell identity [69]. Mutations in GATA3 can cause breast cancer [69]. GATA3 misexpression is correlated with poor prognosis in breast cancer [69]. GATA3 expression demotes EMT and metastasis [69]. Different classes of mutations within the various domains of the GATA3 protein lead to different subtypes of luminal breast cancer [69]. GATA3 expression is critical to the binding site selection of estrogen receptors for activating many other genes important for luminal development [69]. Concerning its prominent role in normal mammary gland development, mutations in GATA3 are risky for breast cancer development [69]. GATA3's influence on the tumor microenvironment can affect tumor progression and metastasis [70]. Understanding more about the GATA3 pathway would help demystify poorly differentiated breast cancers [70].

1.33. GHITM: GROWTH HORMONE INDUCIBLE TRANSMEMBRANE PROTEIN CHROMOSOME 10; 10q23.1

GHITM is a member of the Bax inhibitory [BI-1] family [71]. BI-1 is over-expressed in many tumors, such as lung adenocarcinoma, lymphoma, breast cancer, and lymphoma [71]. GHITM is found to be expressed in many cancer cell lines [71]. GHITM is evolutionarily conserved [72]. GHITM is shown to be downregulated in many types of cancer [72]. GHITM itself is TMBIM5 and belongs to the TMBIM family [72]. All TMBIM proteins regulate apoptosis [72]. TMBIM members have an anti-apoptotic activity [72]. Therefore, aberrations in GHITM expression levels can dysregulate apoptosis, ultimately leading to cancer [72]. The exact function of GHITM is yet to be elucidated [71, 72].

1.34. GPRIN2: G PROTEIN-REGULATED INDUCER OF NEURITE OUTGROWTH 2 CHROMOSOME 10; 10q11.22

GPRIN2 has been reported very recently in Esophageal squamous cell carcinoma [ESCC] [73]. GPRIN2 mutations have been implicated as novel germ-line mutations in ESCC [73]. GRPIN2 is a mutation in melanoma samples [73]. GPRIN2 controls the glutamate-gated ion channel proteins. GPRIN2 dysre-gulation is documented in many other cancers [73].

1.35. GTPBP4: GUANOSINE TRIPHOSPHATE BINDING PROTEIN 4 CHROMOSOME 10; 10p15.3

GTPBP4 enhances gastric cancer proliferation and attenuates apoptotic signals

[74]. GTPBPP4 knockdown increased apoptosis in gastric cancer cells [74]. GTPBP4 was prominently upregulated in gastric cancer cells relative to the adjacent gastric epithelium. GTPBP4 communicates with p53 in gastric cancer cells [74]. GTPBP4 overexpression enhanced the chemoresistance of tumor cells [74]. GTPBP4 and p53 may bind to each other in gastric cancer cells for modulating apoptotic signals and cell proliferation [74]. GTBPP4-mediated downregulation of apoptosis is p53-dependent [74]. GTPBP4 having a prognostic significance in hepatocellular carcinoma [HCC] has been revealed [75]. GTPBP4 was overexpressed in HCC as well [75].GTPBP4 overexpression is interrelated with lesser survival rates in HCC patients [75]. GTPBP4 could become a valuable biomarker for HCC and gastric cancer, providing validation of its reliability in the upcoming years.

1.36. HELLS: HELICASE, LYMPHOID SPECIFIC CHROMOSOME 10; 10q23.33

HELLS was remarkably upregulated in colorectal cancer [76]. HELLS knock-down induced a cell cycle arrest at the G2 phase [76]. HELLS upregulation was linked with colorectal metastasis [76]. HELLS underexpression blocked cell cycle progression and cell proliferation [76]. HELLS expression levels are of clinical significance in deciding the prognosis of patients. HELLS-mediated epigenetic signature changes have caught significant attention in cancer progression [76]. HELLS overexpression is important for sustaining high rates of tumor cell proliferation [76].

1.37. HKDC1: HEXOKINASE DOMAIN COMPONENT 1 CHROMOSO-ME 10; 10q22.1

HKDC1 is overexpressed in breast tumor tissue [77]. HKDC1 controls glucose metabolism and glucose uptake in cancer cells by regulating the mitochondrial pore opening [77]. PGC1-beta modulates HKDC1 expression in breast cancer cells [77]. HKDC1 promoter has an SREBP1 binding site for PGC1-beta to bind and activate HKDC1 [77]. HKDC1 expression distinctly increased breast cancer cell proliferation and HKDC1 knockdown brought down the cancer cell proliferation rates [77]. HKDC1 interferes with the oxidative stress response mecha-nism in breast cancer cells [77]. HKDC1 overexpression supports metastasis [77]. HKDC1 is approved to be a novel lung cancer drug target [78]. HKDC1 overexpression corresponds to aggressive HCC since HKDC1 expression levels influence the beta-catenin/Wnt signaling [79]. Beta-catenin and c-Myc expression attenuated on HKDC1 knockdown [79].

1.38. KIN17: DNA/RNA BINDING PROTEIN KIN17 CHROMOSOME 10; 10P14

KIN17 is implicated in triple-negative breast cancers [TNBC] as a promoter of high proliferation rates [80]. KIN17 knockdown suppressed cell proliferation and enhanced apoptosis in cancer cell lines [80]. KIN17 normally functions with mRNA processing and DNA replication regulation [80]. Kin17 is a positive regulator of cell proliferation in TNBC.

1.39. MTG1 MITOCHONDRIAL RIBOSOME-ASSOCIATED GTPASE 1 CHROMOSOME 10;

Bioinformatics analysis has predicted MTG1 to be a central cancer-causing gene [81]. MTG gene is mutated in lung adenocarcinoma [81]. More research is yet to be performed to validate MTG1 mutations playing a role in oncogenesis. It's safe to presume that MTG1 mutations promote oncogenesis since many other GT-Pases, like Rho GTPases, is significant in cancer deregulations.

1.40. NRBF2: NUCLEAR RECEPTOR-BINDING FACTOR 2 CHROM-OSOME 10; 10q21.3

SNP genotyping of the enhancer-promoter region revealed NBRF1 to have some role in the pathogenesis of breast cancer [82]. iCHAV2 interacts with the promoter region of ZNF365 and NRBF2 in normal and breast cancer cells, but SNP analysis further showed NRBF2 promoter repression in breast cancer cells [82]. The chromosomal band of NRBF2 is susceptible to genomic rearrangements in breast cancer [82].

1.41. OTUD1: OTU DOMAIN-CONTAINING PROTEIN-1/OTU DEUBI-QUITINASE ` CHROMOSOME 10; 10p12.2

OTUD1 prevents the degradation of SMAD7 by cleaving it and thereby inhibiting the ubiquitination of SMAD7 [83]. OTUD1 is deficient in many cancers, and OTUD1 deficiency elevates metastasis rates [83]. OTUD1 upregulation decreases CSC activity and cuts down metastasis [83]. OTUD1 expression reduces breast cancer metastasis by modulating the TGF-beta pathways signaling through its direct interaction with SMAD7 [83]. OTUD1 functions as a metastasis suppressor [83]. OTUD1 modulation of the TGF-beta pathway further inhibits EMT [83].

1.42. PCDH15: PROTOCADHERIN 15 CHROMOSOME 10; 10q21.1

PCDH15 (Fig. **1**) is considered to be the next potential marker for T-cell Lymphomas [84]. PCDH15 expression promoted tumor expansion [84]. Only transformed malignant NK cells harbored PCDH15 expression [84]. PCDH15 expre-ssion in only malignant cells makes it a suitable target for drugs and biomarker development.

1.43. PI4K2A: PHOSPHATIDYLINOSITOL 4-KINASE 2-ALPHA CHRO-MOSOME 10; 10q24.2

The PI4K2A-associated complex is disturbed upon Pac1 binding to PI4K2A [85]. This causes cancer cell lysosomes to become unstable and prompts cell death [85]. PI4K2A plays a vital role in the lysosome-mediated degradation of mis-folded proteins in cancer cells [85]. PI4K2A is directly linked to the PKR network of lysosome cancer cell lysosomal activity [85]. Pac1 can destabilize PI4K2A to suppress PI4K2A expression, which will dysregulate the lysosomal activity of cancer cells [85]. PI4K2A gene expression was highly upregulated in breast cancer patients with lower survival rates [85]. Since lysosomes hold a prominent status in driving the protein recycling machinery and the cellular energy metabolism in cancer cells, targeting the PKR/PI4K2A axis to destabilize the cancer cell lysosomes for triggering cell death is an effective cancer therapeutic approach [85]. PI4K2A overexpression has been correlated to poor differentiation and active malignant proliferation in hepatocellular carcinoma [HCC] [86].

1.44. PIP4K2A: PHOSPHATIDYLINOSITOL-5-PHOSPHATE 4-KINASE TYPE-2 ALPHA CHROMOSOME 10; 10p12.2

PIP4K2A is involved in highly important basic cellular activities like proli-feration, migration, glucose uptake, and metabolism [87]. PIP4K2A mutation can have pleiotropic effects on manifold tissues [87]. PIP4K2A overexpression has been recurrently observed in leukemias and solid cancers [87]. Current studies have displayed an existing link between ethnicity-specific and cancer-subtype specific PIP4K2A SNPs and cancers [87]. PIP4K2A SNPs could be useful in genotyping and identification of myriad cancer subtypes [87]. PIP4K2A SNPs have been associated with ALL susceptibility [87]. PIP4K2A network is deregulated in B-ALL [87]. PIP4K2A is linked with leukemogenesis [87]. PIP4K2A has been reported in Acute Myeloid Leukemia [AML] [88].

1.45. PLEKHS1: PLECKSTRIN HOMOLOGY DOMAIN-CONTAINING S1 CHROMOSOME 10; 10q25.3

Promoter mutation in the PLEKHS1 gene is a prominent non-coding mutation reported in several cancers [89]. PLEKHS1 promoter is a mutational hotspot for many cancers [90]. 40% of tumors have PLEKHS1 promoter mutations [89]. Promoter mutations in PLEKHS1 could deliver further scope for diagnostic analysis in bladder cancer [89]. Worsened prognosis in bladder cancer patients has been linked to PLEKHS1 promoter mutations and PLEKSH1 overexpression [89]. PLEKHS1 has a role in bladder carcinogenesis, but more studies are yet to elucidate its exact part in pathogenesis [89].

1.46. PLXDC2: PLEXIN DOMAIN-CONTAINING PROTEIN 2 CHROMOSOME 10: 10p12.31

PLXDC2 is a cell surface receptor for PEDF [Pigment Epithelium derive factor] [91]. PEDF suppresses the growth of many cancers, particularly melanoma, gastric carcinoma, chondrosarcoma, glioma, *etc* [91]. Mutations in PEDF and PLXDC2 contribute to many cancers [91]. PEDF binding triggers the disassembly of PLXDC2 and PLXDC1 to initiate downstream signaling for important processes like migration and endothelial angiogenesis [91]. PLXDC2 is a marker for distinguishing between Taxol-resistant and non-resistant Epithelial Ovarian Cancer [EOC] patients [92]. PLXDC2 is prominently upregulated in Taxol-resistant EOC patients [92]. PLXDC2 could become the next approved biomarker for checking chemoresistance in EOC [92].

1.47. PTEN: PHOSPHATASE AND TENSIN HOMOLOG CHROMOSOME 10; 10q23.31

PTEN has a tumor suppressor function [93]. PTEN aberration has been involved in breast carcinogenesis and tumor progression [93]. PTEN depletion has been reported in breast cancer patients [93]. Missense mutations and PTEN promoter methylation are prime factors for PTEN depletion in breast cancers [93, 94]. Apart from breast cancers, PTEN inactivation has been discovered in many malignant tumors such as gliomas, prostate, ovarian, thyroid, *etc*. Loss of Heterozygosity [LOH] at the PTEN locus [94]. PTEN mutations happen the most in the later stages of metastatic breast cancer. PTEN deficiency is linked with negative ER [estrogen receptors] expression in breast cancers [94].

1.48. FGF8: FIBROBLAST GROWTH FACTOR8 CHROMOSOME 10; 10q24.32

FGF8 overexpression can cause EGFR upregulation to provide resistance against EGFR inhibitors in human hepatocellular carcinoma cells [95]. FGF8 overexpression in prostate cancer has been correlated to advanced tumor progression and declining patient survival rates [96]. FGF8 induces EMT to intensify metastasis in colorectal cancer [97]. FGF8-mediated regulation of YAP1's transcriptional network supports EMT and metastasis in colorectal cancer [97]. FGF8 has been identified to play a role in breast cancer progression [98].

1.49. FGFR2: FIBROBLAST GROWTH FACTOR RECEPTOR2 CHROMOSOME 10; 10q26.13

FGFR2 is a receptor tyrosine kinase that controls cell proliferation and migration [99]. Oncogenic FGFR2 mutations have been reported in many cancers. "Switching off" the FGFR2 feedback loop in cancer cells results in FGFR2 hyperactivation that upsurges cancer cells' metastatic invasiveness [99]. FGFR2 mutations can inhibit this negative feedback loop arbitrating through the ERKL1/2 pathway [99]. MAPK inhibition in cancer cells is related to FGFR2 deregulation [99]. TSP4 downregulation through the mTOR pathway by FGFR2 enhances gastric cancer progression [62].

1.50. TACC2: TRANSFORMING ACIDIC COILED-COIL CONTAINING PROTEIN 2 CHROMOSOME 10; 10q26.13

TACC2 protein is highly overexpressed in hepatocellular carcinoma. TACC2's normal function is regulating the microtubule dynamics and spindle stability [100]. TACC2 is a reliable prognostic marker in HCC [100]. TACC expression is distinctly elevated in stages III and IV of HCC [100]. Aberrant expression of TACC and TACC gene fusions can lead to mitotic spindle defects, particularly aneuploidy and chromosomal segregation defects [101]. TACC2 has a role in oncogenic transformation in HCC and various other types of cancer [100]. Markedly high expression of TACC2 in HCC tissues is a salient indicator of poor prognosis and for deciding patient survival rates [100]. TACC2 overexpression in androgen-dependent prostate cancer is required to enhance cell proliferation rates of prostate cancer cells [102].

1.51. CCDC6: COILED -COIL DOMAIN CONTAINING 6 CHROMO-SOME 10; 10q21.2

RET-CCDC6 fusions have been detected in Lung tumors, including patient-derived lung tumor cell lines [103]. RET rearrangements are frequent in lung cancers, especially NSCLC [Non-small Cell Lung Cancer]. CCDC6 is a regular fusion gene partner for RET gene in NSCLC [103]. CCDC6-RET fusion is a driver mutation in ALL [Acute Lymphoblastic Leukemia] [104, 105]. Paracentric inversion in the "q" arm of chromosome 10 results in the CCDC6-RET fusion that has been detected in papillary thyroid carcinoma [PTC] [106, 107]. The CCDC6-RET fusion gene is called the PTC1 [RET-PTC1] oncogene [106]. CCDC6 mutations/gene fusions can disable DNA-damage-induced apoptosis, thereby further complementing rapid tumor cell progression [107]. CCDC6 could be a reliable biomarker for drug resistance [107].

1.52. KIF5B: KINESIN FAMILY MEMBER 5B CHROMOSOME 10; 10p11.22

KIF5B-RET fusions are present in lung adenocarcinomas [108]. KIF5B-MET fusion in NSCLC [110]. Overexpression of KIF5B-MET in cancer cells enhanced the cancer cell proliferation rates [109]. In KIF5B fusions, the coiled-coil domain is fused to the tyrosine kinase domain of the partner fusion gene [109]. This results in constitutive activation of the tyrosine kinase domain through the ligand-independent self-dimerization process. The KIF5B-RET fusion gene was reported in the liver metastasis of NSCLC [110]. KIF5B-RET fusion-positive patients have distinct clinicopathological features, and hence KIF5B-RET fusion gene may help in the molecular characterization of the NSCLC subsets [110]. KIF5B-RET's chimeric tyrosine kinase hyper-activates STAT3 signaling to enhance tumorigenic cell growth [111]. KIF5B-RET fusion is the driver of mutations in non-smoking lung cancer populations [111].

1.53. RET: REARRANGED DURING TRANSFECTION CHROMOSOME 10; 10q11.21

RET is a proto-oncogene coding for a receptor tyrosine kinase. RET fusion in solid tumors is a recurrent genetic event [112]. RET fusions are detected in NSCLC [non-small cell lung cancer] and PTC [papillary thyroid carcinoma] [112]. RET/PTC fusion genes such as CCDC6-RET and NCOA4-RET genes are frequently expressed in Papillary thyroid cancer [PTC] [112]. RET fusions like KIF5B-RE in NSCLC [111, 112]. The 3' RET sequences coding for its tyrosine kinase domain are conjugated to a 5' sequence from another gene that codes for a dimerization coiled-coil domain [112]. RET fusion thus formed leads to oncogenic signaling transduction into the nucleus.

1.54. DKK1: DICKKOPF WNT SIGNALING PATHWAY INHIBITOR 1 CHROMOSOME 10; 10q21.1

DKK1 is a critical inhibitor of the Wnt pathway [113]. DKK1 inhibits the Wnt pathway possibly through 2 mechanisms, the first involving the binding of DKK1 to LRP5/6, and the second is the formation of a ternary complex with Krm1/2 [113]. DKK1 overexpression has been described in hepatocellular carcinoma, chondrosarcoma, pancreatic cancer, bladder cancer, and many other cancer types

[113]. In contrast, DKK1 underexpression has been discovered in papillary thyroid cancer and colorectal adenocarcinoma [113]. DKK1 expression is asso-ciated with Cancer stem Cell activity in hepatocellular carcinoma since some microRNAs targeting DKK1 regulate the CSC expression through the Wnt pathway [114].

1.55. VTI1A: VESICLE TRANSPORT THROUGH INTERACTION WITH T-SNARES 1A CHROMOSOME 10; 10q25.2

VTI1A forms a fusion protein with truncated TCF4 in cancer [115]. The VTI1-TCF4 fusion protein has been detected in colon cancer [115, 116]. VTI1A-TCF4 is a powerful antagonist of the Wnt signaling pathway [115, 116]. VTI1A gene fusions can trigger oncogenic events leading to colorectal neoplasms [115]. Molecular investigations in colorectal cancer have concluded that VTI1A fusions are frequent in colorectal neoplasms, especially the VTI1A-TCF7L2 fusion in colorectal adenocarcinoma [117]. Intestinal homeodomain factor CDX2 interacts with VTIA-TCF4 and regulates its expression in colorectal cancers.

1.56. FAS: FAS CELL SURFACE DEATH RECEPTOR CHROMOSOME 10; 10q23.31

FAS is a transmembrane receptor belonging to the TNF [tumor necrosis factor] receptor family and is an apoptosis-regulating protein [118]. The FAS ligand-receptor system is an important entity of our immune system in killing tumor cells [119]. Mutations in FAS can lead to promoting tumor cell progression [119]. FAS is downregulated in the colon epithelium during oncogenic transformation in colon cancers [120]. Epigenetic silencing can cause Fas downregulation in colon cancers [120]. Fas mutations result in Fas resistance that promotes tumorigenesis in gastric cancer [118].

1.57. ZEB1: ZINC FINGER E-BOX BINDING HOMEOBOX 1 CHROMOSOME 10; 10p11.22

ZEB is a crucial decider in EMT [Epithelial Mesenchymal Transition] [121]. ZEB1 overexpression causes EMT and aggrandizes metastasis [121]. ZEB1 is overexpressed in rapidly dividing cancer cells [121]. ZEB1 drives EMT through the epigenetic silencing of E-cadherin [121]. ZEB1 plays a key role in the chemoresistance of metastatic cells [122]. ZEB1 has a prominent role in regulating chief cell cycles processes like senescence and apoptosis. ZEB1 activation functions together with the mutated oncogenes for cancer cells to overcome apoptosis [121]. ZEB1 protein modulates the p53 activity in cancer cells to promote cancer progression [121].

1.58. NODAL: NODAL GROWTH DIFFERENTIATION FACTOR CHROMOSOME 10; 10q22.1

NODAL is an important morphogen in the nucleus conveying signals through the TGF-beta pathway [123]. The NODAL expression has been correlated to cancer stem cell expression, particularly colon CSC and in testicular germ cell cancers [123]. NODAL expression is directly proportional to the tumorigenicity and metastasis of breast cancer cells [123]. NODAL expression is associated with invasiveness and proliferation rates in gliomas and breast cancers. A decrease in NODAL expression can bring down the rapid proliferation rates in breast cancer cells [123]. Elevated NODAL expression levels are associated with aggressively malignant tumors in breast, melanoma, and prostate cancers [124].

1.59. PRINS: PSORIASIS-ASSOCIATED NON-PROTEIN CODING RNA INDUCED BY STRESS CHROMOSOME 10; 10p12.1

PRINS is a long non-coding RNA discovered in the pathogenesis of psoriasis [125]. PRINS controls G1P3 expression [125]. PRINS misexpression caused by its deregulation leads to psoriasis [125]. PRINS deregulation has been confirmed in aggressively malignant adrenocortical carcinoma [ACC] [126]. ACC relapse is related to PRINS underexpression [126]. Research is yet to unfold whether PRINS functions as a tumor suppressor or oncogene in the pathogenesis of cancers [126].

1.60. VIM: VIMENTIN CHROMOSOME 10; 10p13

Vimentin is a vital EMT [Epithelial Mesenchymal Transition] marker [127]. Vimentin overexpression in cancer cells has been linked to metastasis and increased tumor invasion [127]. Vimentin complexes with beclin1 block autophagy in cancer cells through the AKT pathway [128]. Vimentin transcriptional program is controlled through HIF-1 [Hypoxia inducible factor]. Slug-induced EMT is based on Vimentin upregulation [128]. Vimentin has been relevantly connected with metastatic cascade and EMT [128]. Vimentin is a mesenchymal marker [128]. Vimentin controls cell motility and cellular migration [128]. Vimentin expression pattern will convey the cancer cell's metastatic potential [128].

1.61. MAPK8: MITOGEN-ACTIVATED PROTEIN KINASE 8/ JNK1 CHROMOSOME 10; 10q11.22

MAPK8 [JNK1] mediates signal transduction of growth factors and cytokines through phosphorylation pathways to effectuate corresponding intracellular events [129]. Sulindac is an NSAID that depends on JNK1 expression to block proliferation in colon cancer cells and bring about apoptosis [130]. MAPK1 can save us from skin cancer after UV irradiation by associating with Myt1 to induce apoptosis [129]. MAPK1 and its closely related proteins belonging to the same family have a role in the pathogenesis of many cancers [129].

1.62. PAX2: PAIRED BOX 2 CHROMOSOME 10; 10q24.31

PAX2-estrogen receptor [ER-PAX2] complex is formed in breast tumor cells that modulate HER2 expression and regulates the HER2 response to breast cancer drugs such as tamoxifen [131]. PAX2 aberration has been reported in prostate cancer [131]. PAX2 can provide apoptosis resistance in Kaposi sarcoma cells [131]. PAX2 expression supports tumor cell survival in ovarian cancers, renal cell carcinomas, and bladder carcinomas [131]. VHL deficiency in cancer cells supports PAX2 expression for further enhancing tumor cell survival [131]. PAX2 upregulation supports the metastasis of esophageal cancer [132].

1.63. TCF7L2: TRANSCRIPTION FACTOR 7 LIKE 2: CHROMOSOME 10; 10q25.2-q25.3

TCF7L2 is associated with the Wnt signaling pathway [132]. Investigations correlating TCF7L2 polymorphisms with colon, endometrial, and breast cancer have been conducted [132]. Such studies have revealed the TCF7L2 poly-morphisms to be connected with endometrial cancers and breast cancers [132] TCF7L2 undergoes gene fusions with other genes to drive oncogenesis as the fusion protein deregulates important cell signaling pathways [134]. VTI1A-TCF7L2 is a persistently detected fusion protein in colon cancer [114, 134].

1.64. TET1: TET-METHYLCYTOSINE DIOXYGENASE 1 /TEN ELEVEN TRANSLOCATION CHROMOSOME 10; 10q21.3

TET1 overexpression caused apoptosis [133]. TET1 contributes to carcinogenesis [133]. TET1 expression influences the cell cycle [133]. TET overexpression reduced cell proliferation [133]. Anti-cancer molecules like Hydroxyurea [HU] support TET1 expression to cause apoptosis in osteosarcoma [133]. TET1 induces epigenetic changes in hepatocarcinoma cells [133]. TET1 underexpression has been noted in breast cancer and prostate cancer tissues [134]. TET1 expression decides the metastatic cell migration in papillary thyroid carcinoma [134].

1.65. KLF6: KRUPPEL-LIKE FACTOR 6 CHROMOSOME 10; 10p15.2

KLF6 is a tumor suppressor gene [135, 136]. KLF6 codes for a zinc finger transcription factor [139]. KLF6 is frequently mutated in prostate cancer [135, 136]. Mutational inactivation of KLF6 by a deletion in IBD [inflammatory bowel disease] related cancers was discovered [135]. KLF6 aberration can contribute to colorectal carcinogenesis [135]. KLF6 mutations are the pioneer in the formation of non-polypoid colorectal carcinomas [137]. KLF6 is underexpressed in human cancers to promote metastasis [138]. KLF6 overexpression in oral cancer cells inhibited the migratory and invasive potential [138]. Oncogenic HER2 over-expression is strongly correlated to nuclear KLF6 expression in ductal breast carcinomas [139].

1.66. MLLT10: MLLT10 HISTONE LYSINE METHYLTRANSFERASE DOT1L COFACTOR CHROMOSOME 10 ; 10p12.31

MLLT10 has been implicated in colorectal cancer with strongly enhancing tumor migration and subsequent metastasis [140]. MLLT10 expression is significantly higher in colorectal cancer tissues [140]. MLLT10 promotes metastasis of colorectal cancer *via* EMT regulation [140]. MLLT10 rearrangements have been reported in ALL [141].

1.67. MGMT: O-6-METHYLGUANINE-DNA METHYLTRANSFERASE CHROMOSOME 10; 10q26.3

MGMT gene codes for an enzyme that functions in the DNA repair process [142]. MGMT gene silencing *via* epigenetic promoter methylation occurs in highly malignant gliomas [142]. MGMT promoter methylation weakens the DNA repair mechanism because the MGMT enzyme is inoperative [142]. MGMT methylation status and gene product function could be predictive biomarkers for many gliomas and their subtypes [143].

MGMT promoter methylation has become a reliable laboratory test to be asked for in neuro-oncology labs [142].

1.68. BAG3: BCL-2 ASSOCIATED ATHANOGENE 3 CHROMOSOME 10; 10q26.11

BAG3 usually supports tumor proliferation and tumor invasion, as in the case of breast cancer and colorectal cancer [144]. BAG3 is overexpressed in multiple solid tumors involving prostate cancer, ovarian cancer, and glioblastoma. BAG3 is an anti-apoptosis protein [145]. BAG3 interacts with Hsp70 in many pathways [144, 145]. BAG3 is overexpressed in colorectal cancer. BAG3 promotes colorectal cancer cell growth and cell migration *in-vitro* [145]. BAG3 also supports cancer cell growth in breast cancer [144].

1.69. BTRC: BETA-TRANSDUCIN REPEAT CONTAINING E3 UBIQUITIN PROTEIN LIGASE CHROMOSOME 10; 10q24.32

BTRC codes for the beta TCP protein, which is a part of the ubiquitin complex operating in the Wnt pathway [146]. BTRC mutations have been implicated in gastric cancer and lung cancer [146, 148]. Beat-TrCP forms an oncogene-tumor suppressor signaling cascade with FBXW2 and SKP2 to modulate tumor growth [146]. In this axis, these 3 proteins target each other for degradation and their degradation levels determine the survival of lung cancer cells [146, 147].

1.70. POLL: DNA POLYMERASE LAMBDA CHROMOSOME 10; 10q24.32

POLL codes for a DNA Polymerase lambda enzyme which functions in base excision repair [149]. Mutations in POLL cause errors in DNA replication and repair [150]. Such mutations cause cancer [150]. POLL knockout mice showed decreased variation in the VJD junction [150]. Specific mutations, like the R438W [arginine to tryptophan], have promoted cellular transformation and chromosomal defects in breast cancer cells [149]. Estrogen endocrine therapy in R438W[+] POLL mutated breast cancer cells rapidly augmented the oncogenic transformation [149].

CONCLUSION

Given the fact that some of the key genes that chiefly influence the diverse cellular processes are present on chromosome 10, genes on chromosome 10 have received significant limelight among investigators in cancer research. Interestingly, chromosome 10 may come under even more focus in the upcoming years. Genetic abnormalities on chromosome 10 have been prominently correlated with many tumors. Loss of genetic material from chromosome 10 is found in brain cancers, whereas translocation with genes on other chromosomes is found in leukemias. Based on the frequently detected occurrence of chromosome 10's genes in cancer progression, this chapter will provide a thorough recap for researchers in interpreting the roles of these genes.

REFERENCES

[1]   Cimino G, Rapanotti MC, Sprovieri T, Elia L. ALL1 gene alterations in acute leukemia: biological and clinical aspects. Haematologica 1998; 83(4): 350-7.
        [PMID: 9592986]

[2]   Caligiuri MA, Strout MP, Oberkircher AR, Yu F, de la Chapelle A, Bloomfield CD. The partial tandem duplication of *ALL1* in acute myeloid leukemia with normal cytogenetics or trisomy 11 is restricted to one chromosome. Proc Natl Acad Sci USA 1997; 94(8): 3899-902.
        [http://dx.doi.org/10.1073/pnas.94.8.3899] [PMID: 9108076]

[3]   Croce CM. Role of TCL1 and ALL1 in human leukemias and development. Cancer Research; 59.

[4]   Neutrophils Promote ALOX5-Dependent Breast Cancer Lung Metastasis. Cancer Discovery 2016; 6: OF7–OF7.

[5]   Chen Y, Li D, Li S. The Alox5 gene is a novel therapeutic target in cancer stem cells of chronic myeloid leukemia. Cell Cycle 2009; 8(21): 3488-92.
        [http://dx.doi.org/10.4161/cc.8.21.9852] [PMID: 19823023]

[6]   Poczobutt JM, Nguyen TT, Hanson D, *et al.* Deletion of 5-Lipoxygenase in the Tumor Microenvironment Promotes Lung Cancer Progression and Metastasis through Regulating T Cell Recruitment. J Immunol 2016; 196(2): 891-901.
        [http://dx.doi.org/10.4049/jimmunol.1501648] [PMID: 26663781]

[7]   Bergamaschi A, Kim YH, Kwei KA, *et al. CAMK1D* amplification implicated in epithelial-mesenchymal transition in basal-like breast cancer. Mol Oncol 2008; 2(4): 327-39.
        [http://dx.doi.org/10.1016/j.molonc.2008.09.004] [PMID: 19383354]

[8]   Kahl CR, Means AR. Regulation of cyclin D1/Cdk4 complexes by calcium/calmodulin-dependent protein kinase I. J Biol Chem 2004; 279(15): 15411-9.
        [http://dx.doi.org/10.1074/jbc.M312543200] [PMID: 14754892]

[9]   Rodriguez-Mora OG, LaHair MM, McCubrey JA, Franklin RA. Calcium/calmodulin-dependent kinase I and calcium/calmodulin-dependent kinase kinase participate in the control of cell cycle progression in MCF-7 human breast cancer cells. Cancer Res 2005; 65(12): 5408-16.
        [http://dx.doi.org/10.1158/0008-5472.CAN-05-0271] [PMID: 15958590]

[10]   Herber B, Truss M, Beato M, Müller R. Inducible regulatory elements in the human cyclin D1 promoter. Oncogene 1994; 9(4): 1295-304.
        [PMID: 8134134]

[11]   Al-absi B, Noor SM, Saif-Ali R, *et al.* Association of ARID5B gene variants with acute lymphoblastic leukemia in Yemeni children. Tumour Biol 2017; 39(4)
        [http://dx.doi.org/10.1177/1010428317697573] [PMID: 28381164]

[12]   Kreile M, Rots D, Zarina A, *et al.* Association of ARID5B Genetic Variants with Risk of Childhood B Cell Precursor Acute Lymphoblastic Leukaemia in Latvia. APJCP 2018; 19(1): 91-5.
        [PMID: 29373897]

[13]   Gutiérrez-Camino Á, López-López E, Martín-Guerrero I, *et al.* Intron 3 of the ARID5B gene: a hot spot for acute lymphoblastic leukemia susceptibility. J Cancer Res Clin Oncol 2013; 139(11): 1879-86.
        [http://dx.doi.org/10.1007/s00432-013-1512-3] [PMID: 24013273]

[14]   Rudant J, Orsi L, Bonaventure A, *et al.* ARID5B, IKZF1 and non-genetic factors in the etiology of childhood acute lymphoblastic leukemia: the ESCALE study. PLoS One 2015; 10(3): e0121348.
        [http://dx.doi.org/10.1371/journal.pone.0121348] [PMID: 25806972]

[15]   Leong WZ, Tan SH, Ngoc PCT, *et al.* ARID5B as a critical downstream target of the TAL1 complex that activates the oncogenic transcriptional program and promotes T-cell leukemogenesis. Genes Dev 2017; 31(23-24): 2343-60.
[http://dx.doi.org/10.1101/gad.302646.117] [PMID: 29326336]

[16]   Lazarini M, Traina F, Machado-Neto JA, *et al.* ARHGAP21 is a RhoGAP for RhoA and RhoC with a role in proliferation and migration of prostate adenocarcinoma cells. Biochim Biophys Acta Mol Basis Dis 2013; 1832(2): 365-74.
[http://dx.doi.org/10.1016/j.bbadis.2012.11.010] [PMID: 23200924]

[17]   Rosa LRO, Soares GM, Silveira LR, Boschero AC, Barbosa-Sampaio HCL. ARHGAP21 as a master regulator of multiple cellular processes. J Cell Physiol 2018; 233(11): 8477-81.
[http://dx.doi.org/10.1002/jcp.26829] [PMID: 29856495]

[18]   Barcellos KSA, Bigarella CL, Wagner MV, *et al.* ARHGAP21 protein, a new partner of α-tubulin involved in cell-cell adhesion formation and essential for epithelial-mesenchymal transition. J Biol Chem 2013; 288(4): 2179-89.
[http://dx.doi.org/10.1074/jbc.M112.432716] [PMID: 23235160]

[19]   Bai XH, Cho HR, Moodley S, Liu M. XB130—A Novel Adaptor Protein: Gene, Function, and Roles in Tumorigenesis. Scientifica (Cairo) 2014; 2014: 1-9.
[http://dx.doi.org/10.1155/2014/903014] [PMID: 24995146]

[20]   Shi M, Huang W, Lin L, *et al.* Silencing of XB130 is associated with both the prognosis and chemosensitivity of gastric cancer. PLoS One 2012; 7(8): e41660.
[http://dx.doi.org/10.1371/journal.pone.0041660] [PMID: 22927913]

[21]   Lodyga M, Bai X, Kapus A, Liu M. Adaptor protein XB130 is a Rac-controlled component of lamellipodia that regulates cell motility and invasion. J Cell Sci 2010; 123(23): 4156-69.
[http://dx.doi.org/10.1242/jcs.071050] [PMID: 21084565]

[22]   Emaduddin M, Edelmann MJ, Kessler BM, Feller SM. Odin (ANKS1A) is a Src family kinase target in colorectal cancer cells. Cell Commun Signal 2008; 6(1): 7.
[http://dx.doi.org/10.1186/1478-811X-6-7] [PMID: 18844995]

[23]   Zhang XF, An MZ, Ma YP, Lu YM. Regulatory effects of CCDC3 on proliferation, migration, invasion and EMT of human cervical cancer cells. Eur Rev Med Pharmacol Sci 2019; 23(8): 3217-24.
[PMID: 31081073]

[24]   Liao W, Liu H, Zhang Y, *et al.* Ccdc3: A New P63 Target Involved in Regulation Of Liver Lipid Metabolism. Sci Rep 2017; 7(1): 9020.
[http://dx.doi.org/10.1038/s41598-017-09228-8] [PMID: 28827783]

[25]   Azad AK, Chakrabarti S, Xu Z, Davidge ST, Fu Y. Coiled-coil domain containing 3 (CCDC3) represses tumor necrosis factor-α/nuclear factor κB-induced endothelial inflammation. Cell Signal 2014; 26(12): 2793-800.
[http://dx.doi.org/10.1016/j.cellsig.2014.08.025] [PMID: 25193116]

[26]   Yue W, Zhao X, Zhang L, *et al.* Cell cycle protein cyclin Y is associated with human non-small-cell lung cancer proliferation and tumorigenesis. Clin Lung Cancer 2011; 12(1): 43-50.
[http://dx.doi.org/10.3816/CLC.2011.n.006] [PMID: 21273179]

[27]   Yan F, Wang X, Zhu M, Hu X. RNAi-mediated downregulation of cyclin Y to attenuate human breast cancer cell growth. Oncol Rep 2016; 36(5): 2793-9.
[http://dx.doi.org/10.3892/or.2016.5126] [PMID: 27666310]

[28]   Adélaïde J, Finetti P, Bekhouche I, *et al.* Integrated profiling of basal and luminal breast cancers. Cancer Res 2007; 67(24): 11565-75.
[http://dx.doi.org/10.1158/0008-5472.CAN-07-2536] [PMID: 18089785]

[29]   Sannigrahi MK, Srinivas CS, Deokate N, Rakshit S. The strong propensity of Cadherin-23 for aggregation inhibits cell migration. Mol Oncol 2019; 13(5): 1092-109.

[http://dx.doi.org/10.1002/1878-0261.12469] [PMID: 30747484]

[30]   Zhang Q, Peng C, Song J, *et al.* Germline Mutations in CDH23, Encoding Cadherin-Related 23, Are Associated with Both Familial and Sporadic Pituitary Adenomas. Am J Hum Genet 2017; 100(5): 817-23.
       [http://dx.doi.org/10.1016/j.ajhg.2017.03.011] [PMID: 28413019]

[31]   Muthu M, Cheriyan VT, Rishi AK. CARP-1 / CCAR1: A biphasic regulator of cancer cell growth and apoptosis. Oncotarget 2015; 6(9): 6499-510.
       [http://dx.doi.org/10.18632/oncotarget.3376] [PMID: 25894788]

[32]   Rishi AK, Zhang L, Yu Y, *et al.* Cell cycle- and apoptosis-regulatory protein-1 is involved in apoptosis signaling by epidermal growth factor receptor. J Biol Chem 2006; 281(19): 13188-98.
       [http://dx.doi.org/10.1074/jbc.M512279200] [PMID: 16543231]

[33]   Kim JH, Yang CK, Heo K, Roeder RG, An W, Stallcup MR. CCAR1, a key regulator of mediator complex recruitment to nuclear receptor transcription complexes. Mol Cell 2008; 31(4): 510-9.
       [http://dx.doi.org/10.1016/j.molcel.2008.08.001] [PMID: 18722177]

[34]   Lu C, Li J-Y, Ge Z, Zhang L, Zhou G-P. Par-4/THAP1 complex and Notch3 competitively regulated pre-mRNA splicing of CCAR1 and affected inversely the survival of T-cell acute lymphoblastic leukemia cells. Oncogene 2013; 32(50): 5602-13.
       [http://dx.doi.org/10.1038/onc.2013.349] [PMID: 23975424]

[35]   Muthu M, Cheriyan VT, Munie S, *et al.* Mechanisms of neuroblastoma cell growth inhibition by CARP-1 functional mimetics. PLoS One 2014; 9(7): e102567.
       [http://dx.doi.org/10.1371/journal.pone.0102567] [PMID: 25033461]

[36]   Umbreen S, Banday MM, Jamroze A, *et al. COMMD3:BMI1* Fusion and COMMD3 Protein Regulate *C-MYC* Transcription: Novel Therapeutic Target for Metastatic Prostate Cancer. Mol Cancer Ther 2019; 18(11): 2111-23.
       [http://dx.doi.org/10.1158/1535-7163.MCT-19-0150] [PMID: 31467179]

[37]   Zhou W, Guo S, Liu M, Burow ME, Wang G. Targeting CXCL12/CXCR4 Axis in Tumor Immunotherapy. Curr Med Chem 2019; 26(17): 3026-41.
       [http://dx.doi.org/10.2174/0929867324666170830111531] [PMID: 28875842]

[38]   Meng W, Xue S, Chen Y. The role of CXCL12 in tumor microenvironment. Gene 2018; 641: 105-10.
       [http://dx.doi.org/10.1016/j.gene.2017.10.015] [PMID: 29017963]

[39]   Larzabal L, El-Nikhely N, Redrado M, Seeger W, Savai R, Calvo A. Differential effects of drugs targeting cancer stem cell (CSC) and non-CSC populations on lung primary tumors and metastasis. PLoS One 2013; 8(11): e79798.
       [http://dx.doi.org/10.1371/journal.pone.0079798] [PMID: 24278179]

[40]   Koso H, Yi H, Sheridan P, *et al.* Identification of RNA-Binding Protein LARP4B as a Tumor Suppressor in Glioma. Cancer Res 2016; 76(8): 2254-64.
       [http://dx.doi.org/10.1158/0008-5472.CAN-15-2308] [PMID: 26933087]

[41]   Blagden S, Schneider C, Fischer U. Loss of LARP4B, an early event in the tumorigenesis of brain cancer? Transl Cancer Res 2016; 5(S6): S1196-9.
       [http://dx.doi.org/10.21037/tcr.2016.11.33]

[42]   Watanabe H, Nonoguchi K, Sakurai T, et al. A novel protein Depp, which is induced by progesterone in human endometrial stromal cells activates Elk-1 transcription factor. MHR: Basic science of reproductive medicine 2005; 11: 471–476.

[43]   Su MQ, Zhou YR, Rao X, *et al.* Baicalein induces the apoptosis of HCT116ï¿½human colon cancer cells *via* the upregulation of DEPP/Gadd45a and activation of MAPKs. Int J Oncol 2018; 53(2): 750-60.
       [http://dx.doi.org/10.3892/ijo.2018.4402] [PMID: 29749481]

[44]   Lin H, Liu W, Fang Z, *et al.* Overexpression of DHX32 contributes to the growth and metastasis of

colorectal cancer. Sci Rep 2015; 5(1): 9247.
[http://dx.doi.org/10.1038/srep09247] [PMID: 25782664]

[45]   Gregory KJ, Morin SM, Schneider SS. Regulation of early growth response 2 expression by secreted frizzled related protein 1. BMC Cancer 2017; 17(1): 473.
[http://dx.doi.org/10.1186/s12885-017-3426-y] [PMID: 28687085]

[46]   Unoki M, Nakamura Y. EGR2 induces apoptosis in various cancer cell lines by direct transactivation of BNIP3L and BAK. Oncogene 2003; 22(14): 2172-85.
[http://dx.doi.org/10.1038/sj.onc.1206222] [PMID: 12687019]

[47]   Dillon RL, Brown ST, Ling C, Shioda T, Muller WJ. An EGR2/CITED1 transcription factor complex and the 14-3-3sigma tumor suppressor are involved in regulating ErbB2 expression in a transgenic-mouse model of human breast cancer. Mol Cell Biol 2007; 27(24): 8648-57.
[http://dx.doi.org/10.1128/MCB.00866-07] [PMID: 17938205]

[48]   Dey P, Rachagani S, Chakraborty S, *et al.* Overexpression of ecdysoneless in pancreatic cancer and its role in oncogenesis by regulating glycolysis. Clin Cancer Res 2012; 18(22): 6188-98.
[http://dx.doi.org/10.1158/1078-0432.CCR-12-1789] [PMID: 22977192]

[49]   Kim JH, Gurumurthy CB, Naramura M, *et al.* Role of mammalian Ecdysoneless in cell cycle regulation. J Biol Chem 2009; 284(39): 26402-10.
[http://dx.doi.org/10.1074/jbc.M109.030551] [PMID: 19640839]

[50]   Wang Y, Alla V, Goody D, *et al.* Epigenetic factor EPC1 is a master regulator of DNA damage response by interacting with E2F1 to silence death and activate metastasis-related gene signatures. Nucleic Acids Res 2016; 44(1): 117-33.
[http://dx.doi.org/10.1093/nar/gkv885] [PMID: 26350215]

[51]   Dickson BC, Lum A, Swanson D, *et al.* Novel *EPC1* gene fusions in endometrial stromal sarcoma. Genes Chromosomes Cancer 2018; 57(11): 598-603.
[http://dx.doi.org/10.1002/gcc.22649] [PMID: 30144186]

[52]   Lin Z, Zhang X, Tuo J, *et al.* A variant of the Cockayne syndrome B geneERCC6 confers risk of lung cancer. Hum Mutat 2008; 29(1): 113-22.
[http://dx.doi.org/10.1002/humu.20610] [PMID: 17854076]

[53]   Nakajima H, Koizumi K, Tanaka T, *et al.* Loss of HITS (FAM107B) expression in cancers of multiple organs: tissue microarray analysis. Int J Oncol 2012; 41(4): 1347-57.
[http://dx.doi.org/10.3892/ijo.2012.1550] [PMID: 22825356]

[54]   Burdelski C, Borcherding L, Kluth M, *et al.* Family with sequence similarity 13C (FAM13C) overexpression is an independent prognostic marker in prostate cancer. Oncotarget 2017; 8(19): 31494-508.
[http://dx.doi.org/10.18632/oncotarget.16357] [PMID: 28415558]

[55]   Falcon T, Freitas M, Mello AC, Coutinho L, Alvares-da-Silva MR, Matte U. Analysis of the Cancer Genome Atlas Data Reveals Novel Putative ncRNAs Targets in Hepatocellular Carcinoma. BioMed Res Int 2018; 2018: 1-9.
[http://dx.doi.org/10.1155/2018/2864120] [PMID: 30046591]

[56]   FAM188A gene, http://www.ncbi.nlm.nih.gov/entrez/query.fcgi?db=gene&cmd=Retrieve&dopt=full _report&list_uids=80013.

[57]   Chen YF, Yang CC, Kao SY, Liu CJ, Lin SC, Chang KW. MicroRNA-211 enhances the oncogenicity of carcinogen-induced oral carcinoma by repressing TCF12 and increasing antioxidant activity. Cancer Res 2016; 76(16): 4872-86.
[http://dx.doi.org/10.1158/0008-5472.CAN-15-1664] [PMID: 27221705]

[58]   Sayad A, Hajifathali A, Hamidieh AA, Esfandi F, Taheri M. Fas-antisense long noncoding RNA and acute myeloid leukemia: Is there any relation? Asian Pac J Cancer Prev 2018; 19(1): 45-8.
[PMID: 29373891]

[59] Esfandi F, Taheri M, Omrani MD, *et al.* Expression of long non-coding RNAs (lncRNAs) has been dysregulated in non-small cell lung cancer tissues. BMC Cancer 2019; 19(1): 222.
[http://dx.doi.org/10.1186/s12885-019-5435-5] [PMID: 30866866]

[60] Szybowska P, Kostas M, Wesche J, et al. Cancer Mutations in FGFR2 Prevent a Negative Feedback Loop Mediated by the ERK1/2 Pathway. Cells; 8; 1; 2019.

[61] Kim HS, Kim JH, Jang HJ, Han B, Zang DY. Pathological and Prognostic Impacts of FGFR2 Overexpression in Gastric Cancer: A Meta-Analysis. J Cancer 2019; 10(1): 20-7.
[http://dx.doi.org/10.7150/jca.28204] [PMID: 30662521]

[62] Huang T, Liu D, Wang Y, *et al.* FGFR2 Promotes Gastric Cancer Progression by Inhibiting the Expression of Thrombospondin4 *via* PI3K-Akt-Mtor Pathway. Cell Physiol Biochem 2018; 50(4): 1332-45.
[http://dx.doi.org/10.1159/000494590] [PMID: 30355943]

[63] Lu Y, Li J, Cheng J, Lubahn DB. Messenger RNA profile analysis deciphers new Esrrb responsive genes in prostate cancer cells. BMC Mol Biol 2015; 16(1): 21.
[http://dx.doi.org/10.1186/s12867-015-0049-1] [PMID: 26627478]

[64] Saitoh T, Katoh M. FRAT1 and FRAT2, clustered in human chromosome 10q24.1 region, are up-regulated in gastric cancer. Int J Oncol 2001; 19(2): 311-5.
[http://dx.doi.org/10.3892/ijo.19.2.311] [PMID: 11445844]

[65] Zhu K, Guo J, Wang H, Yu W. FRAT1 expression regulates proliferation in colon cancer cells. Oncol Lett 2016; 12(6): 4761-6.
[http://dx.doi.org/10.3892/ol.2016.5300] [PMID: 28101222]

[66] van Amerongen R, Nawijn MC, Lambooij JP, Proost N, Jonkers J, Berns A. Frat oncoproteins act at the crossroad of canonical and noncanonical Wnt-signaling pathways. Oncogene 2010; 29(1): 93-104.
[http://dx.doi.org/10.1038/onc.2009.310] [PMID: 19802005]

[67] Bhalla S, Chaudhary K, Kumar R, *et al.* Gene expression-based biomarkers for discriminating early and late stage of clear cell renal cancer. Sci Rep 2017; 7(1): 44997.
[http://dx.doi.org/10.1038/srep44997] [PMID: 28349958]

[68] Stenzel N, Fetzer CP, Heumann R, Erdmann KS. PDZ-domain-directed basolateral targeting of the peripheral membrane protein FRMPD2 in epithelial cells. J Cell Sci 2009; 122(18): 3374-84.
[http://dx.doi.org/10.1242/jcs.046854] [PMID: 19706687]

[69] Takaku M, Grimm SA, Wade PA. GATA3 in Breast Cancer: Tumor Suppressor or Oncogene? Gene Expr 2015; 16(4): 163-8.
[http://dx.doi.org/10.3727/105221615X14399878166113] [PMID: 26637396]

[70] Chou J, Provot S, Werb Z. GATA3 in development and cancer differentiation: Cells GATA have it! J Cell Physiol 2010; 222(1): 42-9.
[http://dx.doi.org/10.1002/jcp.21943] [PMID: 19798694]

[71] Reimers K, Choi CYU, Bucan V, Vogt PM. The Growth-hormone inducible transmembrane protein (Ghitm) belongs to the Bax inhibitory protein-like family. Int J Biol Sci 2007; 3(7): 471-6.
[http://dx.doi.org/10.7150/ijbs.3.471] [PMID: 18071587]

[72] Rojas-Rivera D, Hetz C. TMBIM protein family: ancestral regulators of cell death. Oncogene 2015; 34(3): 269-80.
[http://dx.doi.org/10.1038/onc.2014.6] [PMID: 24561528]

[73] Khalilipour N, Baranova A, Jebelli A, Heravi-Moussavi A, Bruskin S, Abbaszadegan MR. Familial Esophageal Squamous Cell Carcinoma with damaging rare/germline mutations in KCNJ12/KCNJ18 and GPRIN2 genes. Cancer Genet 2018; 221: 46-52.
[http://dx.doi.org/10.1016/j.cancergen.2017.11.011] [PMID: 29405996]

[74] Li L, Pang X, Zhu Z, *et al.* GTPBP4 promotes gastric cancer progression *via* regulating P53 activity.

Cell Physiol Biochem 2018; 45(2): 667-76.
[http://dx.doi.org/10.1159/000487160] [PMID: 29408813]

[75]   Liu WB, Jia WD, Ma JL, *et al.* Knockdown of GTPBP4 inhibits cell growth and survival in human hepatocellular carcinoma and its prognostic significance. Oncotarget 2017; 8(55): 93984-97.
[http://dx.doi.org/10.18632/oncotarget.21500] [PMID: 29212203]

[76]   Liu X, Hou X, Zhou Y, *et al.* Downregulation of the Helicase Lymphoid-Specific (HELLS) Gene Impairs Cell Proliferation and Induces Cell Cycle Arrest in Colorectal Cancer Cells. OncoTargets Ther 2019; 12: 10153-63.
[http://dx.doi.org/10.2147/OTT.S223668] [PMID: 32063710]

[77]   Chen X, Lv Y, Sun Y, *et al.* PGC1β Regulates Breast Tumor Growth and Metastasis by SREBP1-Mediated HKDC1 Expression. Front Oncol 2019; 9: 290.
[http://dx.doi.org/10.3389/fonc.2019.00290] [PMID: 31058090]

[78]   Li GH, Huang JF. Inferring therapeutic targets from heterogeneous data: HKDC1 is a novel potential therapeutic target for cancer. Bioinformatics 2014; 30(6): 748-52.
[http://dx.doi.org/10.1093/bioinformatics/btt606] [PMID: 24162464]

[79]   Zhang Z, Huang S, Wang H, *et al.* High expression of hexokinase domain containing 1 is associated with poor prognosis and aggressive phenotype in hepatocarcinoma. Biochem Biophys Res Commun 2016; 474(4): 673-9.
[http://dx.doi.org/10.1016/j.bbrc.2016.05.007] [PMID: 27155152]

[80]   Gao X, Liu Z, Zhong M, *et al.* Knockdown of DNA/RNA-binding protein KIN17 promotes apoptosis of triple-negative breast cancer cells. Oncol Lett 2018; 18
[http://dx.doi.org/10.3892/ol.2018.9597] [PMID: 30655766]

[81]   Liu X, Pan L. Predicating Candidate Cancer-Associated Genes in the Human Signaling Network Using Centrality. Curr Bioinform 2016; 11(1): 87-92.
[http://dx.doi.org/10.2174/1574893611888160106154456]

[82]   Darabi H, McCue K, Beesley J, *et al.* Polymorphisms in a Putative Enhancer at the 10q21.2 Breast Cancer Risk Locus Regulate NRBF2 Expression. Am J Hum Genet 2015; 97(1): 22-34.
[http://dx.doi.org/10.1016/j.ajhg.2015.05.002] [PMID: 26073781]

[83]   Zhang Z, Fan Y, Xie F, *et al.* Breast cancer metastasis suppressor OTUD1 deubiquitinates SMAD7. Nat Commun 2017; 8(1): 2116.
[http://dx.doi.org/10.1038/s41467-017-02029-7] [PMID: 29235476]

[84]   Rouget-Quermalet V, Giustiniani J, Marie-Cardine A, *et al.* Protocadherin 15 (PCDH15): a new secreted isoform and a potential marker for NK/T cell lymphomas. Oncogene 2006; 25(19): 2807-11.
[http://dx.doi.org/10.1038/sj.onc.1209301] [PMID: 16369489]

[85]   Pataer A, Ozpolat B, Shao R, *et al.* Therapeutic targeting of the PI4K2A/PKR lysosome network is critical for misfolded protein clearance and survival in cancer cells. Oncogene 2020; 39(4): 801-13.
[http://dx.doi.org/10.1038/s41388-019-1010-4] [PMID: 31554935]

[86]   Ilboudo A, Nault JC, Dubois-Pot-Schneider H, *et al.* Overexpression of phosphatidylinositol 4-kinase type IIIα is associated with undifferentiated status and poor prognosis of human hepatocellular carcinoma. BMC Cancer 2014; 14(1): 7.
[http://dx.doi.org/10.1186/1471-2407-14-7] [PMID: 24393405]

[87]   Zhang S, Li Z, Yan X, *et al.* Regulatory network and prognostic effect investigation of PIP4K2A in leukemia and solid cancers. Front Genet 2019; 9: 721.
[http://dx.doi.org/10.3389/fgene.2018.00721] [PMID: 30697230]

[88]   Lima K, Coelho-Silva JL, Kinker GS, et al. PIP4K2A and PIP4K2C transcript levels are associated with cytogenetic risk and survival outcomes in acute myeloid leukemia. Cancer Genetics 2019; 233–234: 56–66.

[89]   Pignot G, Le Goux C, Vacher S, *et al. PLEKHS1*: A new molecular marker predicting risk of

progression of non-muscle-invasive bladder cancer. Oncol Lett 2019; 18(4): 3471-80.
[http://dx.doi.org/10.3892/ol.2019.10706] [PMID: 31516565]

[90] Weinhold N, Jacobsen A, Schultz N, Sander C, Lee W. Genome-wide analysis of noncoding regulatory mutations in cancer. Nat Genet 2014; 46(11): 1160-5.
[http://dx.doi.org/10.1038/ng.3101] [PMID: 25261935]

[91] Cheng G, Zhong M, Kawaguchi R, *et al*. Identification of PLXDC1 and PLXDC2 as the transmembrane receptors for the multifunctional factor PEDF. eLife 2014; 3: e05401.
[http://dx.doi.org/10.7554/eLife.05401] [PMID: 25535841]

[92] Wang Y, Li H. Identification of proteins associated with paclitaxel resistance of epithelial ovarian cancer using iTRAQ-based proteomics. Oncol Lett 2018; 15(6): 9793-801.
[http://dx.doi.org/10.3892/ol.2018.8600] [PMID: 29928353]

[93] Chen CY, Chen J, He L, Stiles BL. PTEN: Tumor Suppressor and Metabolic Regulator. Front Endocrinol (Lausanne) 2018; 9: 338.
[http://dx.doi.org/10.3389/fendo.2018.00338] [PMID: 30038596]

[94] Zhang HY, Liang F, Jia ZL, Song ST, Jiang ZF. *PTEN* mutation, methylation and expression in breast cancer patients. Oncol Lett 2013; 6(1): 161-8.
[http://dx.doi.org/10.3892/ol.2013.1331] [PMID: 23946797]

[95] Pei Y, Sun X, Guo X, *et al*. FGF8 promotes cell proliferation and resistance to EGFR inhibitors *via* upregulation of EGFR in human hepatocellular carcinoma cells. Oncol Rep 2017; 38(4): 2205-10.
[http://dx.doi.org/10.3892/or.2017.5887] [PMID: 28791365]

[96] Dorkin TJ, Robinson MC, Marsh C, Bjartell A, Neal DE, Leung HY. FGF8 over-expression in prostate cancer is associated with decreased patient survival and persists in androgen independent disease. Oncogene 1999; 18(17): 2755-61.
[http://dx.doi.org/10.1038/sj.onc.1202624] [PMID: 10348350]

[97] Liu R, Huang S, Lei Y, *et al*. FGF8 promotes colorectal cancer growth and metastasis by activating YAP1. Oncotarget 2015; 6(2): 935-52.
[http://dx.doi.org/10.18632/oncotarget.2822] [PMID: 25473897]

[98] Marsh SK, Bansal GS, Zammit C, *et al*. Increased expression of fibroblast growth factor 8 in human breast cancer. Oncogene 1999; 18(4): 1053-60.
[http://dx.doi.org/10.1038/sj.onc.1202392] [PMID: 10023681]

[99] Szybowska P, Kostas M, Wesche J, Wiedlocha A, Haugsten EM. Cancer Mutations in FGFR2 Prevent a Negative Feedback Loop Mediated by the ERK1/2 Pathway. Cells 2019; 8(6): 518.
[http://dx.doi.org/10.3390/cells8060518] [PMID: 31146385]

[100] Shakya M, Zhou A, Dai D, *et al*. High expression of TACC2 in hepatocellular carcinoma is associated with poor prognosis. Cancer Biomark 2018; 22(4): 611-9.
[http://dx.doi.org/10.3233/CBM-170091] [PMID: 29843208]

[101] Singh D, Chan JM, Zoppoli P, *et al*. Transforming fusions of FGFR and TACC genes in human glioblastoma. Science 2012; 337(6099): 1231-5.
[http://dx.doi.org/10.1126/science.1220834] [PMID: 22837387]

[102] Takayama K, Horie-Inoue K, Suzuki T, *et al*. TACC2 is an androgen-responsive cell cycle regulator promoting androgen-mediated and castration-resistant growth of prostate cancer. Mol Endocrinol 2012; 26(5): 748-61.
[http://dx.doi.org/10.1210/me.2011-1242] [PMID: 22456197]

[103] Matsubara D, Kanai Y, Ishikawa S, *et al*. Identification of CCDC6-RET fusion in the human lung adenocarcinoma cell line, LC-2/ad. J Thorac Oncol 2012; 7(12): 1872-6.
[http://dx.doi.org/10.1097/JTO.0b013e3182721ed1] [PMID: 23154560]

[104] Mejia Saldarriaga M, Steinberg A, Severson EA, Binder A. A Case of *CCDC6-RET* Fusion Mutation in Adult Acute Lymphoblastic Leukemia (ALL), a Known Activating Mutation Reported in ALL.

Front Oncol 2019; 9: 1303.
[http://dx.doi.org/10.3389/fonc.2019.01303] [PMID: 31850206]

[105] Santoro M, Carlomagno F. Central role of RET in thyroid cancer. Cold Spring Harb Perspect Biol 2013; 5(12): a009233-3.
[http://dx.doi.org/10.1101/cshperspect.a009233] [PMID: 24296167]

[106] Cerrato A, Merolla F, Morra F, Celetti A. CCDC6: the identity of a protein known to be partner in fusion. Int J Cancer 2018; 142(7): 1300-8.
[http://dx.doi.org/10.1002/ijc.31106] [PMID: 29044514]

[107] Yokota K, Sasaki H, Okuda K, *et al.* KIF5B/RET fusion gene in surgically-treated adenocarcinoma of the lung. Oncol Rep 2012; 28(4): 1187-92.
[http://dx.doi.org/10.3892/or.2012.1908] [PMID: 22797671]

[108] Gow CH, Liu YN, Li HY, *et al.* Oncogenic Function of a KIF5B-MET Fusion Variant in Non-Small Cell Lung Cancer. Neoplasia 2018; 20(8): 838-47.
[http://dx.doi.org/10.1016/j.neo.2018.06.007] [PMID: 30015159]

[109] Cong XF, Yang L, Chen C, Liu Z. KIF5B-RET fusion gene and its correlation with clinicopathological and prognosis features in lung cancer: a meta-analysis. OncoTargets Ther 2019; 12: 4533-42.
[http://dx.doi.org/10.2147/OTT.S186361] [PMID: 31289444]

[110] Qian Y, Chai S, Liang Z, *et al.* KIF5B-RET fusion kinase promotes cell growth by multilevel activation of STAT3 in lung cancer. Mol Cancer 2014; 13(1): 176.
[http://dx.doi.org/10.1186/1476-4598-13-176] [PMID: 25047660]

[111] Li AY, McCusker MG, Russo A, *et al.* RET fusions in solid tumors. Cancer Treat Rev 2019; 81: 101911.
[http://dx.doi.org/10.1016/j.ctrv.2019.101911] [PMID: 31715421]

[112] Shao Y-C, Wei Y, Liu J-F, Xu XY. The role of Dickkopf family in cancers: from Bench to Bedside. Am J Cancer Res 2017; 7(9): 1754-68.
[PMID: 28979801]

[113] Jiang C, Yu M, Xie X, *et al.* miR-217 targeting DKK1 promotes cancer stem cell properties *via* activation of the Wnt signaling pathway in hepatocellular carcinoma. Oncol Rep 2017; 38(4): 2351-9.
[http://dx.doi.org/10.3892/or.2017.5924] [PMID: 28849121]

[114] Bass AJ, Lawrence MS, Brace LE, *et al.* Genomic sequencing of colorectal adenocarcinomas identifies a recurrent VTI1A-TCF7L2 fusion. Nat Genet 2011; 43(10): 964-8.
[http://dx.doi.org/10.1038/ng.936] [PMID: 21892161]

[115] Davidsen J, Larsen S, Coskun M, *et al.* The VTI1A-TCF4 colon cancer fusion protein is a dominant negative regulator of Wnt signaling and is transcriptionally regulated by intestinal homeodomain factor CDX2. PLoS One 2018; 13(7): e0200215.
[http://dx.doi.org/10.1371/journal.pone.0200215] [PMID: 29975781]

[116] Nome T, Hoff AM, Bakken AC, Rognum TO, Nesbakken A, Skotheim RI. High frequency of fusion transcripts involving TCF7L2 in colorectal cancer: novel fusion partner and splice variants. PLoS One 2014; 9(3): e91264.
[http://dx.doi.org/10.1371/journal.pone.0091264] [PMID: 24608966]

[117] Sang Park W, Ra Oh R, Sil Kim Y, *et al.* Somatic mutations in the death domain of theFas (Apo-1/CD95) gene in gastric cancer. J Pathol 2001; 193(2): 162-8.
[http://dx.doi.org/10.1002/1096-9896(2000)9999:9999<::AID-PATH759>3.0.CO;2-A]   [PMID: 11180161]

[118] Hashemi M, Fazaeli A, Ghavami S, *et al.* Functional polymorphisms of FAS and FASL gene and risk of breast cancer - pilot study of 134 cases. PLoS One 2013; 8(1): e53075.
[http://dx.doi.org/10.1371/journal.pone.0053075] [PMID: 23326385]

[119] Butler LM, Hewett PJ, Butler WJ, Cowled PA. Down-regulation of Fas gene expression in colon cancer is not a result of allelic loss or gene rearrangement. Br J Cancer 1998; 77(9): 1454-9. [http://dx.doi.org/10.1038/bjc.1998.239] [PMID: 9652761]

[120] Liu Y, El-Naggar S, Darling DS, Higashi Y, Dean DC. Zeb1 links epithelial-mesenchymal transition and cellular senescence. Development 2008; 135(3): 579-88. [http://dx.doi.org/10.1242/dev.007047] [PMID: 18192284]

[121] Zhang Y, Xu L, Li A, Han X. The roles of ZEB1 in tumorigenic progression and epigenetic modifications. Biomed Pharmacother 2019; 110: 400-8. [http://dx.doi.org/10.1016/j.biopha.2018.11.112] [PMID: 30530042]

[122] Bodenstine TM, Chandler GS, Seftor REB, Seftor EA, Hendrix MJC. Plasticity underlies tumor progression: role of Nodal signaling. Cancer Metastasis Rev 2016; 35(1): 21-39. [http://dx.doi.org/10.1007/s10555-016-9605-5] [PMID: 26951550]

[123] Kalyan A, Carneiro BA, Chandra S, *et al.* Nodal signaling as a developmental therapeutics target in oncology. Mol Cancer Ther 2017; 16(5): 787-92. [http://dx.doi.org/10.1158/1535-7163.MCT-16-0215] [PMID: 28468864]

[124] Széll M, Danis J, Bata-Csörgő Z, Kemény L. PRINS, a primate-specific long non-coding RNA, plays a role in the keratinocyte stress response and psoriasis pathogenesis. Pflugers Arch 2016; 468(6): 935-43. [http://dx.doi.org/10.1007/s00424-016-1803-z] [PMID: 26935426]

[125] Glover AR, Zhao JT, Ip JC, *et al.* Long noncoding RNA profiles of adrenocortical cancer can be used to predict recurrence. Endocr Relat Cancer 2015; 22(1): 99-109. [http://dx.doi.org/10.1530/ERC-14-0457] [PMID: 25595289]

[126] Satelli A, Li S. Vimentin in cancer and its potential as a molecular target for cancer therapy. Cell Mol Life Sci 2011; 68(18): 3033-46. [http://dx.doi.org/10.1007/s00018-011-0735-1] [PMID: 21637948]

[127] Kidd ME, Shumaker DK, Ridge KM. The Role of Vimentin Intermediate Filaments in the Progression of Lung Cancer. Am J Respir Cell Mol Biol 2013; 130827094923003. [PMID: 23980547]

[128] Bubici C, Papa S. JNK signalling in cancer: in need of new, smarter therapeutic targets. Br J Pharmacol 2014; 171(1): 24-37. [http://dx.doi.org/10.1111/bph.12432] [PMID: 24117156]

[129] Song Z, Tong C, Liang J, *et al.* JNK1 is required for sulindac-mediated inhibition of cell proliferation and induction of apoptosis *in vitro* and *in vivo*. Eur J Pharmacol 2007; 560(2-3): 95-100. [http://dx.doi.org/10.1016/j.ejphar.2007.01.020] [PMID: 17292881]

[130] Li CG, Eccles MR. PAX Genes in Cancer; Friends or Foes? Front Genet 2012; 3: 6. [http://dx.doi.org/10.3389/fgene.2012.00006] [PMID: 22303411]

[131] Liu P, Gao Y, Huan J, *et al.* Upregulation of PAX2 promotes the metastasis of esophageal cancer through interleukin-5. Cell Physiol Biochem 2015; 35(2): 740-54. [http://dx.doi.org/10.1159/000369734] [PMID: 25613757]

[132] Slattery ML, Folsom AR, Wolff R, Herrick J, Caan BJ, Potter JD. Transcription factor 7-like 2 polymorphism and colon cancer. Cancer Epidemiol Biomarkers Prev 2008; 17(4): 978-82. [http://dx.doi.org/10.1158/1055-9965.EPI-07-2687] [PMID: 18398040]

[133] Teng S, Ma C, Yu Y, Yi C. Hydroxyurea promotes TET1 expression and induces apoptosis in osteosarcoma cells. Biosci Rep 2019; 39(5): BSR20190456. [http://dx.doi.org/10.1042/BSR20190456] [PMID: 30988069]

[134] Yu S, Yin Y, Hong S, *et al.* TET1 is a Tumor Suppressor That Inhibits Papillary Thyroid Carcinoma Cell Migration and Invasion. Int J Endocrinol 2020; 2020: 1-9.

[http://dx.doi.org/10.1155/2020/3909610] [PMID: 32089682]

[135] Reeves HL, Narla G, Ogunbiyi O, *et al.* Kruppel-like factor 6 (KLF6) is a tumor-suppressor gene frequently inactivated in colorectal cancer. Gastroenterology 2004; 126(4): 1090-103.
[http://dx.doi.org/10.1053/j.gastro.2004.01.005] [PMID: 15057748]

[136] Narla G, Heath KE, Reeves HL, *et al.* KLF6, a candidate tumor suppressor gene mutated in prostate cancer. Science 2001; 294(5551): 2563-6.
[http://dx.doi.org/10.1126/science.1066326] [PMID: 11752579]

[137] Mukai S, Hiyama T, Tanaka S, Yoshihara M, Arihiro K, Chayama K. Involvement of Krüppel-like factor 6 (*KLF6*) mutation in the development of nonpolypoid colorectal carcinoma. World J Gastroenterol 2007; 13(29): 3932-8.
[http://dx.doi.org/10.3748/wjg.v13.i29.3932] [PMID: 17663506]

[138] Hsu LS, Huang RH, Lai HW, *et al.* KLF6 inhibited oral cancer migration and invasion *via* downregulation of mesenchymal markers and inhibition of MMP-9 activities. Int J Med Sci 2017; 14(6): 530-5.
[http://dx.doi.org/10.7150/ijms.19024] [PMID: 28638268]

[139] Gehrau RC, D'Astolfo DS, Dumur CI, Bocco JL, Koritschoner NP. Nuclear expression of KLF6 tumor suppressor factor is highly associated with overexpression of ERBB2 oncoprotein in ductal breast carcinomas. PLoS One 2010; 5(1): e8929.
[http://dx.doi.org/10.1371/journal.pone.0008929] [PMID: 20126619]

[140] Jing X, Wu H, Cheng X, *et al.* MLLT10 promotes tumor migration, invasion, and metastasis in human colorectal cancer. Scand J Gastroenterol 2018; 53(8): 964-71.
[http://dx.doi.org/10.1080/00365521.2018.1481521] [PMID: 30102091]

[141] Hiwatari M, Seki M, Akahoshi S, *et al.* Molecular studies reveal *MLL-MLLT10/AF10* and *ARID5B-MLL* gene fusions displaced in a case of infantile acute lymphoblastic leukemia with complex karyotype. Oncol Lett 2017; 14(2): 2295-9.
[http://dx.doi.org/10.3892/ol.2017.6430] [PMID: 28781666]

[142] Wick W, Weller M, van den Bent M, *et al.* MGMT testing—the challenges for biomarker-based glioma treatment. Nat Rev Neurol 2014; 10(7): 372-85.
[http://dx.doi.org/10.1038/nrneurol.2014.100] [PMID: 24912512]

[143] Hegi ME, Diserens AC, Gorlia T, *et al.* MGMT gene silencing and benefit from temozolomide in glioblastoma. N Engl J Med 2005; 352(10): 997-1003.
[http://dx.doi.org/10.1056/NEJMoa043331] [PMID: 15758010]

[144] Shields S, Conroy E, O'Grady T, *et al.* BAG3 promotes tumour cell proliferation by regulating EGFR signal transduction pathways in triple negative breast cancer. Oncotarget 2018; 9(21): 15673-90.
[http://dx.doi.org/10.18632/oncotarget.24590] [PMID: 29644001]

[145] Li N, Chen M, Cao Y, *et al.* Bcl-2-associated athanogene 3(BAG3) is associated with tumor cell proliferation, migration, invasion and chemoresistance in colorectal cancer. BMC Cancer 2018; 18(1): 793.
[http://dx.doi.org/10.1186/s12885-018-4657-2] [PMID: 30081850]

[146] Xu J, Zhou W, Yang F, *et al.* The β-TrCP-FBXW2-SKP2 axis regulates lung cancer cell growth with FBXW2 acting as a tumour suppressor. Nat Commun 2017; 8(1): 14002.
[http://dx.doi.org/10.1038/ncomms14002] [PMID: 28090088]

[147] Kim CJ, Song JH, Cho YG, *et al.* Somatic mutations of the? -TrCP gene in gastric cancer. Acta Pathol Microbiol Scand Suppl 2007; 115(2): 127-33.
[http://dx.doi.org/10.1111/j.1600-0463.2007.apm_562.x] [PMID: 17295679]

[148] He N, Li C, Zhang X, *et al.* Regulation of lung cancer cell growth and invasiveness by? -TRCP. Mol Carcinog 2005; 42(1): 18-28.
[http://dx.doi.org/10.1002/mc.20063] [PMID: 15536641]

[149] Nemec AA, Bush KB, Towle-Weicksel JB, *et al.* Estrogen Drives Cellular Transformation and Mutagenesis in Cells Expressing the Breast Cancer–Associated R438W DNA Polymerase Lambda Protein. Mol Cancer Res 2016; 14(11): 1068-77.
[http://dx.doi.org/10.1158/1541-7786.MCR-16-0209] [PMID: 27621267]

[150] Lange SS, Takata K, Wood RD. DNA polymerases and cancer. Nat Rev Cancer 2011; 11(2): 96-110.
[http://dx.doi.org/10.1038/nrc2998] [PMID: 21258395]

CHAPTER 11

Chromosome 11

Harini Hariharan[1], **Saurav Panicker**[1] and **Satish Ramalingam**[1,*]

[1] *Department of Genetic Engineering, School of Bioengineering, SRM Institute of Science and Technology, Kattankulathur, India*

Abstract: Over the years, many scientists and doctors have been treating the deadly cancer disease but cannot find a permanent treatment for this disease. Also, sometimes it becomes tough to understand the mechanisms and causes of cancer as it is a very complex disease that involves many biological processes. Due to the redundancy in our biological system, cancer progression becomes very easy, thus making it difficult to cure. To find the root cause of this disease, we should know what genetic alterations are causing cancer progress and who is participating in these alterations, like proteins, signaling pathways, or genes. Cancer is caused due to various reasons; it can be due to genetics but primarily due to carcinogens, causing mutations in the genes, thereby making them an oncogene. The Proto-oncogenes are those genes that usually assist the growth of tumor cells. The alteration, mutation, or increased copy number of a particular gene may turn into a proto-oncogene, which could end up completely activated or turned on. Many Tumor-causing alterations or mutations related to oncogenes are usually acquired and not inherited. These tumor-causing mutations often actuate oncogenes *via* chromosomal rearrangement or changes in the chromosome, which sequestrates one gene after another, thereby permitting the first gene to prompt the alternative. Search which genes are involved in different cancer types would help scientists proceed with new methods for finding a cure for this disease. This article will depict which genes and their location on which chromosomes, specifically on chromosome 11, are related to different types of cancer.

Keywords: Cancer, Chromosome 11, Chromosome Rearrangements, Gene Duplication, Mutation, Oncogene, Proto-oncogene.

1.1. GENE - NUP98; NUCLEOPORIN 98. LOCATION - 11p15.4.

NPCs alter the shipping of macromolecules among the cytoplasm and nucleus and are made up of several polypeptide subunits, many of which belong to the nucleoporin class or family. NPCs belong to the nucleoporin family that codes for 186-

* **Corresponding author Satish Ramalingam**: Department of Genetic Engineering, School of Bioengineering, SRM Institute of Science and Technology, Kattankulathur, India; E-mail: rsatish76@gmail.com

kDa precursor-protein that encountersautoproteolytic-cleavage toform a 98kDa and 96kDa nucleoporin. The ninety-eight kDa nucleoporin includes a repetition of the Gly-Leu-Phe-Gly (GLGF) domain and indulges in many cellular mechanisms, such as nuclear export, mitotic progression, nuclear import, and activation of gene expression. The 96kDa nucleoporin is more or less a scaffold factor of NPC. Proteolytic cleavage is critical for targeting the proteins to NPC. Translocations among the NPC gene and many companion genes have been located in several leukemias. Rearrangements commonly bring chimeras with the N-terminal GLGF area of this NPC gene to the C terminus of the companion gene. The alternative-splicing consequences in a couple of transcript mutations or variants encoding several isoforms, as a minimum of 2 that are proteolytically-processed. Some variants here lack the area that encodes for the ninety-six kDa nucleoporin. The mammalian genes have been established to amalgamate several genes following chromosome translocations in T-cell acute-lymphocytic leukemia and acute-myelogenous leukemia. The NUP98 gene is among numerous genes placed within the imprinted-gene area of 11p15.5, an important tumor-suppressor gene area. The alterations in this area are usually correlated with adrenocortical carcinoma, Wilms tumor, ovarian tumor, Beck with-Wiedemann syndrome, breast cancer, rhabdomyosarcoma and lung cancer. The study of AML childhood suf-ferers from Austria diagnosed one NUP98 gene rearrangement in fifty-nine unselected instances. A study intended to identify the NUP98-HOXA9 fusion found that three of two hundred and eight unselected acute-myelogenous cases of leukemia had NUP98-HOXA9 fusion in the Asian group population [1, 2]. Fusion, NUP98-HOXA9 was diagnosed in sufferers with CML-bc (Ph+), and the combined nature of BCR-ABL and NUP98-HOXA9 fusions was established in the experimental mouse model [3, 4].

1.2. GENE - CCND1; CYCLIN D1 LOCATION - 11q13.3

The protein coded through CCND1-gene belongs to the cyclin family, which is notably very conserved. Its contributors are often characterized by elevated protein abundance during the cycle. Cyclins usually function as actuators of CDK kinases. Various cyclins showcase defined patterns of degradation and expres-sions that contribute to the temporal coordination of every mitotic event. The cyclin D1 configures a complex and actuates as a regulatory or activation subunit of CDK6 or CDK4, whose activation is essential and, indeed, required for the transition phase of the cell cycle (G1/S phase). The protein-CCND1 has been demonstrated to interact with Rb protein, a tumor suppressor. The over-expression, alteration, and mutations of CCND1 involved in the alteration of cell cycle progression are majorly found in several types of cancers, which further contribute to tumorigenesis and oncogenesis. CCND1 actuates as an oncogene and is frequently over-expressed in many cancers through gene rearrangement or amplification [5 - 7]. The CCND1 alterations inhibiting ubiquitin-mediated degradation, nuclear export, and Thr286 phosphorylation *via* the proteasome have activated the CDK6/4 network, thereby enhancing the malignant transformation and cellular proliferation both *in vivo* and *in vitro* [8 - 10].

1.3. GENE -BIRC3; BACULOVIRAL-IAP REPEAT CONTAINING-3. LOCATION - 11q22.2

BIRC3 gene codes a particular member of the IAP family of proteins that inhibits apoptosis by forming a complex with tumor-necrosis factor receptor-associated elements TRAF2 and TRAF1, possibly *via* interfering with the actuation of ICE-like proteases. The encoded protein hinders apoptosis through the means of serum deprivation; however now no longer affects apoptosis as a consequence of exposure to menadione, a vigorous inducer of free radicals. It incorporates three baculovirus repeats of IAP and a ring-finger domain. Transcript-variants coding the identical isoform had been identified. BIRC3 can potentially enhance the therapeutic resistance in Glioblastoma [11]. GBM survival is enhanced by the functional contribution of BIRC3 *via* its mechanism in hindering the actuation of caspases [12, 13]. Still, it promotes inflammatory techniques *via* the mediation of tumor-necrosis-factor α signaling [14 - 18].

1.4. GENE - POU2AF1; POU-CLASS 2 HOMEOBOX-ASSOCIATING FACTOR 1 LOCATION - 11q23.1

The protein is likewise termed as an Oct co-activator from B cells, aka Oct binding complex, and as generally discovered withinside the literature, BOB1. BOB1 is a transcriptional co-activator expressed basically *via* B-cell lymphocytes and mastery of immunoglobulin and different genes essential for those cell's expressions of CRISP-3, CD20, and CD36 [19]. The regulation of BOB1 has been verified beneficial for figuring out positive lymphomas, such as B-cell lymphomas, as typified in research that uses BAB1 expression to assist perceive lymphomas [19]. The increase in copy number of POU2AF1 was identified in 3 out of 23 patients, informing that the POU2AF1 amplification is not the artifact obtained at the time of establishing a cell line. However, an infrequent POU2AF1 amplification was detected in a small range of cases. However, the frequent amplification of the POU2AF1 gene in MM isn't so low as compared with different gene amplification activities: for instance, the MYCN amplification, one of the essential genetic activities figuring out analysis in neuroblastoma, is thought to be located in much less than 20% on this disease [20].

Chromosome 11

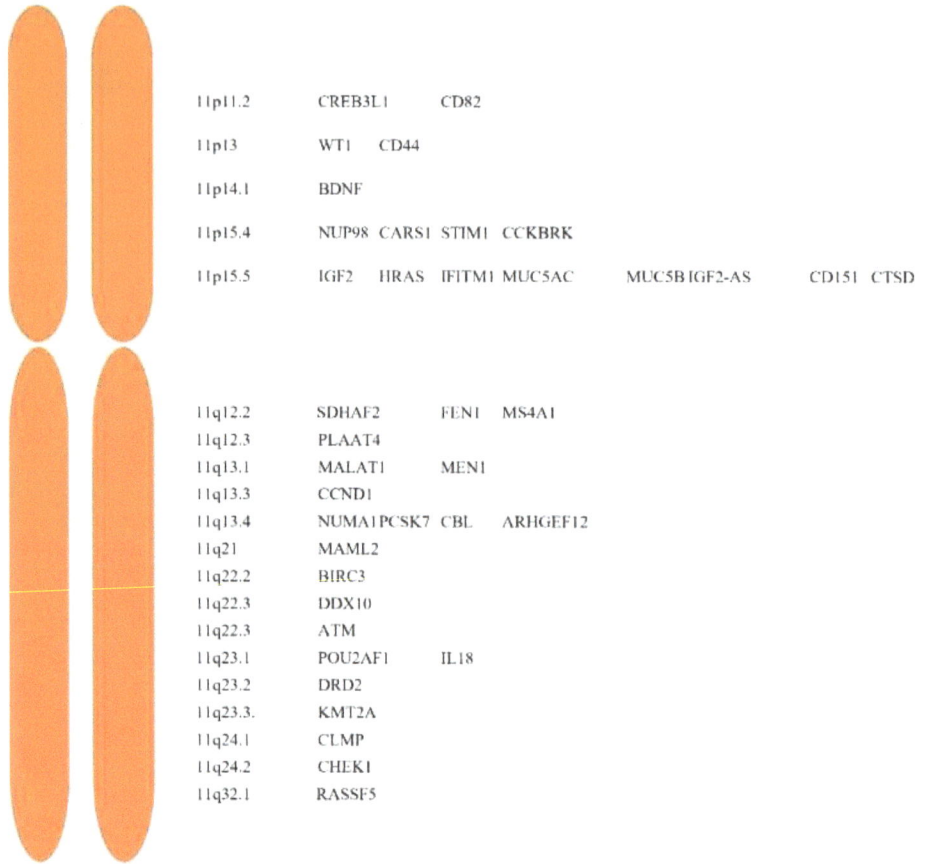

11p11.2	CREB3L1	CD82
11p13	WT1 CD44	
11p14.1	BDNF	
11p15.4	NUP98 CARS1 STIM1 CCKBRK	
11p15.5	IGF2 HRAS IFITM1 MUC5AC MUC5B IGF2-AS CD151 CTSD	

11q12.2	SDHAF2	FEN1 MS4A1
11q12.3	PLAAT4	
11q13.1	MALAT1	MEN1
11q13.3	CCND1	
11q13.4	NUMA1PCSK7 CBL ARHGEF12	
11q21	MAML2	
11q22.2	BIRC3	
11q22.3	DDX10	
11q22.3	ATM	
11q23.1	POU2AF1	IL18
11q23.2	DRD2	
11q23.3.	KMT2A	
11q24.1	CLMP	
11q24.2	CHEK1	
11q32.1	RASSF5	

Fig. (1). This figure displays the loci of the genes from Chromosome 11 whose role in cancer has been explained in this chapter. Sayooj Madhusoodanan designs this diagram.

1.5. GENE -KMT2A; LYSINE-METHYLTRANSFERASE 2 A. LOCATION - 11q23.3.

This gene codes a transcriptional coactivator critical in regulating gene expression during early improvement and hematopoiesis. The coded protein carries a couple of conserved purposeful domains. One of those domains, the SET domain, is chargeable for its H3K4-methyltransferase activity that regulates chromatin changes related to epigenetic-transcriptional activation. The protein is known to be processed *via* the enzyme Taspase-1 into two fragments, MLL-N and MLL-C. These fragments further reassociate and similarly gather into exclusive multi-protein complexes that further alter the transcription of targeted genes, such as a number of the HOX genes. Multiple chromosomal translocations concerning this gene are the leading cause of ALL and AML. KMT2A, called mixed-lineage leukemia or acute-lymphoblastic leukemia 1 (ALL-1), is known as a transcriptional co-activator mediating gene expression for the duration of hematopoiesis and early development [21, 22]. Since KMT2A has stated to modify the regulation and expression of its targeted genes on their promoter region, the studies have tested whether or not it directly altered the gene expression involved in melanoma's growth. hTERT opposes cell senescence and is tremendously expressed in 90% of mammalian cancers, with a pivotal function in cancer progression [23, 24].

1.6. GENE -CREB3L1; CAMP-RESPONSIVE ELEMENT-BINDING PROTEIN3 LIK1. LOCATION - 11p11.2

The protein coded *via* this gene, CREB3L1, is usually located within the ER membrane (endoplasmic reticulum). However, the coded protein clears upon strain and stress given to the endoplasmic reticulum, and the launched cytoplasmic transcription factor translocates to the nucleus. There it turns on the transcription of targeted genes *via* its binding ability to the box-B elements. CREB3L1 gene is localized to endoplasmic reticulum membranes and may migrate to the nucleus to prompt transcription. The nuclear migration is triggered through cleavage by S1P (site 1 Proteases) and S2P (site 2 Proteases), which produces a truncated and actuated form of the CREB2L124 gene. The truncated-CREB2L124 gene is set free to move inside the nucleus and prompt transcription [25]. CREB3L1 is needed for metastatic dissemination in breast cancer animal-model and is up-regulated withinside the breast tumors of sufferers as they develop in the direction of metastatic disease [26].

1.7. GENE - CARS1; CYSTEINYL-TRNA SYNTHETASE 1. LOCATION - 11p15.4

This gene codes a category one aminoacyl tRNA synthetase, cysteinyl tRNA synthetase. This gene is one in every of numerous positioned close to the imprinted-gene domain on chromosome 11 p15.5, an important tumor-suppressor gene place. Alterations in this place were related to Wilms tumor, Beckwith-Wiedemann syndrome, adrenocortical carcinoma, rhabdomyosarcoma, and ovarian, lung and breast cancers. Early CAR - T cell studies have targeted blood tumors. The first authorized remedies use CARs that concentrate on the antigen CD19, found in B-cell-derived tumors with acute-lymphoblastic leukemia and DLBCL (diffuse large B-cell-lymphoma) [27, 28]. CAR-T cells are no longer trafficked expeditiously into the center point of solid-tumor mass, and the antagonistic cancer microenvironment suppresses T-cell activity [29].

1.8.   GENE - MALAT1; METASTASIS-ASSOCIATED LUNG ADENO-CARCINOMA TRANSCRIPT 1. LOCATION - 11q13.1

The MALAT1 gene forms a precursor-transcript from where the long ncRNA is created by the mascRNA (RNase P-cleavage of transfer RNA like small noncoding RNA) at its 3' end. As a result, the mature transcript is observed with the lack of Poly A tailing but stabilized and enriched by a triple helical 3' structure. The mature transcript is hypothesized to produce molecular scaffolding for ribonucleoprotein complexes inside the nucleus, where it is retained. It may actuate as a cell cycle regulator and a transcriptional lever for many genes, including those involved in tumor migration and metastasis. The upregulation of the MALAT1 gene in several cancerous tissues has been connected with the metastasis and proliferation of cancer cells. The inference of MALAT1-RNA withinside the pathology of diverse cancers has been registered. Heightened MALAT1 expression is interrelated with poor overall survival (OS) in several tumors, suggesting that MALAT-1 is a prognosticative factor for various tumors [30 - 32]. The association of the MALAT1 gene is observed in the formation of oncogenesis in various cancers, including pancreatic cancer, lung cancer, and cervical cancer. In these cases, Malat1 ASOs could be used as a potential therapy to inhibit the growth of such malignancies [32].

1.9.   GENE -NUMA1; NUCLEAR-MITOTIC APPARATUS PROTEIN1. LOCATION - 11q13.4

NUMA1 is a gene that codes for a protein involved in forming a structural constituent of the nuclear matrix. The large protein encoded by the NUMA1 gene meticulously communicates with the microtubules and plays a vital role in developing and organizing the mitotic spindle during cell division. The chromosomal translocation of the NUMA1 gene with retinoic-acid receptor α gene (RARA) on chromosome 17 is widely observed in sufferers with acute promyelocytic leukemia. NuMA gene levels in previous studies were observed to be highest in type-I low-grade-serous and mucinous tumors (EOCs), thus suggesting that NuMA overexpression is probably an early process in carcinogenesis [33]. Alternatively, NuMA communicates with dynein, a motor protein, during the process of mitosis. It is indicated that the saturation of this motor protein activity by heightened NuMA may antagonize the pathways that tumor cells utilize to resolve issues like multipolar spindles. These generally rise because of the presence of supernumerary centrosomes, leading to a growth in genomic instability driven by mitotic instability [34].

1.10. GENE - MAML2; MASTERMIND-LIKE TRANSCRIPTIONAL CO-ACTIVATOR2 LOCATION - 11q21

The protein coded using the MAML2 gene is a member of the Mastermind-like family of proteins. All family members are proline and glutamine-rich and contain a conserved basic domain that binds the ankyrin repeat domain of the intracellular domain of the Notch receptors (ICN1-4) in their N-terminus, and a transcriptional activation domain in their C-terminus. This protein integrates to a long groove which is fashioned with the communication of CBF1, LAG-1 (CSL) with ICN, Suppressor-of-Hairless, and forwardly regulates Notch-signaling. High or elevated expression levels of the MAML2 gene were determined in numerous B cell-derived-lymphomas. Translocations ensuing in the fusion proteins with each CRTC3 and CRTC1 were implicated within side the improvement development of mucoepidermoid-carcinomas. In contrast, a translocation with the CXCR4 gene has been related to CLL (chronic lymphocytic leukemia). In the previous study, researchers have focused on the CRTC1/MAML2 fusion oncogene, which is encoded with the recurrent chromosomal-translocation t (11;19) (q14-21;p12-13) in mucoepidermoid-carcinomas (MEC) [35 - 39].

1.11. GENE -DDX10; DEAD BOX HELICASE10. LOCATION - 11q22.3

DEAD-box proteins, characterized with the aid of using the conserved motif Asp-Glu-Ala-Asp, are RNA helicases. They are involved in several cellular processes like alteration of the secondary structure of RNA such as translation-initiation, mitochondrial and nuclear splicing, and spliceosome and ribosome assembly. Based on their patterning of distribution, a few contributors of this own family are thereby believed to be concerned with spermatogenesis, cellular division, cellular growth, and embryogenesis. DDX10 codes for DEAD-box protein and can be concerned with ribosome assembly. The nucleoporin gene (NUP98) and DDX10 gene fusion by inversion 11(p15q22) chromosomal translocation are observed in sufferers with therapy-related and de novo myeloid malignancies. As described earlier, the effectiveness of the NUP98-DDX10 fusion gene on the proliferation and differentiation of human CD34+ cells are exceptionally the same as those described for HOXA9-NUP98 fusion genes beneath the identical conditions as described previously [40, 41]. The induction of numerous homeobox genes using each NUP98-DDX10 and NUP98-HOXA9 indicates that homeobox genes have a crucial position in leukemic transformation using NUP98 fusions. This latest remark supports this belief that homeobox is up gene regulated in murine bone-marrow cells expressing different leukemogenic NUP98-fusions, including NUP98-PMX1, NUP98-HOXD13, NUP98-HHEX and NUP98-NSD1 [42 - 46].

1.12. GENE - PCSK7; PROPROTEIN CONVERTASE SUBTILISIN/ KEXIN TYPE 7. LOCATION - 11q23.3

This gene encodes a subtilisin-like proprotein convertase family member, which includes proteases that process protein and peptide precursors trafficking through regulated or constitutive branches of the secretory pathway. It encodes a type 1 membrane-bound protease in many tissues, including neuroendocrine, liver, gut, and brain. The encoded protein undergoes an initial autocatalytic processing event in the ER. It then sorts to the trans-Golgi network through endosomes, where a second autocatalytic event occurs, and the catalytic activity is acquired. This gene encodes one of the seven essential amino acid-specific members, which cleave their substrates at single or paired basic residues. It can process pro-albumin and is thought to be responsible for activating HIV envelope glycoproteins gp160 and gp140. This gene has been implicated in the transcriptional regulation of house-keeping genes and plays a role in regulating iron metabolism. A t(11;14) (q23;q32) chromosome translocation associated with B-cell lymphoma occurs between this gene and its inverted counterpart. The cytoskeletal extensions observed upon overexpression of CASC4 in Hela cells and the correlation between PCSK7-CASC4 mRNA levels with breast cancer patient's survival [47]. Our METABRIC data indicated that patients with high PCSK7 and high CASC4 had a significantly worse prognosis than those with high CASC4 but low PCSK7 [47].

1.13. GENE - CBL; CBL PROTO-ONCOGENE. LOCATION - 11q23.3

Cbl is a mammalian gene coding protein called CBL, an E3ubiquitin-protein ligase concerned with cellular signaling and protein-ubiquitination. Mutations in this gene have been implicated in some human cancers, especially AML. This gene codes a RING-finger E3-ubiquitin ligase. The encoded domain is one of the enzymes required for concentrated on substrates for degradation with the aid of using the proteasome. This protein majorly mediates the switch of ubiquitin from ubiquitin-conjugating enzymes (E2) to specific substrates. This protein additionally consists of an N-terminal known as a phosphor-tyrosine binding area that permits it to engage with several tyrosine-phosphorylated substrates and goal them for proteasome-degradation. As such, its capabilities as a poor regulator of many sign transduction pathways. This gene is located to be mutated or translocated in many cancers, including AML, and the enlargement of CGG repeats within the 5' UTR has been related to Jacobsen syndrome. Mutations on this gene also are the purpose of Noonan-syndrome-like disorder. c-Cbl is a RING-area containing E3-ubiquitin ligase significantly studied in myeloid malignancies and myeloid cells [48, 49]. The expression and activation of c-Cbl in human-CRC tumors are inversely interrelated with β-catenin and the general survival of metastatic CRC [50 - 52].

1.14. GENE -ARHGEF12; RHO-GUANINE NUCLEOTIDE-EXCHANGE FACTOR12. LOCATION - 11q23.3.

This protein is likewise known as RhoGEF12/ Leukemia-associated Rho-guanine nucleotide-exchange factor (LARG). Rho GTPases had an essential function in several cellular processes, which might be initiated through extracellular stimuli operating *via* G protein-coupled receptors (GPCR). The coded protein may also form a fusion complex with G proteins and enhance Rio-established signals. This protein is said to form a lymphoid/myeloid fusion partner in AML. To have a look at if ARHGEF12 polymorphism-related anemia after exposure to chemotherapy in people living with acute lymphoid leukemia might also additionally interact with the p38-pathway, previous studies have measured the p38-phosphorylation in erythroid-cells in seven remission-associated bone-merpeople living with people living with acute lymphoid leukemia at some point of protection remedy through phospho-flow [53]. ARHGEF12 codes for a RhoA-specified guanine-nucleotide exchange factor that positively activates the RhoA GTP/GDP exchange reaction. ARHGEF12 performs essential roles in invasion and cell migration, reorientating stress fiber responses, mesenchymal stem-cell fate, and cyclic-stretch-induced cell by activating the RhoA activity [54 - 56].

1.15. GENE - RASSF5; RAS ASSOCIATION DOMAIN FAMILY MEMBER 5, LOCATION - 11q32.1

This RASSF5 is a group of the Ras association family. It features as a tumor suppressor and is not activated in quite a few cancers. The coded protein localizes to the microtubules and centrosomes and inter-associates with the GTP-activated sorts of Rap1, Raps, and numerous das-like small GTPases. The protein mediates lymphocyte adhesion and supports cellular growth in reaction to activated Rap1 or Ras. Recent studies have indicated that each RASSF5C and RASSF5A have growth-suppression characteristics *via* cellular growth inhibition, colony forma-tion of cancer cells, and improvement of cellular responses to apoptosis [57]. The evaluation of a massive panel of HCC samples shows that the expression stages of RASSF5A are prominently lower in HCC, characterized by a poorer analysis than that of a higher outcome [58].

1.16. GENE -IGF2; INSULIN-LIKE GROWTH FACTOR 2. LOCATION - 11p15.5

IGF2 codes for insulin-polypeptide GFs, which are related to growth and development. It is called an imprinted gene expressed from the paternal allele, and numerous epigenetic modifications on the locus of this gene are extensively related to Beckwith-Wiedemann syndrome, Wilms tumor, Silver-Russell syndrome, and rhabdomyosarcoma. A read-*via*, INS-IGF2 gene exists, whose 5' area overlaps the INS gene, and the 3' area overlaps this gene. It is sometimes produced in greater islet and non-islet hypoglycemic cell tumors, causing hypoglycemia. Doege-Potter syndrome is a paraneoplastic syndrome [59]. Preeclampsia induces a decrease in methylation degree at IGF2 demethylated area. These various mechanisms are in the back of the association between intrauterine exposure to preeclampsia and an immoderate chance for metabolic diseases within the infants' later existence [60].

1.17. GENE - WT1; WT1 TRANSCRIPTION FACTOR. LOCATION - 11p13.

This gene codes for a transcription factor incorporating four zinc-finger motifs on the C-terminus and a proline-glutamine-rich DNA binding area on the N-terminus. This gene plays a vital role in the ordinary improvement of the urogenital system and is highly mutated or expressed in a small subset of sufferers with Wilms tumor. This gene well-known shows complicated tissue-particular and polymorphic-imprinting patterns, with monoallelic and biallelic expression from both paternal and maternal alleles in exclusive tissues. Multiple transcript variations were described. In numerous variations, there's proof for using a non-AUG translation-initiation (CUG) codon which is upstream of, and in frame with the primary AUG. Mostly qPCR is used to set up the ranges of WT1-expression. The growing degree of WT1 expression is notably related to sickness development and relapse of other proliferative disorders [61]. Despite the terminology, WT1-mutation is discovered in the most effective in approximately five-ten percent of Wilms-Tumor cases [62].

1.18. GENE - HRAS; H-RAS PROTO-ONCOGENE, GTPASE. LOCATION - 11p15.5

HRAS gene belongs to the Ras-oncogene family, under whose contributors are related to the transforming genes of mammalian-sarcoma-retroviruses. Products coded through these genes predominantly feature in the signal-transduction pathways. The proteins usually bind GTP and GDP, and hence they have got intrinsic GTPase activity. This protein majorly undergoes a non-forestall cycle of re- and de-palmitoylation, which activates and regulates its rapid exchange of a number of the Golgi apparatus and the plasma membrane. Mutations in this gene purpose Costello syndrome, a disorder characterized by an accelerated increase at the prenatal stage, development deficiency at the cognitive disability, post-natal stage, predisposition to cancer formation, skin, pores, and other musculoskeletal abnormalities, unique facial appearance, and cardiovascular abnormalities. Defects in this gene are mainly implicated in several cancers, including oral squamous cell carcinoma, follicular-thyroid cancer, and bladder cancer. Somatic mutations withinside the HRAS gene are likely indulged in the improvement of numerous different sorts of tumors. These mutations result in an HRAS protein that usually activates and may direct cells to develop and divide without control. Recent research endorses that the mutations of HRAS are not unusual to place in kidney cancers, salivary-duct carcinoma [63], thyroid, and epithelial-myoep--thelial carcinoma [63]. DNA copy number gain of a section containing the HRAS gene is covered in a genome-wide pattern, which changed into determined to be interrelated with an astrocytoma patient's outcome [64].

1.19. GENE - MEN1; MENIN 1 LOCATION - 11q13.1

This gene codes for menin, which is a tumor-suppressor related to a syndrome called multiple endocrine neoplasia type1. Menin is known as a scaffold protein that features histone change and epigenetic-gene regulation. It is a concept to alter numerous pathways and procedures with the aid of using changing chromatin shape through the change of histones. Menin, the epigenetic regulator, also known as the product of the MEN1 gene, is correlated with the inherited-tumor syndrome multiple endocrine-neoplasia type1 [65]. In PanNETs, the MEN1-gene undergoes some somatic-inactivating mutations with excessive frequency [66].

1.20. GENE -ATM; ATM-SERINE/THREONINE-KINASE. LOCATION - 11q22.3

The protein coded through this gene belongs to the PI3/ PI4- kinase family. This protein ATM is a critical cell-cycle checkpoint kinase that phosphorylates; hence, it has capabilities as an activator of an extensive style of downstream proteins, along with tumor-suppressor proteins like BRCA1 and p53, checkpoint-kinase CHK2, checkpoint-proteins RAD9, and RAD17, and DNA restore protein NBS1.

ATM-protein and the intently associated kinase-ATR are notions of being grasp controllers of cell-cycle checkpoint signaling pathways which might be required and responsible for Genome-stability and DNA damage. Mutations in this gene are related to ataxia telangiectasia. Ataxia-telangiectasia is a rare human disease characterized through manner of way of excessive-cell sensitivity to external factors like radiation, cerebellar degeneration, and a pre-disposition to several cancers. All AT patients contain mutations withinside the ATM gene. Most distinctive AT-like issues are defective in genes encoding the MRN protein complex. One feature of the ATM protein is its speedy boom in kinase hobby proper away following double-strand harm formation [67, 68]. AT patients have an extended hazard for breast cancers that have been ascribed to ATM's interaction and phosphorylation of BRCA1 and its associated proteins following DNA harm [69].

1.21. GENE -SDHAF2; SUCCINATE-DEHYDROGENASE COMPLEX-ASSEMBLY FACTOR2 LOCATION - 11q12.2

Succinate-dehydrogenase complex-assembly factor2, previously referred to as SDH5 and also referred to as SDH assembly factor2, is a protein coded by the SDHAF2-gene. This gene codes a mitochondrial protein which is required for flavination of the succinate-dehydrogenase complex-subunit, required for the activity and regulation of the complex. Mutations in this gene are related to paraganglioma and pheochromocytoma. SDHAF2 is known to be a tumor-suppressor gene. Several constitutional mutations on this gene motive hereditary paraganglioma, neuroendocrine cancer previously recognized to be connected to the SDH-subunit variant. Paraganglioma is known as a neural-crest tumor normally associated with the chemoreceptor tissue of the paraganglion. It can broaden at diverse frame sites, consisting of the neck, head, abdomen, and thorax. In instances of extra-adrenal localization, cancer can also additionally flip aggressive and metastatic. Loss of this gene has been recognized to be the cause of paraganglioma [70 - 72].

1.22. GENE - BDNF; BRAIN-DERIVED NEUROTROPHIC FACTOR LOCATION - 11p14.1

BDNF codes a group of never-growth-factor families of proteins. Alternative-splicing outcomes in a couple of transcript-variants, one of which codes a pre-proprotein that is proteolytically regulated to form the mature protein. Expression of BDNF is decreased in Parkinson's, Alzheimer's, and Huntington's-disease patients. BDNF gene may also play a function in the activation and regulation of stress responses and other mood disorders. BDNF has additionally been implicated in regulating oncogenic transformation [73, 74] and tumor relapse [75] after being intended as a hit remedy for cancer.

1.23. GENE - CD44; CD44 MOLECULE (INDIAN BLOOD GROUP) LOCATION - 11p13

The protein coded by the CD44 gene is a cellular glycoprotein concerned with cell/cell interactions, cell migration, and adhesion. It is a receptor for hyaluronic acid (HA) and also can interact with different ligands, inclusive of osteopontin, collagens, and matrix metalloproteinases (MMPs). This protein participates in a huge type of cell features consisting of lymphocyte activation, recirculation and homing, hematopoiesis, and tumor metastasis. Transcripts for this gene go through complicated opportunity splicing that outcome in lots of functionally variant isoforms, however, the full-period nature of a number of those editions has now no longer been determined. Alternative splicing is the idea for this protein's structural and purposeful range and can be associated with tumor metastasis. High levels of the adhesion molecule CD44 on leukemic cells are essential to generate leukemia [76]. Furthermore, due to alternative-splicing and post-translational modifications that generate many specific CD44 sequences involving some tumor-specific sequences, the formation of anti-CD44 tumor specific-agents might be a sensible healing and realistic approach for treating cancers [77].

1.24. GENE - CD82; CD82 MOLECULE LOCATION - 11p11.2

The metastasis-suppressor gene outcome is a membrane-glycoprotein that could be a member of the trans-membrane four superfamilies. Expression and mutation of this gene are proven to be down-regulated in tumor development of human tumors and may be activated and regulated by p5 *via* a consensus-binding sequence at the promotor region. Two alternatively-spliced transcript variants coding the distinct isoforms are found for this gene. CD82, additionally called KAI1, mainly belong to the tetraspanin family related to both pathological and physiological processes of tumors, including cancer metastasis and cancer invasion [78, 79]. Its differential expressions are majorly found in several malignant and normal tissues, which suggests that CD82 may have a significant role in cancer progression, cancer growth, cancer metastasis, invasion, and motility [80 - 82].

1.25. GENE - NOX4 LOCATION - 11q14.3

NOX4 gene codes a member of the NOX family that regulates and functions as a catalytic subunit of the NADPH-oxidase complex. The ROS formed by the NOX4 protein was implicated in several biological functions like tumor cell growth, cellular differentiation, and signal transduction. As an essential source of ROS generation, the NADPH-oxidase family (NOX), including the members DUOX1-2 and NOX1-5, is highly intended to correlate with tumor progression and cancer development [83]. NOX1 is critical for oncogenic-Ras transformation [84], and NOX-5 is indulged in the cellular viability of prostate tumor cells [84].

1.26. GENE - CHEK1; CHECKPOINT KINASE 1. LOCATION - 11q24.2

The protein coded using this gene belongs to the Ser/Thr protein kinase family. It is needed for checkpoint-mediated cellular cycle arrest in reaction to DNA damage or the presence of un-replicated DNA. This protein combines signals from ATM and ATR, cell cycle proteins indulged in DNA-damage responses that still accomplice with chromatin in meiotic prophase I. Phosphorylation of CDC25A protein phosphatase with the aid of using this protein is needed for cells to put off cell-cycle development in reaction to double-strand DNA breaks. Several instead spliced transcript variations were discovered for this gene. Initially, Chk1 was thought to function as a tumor suppressor due to the regulatory role it serves amongst cells with DNA damage. However, there has been no evidence of homozygous loss of function mutants for Chk1 in human tumors. Instead, the Chk1 gene is over-expressed in numerous tumors, including liver, colon, breast, nasopharyngeal and gastric carcinoma [85].

1.27. GENE -STIM1; STROMAL-INTERACTION MOLECULE1. LOCATION - 11p15.4

This gene codes for type1 trans-membrane protein which mediates Ca^{2+}-influx after the depletion of intracellular Ca^{2+}-stores by gating SOCs. It is considered one among numerous genes placed within the imprinted gene region of 11p15.5, an important tumor suppressor gene location. This area's alteration was related to the Wilms tumor, Beckwith-Wiedemann syndrome, adrenocortical carcinoma, rhabdomyosarcoma, and breast, ovarian, and lung cancer. This gene may also play a position in malignancies and ailments that contain this region, in addition to early hematopoiesis, through mediating attachment to the stromal cells. Aberrations or mutations on this gene are related to deadly Kaposi-sarcoma and immuno-deficiency because of defects in SOCE in tubular-aggregate myopathy, ectodermal dysplasia, and fibroblasts. This gene is orientated in a head-to-tail configuration with the ribonucleotide-reductase-1 gene. Alternative splicing of this gene outcomes in a couple of transcript variants. Studies have moreover implicated a role for Orai1 and STIM1 in the EMT of breast cancer cells, an important step in tumor metastasis [86, 87].

1.28. GENE - CCKBR; CHOLECYSTOKININ B RECEPTOR LOCATION - 11p15.4

CCKBR gene codes for a G protein-coupled- receptor for cholecystokinin and gastrin, also known as regulatory peptides of the GI tract and brain. CCKBR protein, also known as B-gastrin receptor, has an extreme affinity for every non-sulfated and sulfated CCK-analogs and is discovered basically within the significant machine and the GI tract. The alternative-splicing outcomes in a couple of transcript-variants. A miss-spliced variation in the transcript has been established in the cells derived from pancreatic and colorectal tumors. Over-expression of the CCKBR gene was reported in various types of tumors, leading to the progression of CCKBR-targeted therapeutic agents. No successful clinical trials have been reported to date [86].

1.29. GENE - IFITM1; INTERFERON-INDUCED TRANSMEMBRANE PROTEIN 1 LOCATION - 11p15.5

Interferon-triggered transmembrane protein 1 is a protein that, in people, is encoded with the aid of using the IFITM1 gene. IFITM1 has additionally lately been specified CD225 (cluster of differentiation 225). IFITM proteins have a brief N-terminal and C-terminal domain, transmembrane domains (TM1 and TM2), and a brief cytoplasmic domain. Interestingly, over the past decade, increasing evidence has shown that IFITM1 is overexpressed in a large number of solid human tumors. Yu *et al* . determined that blocking of IFITM1 expression inhi-bited the proliferation of glioma cells and thereby caused the cell-cycle arrest, followed with the aid of using a discount of cyclin B1, cyclin E, cyclin D1, cyclin A, CDK4, and CDK2, and up-regulation of p27kip1 [88].

1.30. GENE -MUC5AC; MUCIN5AC, OLIGOMERIC-MUCUS/GE--FORMING. LOCATION - 11p15.5

MUC5AC is a Protein Coding-gene. Diseases related to MUC5AC include Biliary Papillomatosis and Barrett Esophagus. Its associated pathways are Defective-C1GALT1C1 causes TNPS and the Metabolism of certain proteins. NPC-1C gene actuates and reacts with specific epitopes expressed by the colorectal and pancreatic tumor-related MUC5AC [89].

1.31. GENE -MUC5B; MUCIN5B, OLIGOMERIC-MUCUS/GE--FORMING. LOCATION - 11p15.5

This gene codes a member of the mucin family, which can be highly gly-cosylated-macromolecular components of mucus secretions. This member of the family is the important gel-forming mucin in the mucus. It is a first-rate contributor to certain properties including the viscoelastic and lubricating functions of whole saliva, cervical mucus, and normal-lung mucus. This gene up-regulates several human diseases like sinus mucosa of CRS, COPD, nasal polyps with CRS, and H pylori-related gastric disease. Mucins are involved in most tumors by regulating cell signaling, cell adhesion, cellular apoptosis, and cellular growth. The secreted pr formed mucin -MUC5B, the crucial issue of the breathing tract mucus, is highly expressed in breast cancers, in which it can constitute a tumor biomarker [90].

1.32. GENE - FEN1; FLAP STRUCTURE-SPECIFIC ENDONUCLEASE LOCATION - 11q12.2

The protein coded by the FEN1 gene detaches the 5' overhanging flaps in the DNA repair mechanism and helps process the 5'-ends of Okazaki fragments in the lagging strands of DNA synthesis. The physical interaction betwixt FEN1 protein and AP-endonuclease1 at the time of long patch base-excision repair results in a sequestrated loading of certain proteins onto the substrate, thereby passing the substrate sequentially from one enzyme to another enzyme. FEN1 is a group of RAD2/XPG endonuclease-family and is 1 in 10 proteins that are essential for cell-free DNA replication. The secondary structure of the DNA can forestall and inhibit the process of flap mechanism at trinucleotide repeats by blocking out the 5'-end of the flap, which is required for cleaving and binding by the FEN1 protein coded by this gene. Therefore, the secondary structure can deter the protective function of this protein, leading to site-specific trinucleotide expansions. Previous observations have concluded that FEN1 SNPs are indulged in several tumor developments, including lung cancer, esophageal cancer, hepatocellular carcinoma, gastric cancer, breast cancer, and glioma [91-97].

1.33. GENE - PLAAT4; PHOSPHOLIPASE A AND ACYLTRANSFERASE 4 OR RARRES3 (RETINOIC ACID RECEPTOR RESPONDER PROTEIN 3). LOCATION - 11q12.3

Retinoids employ certain biologic effects, including cell-differentiation activities and growth-inhibitory factors that are mainly used in treating hyperproliferative-dermatological diseases. These effects are regulated by particular nuclear-receptor proteins which are known to be a member of the thyroid and steroid hormone-receptor family of transcriptional activators. RARRES3, RARRES2, and RARRES1 genes are highly upregulated *via* the synthetic retinoid-tazarotene. In many instances, RARRES3 either acts as a growth regulator or a tumor suppressor. Combined activation and expression of specific subunits of immunoproteasomes like PSMB8, PSMB10, RARRES3, and PSMB9 are observed in a BM-MSC-networking and are conserved in the datasets presenting the breast cancer cells and tissues [25].

1.34. GENE- IGF2-AS; IGF2 ANTISENSE RNA LOCATION - 11p15.5

The IGF2-AS gene is expressed in an antisense form to the IGF2 gene and is paternally expressed and imprinted. It is believed to be non-coding as the putative protein here is not conserved, and the translation is forecasted to trigger nonsense-mediated decay. The transcripts from the IGF2-AS gene are yielded in cancer and may actuate to suppress cellular growth. The activation of IR-A and its mechanism with IGF2 have some mitogenic effects and may enhance tumori-genesis compared with the action of insulin, the action of IGF2 through IR-A differentially influences the gene expression that is acting through the same receptor [60].

1.35. GENE -MS4A1; MEMBRANE-SPANNING 4-DOMAINS A1 LOCATION - 11q12.2

This gene encodes a member of the membrane-spanning 4A gene family. Members of this nascent protein family are characterized by common structural features and similar intron/exon splice boundaries and display unique expression patterns among hematopoietic cells and nonlymphoid tissues. This gene encodes a B-lymphocyte surface molecule which plays a role in the development and differentiation of B-cells into plasma cells. This family member is localized to 11q12, among a cluster of family members. Because MS4A1 encodes the CD20 B lymphocyte marker, the origin of its up-regulation in ARLC-SCC, which comprises primary tumor cells as wand stroma, was explored using immuno-histochemistry to determine if deregulation was due to stromal lymphocytes rather than lung tumor cells [96].

1.36. GENE -CD151; CD151-MOLECULE (RAPH BLOOD-GROUP) LOCATION - 11p15.5

The protein encoded by this gene is a member of the transmembrane 4 superfamilies, also known as the tetraspanin family. Most of these members are cell-surface proteins that are characterized by the presence of four hydrophobic domains. The proteins mediate signal transduction events that play a role in the regulation of cell development, activation, growth, and motility. This encoded protein is a cell surface glycoprotein that is known to be complex with integrins and other transmembrane 4 superfamily proteins. It is involved in cellular processes, including cell adhesion and may regulate integrin trafficking and/or function. This protein enhances cell motility, invasion, and metastasis of cancer cells. Multiple alternatively spliced transcript variants that encode the same protein have been described for this gene (19). *Li et al.* assessed the mechanism of the CD151 gene in de-novo tumorigenesis, the progression of SCC, and its multiplicity in juxtaposition with normal cells [98]. Over-expression of the CD151 gene was also reported to associate with poor prognosis of lung, colon, esophageal, pancreatic, and endometrial cancers [91, 99, 100].

1.37. GENE - CTSD; CATHEPSIN D LOCATION - 11p15.5

This gene codes for the A1 peptidase's family. The encoded pre-proprotein is proteolytically regulated to generate more than one protein product. These products consist of the cathepsin-D heavy and light chains, that heterodimerize to produce the mature enzymes. This enzyme reveals a pepsin-like mechanism and performs a function in protein turnover and withinside the proteolytic regulation of certain growth factors and hormones. Mutations on this gene play a critical function in neuronal-ceroid lipofuscinosis-10 and can be concerned withinside the pathogenesis of numerous different diseases, which include breast tumors and likely Alzheimer's disease. In breast tumors, the protease is known to be an individualistic marker of poor prognosis, which represents an up-regulation of CTSD-mRNA and shows a tissue marker with a high risk of tumor metastasis [101 - 103].

1.38. GENE - IL18; INTERLEUKIN 18 LOCATION - 11q23.1

The protein coded through this gene is a proinflammatory-cytokine that augments NK cellular activity in the spleen cells and enhances interferon-gamma formulation in T-type helper cells. Several cellular types, both non-hematopoietic and hematopoietic cells, can form IL-18. Of note, metastasis may be facilitated through IL-18 *via* up-regulation of CD44 and VEGF [18]. The potential of IL-18 to stimulate angiogenesis may be a concern in tumor development and metastasis [104].

1.39. GENE - DRD2; DOPAMINE-RECEPTORD2 LOCATION - 11q23.2

This gene codes the D2 subtype of the dopamine receptor. The G-protein coupled receptor (GPCR) inhibits adenylyl-cyclase activity. A missense mutation on this gene reasons myoclonus dystonia; different mutations were related to schizophrenia. Alternative splicing of this gene consequences in transcript editions encoding exclusive isoforms. A 3rd variation has been described; however, it has now no longer been decided whether the form is either normal or due to aberrant splicing. As the regulation and expression of DRD2 correlated with the survival of sufferers with gastric tumors, it might actuate in tumor cell survival. Developing small-molecule drugs to treat and target DRD2 can provide anti-tumor effects [105].

1.40. GENE -CLMP; CXADR-LIKE MEMBRANE PROTEIN LOCATION - 11q24.1

This gene codes a type1 transmembrane protein localized to junctional complexes among epithelial and endothelial cells and might have a position in cell/cell adhesion. Expression or regulation of this gene in the white-adipose tissue is involved in adipocyte development and maturation of obesity. This gene is likewise critical for everyday intestinal improvement, and mutations withinside the gene are related to congenital brief bowel syndrome. This latter discovery does now not contradict a predicted CLMP enrichment because of the truth that their desire for a baseline tissue became a mouse P5-cerebellum, an early diploma of proliferation that expresses the genes of cerebellar improvement [106].

1.41. GENE -KCNQ1OT1; KCNQ1 OPPOSITE-STRAND/ANTISENSE TRANSCRIPT1 LOCATION - 11p15.5

Human chromosomal vicinity 11p15.5 includes clusters of epigenetically-activated genes that might be expressed from one chromosome in a parent-of - foundation manner. A functionally independent imprinting-control region activates each cluster. The human KCNQ1OT1/ CDKN1C region is activated *via* a particular way of means of an ICR-positioned in an intron region of the KCNQ1 gene. It includes a minimum of eight genes that might be expressed preferentially and entirely from the maternally inherited allele. The ICR involves the promoter of the KCNQ1OT1-gene, which is wholly expressed from the paternal allele. The KCNQ1OT1 transcript is the anti-sense to the KCNQ1 gene and is an unspliced lengthy non-coding RNA. It interacts and communicates with chromatin and activates the transcription of a couple of genes *via* a few epigenetic modifications. The transcript is abnormally expressed from each chromosome in maximum sufferers with Beckwith-Wiedemann syndrome, and the transcript additionally performs a crucial function in colorectal carcinogenesis. Of the many cancer-associated lncRNAs, it was reported that lncRNA of KCNQ1 opposite strand/antisense transcript 1 (KCNQ1OT1) is upregulated in several human tumors, and regulates cancer cell epigenetics [107].

CONCLUSION

Cancer has become a great challenge daily, and locating a particular and everlasting remedy for that is an even greater difficulty. This database of most cancer genes and their function in exclusive kinds of cancers will subsequently assist scientists to study and work on new therapeutics, thereby enabling them to come up with new strategies to combat several cancers.

REFERENCES

[1] Nebral K, König M, Schmidt HH, *et al.* Screening for NUP98 rearrangements in hematopoietic malignancies by fluorescence *in situ* hybridization. Haematologica 2005; 90(6): 746-52.
[PMID: 15951287]

[2] Kwong YL, Pang A. Low frequency of rearrangements of the homeobox geneHOXA9/t(7;11) in adult acute myeloid leukemia. Genes Chromosomes Cancer 1999; 25(1): 70-4.
[http://dx.doi.org/10.1002/(SICI)1098-2264(199905)25:1<70::AID-GCC11>3.0.CO;2-E] [PMID: 10221343]

[3] Ahuja HG, Popplewell L, Tcheurekdjian L, Slovak ML. NUP98 gene rearrangements and the clonal evolution of chronic myelogenous leukemia. Genes Chromosomes Cancer 2001; 30(4): 410-5.
[http://dx.doi.org/10.1002/1098-2264(2001)9999:9999<::AID-GCC1108>3.0.CO;2-9] [PMID: 1124-1795]

[4] Dash AB, Williams IR, Kutok JL, *et al.* A murine model of CML blast crisis induced by cooperation between BCR/ABL and NUP98/HOXA9. Proc Natl Acad Sci USA 2002; 99(11): 7622-7.
[http://dx.doi.org/10.1073/pnas.102583199] [PMID: 12032333]

[5] Diehl JA. Cycling to cancer with cyclin D1. Cancer Biol Ther 2002; 1(3): 226-31.
[http://dx.doi.org/10.4161/cbt.72] [PMID: 12432268]

[6] Hardisson D. Molecular pathogenesis of head and neck squamous cell carcinoma. Eur Arch Otorhinolaryngol 2003; 260(9): 502-8.
[http://dx.doi.org/10.1007/s00405-003-0581-3] [PMID: 12736744]

[7] Lukas J, Jadayel D, Bartkova J, *et al.* BCL-1/cyclin D1 oncoprotein oscillates and subverts the G1 phase control in B-cell neoplasms carrying the t(11;14) translocation. Oncogene 1994; 9(8): 2159-67.
[PMID: 8036001]

[8] Alt JR, Cleveland JL, Hannink M, Diehl JA. Phosphorylation-dependent regulation of cyclin D1 nuclear export and cyclin D1-dependent cellular transformation. Genes Dev 2000; 14(24): 3102-14.
[http://dx.doi.org/10.1101/gad.854900] [PMID: 11124803]

[9] Gladden AB, Woolery R, Aggarwal P, Wasik MA, Diehl JA. Expression of constitutively nuclear cyclin D1 in murine lymphocytes induces B-cell lymphoma. Oncogene 2006; 25(7): 998-1007.
[http://dx.doi.org/10.1038/sj.onc.1209147] [PMID: 16247460]

[10] Lin DI, Lessie MD, Gladden AB, Bassing CH, Wagner KU, Diehl JA. Disruption of cyclin D1 nuclear export and proteolysis accelerates mammary carcinogenesis. Oncogene 2008; 27(9): 1231-42.
[http://dx.doi.org/10.1038/sj.onc.1210738] [PMID: 17724472]

[11] Wang D, Berglund A, Kenchappa RS, Forsyth PA, Mulé JJ, Etame AB. BIRC3 is a novel driver of therapeutic resistance in Glioblastoma. Sci Rep 2016; 6(1): 21710.
[http://dx.doi.org/10.1038/srep21710] [PMID: 26888114]

[12] Vucic D, Dixit VM, Wertz IE. Ubiquitylation in apoptosis: a post-translational modification at the edge of life and death. Nat Rev Mol Cell Biol 2011; 12(7): 439-52.

[http://dx.doi.org/10.1038/nrm3143] [PMID: 21697901]

[13] Vaux DL, Silke J. Mammalian mitochondrial IAP binding proteins. Biochem Biophys Res Commun 2003; 304(3): 499-504.
      [http://dx.doi.org/10.1016/S0006-291X(03)00622-3] [PMID: 12729584]

[14] Mahoney DJ, Cheung HH, Mrad RL, *et al.* Both cIAP1 and cIAP2 regulate TNFα-mediated NF-κB activation. Proc Natl Acad Sci USA 2008; 105(33): 11778-83.
      [http://dx.doi.org/10.1073/pnas.0711122105] [PMID: 18697935]

[15] Zhao X, Laver T, Hong SW, *et al.* An NF-κB p65-cIAP2 link is necessary for mediating resistance to TNF-α induced cell death in gliomas. J Neurooncol 2011; 102(3): 367-81.
      [http://dx.doi.org/10.1007/s11060-010-0346-y] [PMID: 21279667]

[16] Rothe M, Pan MG, Henzel WJ, Ayres TM, Goeddel DV. The TNFR2-TRAF signaling complex contains two novel proteins related to baculoviral inhibitor of apoptosis proteins. Cell 1995; 83(7): 1243-52.
      [http://dx.doi.org/10.1016/0092-8674(95)90149-3] [PMID: 8548810]

[17] Shu HB, Takeuchi M, Goeddel DV. The tumor necrosis factor receptor 2 signal transducers TRAF2 and c-IAP1 are components of the tumor necrosis factor receptor 1 signaling complex. Proc Natl Acad Sci USA 1996; 93(24): 13973-8.
      [http://dx.doi.org/10.1073/pnas.93.24.13973] [PMID: 8943045]

[18] Zarnegar BJ, Wang Y, Mahoney DJ, *et al.* Noncanonical NF-κB activation requires coordinated assembly of a regulatory complex of the adaptors cIAP1, cIAP2, TRAF2 and TRAF3 and the kinase NIK. Nat Immunol 2008; 9(12): 1371-8.
      [http://dx.doi.org/10.1038/ni.1676] [PMID: 18997794]

[19] Zhao C, Inoue J, Imoto I, *et al.* POU2AF1, an amplification target at 11q23, promotes growth of multiple myeloma cells by directly regulating expression of a B-cell maturation factor, TNFRSF17. Oncogene 2008; 27(1): 63-75.
      [http://dx.doi.org/10.1038/sj.onc.1210637] [PMID: 17621271]

[20] Moreau LA, McGrady P, London WB, *et al.* Does MYCN amplification manifested as homogeneously staining regions at diagnosis predict a worse outcome in children with neuroblastoma? A Children's Oncology Group study. Clin Cancer Res 2006; 12(19): 5693-7.
      [http://dx.doi.org/10.1158/1078-0432.CCR-06-1500] [PMID: 17020972]

[21] Liu H, Cheng EHY, Hsieh JJD. MLL fusions: Pathways to leukemia. Cancer Biol Ther 2009; 8(13): 1204-11.
      [http://dx.doi.org/10.4161/cbt.8.13.8924] [PMID: 19729989]

[22] Zhang P, Bergamin E, Couture JF. The many facets of MLL1 regulation. Biopolymers 2013; 99(2): 136-45.
      [http://dx.doi.org/10.1002/bip.22126] [PMID: 23175388]

[23] Akincilar SC, Unal B, Tergaonkar V. Reactivation of telomerase in cancer. Cell Mol Life Sci 2016; 73(8): 1659-70.
      [http://dx.doi.org/10.1007/s00018-016-2146-9] [PMID: 26846696]

[24] Ohira T, Naohiro S, Nakayama Y, *et al.* miR-19b regulates hTERT mRNA expression through targeting PITX1 mRNA in melanoma cells. Sci Rep 2015; 5(1): 8201.
      [http://dx.doi.org/10.1038/srep08201] [PMID: 25643913]

[25] Murakami T, Kondo S, Ogata M, *et al.* Cleavage of the membrane-bound transcription factor OASIS in response to endoplasmic reticulum stress. J Neurochem 2006; 96(4): 1090-100.
      [http://dx.doi.org/10.1111/j.1471-4159.2005.03596.x] [PMID: 16417584]

[26] Feng YX, Jin DX, Sokol ES, Reinhardt F, Miller DH, Gupta PB. Cancer-specific PERK signaling drives invasion and metastasis through CREB3L1. Nat Commun 2017; 8(1): 1079.
      [http://dx.doi.org/10.1038/s41467-017-01052-y] [PMID: 29057869]

[27]   Kochenderfer JN, Wilson WH, Janik JE, *et al.* Eradication of B-lineage cells and regression of lymphoma in a patient treated with autologous T cells genetically engineered to recognize CD19. Blood 2010; 116(20): 4099-102.
[http://dx.doi.org/10.1182/blood-2010-04-281931] [PMID: 20668228]

[28]   Kochenderfer JN, Dudley ME, Kassim SH, *et al.* Chemotherapy-refractory diffuse large B-cell lymphoma and indolent B-cell malignancies can be effectively treated with autologous T cells expressing an anti-CD19 chimeric antigen receptor. J Clin Oncol 2015; 33(6): 540-9.
[http://dx.doi.org/10.1200/JCO.2014.56.2025] [PMID: 25154820]

[29]   Schultz L, Mackall C. Driving CAR T cell translation forward. Sci Transl Med 2019; 11(481): eaaw2127.
[http://dx.doi.org/10.1126/scitranslmed.aaw2127] [PMID: 30814337]

[30]   Yoshimoto R, Mayeda A, Yoshida M, Nakagawa S. MALAT1 long non-coding RNA in cancer. Biochim Biophys Acta Gene Regul Mech 2016; 1859(1): 192-9.
[http://dx.doi.org/10.1016/j.bbagrm.2015.09.012] [PMID: 26434412]

[31]   Tian X, Xu G. Clinical value of lncRNA MALAT1 as a prognostic marker in human cancer: systematic review and meta-analysis. BMJ Open 2015; 5(9): e008653.
[http://dx.doi.org/10.1136/bmjopen-2015-008653] [PMID: 26423854]

[32]   Wei Y, Niu B. Role of MALAT1 as a Prognostic Factor for Survival in Various Cancers: A Systematic Review of the Literature with Meta-Analysis 2015.
[http://dx.doi.org/10.1155/2015/164635]

[33]   Brüning-Richardson A, Bond J, Alsiary R, *et al.* NuMA overexpression in epithelial ovarian cancer. PLoS One 2012; 7(6): e38945.
[http://dx.doi.org/10.1371/journal.pone.0038945] [PMID: 22719996]

[34]   Quintyne NJ, Reing JE, Hoffelder DR, *et al.* Spindle multipolarity is prevented by centrosomal clustering 2005.
[http://dx.doi.org/10.1126/science.1104905]

[35]   O'Neill ID. New insights into the nature of Warthin's tumour. J Oral Pathol Med 2009; 38(1): 145-9.
[http://dx.doi.org/10.1111/j.1600-0714.2008.00676.x] [PMID: 18647217]

[36]   O'Neill ID. t(11;19) translocation and CRTC1-MAML2 fusion oncogene in mucoepidermoid carcinoma. Oral Oncol 2009; 45(1): 2-9.
[http://dx.doi.org/10.1016/j.oraloncology.2008.03.012] [PMID: 18486532]

[37]   Behboudi A, Enlund F, Winnes M, *et al.* Molecular classification of mucoepidermoid carcinomas—Prognostic significance of theMECT1-MAML2 fusion oncogene. Genes Chromosomes Cancer 2006; 45(5): 470-81.
[http://dx.doi.org/10.1002/gcc.20306] [PMID: 16444749]

[38]   Enlund F, Behboudi A, Andrén Y, *et al.* Altered Notch signaling resulting from expression of a WAMTP1-MAML2 gene fusion in mucoepidermoid carcinomas and benign Warthin's tumors. Exp Cell Res 2004; 292(1): 21-8.
[http://dx.doi.org/10.1016/j.yexcr.2003.09.007] [PMID: 14720503]

[39]   Tonon G, Modi S, Wu L, *et al.* t(11;19)(q21;p13) translocation in mucoepidermoid carcinoma creates a novel fusion product that disrupts a Notch signaling pathway. Nat Genet 2003; 33(2): 208-13.
[http://dx.doi.org/10.1038/ng1083] [PMID: 12539049]

[40]   Yassin ER, Sarma NJ, Abdul-Nabi AM, *et al.* Dissection of the transformation of primary human hematopoietic cells by the oncogene NUP98-HOXA9. PLoS One 2009; 4(8): e6719.
[http://dx.doi.org/10.1371/journal.pone.0006719] [PMID: 19696924]

[41]   Takeda A, Goolsby C, Yaseen NR. NUP98-HOXA9 induces long-term proliferation and blocks differentiation of primary human CD34+ hematopoietic cells. Cancer Res 2006; 66(13): 6628-37.
[http://dx.doi.org/10.1158/0008-5472.CAN-06-0458] [PMID: 16818636]

[42] Palmqvist L, Pineault N, Wasslavik C, Humphries RK. Candidate genes for expansion and transformation of hematopoietic stem cells by NUP98-HOX fusion genes. PLoS One 2007; 2(8): e768. [http://dx.doi.org/10.1371/journal.pone.0000768] [PMID: 17712416]

[43] Pineault N, Buske C, Feuring-Buske M, *et al.* Induction of acute myeloid leukemia in mice by the human leukemia-specific fusion gene NUP98-HOXD13 in concert with Meis1. Blood 2003; 101(11): 4529-38. [http://dx.doi.org/10.1182/blood-2002-08-2484] [PMID: 12543865]

[44] Jankovic D, Gorello P, Liu T, *et al.* Leukemogenic mechanisms and targets of a NUP98/HHEX fusion in acute myeloid leukemia. Blood 2008; 111(12): 5672-82. [http://dx.doi.org/10.1182/blood-2007-09-108175] [PMID: 18388181]

[45] Hirose K, Abramovich C, Argiropoulos B, Humphries RK. Leukemogenic properties of NUP98-PMX1 are linked to NUP98 and homeodomain sequence functions but not to binding properties of PMX1 to serum response factor. Oncogene 2008; 27(46): 6056-67. [http://dx.doi.org/10.1038/onc.2008.210] [PMID: 18604245]

[46] Wang GG, Cai L, Pasillas MP, Kamps MP. NUP98-NSD1 links H3K36 methylation to Hox-A gene activation and leukaemogenesis. Nat Cell Biol 2007; 9(7): 804-12. [http://dx.doi.org/10.1038/ncb1608] [PMID: 17589499]

[47] Duval S, Abu-Thuraia A, Elkholi IE, *et al.* Shedding of cancer susceptibility candidate 4 by the convertases PC7/furin unravels a novel secretory protein implicated in cancer progression. Cell Death Dis 2020; 11(8): 665. [http://dx.doi.org/10.1038/s41419-020-02893-0] [PMID: 32820145]

[48] Thien CBF, Langdon WY. Cbl: many adaptations to regulate protein tyrosine kinases. Nat Rev Mol Cell Biol 2001; 2(4): 294-307. [http://dx.doi.org/10.1038/35067100] [PMID: 11283727]

[49] Schmidt MHH, Dikic I. The Cbl interactome and its functions. Nat Rev Mol Cell Biol 2005; 6(12): 907-19. [http://dx.doi.org/10.1038/nrm1762] [PMID: 16227975]

[50] Kumaradevan S, Lee SY, Richards S, *et al.* c-Cbl Expression Correlates with Human Colorectal Cancer Survival and Its Wnt/β-Catenin Suppressor Function Is Regulated by Tyr371 Phosphorylation. Am J Pathol 2018; 188(8): 1921-33. [http://dx.doi.org/10.1016/j.ajpath.2018.05.007] [PMID: 30029779]

[51] Shashar M, Siwak J, Tapan U, *et al.* c-Cbl mediates the degradation of tumorigenic nuclear β-catenin contributing to the heterogeneity in Wnt activity in colorectal tumors. Oncotarget 2016; 7(44): 71136-50. [http://dx.doi.org/10.18632/oncotarget.12107] [PMID: 27661103]

[52] Chitalia V, Shivanna S, Martorell J, Meyer R, Edelman E, Rahimi N. c-Cbl, a ubiquitin E3 ligase that targets active β-catenin: a novel layer of Wnt signaling regulation. J Biol Chem 2013; 288(32): 23505-17. [http://dx.doi.org/10.1074/jbc.M113.473801] [PMID: 23744067]

[53] Perez OD, Mitchell D, Campos R, *et al.* Multiparameter analysis of intracellular phosphoepitopes in immunophenotyped cell populations by flow cytometry. 2005. [http://dx.doi.org/10.1002/0471142956.cy0620s32]

[54] Thompson WR, Yen SS, Uzer G, *et al.* LARG GEF and ARHGAP18 orchestrate RhoA activity to control mesenchymal stem cell lineage. Bone 2018; 107: 172-80. [http://dx.doi.org/10.1016/j.bone.2017.12.001] [PMID: 29208526]

[55] Abiko H, Fujiwara S, Ohashi K, *et al.* Rho-guanine nucleotide exchange factors involved in cyclic stretch-induced reorientation of vascular endothelial cells. J Cell Sci 2015; 128(9): jcs.157503. [http://dx.doi.org/10.1242/jcs.157503] [PMID: 25795300]

[56] Shi GX, Yang WS, Jin L, Matter ML, Ramos JW. RSK2 drives cell motility by serine phosphorylation of LARG and activation of Rho GTPases. Proc Natl Acad Sci USA 2018; 115(2): E190-9.
[http://dx.doi.org/10.1073/pnas.1708584115] [PMID: 29279389]

[57] Lee CK, Lee JH, Lee MG, *et al.* Epigenetic inactivation of the NORE1gene correlates with malignant progression of colorectal tumors. BMC cancer. 2010; 10(1): 1-5.

[58] Calvisi DF, Ladu S, Gorden A, *et al.* Ubiquitous activation of Ras and Jak/Stat pathways in human HCC. Gastroenterology 2006; 130(4): 1117-28.
[http://dx.doi.org/10.1053/j.gastro.2006.01.006] [PMID: 16618406]

[59] Reuvers JRD, van Dorp M, Van Schil PE. Solitary fibrous tumor of the pleura with associated Doege-Potter syndrome. Acta Chir Belg 2016; 116(6): 386-7.
[http://dx.doi.org/10.1080/00015458.2016.1171079] [PMID: 27376978]

[60] He J, Zhang A, Fang M, *et al.* Methylation levels at IGF2 and GNAS DMRs in infants born to preeclamptic pregnancies. BMC Genomics 2013; 14(1): 472.
[http://dx.doi.org/10.1186/1471-2164-14-472] [PMID: 23844573]

[61] Candoni A, Toffoletti E, Gallina R, *et al.* Monitoring of minimal residual disease by quantitative WT1 gene expression following reduced intensity conditioning allogeneic stem cell transplantation in acute myeloid leukemia. Clin Transplant 2011; 25(2): 308-16.
[http://dx.doi.org/10.1111/j.1399-0012.2010.01251.x] [PMID: 20412098]

[62] Halachmi S. Wilms' tumor. Harefuah 2003; 142: 438-441, 485.

[63] Chiosea SI, Williams L, Griffith CC, *et al.* Molecular characterization of apocrine salivary duct carcinoma. Am J Surg Pathol 2015; 39(6): 744-52.
[http://dx.doi.org/10.1097/PAS.0000000000000410] [PMID: 25723113]

[64] Aiello KA, Alter O. Platform-independent genome-wide pattern of DNA copy-number alterations predicting astrocytoma survival and response to treatment revealed by the GSVD formulated as a comparative spectral decomposition. PLoS One 2016; 11(10): e0164546.
[http://dx.doi.org/10.1371/journal.pone.0164546] [PMID: 27798635]

[65] Chandrasekharappa SC, Guru SC, Manickam P, *et al.* Positional cloning of the gene for multiple endocrine neoplasia-type 1. Science (80-) 1997; 276: 404–406.

[66] Y. J, C. S, B.H. E, *et al.* DAXX/ATRX, MEN1, and mTOR pathway genes are frequently altered in pancreatic neuroendocrine tumors. Science (80-) 2011; 331: 1199–1203.

[67] Banin S, Shieh SY, Taya Y, *et al.* Enhanced Phosphorylation of p53 by ATM in Response to DNA Damage 1998.
[http://dx.doi.org/10.1126/science.281.5383.1674]

[68] Canman CE, Lim DS. The role of ATM in DNA damage responses and cancer. Oncogene 1998; 17(25): 3301-8.
[http://dx.doi.org/10.1038/sj.onc.1202577] [PMID: 9916992]

[69] Hao HX, Khalimonchuk O, Schraders M, *et al.* SDH5, a gene required for flavination of succinate dehydrogenase, is mutated in paraganglioma 2009.
[http://dx.doi.org/10.1126/science.1175689]

[70] Kugelberg J, Welander J, Schiavi F, *et al.* Role of SDHAF2 and SDHD *in von* Hippel-Lindau associated pheochromocytomas. World J Surg 2014; 38(3): 724-32.
[http://dx.doi.org/10.1007/s00268-013-2373-2] [PMID: 24322175]

[71] Bayley JP, Kunst HPM, Cascon A, *et al.* SDHAF2 mutations in familial and sporadic paraganglioma and phaeochromocytoma. Lancet Oncol 2010; 11(4): 366-72.
[http://dx.doi.org/10.1016/S1470-2045(10)70007-3] [PMID: 20071235]

[72] Yin B, Ma ZY, Zhou ZW, *et al.* The TrkB+ cancer stem cells contribute to post-chemotherapy recurrence of triple-negative breast cancers in an orthotopic mouse model. Oncogene 2015; 34(6):

761-70.
[http://dx.doi.org/10.1038/onc.2014.8] [PMID: 24531713]

[73] Lawn S, Krishna N, Pisklakova A, *et al*. Neurotrophin signaling *via* TrkB and TrkC receptors promotes the growth of brain tumor-initiating cells. J Biol Chem 2015; 290(6): 3814-24.
[http://dx.doi.org/10.1074/jbc.M114.599373] [PMID: 25538243]

[74] Zhang S yang, Hui L ping, Li C yan, *et al*. More expression of BDNF associates with lung squamous cell carcinoma and is critical to the proliferation and invasion of lung cancer cells. BMC Cancer; 16. Epub ahead of print 2016.
[http://dx.doi.org/10.1186/s12885-016-2218-0]

[75] Quere R, Andradottir S, Brun A, *et al*. High Levels of the Adhesion Molecule CD44 on Leukemic Cells Generate Acute Myeloid Leukemia Relapse After Withdrawal of the Initial Transforming Event. Blood 2010; 116(21): 3154-4.
[http://dx.doi.org/10.1182/blood.V116.21.3154.3154] [PMID: 21116281]

[76] Eibl RH, Pietsch T, Moll J, *et al*. Expression of variant CD44 epitopes in human astrocytic brain tumors. J Neurooncol 1995; 26(3): 165-70.
[http://dx.doi.org/10.1007/BF01052619] [PMID: 8750182]

[77] Yang YG, Sari IN, Zia MF, Lee SR, Song SJ, Kwon HY. Tetraspanins: Spanning from solid tumors to hematologic malignancies. Exp Hematol 2016; 44(5): 322-8.
[http://dx.doi.org/10.1016/j.exphem.2016.02.006] [PMID: 26930362]

[78] You J, Madigan MC, Rowe A, Sajinovic M, Russell PJ, Jackson P. An inverse relationship between KAI1 expression, invasive ability, and MMP-2 expression and activity in bladder cancer cell lines. Urol Oncol 2012; 30(4): 502-8.
[http://dx.doi.org/10.1016/j.urolonc.2010.02.013] [PMID: 20864363]

[79] Richardson MM, Jennings LK, Zhang XA. Tetraspanins and tumor progression. Clin Exp Metastasis 2011; 28(3): 261-70.
[http://dx.doi.org/10.1007/s10585-010-9365-5] [PMID: 21184145]

[80] Christgen M, Christgen H, Heil C, *et al*. Expression of KAI1/CD82 in distant metastases from estrogen receptor-negative breast cancer. Cancer Sci 2009; 100(9): 1767-71.
[http://dx.doi.org/10.1111/j.1349-7006.2009.01231.x] [PMID: 19549254]

[81] Miranti CK. Controlling cell surface dynamics and signaling: How CD82/KAI1 suppresses metastasis. Cell Signal 2009; 21(2): 196-211.
[http://dx.doi.org/10.1016/j.cellsig.2008.08.023] [PMID: 18822372]

[82] Juhasz A, Ge Y, Markel S, *et al*. Expression of NADPH oxidase homologues and accessory genes in human cancer cell lines, tumours and adjacent normal tissues. Free Radic Res 2009; 43(6): 523-32.
[http://dx.doi.org/10.1080/10715760902918683] [PMID: 19431059]

[83] Mitsushita J, Lambeth JD, Kamata T. The superoxide-generating oxidase Nox1 is functionally required for Ras oncogene transformation. Cancer Res 2004; 64(10): 3580-5.
[http://dx.doi.org/10.1158/0008-5472.CAN-03-3909] [PMID: 15150115]

[84] Brar SS, Corbin Z, Kennedy TP, *et al*. NOX5 NAD(P)H oxidase regulates growth and apoptosis in DU 145 prostate cancer cells. Am J Physiol Cell Physiol 2003; 285(2): C353-69.
[http://dx.doi.org/10.1152/ajpcell.00525.2002] [PMID: 12686516]

[85] Zhang Y, Hunter T. Roles of Chk1 in cell biology and cancer therapy. Int J Cancer 2014; 134(5): 1013-23.
[http://dx.doi.org/10.1002/ijc.28226] [PMID: 23613359]

[86] Roy J, Putt KS, Coppola D, *et al*. Assessment of cholecystokinin 2 receptor (CCK2R) in neoplastic tissue. Oncotarget 2016; 7(12): 14605-15.
[http://dx.doi.org/10.18632/oncotarget.7522] [PMID: 26910279]

[87] Davis FM, Peters AA, Grice DM, *et al*. Non-stimulated, agonist-stimulated and store-operated Ca^{2+}

influx in MDA-MB-468 breast cancer cells and the effect of EGF-induced EMT on calcium entry. PLoS One 2012; 7(5): e36923.
[http://dx.doi.org/10.1371/journal.pone.0036923] [PMID: 22666335]

[88] Yu F, Ng SSM, Chow BKC, *et al.* Knockdown of interferon-induced transmembrane protein 1 (IFITM1) inhibits proliferation, migration, and invasion of glioma cells. J Neurooncol 2011; 103(2): 187-95.
[http://dx.doi.org/10.1007/s11060-010-0377-4] [PMID: 20838853]

[89] Patel SP, Bristol A, Saric O, *et al.* Anti-tumor activity of a novel monoclonal antibody, NPC-1C, optimized for recognition of tumor antigen MUC5AC variant in preclinical models. Cancer Immunol Immunother 2013; 62(6): 1011-9.
[http://dx.doi.org/10.1007/s00262-013-1420-z] [PMID: 23591984]

[90] García EP, Tiscornia I, Libisch G, *et al.* MUC5B silencing reduces chemo-resistance of MCF-7 breast tumor cells and impairs maturation of dendritic cells. Int J Oncol 2016; 48(5): 2113-23.
[http://dx.doi.org/10.3892/ijo.2016.3434] [PMID: 26984395]

[91] Tokuhara T, Hasegawa H, Hattori N, *et al.* Clinical significance of CD151 gene expression in non-small cell lung cancer. Clin Cancer Res 2001; 7(12): 4109-14.
[PMID: 11751509]

[92] Hashida H, Takabayashi A, Tokuhara T, *et al.* Clinical significance of transmembrane 4 superfamily in colon cancer. Br J Cancer 2003; 89(1): 158-67.
[http://dx.doi.org/10.1038/sj.bjc.6601015] [PMID: 12838318]

[93] Zou J, Zhu L, Jiang X, *et al.* Curcumin increases breast cancer cell sensitivity to cisplatin by decreasing FEN1 expression. Oncotarget 2018; 9(13): 11268-78.
[http://dx.doi.org/10.18632/oncotarget.24109] [PMID: 29541412]

[94] Pandini G, Conte E, Medico E, Sciacca L, Vigneri R, Belfiore A. IGF-II binding to insulin receptor isoform A induces a partially different gene expression profile from insulin binding. Ann N Y Acad Sci 2004; 1028(1): 450-6.
[http://dx.doi.org/10.1196/annals.1322.053] [PMID: 15650270]

[95] Kalim KW, Basler M, Kirk CJ, Groettrup M. Immunoproteasome subunit LMP7 deficiency and inhibition suppresses Th1 and Th17 but enhances regulatory T cell differentiation. J Immunol 2012; 189(8): 4182-93.
[http://dx.doi.org/10.4049/jimmunol.1201183] [PMID: 22984077]

[96] Wright CM, Savarimuthu Francis SM, Tan ME, *et al.* MS4A1 dysregulation in asbestos-related lung squamous cell carcinoma is due to CD20 stromal lymphocyte expression. PLoS One 2012; 7(4): e34943.
[http://dx.doi.org/10.1371/journal.pone.0034943] [PMID: 22514692]

[97] Li Q, Yang XH, Xu F, *et al.* Tetraspanin CD151 plays a key role in skin squamous cell carcinoma. Oncogene 2013; 32(14): 1772-83.
[http://dx.doi.org/10.1038/onc.2012.205] [PMID: 22824799]

[98] Voss MA, Gordon N, Maloney S, *et al.* Tetraspanin CD151 is a novel prognostic marker in poor outcome endometrial cancer. Br J Cancer 2011; 104(10): 1611-8.
[http://dx.doi.org/10.1038/bjc.2011.80] [PMID: 21505452]

[99] Suzuki S, Miyazaki T, Tanaka N, *et al.* Prognostic significance of CD151 expression in esophageal squamous cell carcinoma with aggressive cell proliferation and invasiveness. Ann Surg Oncol 2011; 18(3): 888-93.
[http://dx.doi.org/10.1245/s10434-010-1387-3] [PMID: 20978946]

[100] Zhu GH, Huang C, Qiu ZJ, *et al.* Expression and prognostic significance of CD151, c-Met, and integrin alpha3/alpha6 in pancreatic ductal adenocarcinoma. Dig Dis Sci 2011; 56(4): 1090-8.
[http://dx.doi.org/10.1007/s10620-010-1416-x] [PMID: 20927591]

[101] Maynadier M, Farnoud R, Lamy PJ, Laurent-Matha V, Garcia M, Rochefort H. Cathepsin D stimulates the activities of secreted plasminogen activators in the breast cancer acidic environment. Int J Oncol 2013; 43(5): 1683-90.
[http://dx.doi.org/10.3892/ijo.2013.2095] [PMID: 24026424]

[102] Liaudet-Coopman E, Beaujouin M, Derocq D, *et al.* Cathepsin D: newly discovered functions of a long-standing aspartic protease in cancer and apoptosis. Cancer Lett 2006; 237(2): 167-79.
[http://dx.doi.org/10.1016/j.canlet.2005.06.007] [PMID: 16046058]

[103] Shen D, Chang HR, Chen Z, *et al.* Loss of annexin A1 expression in human breast cancer detected by multiple high-throughput analyses. Biochem Biophys Res Commun 2004; 326(1): 218-27.
[http://dx.doi.org/10.1016/j.bbrc.2004.10.214] [PMID: 15567174]

[104] G. P, A. B, S. B, *et al.* Interleukin 18: Friend or foe in cancer. Biochim Biophys Acta - Rev Cancer 2013; 1836: 296–303.

[105] Sachlos E, Risueño RM, Laronde S, *et al.* Identification of drugs including a dopamine receptor antagonist that selectively target cancer stem cells. Cell 2012; 149(6): 1284-97.
[http://dx.doi.org/10.1016/j.cell.2012.03.049] [PMID: 22632761]

[106] Kho AT, Zhao Q, Cai Z, *et al.* Conserved mechanisms across development and tumorigenesis revealed by a mouse development perspective of human cancers. Genes Dev 2004; 18(6): 629-40.
[http://dx.doi.org/10.1101/gad.1182504] [PMID: 15075291]

[107] Gong W, Zheng J, Liu X, *et al.* Knockdown of long non-coding RNA KCNQ1OT1 restrained glioma cell's malignancy by activating miR-370/CCNE2 Axis. Front Cell Neurosci 2017; 11: 84.
[http://dx.doi.org/10.3389/fncel.2017.00084] [PMID: 28381990]

CHAPTER 12

Chromosome 12

Yamini Chandraprakash[1], **Ravi Gor**[1], **Saurav Panicker**[1] and **Satish Ramalingam**[1,*]

[1] *Department of Genetic Engineering, School of Bioengineering, SRM Institute of Science and Technology, Kattankulathur, India*

Abstract: Chromosome 12 spans about 134 million DNA building blocks and represents approximately 4.5 percent of the total cellular DNA. Gene dysregulation from chromosome 12 has triggered a cell to transform into a cancerous cell. Different types of genes are present in chromosome 12 that cause colon cancer, ovarian cancer, prostate cancer, ampulla of Vater cancer (Vater cancer), *etc.* These genes play their role in the development and the progression of cancer into metastasis, Epithelial to mesenchymal transition, and overall cancer growth. In this chapter, we have enlisted the genes responsible for cancer and their short introduction.

Keywords: Cancer, Cancerous Cell, Colon Cancer, Cancer Growth, Downregulated, Epithelial-Mesenchymal, Gene Dysregulation, Metastasis, Ovarian Cancer, Prostate Cancer.

1.1. A2M – ALPHA-2-MACROGLOBULIN, CHROMOSOME 12; 12p13.31

The protein encoded by this gene is a protease inhibitor and cytokine transporter. It uses a bait-and-trap mechanism to inhibit a broad spectrum of proteases, including trypsin, thrombin and collagenase. Downregulated DEGs of *A2M* were significantly associated with the "Complement and coagulation cascades" pathway and the "Ras signaling pathway." Downregulated A2M might contribute to the progression of Bladder Cancer [1]. *A2M* out of the seven predicted gene markers was found to encode proteins secreted into urine, providing potential diagnostic evidence for pancreatic cancer [2].

---

* **Corresponding author Satish Ramalingam**: Department of Genetic Engineering, SRM Institute of Science and Technology, Kattankulathur, India; E-mail: rsatish76@gmail.com

1.2. A2LM1 - ALPHA 2 MICROGLOBULIN LIKE 1 CHROMOSOME 12; 12p13.31

A2ML1, which are under-expressed in the ER+ group and over-expressed in the ER− group. *A2ML1* which encodes the secreted protease inhibitor α-2-M [A2M]-, like-1 activates mutations in signal transducers of the RAS/mitogen-activated protein kinase [MAPK] pathway [3].

1.3. AACS-ACETOACETYL-COA SYNTHETASE CHROMOSOME 12; 12q24.31

Acetoacetyl-CoA synthetase [AACS] is the enzyme responsible for cholesterol and fatty acid synthesis in the cytosol. *AACS* dysregulation by Sp1 has been reported in neuroblastoma cell lines. AACS gene has been reported in Vater cancer. A small opening connecting the pancreas and bile ducts to the duodenum is called the ampulla of Vater. Mutation in the *AACS* gene (Fig. **1**) causes cancer in this Ampulla of Vater. AACS protein is related to Valine, isoleucine, and leucine degradation pathways. AACS protein is also linked to Ketone body metabolism [4].

1.4. ABCB9 - ATP-BINDING CASSETTE, SUBFAMILY B, MEMBER 9 CHROMOSOME 12; 12q24.31

Paclitaxel is widely used in treating breast cancer; drug resistance increases the failure of chemotherapy. Using microRNA target prediction tools, they have identified that *ABCB9* could be one of the target genes of miR-24. miR-24 can also affect the expression of *ABCB9* to regulate the sensitivity toward paclitaxel of breast cancer cells. It was identified that miR-24 could directly bind to the 3′-UTR of ABCB9, thereby inhibiting the translation of *ABCB9* [5].

1.5. ABCC9 - ATP-BINDING CASSETTE, SUBFAMILY C, MEMBER 9 CHROMOSOME 12; 12p12.1

ABC transporters play a major role in prostate cancer [PCa] development, and the *ABC* transporter gene expression was analyzed in PCa and noncancerous prostate tissues [NPT]. ABCA8, ABCB1, ABCC6, ABCC9, ABCC10, ABCD2, ABCG2, and ABCG4 expression of eight ABC transporter genes were down-regulated in the absence of the TMPRSS2- ERG fusion transcript Prostate cancer [PCa] as compared to Noncancerous prostate tissue [NPT], and only two genes [*ABCC4* and *ABCG1*] were up-regulated [6].

1.6. ABCD2 - ATP-BINDING CASSETTE, SUBFAMILY 3, MEMBER 2 CHROMOSOME 12; 12q12

X-linked adrenoleukodystrophy [X-ALD] is a peroxisomal disorder which is caused by mutations in the *ABCD1* gene that encodes the peroxisomal ATP-binding cassette [ABC] transporter subfamily D member 1 protein [ABCD1], which is also referred to as the adrenoleukodystrophy protein [ALDP]. Induction of the *ABCD2* gene, which is closest to ABCD*1*, has a possible therapeutic option for the defective ABCD1 protein in X-ALD. X-ALD is caused by mutations that occurred in the *ABCD1* gene, which is also associated with the accumulation of VLCFAs [Very Long Chain Fatty Acids] in the plasma and tissues of the patients, Induction of *ABCD2* can be a better treatment option for X-ALD because expression of this protein can decrease VLCFAs [Very Long Chain Fatty Acids] levels in fibroblasts [7].

1.7. ACRBP - ACROSIN-BINDING PROTEIN CHROMOSOME 12; 12P13-p 12

Myxoid and round cell liposarcoma are formed in soft and fat tissues. Cancertestis antigens are immunogenic antigens that have an expression restricted to testicular germ cells and malignancies, making them attractive targets for cancer immunotherapy. Gene expression studies reported that expression of various cancer-testis antigens in liposarcoma, with mRNA expression of CTAG1B, CTA-G2, MAGEA9, and PRAME, are described in myxoid and round-cell liposarcoma. Overexpression of *NY-ESO-1* in myxoid and round cell liposarcoma, the expression of cancer-testis antigens evaluated are MAGEA1, ACRBP, PRAME, SSX2, and by immunohistochemistry and PRAME, CTAG2, and MAGEA3 by quantitative real-time PCR [8].

1.8. ACSS3 - ACYL-COA SYNTHETASE SHORT CHAIN FAMILY, MEMBER 3CHROMOSOME 12; 12q21.31

Gastric cancer [GCa] is one of leading cancer in humans. Mitochondrial-derived acetyl-CoA contributing enzymes [acyl-coA synthetase super-family 3; ACSS3] are patient's progression of Gastric Cancer [GCa]. Cholesterol is an essential component for fast-growing cancer cells. The mevalonate pathway is an enzymatic cascade that is responsible for de novo cholesterogenesis. *ACSS3* is a landmark cancer progression gene in Gastric Cancer [GCa] patients, which is part of the biochemical process for the mitochondrial production of acetyl-CoA [9].

1.9. ACTR6 - ACTIN RELATED PROTEIN 6 CHROMOSOME 12; 12q23.1

Testicular Germ Cell Tumors [TGCTs] are the most common neoplasm among young adult Caucasian men; Research is done on the role of DNA methyl-transferases [*DNMTs*] and DNA demethylases [*TETs*]. DNA and Histone Modi-fying Enzymes and Chromatin Remodelling Complexes cause Testicular Germ Cell Tumors [TGCTs]. The most commonly deregulated enzyme is *ARP6/ACTR6,* and there were no significant co-occurrent or mutually exclusive pairs [10].

1.10. ACVR1B - ACTIVIN A RECEPTOR, TYPE IB CHROMOSOME 12; 12q13.13

Pancreatic Cancer is one of the leading cancers in the Pancreatic region. Four genes were analyzed MAP2K4; 4, MADH4 [SMAD4/DAC4], ACVR1B, and BRCA2. Each tumor suppressor gene is known to undergo germ-line or somatic genetic inactivation in sporadic pancreatic cancer. Somatic gene mutations in ACVR1B have been seen in pancreatic tumors, which cause Pancreatic Cancer [11].

1.11. ACVRL1 - ACTIVIN A RECEPTOR, TYPE II-LIKE 1 CHROMOSOME 12;12q13.13

Metastatic colorectal cancer is one cancer that occurs in the colon region; the ACVRL1 gene encodes for the ALK1, which is also a member of the TGF-b receptor family and involves in pathologic angiogenesis. *ACVRL1* gene expression is a prognostic biomarker for metastatic colorectal cancer patients receiving bevacizumab-based chemotherapy [12] (Fig. **1**).

1.12. ADCY6 - ADENYLATE CYCLASE 6 CHROMOSOME 12; 12q13.12

Breast cancer is a malignant tumor that occurs commonly in Females and rarely in Males. DNA methylation, gene expression profile, and the tumor-immune microenvironment of luminal-like breast cancer are identified and studied. The protein-protein interaction [PPI] network was constructed by the String database and Cytoscape software. DNA methylation regulated the cellular pathways of luminal-like breast cancer immune cell infiltration. And ADCY6 was found as a part to be a prognostic factor in the DNA methylation-regulated immune pro-cesses in luminal-like breast cancer [13].

1.13. ADGRD1 - ADHESION G PROTEIN-COUPLED RECEPTOR D1 CHROMOSOME 12; 12q24.33

Metastatic growth is a rate-limiting step in cancer progression; metastatic growth requires a supportive microenvironment, the extracellular matrix [ECM]. *ADGRG1* is downregulated in metastatic melanoma and inhibits the growth and metastasis of the human melanoma cell line, MC-1. ADGRG1 does not affect the formation of lung micrometastases but inhibits the expansion of micrometastases into macro metastases. *ADGRG1* is downregulated in metastatic melanoma cells, so the expression levels in metastases serve as a prognostic marker for the metastatic potential of the tumors [14].

1.14. ADIPOR2 - ADIPONECTIN RECEPTOR 2 CHROMOSOME 12;12 p13.33

Adiponectin is a hormone in the human plasma. It is present in a decreased amount in patients with cancer, which results in adiposity carcinogenesis, and this is mostly seen in Gastric cancer. They bind to receptors like ADIPOR1 and ADIPOR2, which causes the progression of Gastric cancer [15] (Fig. **1**).

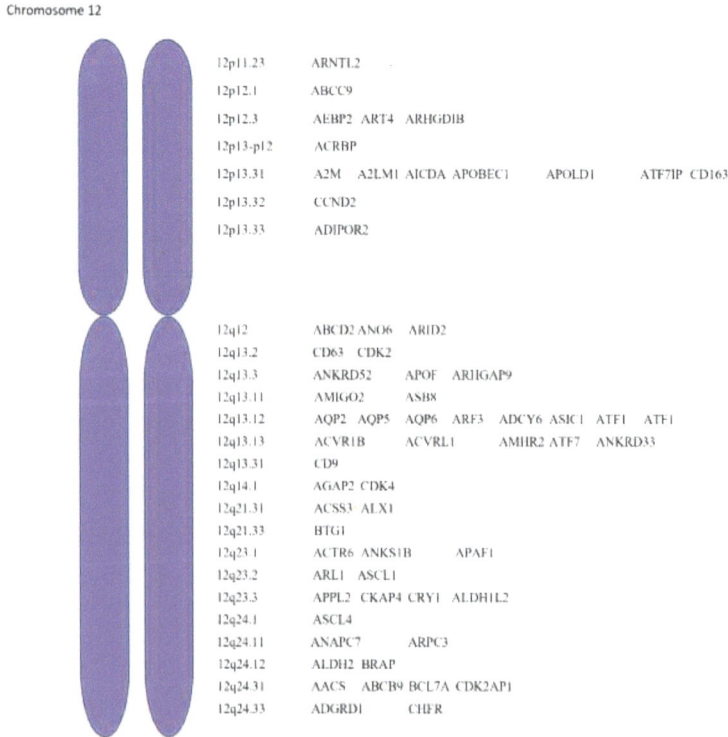

Fig. (1). This figure displays the loci of the genes from Chromosome 12 whose roles in cancer have been explained in this chapter. Sayooj Madhusoodanan designed this diagram.

1.15. AEBP2 - AE-BINDING PROTEIN 2 CHROMOSOME 12; 12p12.3

The Polycomb group proteins [PcGs] are important regulators of epigenetic changes in living species. The Polycomb-repressive complex 2 subunits [EZH2] affect the expression of protein-coding genes, form feedback network and autoregulatory loops, form networks with important upstream and downstream factors, and stabilizes the factor of the pathway. And these non-coding RNAs affect the epigenetic modifications, which lead to malignant transformation. AEBP2 (Fig. **1**) are cofactors and PRC2 enzymatic activity modulators. MicroRNAs [miRNAs] and Long non-coding RNAs [lncRNAs] are involved in cellular homeostasis affecting cell proliferation, cell growth, differentiation, and apoptosis. At the same time, their disruption leads to malignant transformation of the cells [16].

1.16. AGAP2 - ARF GTPASE-ACTIVATING PROTEIN WITH GTPASE DOMAIN, ANKYRIN REPEAT, AND PLECKSTRIN HOMOLOGY DOMAIN 2 CHROMOSOME 12; 12q14.1

Long noncoding RNAs [lncRNAs] are essential regulators of tumorigenesis and cancer progression. *AGAP2-AS1* is identified as an oncogenic Long noncoding RNA [lncRNA] in human non-small cell lung cancer [NSCLC], and higher expression will lead to human non-small cell lung cancer [NSCLC] development and progression. *AGAP2-AS1* upregulated by SP1 plays a major role in Gastric Cancer [GC] development and progression and suppressing P21 and E-cadherin. *AGAP2-AS1* is a potential diagnostic marker and therapeutic target for Gastric Cancer [GC] patients [17].

1.17. AICDA - ACTIVATION-INDUCED CYTIDINE DEAMINASE CHROMOSOME 12; 12p13.31

Lung cancer is commonly treated with EGFR Tyrosine Kinase Inhibitors [TKI] and develops resistance to this treatment. A single base transition mutation of the *EGFR T790M* at position c.2369 is the most frequent resistance to EGFR Tyrosine Kinase Inhibitors [TKI]. Treatment with EGFR Tyrosine Kinase Inhibitors [TKI] leads to the activation of the NFκB pathway, which induces the expression of Activation Induced Cytidine Deaminase [AICDA]. Activation Induced Cytidine Deaminase [AICDA] causes the deamination of 5-methylcytosine to thymine at position c.2369 to generate the *T790M* mutation. The patients who are treated with first-line EGFR Tyrosine Kinase Inhibitors [TKI] show an increased expression of Activation Induced Cytidine Deaminase [AICDA] and detection of the T790M mutation upon progression [18].

1.18. ALDH1L2 - ALDEHYDE DEHYDROGENASE 1 FAMILY, MEMBER L2 CHROMOSOME 12; 12q23.3

Folate plays an important role in one-carbon metabolism and is needed for methylation reactions, nucleotide synthesis, and DNA repair. The expression of three mitochondrial folate metabolic enzymes, Serine Hydroxyethyl Transferase [SHMT2], Methylene Tetra Hydro Folate Dehydrogenase [MTHFD2], and Aldehyde Dehydrogenase 1 family member L2 [ALDH1L2], are upregulated in Human Colorectal Tumour tissues compared to normal tissues. Rates of recurrence-free survival [RFS] and overall survival [OS]. The expression levels of the mitochondrial folate metabolic enzymes, such as Serine Hydroxyethyl Transferase [SHMT2], Methylene Tetra Hydro Folate Dehydrogenase [MTHFD2], and Aldehyde Dehydrogenase 1 family member L2 [ALDH1L2], was upregulated in humans, Colorectal Tumor tissues were seen in patients [19].

1.19. ALDH2 - ALDEHYDE DEHYDROGENASE 2 FAMILY CHROMOSOME 12;12q24.12

ALDH2 is involved in oesophageal cancer in humans, ALDH2 genes form an inactive subunit that inactivates the protein, which is unable the metabolization of acetaldehyde, and these are seen in alcohol consumption patients, first due to alcohol, there is a high risk of cancer and secondly the changes in the acetaldehyde levels, thus involve the formation of oesophageal cancer in humans [20].

1.20. ALX1 - ARISTALESS-LIKE HOMEOBOX 1 CHROMOSOME 12; 12q21.31

Ovarian cancer is one of the highly metastatic cancers, Epithelial-to-Mesenchymal Transition [EMT] is a complex multi-step process that occurs during embryonic development, tumor progression, and tissue fibrosis. During this Epithelial-to-Mesenchymal Transition [EMT] process, the Epithelial cells will lose many of their epithelial characteristics mesenchymal-like cells, and have mesenchymal characteristics, such as increased motility and invasiveness. Epithelial-to-Mesenchymal Transition [EMT] is triggered by extracellular stimuli, such as TGF-b, fibroblast growth factor, hepatocyte growth factor, and endothelin-1. The signaling pathways activated by these factors will induce changes in cytoskeletal organization and disrupt the cell-cell junctions. Snail is a zinc-finger transcription factor that binds to the E-box sequences which are present in the promoter regions of the target genes. siRNA screening was done, and they found that Aristaless-like homeobox1 [ALX1], also known as Cart1 is an important factor for inducing the morphologic changes in ovarian cancer cells. Aristaless-like homeobox1 [ALX1] induces Epithelial-to-Mesenchymal Transition [EMT] and cell invasion in ovarian cancer cells by promoting the expression of Snails [21] (Fig. **1**).

1.21. AMHR2 - ANTI-MULLERIAN HORMONE TYPE II RECEPTOR CHROMOSOME 12; 12q13.13

Lung cancer is one of the leading cancers; in Non-Small Cell Lung Cancer [NSCLC], the molecular chaperone Heat Shock Protein 90 [HSP90] helps to act against the high rates of protein misfolding, clusters of rapidly and abnormally proliferating cells. Heat Shock Protein 90 [HSP90] binds and activates the proteins, including EGFR, ERBB2/HER2, c-MET, RAF, EML4-ALK, and SRC family kinases which involves in the oncogenic and drug resistance pathways. Anti-Mullerian hormone [AMH] and its type II receptor, AMHR2, are involved in potent regulators of transforming growth factor [TGF-b]/bone morphogenetic protein [BMP] signaling and Epithelial-Mesenchymal Transition [EMT] in lung cancer and influences BMP-dependent signaling in Non-Small Cell Lung Cancer [NSCLC]. *AMH* and *AMHR2* are selectively expressed in epithelial *versus* mesenchymal cells, and loss of expression in AMH/AMHR2 induces Epithelial-Mesenchymal Transition [EMT] [22].

1.22. AMIGO2 - ADHESION MOLECULE WITH IG-LIKE DOMAIN 2 CHROMOSOME 12; 12q13.11

Human Gastric Adeno carcinomas [AGS] are found in the stomach in humans; AMIGO2 is a leucine-rich repeat-containing cell adhesion molecule implicated in axon tract development. Stable expression of a DEGA/AMIGO-2 antisense which is constructed in the gastric adenocarcinoma cell line [AGS], leads to altered morphology, increased ploidy, chromosomal instability, decreased cell adhesion, and migration. This involves the potential role of DEGA/AMIGO-2 in gastric adenocarcinoma [23].

1.23. ANAPC7 - ANAPHASE-PROMOTING COMPLEX, SUBUNIT 7 CHROMOSOME 12; 12q24.11

Acute myeloid leukemia [AML] is a type of cancer that occurs in blood; Circular RNAs [circRNAs] are a family of novel non-coding RNAs which involves in cancer and have a regulatory role for protein-coding genes in the tumorigenesis, maintenance, and progression of Acute myeloid leukemia [AML], circ-*ANAPC7* is a promising biomarker for Acute myeloid leukemia [AML], which involves in the pathogenesis of AML by acting as a sponge for the miR-181 family [24].

1.24. ANKRD33 - ANKYRIN REPEAT DOMAIN 33 CHROMOSOME 12; 12q13.13

Gastric cancer is the fourth most common cancer in the world; Ankyrin Repeat Domain 33 [*ANKRD33*] is a gene encoding an ankyrin repeat-containing protein, that functions as a repressor for transcription of CRX-regulated photoreceptor genes. The ankyrin repeat was found in signaling proteins Cdc10, and Drosophila Notch in yeast. Expression of Ankyrin Repeat Domain 33 [*ANKRD33*] in gastric adenocarcinoma was upregulated and compared to that in normal tissues, indicating that Ankyrin Repeat Domain 33 [*ANKRD33*] can be a promoter in gastric adenocarcinoma development. Knockdown of Ankyrin Repeat Domain 33 [*ANKRD33*] suppressed the proliferation and migration of gastric adenocarcinoma cells by modulating the PI3K signaling pathway. Ankyrin Repeat Domain 33 [ANKRD33] acts as a promising biomarker for gastric adenocarcinoma diagnosis and treatment [25].

1.25. ANKRD52 - ANKYRIN REPEAT DOMAIN 52 CHROMOSOME 12; 12q13.3

Ankyrin repeat domain 52 [ANKRD52] has been involved in the regulation of lung adenocarcinoma metastasis. Ankyrin repeat proteins have a function for protein-protein interactions, and Ankyrin repeat domain 52 [ANKRD52] interacts with protein phosphatase 6 [PP6]. Immunohistochemistry staining in lung cancer tissue shows prolonged disease-free survival in the high Ankyrin repeat domain 52 [*ANKRD52*] expressing cases. In Lung cancer cell lines, Ankyrin repeat domain 52 [*ANKRD52*] knockdowns show increased cell mobility, while forced expressed Ankyrin repeat domain 52 [*ANKRD52*] shows decreased cell mobility. Mass spectrometry analysis shows that p21-activated kinases [PAK1] were found to interact with Ankyrin repeat domain 52 [ANKRD52] [26].

1.26. ANKS1B - ANKYRIN REPEAT AND STERILE ALPHA MOTIF DOMAINS-CONTAINING PROTEIN 1B CHROMOSOME 12;12q23.1

Cigarette smoking is involved in the development of clear cell renal cell carcinoma [ccRCC]. Ankyrin repeat and sterile alpha motif domain-containing protein 1B, [ANKS1B] is a tyrosine kinase signal transduction gene that is expressed in the brain and testis. The expression of the Ankyrin repeats and sterile alpha motif domain-containing protein 1B [ANKS1B] gene is associated with smoking-related cell renal cell carcinoma [ccRCC] development. Ankyrin repeat and sterile alpha motif domain-containing protein 1B [ANKS1B] is involved in apoptosis and plays a role in cancer development. Ankyrin repeat and sterile alpha motif domain-containing protein 1B [ANKS1B] is up-regulated in smokers relative to non-smokers in normal kidney tissue. Ankyrin repeat and sterile alpha motif domain-containing protein 1B [ANKS1B] expression is associated with smoking-related clear cell renal cell carcinoma [ccRCC] [27].

1.27. ANO6 - ANOCTAMIN 6 CHROMOSOME 12; 12q12

Cell migration plays an important role in embryogenesis to tumor metastases. TMEM16A[ANO1] and TMEM16F [ANO6] are channels which have the highest expression of TMEM16 channels in Ehrlich Lettre ascites [ELA] cells. TMEM16A [ANO1] has expression in directional migration, and TMEM16F [ANO6] has expression in determination of the speed of migration. TMEM16F [ANO6] is involved in Ca^{2+}-activation Cl^- channel with delayed Ca^{2+} activation [28].

1.28. APAF1 - APOPTOTIC PROTEASE ACTIVATING FACTOR 1 CHROMOSOME 12;12q23.1

Epithelial ovarian cancer is ovarian cancer in human beings. microRNA-21 [miR21] is miRNAs in exosomes, and tissue lysates are isolated from cancer-associated adipocytes [CAAs] and fibroblasts [CAFs]. miR21 is transferred from cancer-associated adipocytes [CAAs] and fibroblasts [CAFs] to the cancer cells, in which it suppresses ovarian cancer apoptosis and chemoresistance by binding it to the target, which is Apoptotic protease activating factor 1 [APAF1] [29].

1.29. APOBEC1 - APOLIPOPROTEIN B MRNA-EDITING ENZYME, CATALYTIC POLYPEPTIDE 1 CHROMOSOME 12;12p13.31

Apolipoprotein B mRNA editing enzyme, catalytic polypeptide 1 [APOBEC1], are deaminases that act on cytosines-linked pathways and cause genetic alterations which involve in the progression of cancer. Apolipoprotein B mRNA editing enzyme, catalytic polypeptide 1[APOBEC1], is one of the RNA editing complex regions that deaminates C6666 to U in the transcript of human

Apolipoprotein B. Apolipoprotein B mRNA editing enzyme, catalytic polypeptide 1 [APOBEC1] function is seen in the small intestine in humans, and in the liver in rodents. Apolipoprotein B mRNA editing enzyme, catalytic polypeptide 1 [APOBEC1] expression is linked to cancer in transgenic mice and rabbits in the liver, and they develop hepatocellular carcinoma. Apolipoprotein B mRNA editing enzyme, catalytic polypeptide 1 [APOBEC1] causes human esophageal adenocarcinomas in human beings Apolipoprotein B mRNA editing enzyme, catalytic polypeptide 1 [APOBEC1] can induce mutations in genomic DNA, and also alter several cellular [30].

1.30. APOF - APOLIPOPROTEIN F CHROMOSOME 12; 12q13.3

Apolipoprotein F [ApoF] inhibits the cholesteryl ester transfer protein [CETP] activity in lipid metabolism. The *ApoF* promoter shows higher activities in hepatoma cell lines, the -198 nt to +79 nt promoter region contains the maximum promoter activity, and the promoter region of -198 nt to -2 nt shows four putative binding sites for transcription factors E-twenty-six [ETS]-1/ETS-2 named as EBS-1 to EBS-4 and one for C/EBP. Mutation of EBS-2, EBS4, and the C/EBP binding site removes the promoter activity, and ETS-1/ETS-2 and C/EBPa interact with binding sites. Overexpression of *ETS-1/2* or *C/EBPa* is enhanced and dominant-negative mutants of ETS-1/2 and knockdown of *C/EBPa* are decreased. *ETS-1* and *C/EBPa* are involved in activating *ApoF* transcription. This results in the combined activation of the *ApoF* promoter by liver-enriched and ubiquitous transcription factors. Direct interactions between C/EBPa and ETS-1 are essential for high liver-specific expression of ApoF [31].

1.31. APOLD1 -APOLIPOPROTEIN L DOMAIN-CONTAINING 1 CHROMOSOME 12; 12p13.1

Testicular germ cell tumor [TGCT] is an invasive germ cell tumor that occurs in males and can be classified as seminoma and non-seminoma. Gene expression was expressed in a group of differentially expressed genes regulated by DNA methylation. The genes involved are APOLD1, PCDH10, and RGAGI, and APOLD1 has reported which has been engaged in Testicular germ cell tumors [TGCT]. CpG island hypermethylation results in changes in chromatin accessibility and it represses gene transcription [32].

1.32. APPL2 - ADAPTOR PROTEIN, PHOSPHOTYROSINE INTERAC-TION, PH DOMAIN, AND LEUCINE ZIPPER- CONTAINING PROT-EIN 2 CHROMOSOME 12;12q23.3

Breast cancer is common cancer among the women in the world. Breast cancer forms tumors and shows different behaviours from one person to another, this can be caused by genetic, environmental, and gene alterations. Long non-coding RNAs [lncRNAs] are groups of non-coding RNA molecules, which are involved in gene expression. Overexpression of colon carcinoma is seen ,and screening is done between normal and carcinoma cells. Different mechanisms are involved for the initiation and progression of the breast cancer. OCC-1 and APPL2 neighbouring genes which are related with colorectal cancer. APPL2 protein enhances PI3K/Akt signalling by increasing Akt phosphorylation and PI3K/Akt pathway has a major role in cell cycle progression [33].

1.33. AQP2 - AQUAPORIN 2 CHROMOSOME 12; 12q13.12

Lung cancer is one of the common cancers; Lung cancer can be classified into two types: non-small cell lung cancer [NSCLC] and small cell lung cancer [SCLC]. Cisplatin and carboplatin are commonly used as therapeutic drugs; platinum-based chemotherapy is the common treatment method for lung cancer patients. And 5 transporter genes *OCT2, AQP2, AQP9, MVP* and *TMEM205,* are involved in lung cancers and also with platinum-based chemotherapy response. *AQP2* is associated with resistance of cisplatin and might be a membrane transporter/ binding protein/carrier for it and also involved in lung cancer [34].

1.34. AQP5 - AQUAPORIN 5 CHROMOSOME 12;12q13.12

Cervical cancer is caused in the cervical region of women; the aquaporins [AQPs] are small, integral membrane proteins that selectively transport water across cell plasma membranes. Overexpression of *AQP5* has been involved in many cancers like ovarian cancer, lung cancer gastric carcinoma, and colon and colorectal cancer, and overexpression of *AQP5* is also involved in cell differentiation in cancer cells [35].

1.35. AQP6 - AQUAPORIN 6 CHROMOSOME 12; 12q13.12

AQPs are involved in tumor's occurrence, development, invasion, and metastasis. *AQP6* is expressed in epithelial ovarian tumors and serous ovarian cancers. The down-regulation of *AQP6* is associated with the changes in apoptotic mechanism in serous ovarian cancers. *AQP6* is also involved in the progression of serous ovarian cancers [36].

1.36. ARF3 - ADP-RIBOSYLATION FACTOR 3 CHROMOSOME 12; 12q13.12

ADP-ribosylation factor 3 [ARF3] is a member of the KRAS proto-oncogene, GTPase [Ras] super-family of guanine nucleotide-binding proteins that mediate Golgi-related mitosis; breast cancer is usually found in women, ARF3 plays an important role in the proliferation of human breast cancer cells, *ARF3* expression is also involved in promoting tumor growth and progression of tumor in breast cancer cell [37].

1.37. ARHGAP9 - RHO GTPASE-ACTIVATING PROTEIN 9 CHROMO-SOME 12; 12q13.3

Breast cancer [BC] is common among women, and the biological indicators of Breast cancer [BC], are estrogen receptor [ER] and progesterone receptor [PR] and human epidermal growth factor receptor 2 [HER-2], RhoGAP proteins, consisting of *ARHGAP9* and Silencing of ARHGAP9 will inhibit proliferation, colony-formation, and invasion, and also induces cell cycle arrest and apoptosis of these MCF-7 and MDA-MB-231 cell lines. ARHGAP9 has involved in Breast cancer [BC] tumor genesis, progression, and prognosis [38].

1.38. ARHGDIB - RHO GDP-DISSOCIATION INHIBITOR BETA CHROMOSOME 12;12p12.3

The guanosine triphosphatase [GTPase] inhibitor LyGDI consist of ARHGDIB, Ly/D4-GDI, RhoGDIb, or RhoGDI 2, which is expressed in hematopoietic cells and also involves in apoptosis. The Ras-related small guanosine triphosphate-binding proteins [GTPases] are signaling molecules that are involved in cellular processes like cell growth, cytoskeletal organization, and secretion. Gene expression profiling of Hodgkin cell lines resulted that LyGDI expression being downregulated in Hodgkin cell lines, and was strongly expressed in B-Non-Hodgkin Lymphoma cell lines [39].

1.39. ARID2 - AT-RICH INTERACTION DOMAIN-CONTAINING PROTEIN 2 CHROMOSOME 12;12q12

Hepatocellular Carcinoma [HCC] is one of the types of cancer, which is seen among human beings, ARID2 is associated with other types like Hepatitis C virus [HCV], Hepatitis B virus [HBV], Alcohol-associated Hepatocellular Carcinoma [HCC] and Hepatocellular Carcinoma [HCC] which is associated with unknown factors. ARID2 mutations in Hepatocellular Carcinoma [HCC] were seen in polypeptides with less interaction in the Zn finger motif, ARID2 is involved in the Jak-STAT signaling pathway and which provides the increase for chronic Hepatitis C virus [HCV] during Hepatocellular Carcinoma [HCC] development [40].

1.40. ARL1 - ADP-RIBOSYLATION FACTOR-LIKE 1 CHROMOSOME 12;12Q23.2

ARL1 is involved in Hepatocellular carcinoma [HCC] and liver cancer. *ARL1* gene expression was upregulated in liver cancer cells. The elevation is high, thus with results in liver cancer, and this will increase liver cancer in patients. ARL1 is involved and responsible for the progression of liver cancer [41].

1.41. ARNTL2 - ARYL HYDROCARBON RECEPTOR NUCLEAR TRANSLOCATOR-LIKE PROTEINP CHROMOSOME 12;12p11.232

Colorectal cancer is most common in humans, initially occurring in the human colon region. Colorectal cancer can occur due to mutation, metastasis from one region to another region, and mutational pathways such as microsatellite instability [MSI] or chromosomal instability [CIN] can cause colorectal cancer. *ARNTL2* will activate the promoter region of the plasminogen activator inhibitor type-1 [*PAI-1*] gene, and thus this gene is called SERPINE1. ARNTL2 will induce cell proliferation and apoptosis, similar to colorectal cancer cells, and when the expression in ARNTL2 and SERPINE1 is increased, it involves tumor invasion and cancer progression [42].

1.42. ARPC3 - ACTIN-RELATED PROTEIN 2/3 COMPLEX, SUBUNIT 3 CHROMOSOME 12;12q24.11

Actin-related protein 2/3 [ARPC3] complex consists of an actin nucleator that involves cell migration. The expression of *ARPC3* is observed in a pancreatic cancer cell by quantitative RT-PCR. ARP2/3 complex is involved in pancreatic cancer cell migration. Silencing of the *ARPC3* complex subunits results in less cell migration. And thus, silencing of ARPC3 will reduce cancer cell migration and cell proliferation [43].

1.43. ART4 - ADP-RIBOSYLTRANSFERASE 4 CHROMOSOME 12;12 p12.3

Gynaecologic cancer is found in women, such as ovarian, cervical, and endometrial cancer. Genes that encode tumor-rejection antigens are identified as Cytotoxic T Lymphocytes [CTL], and four tumor-rejection antigens such as SART-1259, SART2, SART3, and ART4, which contain tumor epitopes that induce HLA-A2402 which are limited Cytotoxic T Lymphocytes [CTL] in cancer patients. *ART4* is expressed in the majority of gynecologic cancers, such as ovarian, cervical, and endometrial cancer [44].

1.44. ASB8 - ANKYRIN REPEAT- AND SOCS BOX-CONTAINING PROTEIN 8 CHROMOSOME 12;12q13.11

ASB8 is one of the members of the human ankyrin repeat and SOCS box-containing protein family [ASB]. ASB8 has greater expression in lung carcinomas which involve proliferation and growth in the SPC-A1 cell line. *ASB8* has higher expression in lung cancer tissues, and ASB8 is mainly involved in the growth and proliferation of lung cancer and acts as a positive regulator [45].

1.45. ASCL1 - ACHAETE-SCUTE FAMILY BHLH TRANSCRIPTION FACTOR 1 CHROMOSOME 12;12q23.2

Aggressive neuroendocrine lung cancers, which include small cell lung cancer [SCLC] and non-small cell lung cancer [NSCLC], and ASCL1 required for proper development of pulmonary neuroendocrine cells, which is important for the survival of lung cancers like small cell lung cancer [SCLC] and non-small cell lung cancer [NSCLC]. *ASCL1* is found as a lineage oncogene that has therapeutic targets for neuroendocrine lung cancers, and finding these genes can inhibit growth, cell division, and differentiation [46].

1.46. ASCL4 - ACHAETE-SCUTE FAMILY BHLH TRANSCRIPTION FACTOR 4 CHROMOSOME 12; 12q24.1

Lung squamous cell carcinoma is a common type of lung cancer [SQCC] that is caused in regions of the Lungs and this occurs due to the *EGFR* and *KRAS* mutations which lead to Lung Adenocarcinoma. Truncating mutations in *ASCL4* are seen in human lungs, which alters to form cancer and these alterations are seen in *NOTCH1*, *NOTCH2,* and *ASCL4,* which leads to the increase of *TP63* and *SOX* [47].

1.47. ASIC1 - ACID SENSING ION CHANNEL SUBUNIT 1 CHROMOSOME 12; 12q13.12

Pancreatic cancer is a form of cancer that is seen in the pancreatic region and pancreatic cancer metastasizes Epithelial-mesenchymal transition [EMT] involves in tumor invasion, and metastasis process, and this process is done by the signaling molecules called Snail, which involves increases the metastasis of pancreatic cancer [48].

1.48. ATF1 - ACTIVATING TRANSCRIPTION FACTOR 1 CHROMO-SOME 12;12q13.12

Clear cell sarcoma [CCS] is a rare type of melanoma that occurs in soft tissues, these tissues are associated with tendons and aponeuroses and it can occur in other regions like the head, neck, *etc*. This Clear cell sarcoma [CCS] occurs in both young and adults and this is determined by fusion genes *EWS/ATF1,* which forms the chromosomal aberrations and causes translocation, which leads to Clear cell sarcoma [CCS] in Humans [49].

1.49. ATF7 - ACTIVATING TRANSCRIPTION FACTOR 7 CHROMOS-OME 12;12q13.13

Colorectal cancer [CRC] is caused in the colon and rectal region of humans. *ATF7* expression is seen in other tissues, intestines, *etc*. ATF7 is involved in tumor development, invasion, and progression of cancer in a specific region. The activation of *ATF7* will also lead to the formation of tumors and the proliferation of cells [50].

1.50. ATF7IP - ACTIVATING TRANSCRIPTION FACTOR 7- INTERA-CTING PROTEIN CHROMOSOME 12;12p13.1

Testicular germ cell tumor [TGCT] is cancer that occurs in men; this cancer develops in the embryonic germ cells and forms tumors, and this may lead to other defects in men *ATF7IP* is expressed in cancer cells, and these expressions are seen in germ cell lines since these are present in the germ cell which leads to translocation of chromosomes and aberrations which lead to the tumor progression and development [51].

1.51. BCL7A - B-CELL CLL/LYMPHOMA 7A CHROMOSOME 12;12q 24.31

Cutaneous T-cell lymphoma [CTCLs] is also known as extranodal non-Hodgkin's lymphomas obtained from Mature T-cells which are present in the Skin. *BCL7A* is involved in the Silencing of the genes, and this BCL7A is the common recurrent breaking point that leads to the formation of lymphomas and also forms skin lesions [52].

1.52. BRAP - BRCA1-ASSOCIATED PROTEIN CHROMOSOME 12;12q 24.12

BRAP is a protein complex that is associated with BRCA1, which results in breast cancer, these proteins are involved in breast cancer in humans, and defects in this gene can lead to breast cancer formation and skin lesions on the breast surface region. Centrosome dysfunction leads to the formation and proliferation of tumors and lesions on the breast, which is the initial stage of breast cancer [53].

1.53. BTG1 - B-CELL TRANSLOCATION GENE 1 CHROMOSOME 12;12q21.33

BTG1 is involved in the cell cycle process, which inhibits proliferation, induces apoptosis, and forms multiple cell growth. *BTG1* is a translocation partner of a c-Myc gene which involves in promoting and formation of cancer. Overexpression of *BTG1* will inhibit cell proliferation in Breast cancer [54].

1.54. CCND2 - CYCLIN D2 CHROMOSOME 12;12p13.32

CCND2 gene is involved in cell cycle regulation; an aberration in the gene can lead to abnormal proliferation of the cells, which leads to the formation of tumors and cancers like Gastric cancer, Colorectal cancer, and overexpression can form Prostate cancer. MicroRNAs [miRNAs] are used to target the gene expression regions, and it's a direct target gene of miR-154 [55].

1.55. CD163 - CD163 ANTIGEN CHROMOSOME 12;12p13.31

CD163 are scavenger receptor for haptoglobin and hemoglobin complexes, cells obtained from monocyte and macrophage are involved in tumor migration, invasion, and metastasis and the primary breast cancer cells contains macrophages which are related to tumors; *CD163* are also expressed by neoplasms with monocytic and histiocytic differentiation, CD163 positive patients have distant metastasis and shorter survival [56].

1.56. CD63 - CD63 ANTIGEN CHROMOSOME 12;12q13.2

CD63 is involved in the formation of thyroid tumors in humans, and the mRNA and protein expression remains unchanged in thyroid tumors that are caused by CD63. And these expressions are seen in benign goiter and solid tumors, and the first form primary thyroid carcinoma tissues, and further it gets develops into tumors.CD63 is also involved in tumor carcinogenesis [57].

1.57. CD9 - CD9 ANTIGEN CHROMOSOME 12;12q13.31

CD9 is involved in the development of solid tumors and metastasis in Breast cancer. CD9 belongs to the transmembrane 4 superfamilies they also act as a progression for breast cancer. CD9 gene expression is also a good predictor for detecting the recurrence of Breast cancer. CD9 has cell surface membrane glycoproteins which are seen in the epithelial region, so the patients have high-risk chances of formation of new tumors in the same breast tissue region [58].

1.58. CDK2 - CYCLIN-DEPENDENT KINASE 2 CHROMOSOME 12;12q 13.2

Cyclins are kinases that are involved in the cell cycle process and some dysregulation can lead to the overgrowth of cells and thus will disturb the cycle regulation which leads to abnormalities of cell proliferation and involves the development of cancer. And thus, these expressions are seen in benign tumors of ovarian cancer, and CDK2 is involved in metastasis benign tumors in ovarian cancer patients and this mainly occurs due to the loss of control of the cyclin kinases in the cell cycle [59].

1.59. CDK2AP1 - CDK2-ASSOCIATED PROTEIN 1 CHROMOSOME 12;12q24.31

CDK2AP1 are cell cycle regulators which are also involved in the cell cycle process; these expressions are seen in prostate cancer, and these cancers are involved with the androgen receptors, which are essential for the mechanism of prostate glands, the alteration and modification of the structure can lead to cancer progression [60].

1.60. CDK4 - CYCLIN-DEPENDENT KINASE 4 CHROMOSOME 12;12 q14.1

CDK4 is involved in the formation of breast cancer, CDK4 is one of the cyclin kinases which are present in the cell cycle process, the overexpression of ErbB-2 oncogene is seen along with cyclin D, which dependents on this CDK2 for the cell proliferation and overexpression of the breast cancer cells and these kinases are cyclin-dependent and cyclin independent, ErbB-2 are also involved in other malignancy and tumor progression [61].

1.61. CDKN1B - CYCLIN-DEPENDENT KINASE INHIBITOR 1B CHR-OMOSOME 12;12p13.1

CDKN1B is important in the cell cycle family, which is involved in the tumor and cancer progression of prostate cancer, and it is also said that polymorphism of

CDKN1B can involve in the progression of hereditary prostate cancer, which evolves from one family generation to another family generation who have histories of prostate cancer. CDKN1B regulates the region of the chromosome and involves in prostate tumor progression [62].

1.62. CHFR - CHECKPOINT PROTEIN WITH FHA AND RING FINGER DOMAINS CHROMOSOME 12;12q24.33

CHFR genes are involved in lung cancer, and these genes have a hypermethylation process, and they have a loss of expression, which leads to the formation of lung cancer in humans. *CHFR* genes have many checkpoints in their promoter, and when these regions get hypermethylated and cause cancer [63].

1.63. CKAP4 - CYTOSKELETON-ASSOCIATED PROTEIN 4 CHROMOSOME 12;12q23.3

CKAP4 are commonly found and formed in pancreatic and lung cancers. They act as a receptor for Dickkopf-1[DKK-1] in cancer cells; they are secretory protein that acts as an antagonist in the Wnt signaling pathway, abnormal activation of Wnt signaling can lead to tumorigenesis and proliferation of cells in Colon, Breast and hepatocellular carcinomas. Targeting the CKAP4 and DKK-1 signaling pathways can be an effective target therapeutic drug for the cure of many cancers [64].

1.64. CRY1 - CRYPTOCHROME 1 CHROMOSOME 12;12q23.3

Disruption in the circadian cycle can involve the progression of cancer and tumorigenesis, and the gene cryptochrome *CRY1* is involved in the expression of cancer in human colorectal cancer. *CRY1* gene alteration can be seen in colorectal cancer, and gene alteration is seen in patients; this gene alteration differs from gender to gender and the cancer expression also differs in each individual [65].

CONCLUSION

As chromosome 12 genes are looked up for the cancer-causing genes, many of them have been shown to support cancer development in their ways. The genetic abnormalities, including downregulation, overexpression, mutations, gene mutations, *etc*, have made a normal functioning gene into a cancer-developing gene. Mutation in the AACS gene leads to the development of Vater cancer. ABC transporter proteins like ABCB9, ABCC9, *etc*, are also present in this chromosome which is responsible for the chemoresistance of the cancer cells.

Genes from this chromosome also help in the metastasis of cancer like ACVRL1, and downregulation of certain genes turns the normal cells into cancerous cell-like the A2M gene. The detail of the often-involving Chromosome 12 gene and their involvement in cancer will help for better research resources for targeting them for cancer treatment.

REFERENCES

[1]   Liu Y, Xiong S, Liu S, *et al.* Analysis of Gene Expression in Bladder Cancer: Possible Involvement of Mitosis and Complement and Coagulation Cascades Signaling Pathway. J Comput Biol 2020; 27(6): 987-98.
       [http://dx.doi.org/10.1089/cmb.2019.0237] [PMID: 31545079]

[2]   Wang Y, Liu K, Ma Q, *et al.* Pancreatic cancer biomarker detection by two support vector strategies for recursive feature elimination. Biomarkers Med 2019; 13(2): 105-21.
       [http://dx.doi.org/10.2217/bmm-2018-0273] [PMID: 30767554]

[3]   Li Y, Tang XQ, Bai Z, Dai X. Exploring the intrinsic differences among breast tumor subtypes defined using immunohistochemistry markers based on the decision tree. Sci Rep 2016; 6(1): 35773.
       [http://dx.doi.org/10.1038/srep35773] [PMID: 27786176]

[4]   Hasegawa S, Imai M, Yamasaki M, Takahashi N, Fukui T. Transcriptional regulation of acetoacetyl-CoA synthetase by Sp1 in neuroblastoma cells. Biochem Biophys Res Commun 2018; 495(1): 652-8.
       [http://dx.doi.org/10.1016/j.bbrc.2017.11.068] [PMID: 29137983]

[5]   Gong JP, Yang L, Tang JW, *et al.* Overexpression of microRNA-24 increases the sensitivity to paclitaxel in drug-resistant breast carcinoma cell lines *via* targeting ABCB9. Oncol Lett 2016; 12(5): 3905-11.
       [http://dx.doi.org/10.3892/ol.2016.5139] [PMID: 27895747]

[6]   Demidenko R, Razanauskas D, Daniunaite K, Lazutka JR, Jankevicius F, Jarmalaite S. Frequent down-regulation of ABC transporter genes in prostate cancer. BMC Cancer 2015; 15(1): 683.
       [http://dx.doi.org/10.1186/s12885-015-1689-8] [PMID: 26459268]

[7]   Park CY, Kim HS, Jang J, *et al.* ABCD2 is a direct target of β-catenin and TCF-4: implications for X-linked adrenoleukodystrophy therapy. PLoS One 2013; 8(2): e56242.
       [http://dx.doi.org/10.1371/journal.pone.0056242] [PMID: 23437103]

[8]   Hemminger JA, Toland AE, Scharschmidt TJ, Mayerson JL, Guttridge DC, Iwenofu OH. Expression of cancer-testis antigens MAGEA1, MAGEA3, ACRBP, PRAME, SSX2, and CTAG2 in myxoid and round cell liposarcoma. Mod Pathol 2014; 27(9): 1238-45.
       [http://dx.doi.org/10.1038/modpathol.2013.244] [PMID: 24457462]

[9]   Chang WC, Cheng WC, Cheng BH, *et al.* Mitochondrial Acetyl-CoA Synthetase 3 is Biosignature of Gastric Cancer Progression. Cancer Med 2018; 7(4): 1240-52.
       [http://dx.doi.org/10.1002/cam4.1295] [PMID: 29493120]

[10]   Lobo J, Henrique R, Jerónimo C. The Role of DNA/Histone Modifying Enzymes and Chromatin Remodeling Complexes in Testicular Germ Cell Tumors. Cancers (Basel) 2018; 11(1): 6.
       [http://dx.doi.org/10.3390/cancers11010006] [PMID: 30577487]

[11]   Murphy KM, Brune KA, Griffin C, *et al.* Evaluation of candidate genes MAP2K4, MADH4, ACVR1B, and BRCA2 in familial pancreatic cancer: deleterious BRCA2 mutations in 17%. Cancer Res 2002; 62(13): 3789-93.
       [PMID: 12097290]

[12]   Hanna DL, Loupakis F, Yang D, *et al.* Prognostic Value of ACVRL1 Expression in Metastatic Colorectal Cancer Patients Receiving First-line Chemotherapy With Bevacizumab: Results From the Triplet Plus Bevacizumab (TRIBE) Study. Clin Colorectal Cancer 2018; 17(3): e471-88.

[http://dx.doi.org/10.1016/j.clcc.2018.03.006] [PMID: 29636300]

[13] Li W, Sang M, Hao X, *et al.* Gene expression and DNA methylation analyses suggest that immune process-related ADCY6 is a prognostic factor of luminal-like breast cancer 2019.

[14] Millar MW, Corson N, Xu L. The Adhesion G-Protein-Coupled Receptor, GPR56/ADGRG1, Inhibits Cell–Extracellular Matrix Signaling to Prevent Metastatic Melanoma Growth. Front Oncol 2018; 8: 8.
[http://dx.doi.org/10.3389/fonc.2018.00008] [PMID: 29450192]

[15] Ishikawa M, Kitayama J, Yamauchi T, *et al.* Adiponectin inhibits the growth and peritoneal metastasis of gastric cancer through its specific membrane receptors AdipoR1 and AdipoR2. Cancer Sci 2007; 98(7): 1120-7.
[http://dx.doi.org/10.1111/j.1349-7006.2007.00486.x] [PMID: 17459059]

[16] Benetatos L, Voulgaris E, Vartholomatos G, Hatzimichael E. Non-coding RNAs and EZH2 interactions in cancer: Long and short tales from the transcriptome. Int J Cancer 2013; 133(2): 267-74.
[http://dx.doi.org/10.1002/ijc.27859] [PMID: 23001607]

[17] Qi F, Liu X, Wu H, *et al.* Long noncoding AGAP2-AS1 is activated by SP1 and promotes cell proliferation and invasion in gastric cancer. J Hematol Oncol 2017; 10(1): 48.
[http://dx.doi.org/10.1186/s13045-017-0420-4] [PMID: 28209205]

[18] El Kadi N, Wang L, Davis A, *et al.* The EGFR T790M Mutation Is Acquired through AICDA-Mediated Deamination of 5-Methylcytosine following TKI Treatment in Lung Cancer. Cancer Res 2018; 78(24): 6728-35.
[http://dx.doi.org/10.1158/0008-5472.CAN-17-3370] [PMID: 30333118]

[19] Miyo M, Konno M, Colvin H, *et al.* The importance of mitochondrial folate enzymes in human colorectal cancer. Oncol Rep 2017; 37(1): 417-25.
[http://dx.doi.org/10.3892/or.2016.5264] [PMID: 27878282]

[20] Lewis SJ, Davey Smith G. Alcohol, ALDH2, and esophageal cancer: a meta-analysis which illustrates the potentials and limitations of a Mendelian randomization approach. Cancer Epidemiol Biomarkers Prev 2005; 14(8): 1967-71.
[http://dx.doi.org/10.1158/1055-9965.EPI-05-0196] [PMID: 16103445]

[21] Yuan H, Kajiyama H, Ito S, *et al.* ALX1 induces snail expression to promote epithelial-to - mesenchymal transition and invasion of ovarian cancer cells. Cancer Res 2013; 73(5): 1581-90.
[http://dx.doi.org/10.1158/0008-5472.CAN-12-2377] [PMID: 23288509]

[22] Beck TN, Korobeynikov VA, Kudinov AE, *et al.* Anti-Müllerian Hormone Signaling Regulates Epithelial Plasticity and Chemoresistance in Lung Cancer. Cell Rep 2016; 16(3): 657-71.
[http://dx.doi.org/10.1016/j.celrep.2016.06.043] [PMID: 27396341]

[23] Rabenau KE, O'Toole JM, Bassi R, *et al.* DEGA/AMIGO-2, a leucine-rich repeat family member, differentially expressed in human gastric adenocarcinoma: effects on ploidy, chromosomal stability, cell adhesion/migration and tumorigenicity. Oncogene 2004; 23(29): 5056-67.
[http://dx.doi.org/10.1038/sj.onc.1207681] [PMID: 15107827]

[24] Chen H, Liu T, Liu J, *et al.* Circ-ANAPC7 is Upregulated in Acute Myeloid Leukemia and Appears to Target the MiR-181 Family. Cell Physiol Biochem 2018; 47(5): 1998-2007.
[http://dx.doi.org/10.1159/000491468] [PMID: 29969755]

[25] Li QH, Yu M, Ding YL, Chen YX. Retracted: ANKRD33 is overexpressed in gastric adenocarcinoma and predictive for poor prognosis. Biosci Biotechnol Biochem 2019; 83(11): 2075-81.
[http://dx.doi.org/10.1080/09168451.2019.1642100] [PMID: 31314707]

[26] Lin Y-F, Liu Y-P, Lee T-F, *et al.* Abstract 4843: ANKRD52 inhibited tumor metastasis through dephosphorylation of PAK1 in lung adenocarcinoma.Tumor Biology. 4843-3.

[27] Eckel-Passow JE, Serie DJ, Bot BM, Joseph RW, Cheville JC, Parker AS. ANKS1B is a smoking-related molecular alteration in clear cell renal cell carcinoma. BMC Urol 2014; 14(1): 14.
[http://dx.doi.org/10.1186/1471-2490-14-14] [PMID: 24479813]

[28]   Jacobsen KS, Zeeberg K, Sauter DRP, Poulsen KA, Hoffmann EK, Schwab A. The role of TMEM16A (ANO1) and TMEM16F (ANO6) in cell migration. Pflugers Arch 2013; 465(12): 1753-62.
[http://dx.doi.org/10.1007/s00424-013-1315-z] [PMID: 23832500]

[29]   Au Yeung CL, Co NN, Tsuruga T, *et al.* Exosomal transfer of stroma-derived miR21 confers paclitaxel resistance in ovarian cancer cells through targeting APAF1. Nat Commun 2016; 7(1): 11150.
[http://dx.doi.org/10.1038/ncomms11150] [PMID: 27021436]

[30]   Saraconi G, Severi F, Sala C, Mattiuz G, Conticello SG. The RNA editing enzyme APOBEC1 induces somatic mutations and a compatible mutational signature is present in esophageal adenocarcinomas. Genome Biol 2014; 15(7): 417.
[http://dx.doi.org/10.1186/s13059-014-0417-z] [PMID: 25085003]

[31]   Shen XB, Huang L, Zhang SH, *et al.* Transcriptional regulation of the apolipoprotein F (ApoF) gene by ETS and C/EBPα in hepatoma cells. Biochimie 2015; 112: 1-9.
[http://dx.doi.org/10.1016/j.biochi.2015.02.013] [PMID: 25726912]

[32]   Cheung HH, Lee TL, Davis AJ, Taft DH, Rennert OM, Chan WY. Genome-wide DNA methylation profiling reveals novel epigenetically regulated genes and non-coding RNAs in human testicular cancer. Br J Cancer 2010; 102(2): 419-27.
[http://dx.doi.org/10.1038/sj.bjc.6605505] [PMID: 20051947]

[33]   Ghalaei A, Kay M, Zarrinfam S, Hoseinpour P, Behmanesh M, Soltani BM. Overexpressed in colorectal carcinoma gene (OCC-1) upregulation and APPL2 gene downregulation in breast cancer specimens. Mol Biol Rep 2018; 45(6): 1889-95.
[http://dx.doi.org/10.1007/s11033-018-4336-z] [PMID: 30218350]

[34]   Wang Y, Yin JY, Li XP, *et al.* The association of transporter genes polymorphisms and lung cancer chemotherapy response. PLoS One 2014; 9(3): e91967.
[http://dx.doi.org/10.1371/journal.pone.0091967] [PMID: 24643204]

[35]   Zhang T, Zhao C, Chen D, Zhou Z. Overexpression of AQP5 in cervical cancer: correlation with clinicopathological features and prognosis. Med Oncol 2012; 29(3): 1998-2004.
[http://dx.doi.org/10.1007/s12032-011-0095-6] [PMID: 22048942]

[36]   Ma J, Zhou C, Yang J, Ding X, Zhu Y, Chen X. Expression of AQP6 and AQP8 in epithelial ovarian tumor. J Mol Histol 2016; 47(2): 129-34.
[http://dx.doi.org/10.1007/s10735-016-9657-4] [PMID: 26779650]

[37]   Huang D, Pei Y, Dai C, *et al.* Up-regulated ADP-Ribosylation factor 3 promotes breast cancer cell proliferation through the participation of FOXO1. Exp Cell Res 2019; 384(2): 111624.
[http://dx.doi.org/10.1016/j.yexcr.2019.111624] [PMID: 31539530]

[38]   Wang T, Ha M. *Retracted* : Silencing ARHGAP9 correlates with the risk of breast cancer and inhibits the proliferation, migration, and invasion of breast cancer. J Cell Biochem 2018; 119(9): 7747-56.
[http://dx.doi.org/10.1002/jcb.27127] [PMID: 29905031]

[39]   Ma L, Xu G, Sotnikova A, *et al.* Loss of expression of LyGDI (ARHGDIB), a rho GDP-dissociation inhibitor, in Hodgkin lymphoma. Br J Haematol 2007; 139(2): 217-23.
[http://dx.doi.org/10.1111/j.1365-2141.2007.06782.x] [PMID: 17897297]

[40]   Li M, Zhao H, Zhang X, *et al.* Inactivating mutations of the chromatin remodeling gene ARID2 in hepatocellular carcinoma. Nat Genet 2011; 43(9): 828-9.
[http://dx.doi.org/10.1038/ng.903] [PMID: 21822264]

[41]   Jin JF, Yuan LD, Liu L, Zhao ZJ, Xie W. Preparation and characterization of polyclonal antibodies against ARL-1 protein. World J Gastroenterol 2003; 9(7): 1455-9.
[http://dx.doi.org/10.3748/wjg.v9.i7.1455] [PMID: 12854140]

[42]   Mazzoccoli G, Pazienza V, Panza A, *et al.* ARNTL2 and SERPINE1: potential biomarkers for tumor aggressiveness in colorectal cancer. J Cancer Res Clin Oncol 2012; 138(3): 501-11.

[http://dx.doi.org/10.1007/s00432-011-1126-6] [PMID: 22198637]

[43] HANNA E. RAUHALA1,2,3, SUSANNA TEPPO1,2,3, SANNA NIEMELÄ1,2 3 and ANNE KALLIONIEMI. Silencing of the ARP2/3 Complex Disturbs Pancreatic Cancer Cell Migration. Anticancer Res; 33: no. 1 45-52.

[44] Tanaka S, Tsuda N, Kawano K, *et al.* Expression of tumor-rejection antigens in gynecologic cancers. Jpn J Cancer Res 2000; 91(11): 1177-84.
[http://dx.doi.org/10.1111/j.1349-7006.2000.tb00902.x] [PMID: 11092984]

[45] Liu Y-Z, Li J-J, Zhang F-R, *et al.* [Exogenous expression of SOCS box-deficient mutant ASB-8 suppresses the growth of lung adenocarcinoma SPC-A1 cells]. Sheng Wu Hua Xue Yu Sheng Wu Wu Li Xue Bao (Shanghai) 2003; 35(6): 548-53.
[PMID: 12796816]

[46] Augustyn A, Borromeo M, Wang T, *et al.* ASCL1 is a lineage oncogene providing therapeutic targets for high-grade neuroendocrine lung cancers. Proc Natl Acad Sci USA 2014; 111(41): 14788-93.
[http://dx.doi.org/10.1073/pnas.1410419111] [PMID: 25267614]

[47] Hammerman PS, Voet D, Lawrence MS, *et al.* Comprehensive genomic characterization of squamous cell lung cancers. Nature 2012; 489(7417): 519-25.
[http://dx.doi.org/10.1038/nature11404] [PMID: 22960745]

[48] Zhu S, Zhou HY, Deng SC, *et al.* ASIC1 and ASIC3 contribute to acidity-induced EMT of pancreatic cancer through activating Ca^{2+}/RhoA pathway. Cell Death Dis 2017; 8(5): e2806-6.
[http://dx.doi.org/10.1038/cddis.2017.189] [PMID: 28518134]

[49] Panagopoulos I, Mertens F, Dêbiec-Rychter M, *et al.* Molecular genetic characterization of the *EWS/ATF1* fusion gene in clear cell sarcoma of tendons and aponeuroses. Int J Cancer 2002; 99(4): 560-7.
[http://dx.doi.org/10.1002/ijc.10404] [PMID: 11992546]

[50] Guo HQ, Ye S, Huang GL, Liu L, Liu OF, Yang SJ. Expression of activating transcription factor 7 is correlated with prognosis of colorectal cancer. J Cancer Res Ther 2015; 11(2): 319-23.
[http://dx.doi.org/10.4103/0973-1482.148688] [PMID: 26148593]

[51] Turnbull C, Rapley EA, Seal S, *et al.* Variants near DMRT1, TERT and ATF7IP are associated with testicular germ cell cancer. Nat Genet 2010; 42(7): 604-7.
[http://dx.doi.org/10.1038/ng.607] [PMID: 20543847]

[52] van Doorn R, Zoutman WH, Dijkman R, *et al.* Epigenetic profiling of cutaneous T-cell lymphoma: promoter hypermethylation of multiple tumor suppressor genes including BCL7a, PTPRG, and p73. J Clin Oncol 2005; 23(17): 3886-96.
[http://dx.doi.org/10.1200/JCO.2005.11.353] [PMID: 15897551]

[53] Pujana MA, Han JDJ, Starita LM, *et al.* Network modeling links breast cancer susceptibility and centrosome dysfunction. Nat Genet 2007; 39(11): 1338-49.
[http://dx.doi.org/10.1038/ng.2007.2] [PMID: 17922014]

[54] Zhu R, Zou ST, Wan JM, Li W, Li XL, Zhu W. BTG1 inhibits breast cancer cell growth through induction of cell cycle arrest and apoptosis. Oncol Rep 2013; 30(5): 2137-44.
[http://dx.doi.org/10.3892/or.2013.2697] [PMID: 23982470]

[55] Zhu C, Shao P, Bao M, *et al.* miR-154 inhibits prostate cancer cell proliferation by targeting CCND2. Urol Oncol 2014; 32(1): 31.e9-31.e16.
[http://dx.doi.org/10.1016/j.urolonc.2012.11.013] [PMID: 23428540]

[56] Shabo I, Stål O, Olsson H, Doré S, Svanvik J. Breast cancer expression of CD163, a macrophage scavenger receptor, is related to early distant recurrence and reduced patient survival. Int J Cancer 2008; 123(4): 780-6.
[http://dx.doi.org/10.1002/ijc.23527] [PMID: 18506688]

[57] Chen Z, Mustafa T, Trojanowicz B, *et al.* CD82, and CD63 in thyroid cancer. Int J Mol Med 2004;

14(4): 517-27.
[http://dx.doi.org/10.3892/ijmm.14.4.517] [PMID: 15375577]

[58] Huang C, Kohno N, Ogawa E, Adachi M, Taki T, Miyake M. Correlation of reduction in MRP-1/CD9 and KAI1/CD82 expression with recurrences in breast cancer patients. Am J Pathol 1998; 153(3): 973-83.
[http://dx.doi.org/10.1016/S0002-9440(10)65639-8] [PMID: 9736046]

[59] Marone M, Scambia G, Giannitelli C, *et al.* Analysis of cyclin E and CDK2 in ovarian cancer: Gene amplification and RNA overexpression. Int J Cancer 1998; 75(1): 34-9.
[http://dx.doi.org/10.1002/(SICI)1097-0215(19980105)75:1<34::AID-IJC6>3.0.CO;2-2] [PMID: 942-6687]

[60] Zolochevska O, Figueiredo ML. Cell cycle regulator *cdk2ap1* inhibits prostate cancer cell growth and modifies androgen-responsive pathway function. Prostate 2009; 69(14): 1586-97.
[http://dx.doi.org/10.1002/pros.21007] [PMID: 19585490]

[61] Yu Q, Sicinska E, Geng Y, *et al.* Requirement for CDK4 kinase function in breast cancer. Cancer Cell 2006; 9(1): 23-32.
[http://dx.doi.org/10.1016/j.ccr.2005.12.012] [PMID: 16413469]

[62] Chang B, Zheng SL, Isaacs SD, *et al.* A polymorphism in the CDKN1B gene is associated with increased risk of hereditary prostate cancer. Cancer Res 2004; 64(6): 1997-9.
[http://dx.doi.org/10.1158/0008-5472.CAN-03-2340] [PMID: 15026335]

[63] Mizuno K, Hasegawa K, Katagiri T, Ogimoto M, Ichikawa T, Yakura H. MPTP delta, a putative murine homolog of HPTP delta, is expressed in specialized regions of the brain and in the B-cell lineage. Mol Cell Biol 1993; 13(9): 5513-23.
[PMID: 8355697]

[64] Bhavanasi D, Speer KF, Klein PS. CKAP4 is identified as a receptor for Dickkopf in cancer cells. J Clin Invest 2016; 126(7): 2419-21.
[http://dx.doi.org/10.1172/JCI88620] [PMID: 27322056]

[65] Mazzoccoli G, Colangelo T, Panza A, *et al.* Deregulated expression of cryptochrome genes in human colorectal cancer. Mol Cancer 2016; 15(1): 6.
[http://dx.doi.org/10.1186/s12943-016-0492-8] [PMID: 26768731]

SUBJECT INDEX

A

Acid 108, 165, 234, 257, 289, 356
  glutamic 165
  hyaluronic 257, 356
  retinoic 234
  thymidylic 108
Actin-filament-associated proteins (AFAP) 95
Activity 36, 45, 115, 116, 194, 207, 244, 259,
    265, 349
  antioxidant 45, 259
  downregulates macrophage 116
  metastatic 36
  motor protein 349
  protease 244
  telomerase 207, 265
  tumor-associated angiogenic 194
  tumor-suppressing 115
Acute myeloid leukemia (AML) 33, 55, 57,
    90, 160, 162, 249, 251, 253, 307, 324,
    351, 352, 378, 379
Adipogenesis 115, 125
AMP-activated kinase 85
Anchorage-independent growth 53, 79, 170,
    172, 195, 261, 298, 312
Androgen dependent prostate cancer (ADPC)
    81
Angiogenesis 36, 42, 43, 45, 95, 97, 166, 168,
    169, 170, 174, 194, 230, 231, 245, 246,
    374
  inhibitor genes 245
  pathologic 374
  tumor-associated 194
Angiogenic factors 96, 111, 180, 184, 185
Anti-apoptotic proteins 189
Anticancer therapy 103, 107
Apoptosis, cytokine-induced 167
Apoptotic protease 380
Atherosclerosis 261, 287

B

Barrett's adenocarcinoma 184
Beck with-Wiedemann syndrome 345
Brain tumors 59, 227, 231, 252
Breast 95, 160, 168, 179, 188, 199, 325
  carcinogenesis 325
  carcinomas 95, 160, 188, 199
  tumorigenesis 168, 179
Breast cancer 13, 30, 32, 35, 37, 60, 71, 99,
    100, 103, 109, 111, 114, 115, 117, 119,
    120, 123, 160, 166, 173, 174, 193, 196,
    197, 260, 264, 308, 312, 313, 321, 323,
    325, 374, 383, 387
  aggressive 173
  bone metastasis 30
  luminal 312, 321
  metastasis 32, 60, 99, 100, 174, 313, 323
  metastatic 111, 197, 325
  migration 103
  risk 109, 115, 123, 196

C

Cancer(s) 105, 190, 196, 198, 199, 254, 313,
    296, 355, 384
  carcinogen-induced 105
  cell migration 313, 384
  colitis-associated 199
  estrogen-related 198
  nasopharyngeal 254
  neuroendocrine 355
  Hodgkin's lymphoma 190, 196, 296
  risk 190, 196
Carcinogenic 165, 179, 180
Carcinomas 8, 16, 33, 43, 63, 119, 166, 172,
    173, 185, 187, 188, 198, 292, 297, 321,
    325, 357, 382
  esophageal squamous cell 8, 16, 63, 119,
    166, 292, 297, 321
  gallbladder 185
  gastric 43, 173, 325, 357, 382

www.ingramcontent.com/pod-product-compliance
Lightning Source LLC
Chambersburg PA
CBHW050759220326
41598CB00006B/64